Cancer Management

Walter Lawrence, Jr., M.D.

American Cancer Society Professor
of Clinical Oncology
Division of Surgical Oncology
and
Director, Cancer Center
Medical College of Virginia
Virginia Commonwealth University
Richmond, Virginia

Jose J. Terz, M.D.

Professor of Surgery
Division of Surgical Oncology
and
Senior Member, Cancer Center
Medical College of Virginia
Virginia Commonwealth University
Richmond, Virginia

and Contributors

GRUNE & STRATTON

A Subsidiary of Harcourt Brace Jovanovich, Publishers
New York   San Francisco   London

Library of Congress Cataloging in Publication Data

Main entry under title:

Cancer management.

    Bibliography: p.
    Includes index.
    1. Cancer. I. Lawrence, Walter, 1925–
II. Terz, Jose J. [DNLM: 1. Neoplasms—Therapy.
QZ266 C216]
RC262.C293   616.9'94   76-56866
ISBN 0-8089-0985-1

Grune & Stratton, Inc.
111 Fifth Avenue
New York, New York 10003

Distributed in the United Kingdom by
Academic Press, Inc. (London) Ltd.
24/28 Oval Road, London NW 1

Library of Congress Catalog Number 76-56866
International Standard Book Number 0-8089-0985-1

Printed in the United States of America

Contents

Contributors

Paul C. Adkins, M.D., Professor and Chairman Department of Surgery, The George Washington University Medical Center, Washington, D.C.

Hugh R.K. Barber, M.D., Director, Department of Obstetrics and Gynecology; Lenox Hill Hospital, New York City, New York

L. Thompson Bowles, M.D., Associate Professor of Surgery, The George Washington University Medical Center, Washington, D.C.

Tapan Hazra, M.D., Professor and Chairman, Division of Radiation Therapy and Oncology; Senior Member, Cancer Center, Medical College of Virginia, Virginia Commonwealth University, Richmond, Virginia

Warren W. Koontz, M.D., Professor and Chairman, Division of Urology, Medical College of Virginia, Virginia Commonwealth University, Richmond, Virginia

Taehae Kwon, M.D., Fellow in Gynecologic Oncology; University of Mississippi; formerly American Cancer Society Fellow (New York City Division), Lenox Hill Hospital, New York, New York

Harold M. Maurer, M.D., Professor and Chairman, Department of Pediatrics; Senior Member, Cancer Center; Medical College of Virginia, Virginia Commonwealth University, Richmond, Virginia

Nancy B. McWilliams, M.D., Assistant Professor of Pediatrics; Member, Cancer Center; Medical College of Virginia, Virginia Commonwealth University, Richmond, Virginia

Heber H. Newsome, Jr., M.D., Associate Professor of Surgery, Medical College of Virginia, Virginia Commonwealth University, Richmond, Virginia

M. J. Vernon Smith, M.D., Ph.D., Professor of Surgery, Division of Urology, Medical College of Virginia, Virginia Commonwealth University, Richmond, Virginia

Preface

This book has been written to meet the frequently expressed need for a brief, practical book on the management of patients with cancer. In approaching this task, we did not attempt to review exhaustively the diagnosis and treatment of all the various human cancers, but to respond to the clinical management questions that are often raised by the general physician, the general surgeon, or the postgraduate trainee in the various specialities. More detailed and exhaustive reviews on cancer are available and referred to in this text for the reader who wishes to explore the specific problems in greater depth. Our objective is to establish general guidelines for the management of cancer that might be used by the physicians who are first presented with these clinical problems.

The reader will quickly note that the cancers under consideration in this book are limited to "solid tumors" since leukemia is so uniquely different from other cancers in addition to being so well covered in other publications. Primary neoplasms of the central nervous system have been omitted for similar reasons as well as the fact that charting the course of therapy for these lesions is rarely the responsibility of physicians in the general specialities.

Both of the editors are general surgeons who are committed to the management of cancer—now appropriately designated as surgical oncologists. This cannot help but give a surgeon's bias to this practical handbook on cancer care, but we have tried to add some degree of balance by inviting friends and colleagues from other specialties as contributors for certain chapters. The surgical accent of our book has some merit, however, since the general surgeon in the community is frequently the physician responsible for charting the initial therapeutic course of the cancer patient. For this reason we have inserted a few technical aspects of surgical interest, but we have avoided detailed considerations of operative technique as well as precise technical details of radiotherapy or chemotherapy.

We are grateful to many friends and co-workers who played a major role in our ability to complete this project. Both of us had our initial clinical experience in cancer at the Memorial Sloan–Kettering Cancer Center, and we are indebted to H. Thomas Randall, former Clinical Director and Chief of Surgery, the late Gordon P. McNeer, Chief of the Gastric and Mixed Tumor Service during those years, and our many colleagues and friends in all specialties at this institution from whom we learned so much. We are also indebted to the late David M. Hume, the Chairman of Surgery, and Kinloch Nelson, Dean Emeritus, at the Medical College of Virginia, who had the foresight in 1966 to encourage and support us in the initiation of what we believe to be one of the first truly functional division of surgical oncology in a university setting. This has led to the subsequent identification and definition of oncology as a legitimate clinical activity in the other departments at the Medical College of Virginia and has laid the groundwork for the Medical College of Virginia Cancer Center. We are grateful for the valuable support of our teammates, Roger E. King (Morgantown, West Virginia) and Ranes Chakravorty (University of Virginia), who were members of our division in previous years, and Peter W. Brown and J. Shelton Horsley, III, who are our present partners in the Division of Surgical Oncology at the Medical College of Virginia.

Our colleagues in Medical Oncology, Radiation Therapy and Oncology, and Pediatric Oncology at the Medical College of Virginia have given us much clinical information that we have utilized in this presentation, as well as having played a vital role in our own patient management process. We are grateful to them and to Lazar Greenfield and all of our colleagues in the other divisions in the Department of Surgery who have given us enthusiastic support in our attempt to develop this multidisciplinary approach to the cancer patient.

The actual production of this book has required much devoted and loyal help. We are indebted to Kathy Lawson for her major role in secretarial assistance and to Betsy Hyatt, Jackie Young, Sarah Metz, and others who provided valuable and needed help in this area. We are grateful to Dorothy Irwin for her enthusiastic and skillful help in developing the major portion of our illustrative material, and to Susan Lawrence for editing major portions of the manuscript. The expert assistance of Jeff Robbins of Grune & Stratton in the production of this book is also gratefully acknowledged.

Lastly, we are most appreciative to the patients with cancer whom we have had the privilege to treat, as they are the source of any knowledge or understanding that we can now transmit to the reader.

Walter Lawrence, Jr., M.D.
Jose J. Terz, M.D.

To Our Teachers—Our Patients with Cancer

1
Cancer Management—General Concepts

The scope of cancer patient management actually extends from possible prevention of cancer to the final physical and emotional rehabilitation of the patient who has undergone successful treatment of cancer. Between these extremes are early detection, establishing the diagnosis, and the treatment process itself. The practicing physician, however, is primarily challenged with the diagnosis and the treatment decisions that follow the presentation of the clinical problem in a patient with symptoms or findings suggestive of cancer. The purpose of this volume, therefore, is to summarize briefly an approach to the diagnosis and treatment of most human cancers. It is hoped that the family physician, the internist, the pediatrician, or the general surgeon who is presented with these problems can use the principles presented either for his role in management or as a guideline to appropriate patient referral.

DIAGNOSIS OF CANCER

Histologic proof of the diagnosis of cancer is crucial from the standpoint of planning appropriate therapy. Correct interpretation of symptoms and clinical findings is important in any disease, but nowhere is the proof of the diagnosis more important to the subsequent management of the patient than it is with neoplastic disease. Proof is needed to justify both the potential risks of the treatments planned in some patients and the withholding of further attempts at vigorous therapy for others. This point seems elementary, but it deserves emphasis nevertheless. The indications for diagnostic procedures and the methods employed for specific

1

clinical presentations are summarized in the subsequent disease-oriented chapters because accurate diagnosis is the key to appropriate treatment planning.

Early Diagnosis

The ease and high success rate of treatment methods for small, "early" cancers of most anatomic sites have led to an emphasis on the early detection of cancer. The definition of early diagnosis or early detection must be arbitrary, but early detection usually implies the discovery of the cancer before it has reached a stage where medical care is sought spontaneously by the patient. In the biologic sense a small lesion may not be "early" at all, but small lesions are generally more favorable problems to treat for most anatomic sites. For other neoplastic discoveries (e.g., in situ carcinoma discovered by vaginal smear or by xeromammography) the time of diagnosis may have a major impact on the eventual outcome. For these reasons, it is imperative that we minimize both patient and physician delay.

The problem of preclinical detection of cancer in man would be much easier to solve if we had a reliable blood test for this purpose. Actually, the optimal strategy for detecting presymptomatic cancer is far from clear. The widespread use of some examinations (e.g., the "pap" test) is feasible, although selectivity on the basis of "high-risk factors" is essential for more detailed, expensive, and time-consuming examinations (e.g., xeromammography). Despite the problems and disappointments associated with developing a strategy for screening, this approach, plus the exploration of preventive measures, will undoubtedly have a much greater impact on cancer in our population than the therapeutic measures that are the primary focus of this book.

TREATMENT OF CANCER

Philosophy of Cancer Treatment

The philosophy underlying all cancer treatment is to improve the quality and/or length of life of the patient. The ideal is to achieve a long-term "cure," which is possible in some cases, but in many instances the nature and stage of the neoplastic disease clearly preclude this objective. In some other chronic disease processes (heart disease, renal disease, peripheral vascular disease, pulmonary emphysema, cirrhosis) complete cure is never possible. The goals of the treatment of these diseases are effective clinical management of the various disabilities produced by the disease and achievement of the highest quality of life possible despite the limitations of function and decreased life expectancy that the disease will surely cause—a concept of "disease control." Too often, physicians faced with an "incurable" cancer problem do not apply this same concept of "disease control."

From the standpoint of the patient, disease control is as important as the effort to cure it. The physician who develops this philosophy will convey a positive approach to each patient. The cancer patient needs physicians who are anxious to help alleviate his problem, whatever the outcome of the disease process.

Choice of Treatment Method

Most treatment planning requires a thorough knowledge of the expected behavior or natural history of cancers at various sites. Another factor of great importance in the treatment plan is the stage of disease at the time of initial presentation. Past experience has led to accumulation of data supporting one therapeutic plan for the early stages of disease for some cancers, whereas a different approach may be much more effective for more advanced stages. Various patterns of metastatic disease can be recognized also for each individual neoplasm, and knowledge of responses of these patterns will assist in the choice of optimal treatment from specific options that are available. This concept is best illustrated in the discussion of the various patterns of "recurrent" disease in patients with breast cancer (Chap. 7). If benefits from the therapy are to be greater than its disadvantages, the treatment plan for an individual patient should be guided by the specific histologic diagnosis, the extent of the neoplasm at the time of initial presentation, and a thorough understanding of the natural history of the disease.

The major treatment methods used for cancer in past years have been surgical resection and radiation therapy. Many physicians in this country considered surgical resection of most cancers as the primary curative treatment of localized lesions, whereas radiation therapy was more widely used for management of manifestations of the local process when total resection was not feasible. However, appreciation of the effectiveness of radiation therapy as primary treatment for many cancers and major improvements in radiation techniques have led to a much more prominent role for radiation therapy in cancer management. The choice between these techniques of treatment varies with both the individual cancers and the individual patients as outlined in subsequent chapters.

The systemic methods of cancer treatment were considered palliative tools until recently, but chemotherapy has now emerged as a major treatment modality, either alone or in combination with other therapeutic methods. Immunotherapy is still in the investigational stage, just as chemotherapy was in the past, but this approach is certainly one with future potential. The current status of these methods is reviewed in Chapters 2 and 3, and their role in management of cancer of specific sites is noted in other chapters where appropriate. As progress is made in cancer management, these systemic approaches will undoubtedly be the methods responsible for improved results as the maximum benefits of surgery and radiation therapy have been attained.

A detailed description of operative technique, radiation therapy equipment and treatment planning, and the administration of chemotherapeutic agents is beyond the scope of this volume. Some of these technical considerations are alluded to in various sections in order to clarify the treatment plans described, particularly if there are no convenient references for specific procedures that may be of interest to the reader. Our purpose, however, has been to develop general guidelines for the management of "solid tumors" in man.

Interdisciplinary Approach to Cancer

Frequently, optimal treatment planning for the patient with cancer requires a coordination of professional talents that cannot be provided by a single individual. Some patients may be treated by a representative of one discipline, but in other situations the ideal treatment may require a combination of modalities. The focus of most cancer patient care programs is on this vital interdisciplinary concept. Despite the importance of the team approach, however, a primary physician is still needed to maintain continuity of care during the long management process.

One of the most efficient means of achieving multidisciplinary consultation for the purposes listed above is the hospital cancer conference or "tumor board." Although this type of conference is usually designed to function as an educational device, it also plays a vital role in terms of consultative activity for patients with cancer. Many tumor boards are composed of only those physicians available and interested in cancer problems in a community or hospital, but most include a radiologist, a pathologist, an internist, a pediatrician, a surgeon, a gynecologist, and representatives of various other specialities. This wide speciality representation is needed if this type of patient-oriented conference is to provide the team approach to evaluation of patients and treatment planning. Participation of a large portion of a hospital staff is also important for this mechanism to be successful in its educational function. Although the final management recommendation for an individual patient must be made by the physician in whom the patient has placed his trust, this physician is able to provide the best options and care if he or she has the opportunity to exploit the opinions of a team with differing points of view.

THE ONCOLOGIST

The field of oncology has been receiving more emphasis in recent years as the impact of cancer on our population has been more fully appreciated. The radiation therapist has always been an oncologist as the activity of his specialty is virtually confined to cancer problems. Some specialists in other fields, such as pediatrics, internal medicine, gynecology, and surgery, have focused on cancer problems within their own area of specialization. This area of subspecialization has been recognized by some of these fields to the extent that special training programs and certifying board examinations have been developed (e.g., medical oncology, pediatric oncology, and gynecologic oncology). Surgeons who put their major clinical effort into clincial cancer problems are also identified as oncologists (surgical oncology), and training programs are now emerging for surgeons who wish to develop additional experience and competence in the broad field of cancer. It is important to remember, however, that none of these oncology specialists within the various disciplines is able to provide the balanced interdisciplinary view that the team approach achieves.

Each "oncologist" obviously becomes an important participant in the collaborative treatment planning program at his own institution. In addition, his special interest in cancer provides an additional consultative resource for colleagues in his general specialty. The oncologists in the various specialty areas must provide leadership in cancer education and clinical investigation for the much larger group of students and physicians of all specialities who will continue to provide most of the care for the majority of cancer patients.

CLINICAL RESEARCH AND CANCER PATIENT CARE

The development of cancer chemotherapy, as outlined in Chapter 2, has been accompanied by improvement in the capability of the pharmacologic approach to cancer. This progress has been a result of continuing clinical research programs designed to develop the optimal protocols for drugs used alone or in combination with other methods. In many instances, the patient involved in ongoing clinical investigation receives the optimal current treatment. The structure of these investigative programs requires careful planning so that no patient is ever given therapy that is liable to be less effective than the standard established approach. However, it is just as important to test new treatment alternatives by prospective controlled clinical trials, rather than exploit these new clinical ideas without either a solid basis or a hope of compiling reliable new information. The advantages of this general approach to clinical investigation are well demonstrated by the exciting progress that has been made in the treatment of childhood leukemia.

In contrast to many investigative chemotherapeutic programs, much of our current practice in surgery and radiotherapy was developed by trial and error. In many instances the use of a therapeutic procedure was clearly unacceptable because of morbidity greater than the potential advantages to the patient. On the other hand, a number of treatment procedures have been accepted as standard practice without truly objective evidence that they are superior to other, less popular approaches. In some instances, the choice between these alternative methods is of little moment in terms of risk, disability, or cost. In others, there may be a real advantage to challenging the time-honored approach. Unless prospective clinical trials are applied to these treatment plans in the same way that they have been applied to chemotherapeutic trials, we will never be able to justify the use of one therapeutic approach over another. Both surgeons and radiotherapists have come to accept the need for objective clinical data in recent years, and some of our established ideas are now being tested by prospective clinical trials.

Cooperative Clinical Investigation

It is usually necessary to develop cooperative protocols by groups of clinical investigators to obtain the goal of adequate numbers of study patients for obtaining meaningful answers from these prospective clinical trials. One approach for obtaining data of this type is through the cooperative clinical groups sponsored and supported by the National Cancer Institute. Many of these cooperative groups were initiated with the limited goal of improving therapeutic regimes for certain specific categories of malignant disease, and often they included cooperating investigators in only one medical discipline. As it became evident that the range of disease under study required participation by members of all disciplines, the cooperative groups and their institutional members expanded to include representatives of all major disciplines. The studies being performed in this way are a model of the interdisciplinary approach to the treatment of cancer.

Clinical Investigation and
the Practicing Physician

The solitary practicing physician obviously cannot carry out prospective clinical trials with sufficient patient entries to answer these clinical questions with statistical confidence. Other practical features relating to health care delivery also may prevent his participation in organized clinical trials that are actually ongoing in his geographic region. However, the development of coordinated cancer centers, both university and community based, will encourage and assist the involvement of the physician and his patients in forward-looking cooperative clinical studies that are seeking answers regarding optimum treatment plans. This involvement, when feasible, will ensure more rapid accession of clinical knowledge regarding preferred treatment as well as make the currently best treatments available to virtually all patients. One of the most exciting aspects of cancer education in our country is that the majority of physicians now accept controlled clinical investigations of this type as not only appropriate but necessary, if we are to design the best treatment plans for our future patients with cancer.

OTHER RESOURCES FOR THE CANCER PATIENT AND HIS PHYSICIAN

American Cancer Society

The local or regional subsidiary of the American Cancer Society is a prime resource for the physician concerned with cancer patients. Their programs include public education, professional education, research, and services to cancer patients. Through the dedication of the leadership and the vast army of volunteers in this organization have come major contributions that are far in excess of the financial support that has been provided to the activities listed. The role of the American Cancer Society in education of the public and health care professionals is of particular benefit to the practicing physician, and his own involvement as a volunteer is rewarding both to him and to the cause he serves.

On the national scene, the American Cancer Society has become a partner with the federal government in providing needed basic and clinical research support for cancer. Since the society shares all of the goals of cancer center programs, it is often the nucleus for development of this emerging coordinating activity. This society deserves our whole-hearted support.

Hospital Cancer Programs

Hospital programs have been organized and encouraged through the stimulus of the Commission on Cancer of the American College of Surgeons.[1] They vary in both breadth and intensity, depending on the size and overall resources of the individual institution, but the quality of cancer patient care is enhanced by the involvement of physicians and their commitment to these programs. The key features are (a) the appointment in each hospital of an interdisciplinary cancer committee that is responsible for supervising both education and patient management programs in that institution; (b) the development of a functioning interdisciplinary education program that is directed toward improved patient management; and (c) the creation of a well-functioning and up-to-date cancer registry that is used effectively for both patient follow-up and physician education. These components of the program lead to teamwork in developing a broad-based attack on cancer at the institution concerned.

Cancer Registry

The hospital-based cancer registry (or tumor registry) has proven to be a useful mechanism for raising the standards of cancer patient care in individual institutions as well as having other benefits of an epidemiologic nature when efforts are combined in regional registries.

To many physicians the concept of the cancer registry is confusing. Some claim that it is a dusty repository for information that will never be used for the benefit of anyone. Nothing could be further from the truth if the registry has been properly developed. Important information on the natural history of various cancers in a community or region is accumulated. The registry can assist in the follow-up of treated patients and will serve as a reminder to both the physician and the patient that continued follow-up care is the essence of ideal patient management.[2] The registry should also play an important role in postgraduate education in cancer by virtue of periodic reports to the medical staff of an institution or geographic region on the status of their patients. The benefits of the information accumulated in the registry are not fully exploited if the data are not disseminated.

Cancer Centers

The increased interest of the entire nation in upgrading cancer care is well demonstrated by the overall increase in our federal commitment to the cancer problem. There has been an expansion of federal funding, both in research and in patient care programs, as a result of the National Cancer Act. The development of cancer centers as the means of coordinating cancer education, research, and patient care will undoubtedly be one of the more useful recent products of this increased federal emphasis on cancer. The underlying theme of the cancer center concept is to coordinate existing resources and to fill the gaps that exist in a region in order to elevate the level of care of all cancer patients to the maximum obtainable within the framework of our current knowledge. One of the key features of the cancer center is that it must both augment and coordinate the available cancer care resources rather than replace or compete with them.

Virtually all of the cancer centers that have been founded are in established medical centers. Frequently, there has been a historical lack of coordination between many of these medical centers and the other health care providers in the community for virtually all patient care functions. This is probably why the growth of cancer centers has been somewhat slow and awkward in the early stages of their development. The cancer center "system," when fully developed, will raise the level of cancer information of all practitioners by means of educational programs. It will provide specialized consultation and unique services that are requested for patients in a coordinating fashion; it will supplement existing cancer education programs and disseminate knowledge of the available treatment resources; and it will allow both the development and the exploitation of new research advances for all patients at the earliest possible time. To achieve these goals, a cancer center coordinating structure must actively involve all participants in the program, including the public, and the overall direction of the activities must be mutually agreed on by all concerned parties. The necessity of subjugating individual institutional egos to a common goal underlies the "growing pains" of some of these new cancer centers, but it is clear that the underlying concept has merit. Cancer centers may even serve as models for improving health care in other categories of disease.

Other Health Resources

Many important members of the health care team contribute to the improved care of the cancer patient. These include public health and visiting nurse services that are available in many communities for effectively providing the supportive care so important in improving the quality of life. Other voluntary agencies, such as the American Cancer Society, play a major role in cancer patient support in many communities. The social worker is also a key individual in total patient management because cancer patients often have urgent personal problems related to the disease. Rehabilitation services of various kinds are often an integral part of patient treatment, particularly for the patient who needs help in adapting to the disability produced by the primary therapy. Good examples of this are the "Reach to Recovery Program" for postmastectomy breast cancer patients (initiated by the American Cancer Society), societies for rehabilitation of patients who have lost their larynx, programs for amputees, and the "ostomy" clubs. Some of these programs were initiated by patients who wanted to help others with the same disability. Psychologists have also been of great help in improving our understanding of the patient's adjustment to disease and in developing solutions for some of these problems. It is vital for the physician treating patients with cancer to be aware of and willing to use all services available to the patient in his community.

SUMMARY

The problems of cancer management extend from prevention and early detection to the thoughtful management of the patient with advanced or "recurrent" cancer. The physician assuming responsibility for this management process must avail himself of all of the existing resources for diagnosis, treatment planning, and rehabilitation if he is to serve his patient well.

The primary emphasis of this volume will be to summarize briefly the current status of diagnosis and treatment of patients with cancer, but this primary emphasis should not limit our perspective. The future focus of cancer management must be on the beginning and end of the spectrum—prevention and rehabilitation.

REFERENCES

1. Cancer Program Manual. Commission on Cancer, American College of Surgeons, 1974
2. The Patient with Cancer: Guidelines for Follow-up. Commission on Cancer, American College of Surgeons, 1976

2

Principles and Techniques of Cancer Chemotherapy

Cancer chemotherapy with cytotoxic agents began in earnest 30 years ago with the observation by C. P. Rhoads[19] and many others that nitrogen mustard had a significant anticancer effect. Early investigations with alkylating agents were followed by years of relatively empirical trials of several classes of agents that were found to have antitumor activity in animal screening systems. The initial hope was that a "magic bullet" would soon emerge, but real practical clinical benefit was somewhat slower than desired or anticipated. However, we have now entered an era of more sophisticated and effective application of pharmacologic knowledge to clinical cancer problems. Much of this recent progress in cancer chemotherapy is the result of new knowledge from research in cancer cell biology during this same period. Also, new agents have been identified, the mechanisms of action of effective agents have been studied and better understood, and new information has been obtained in terms of cancer cell kinetics. These contributions have all aided our progress, but the major credit for the current status of improved anticancer chemotherapy must go to the persistence of the many clinical investigators who have performed endless controlled therapeutic trials in man. Cancer chemotherapy has advanced so that a few forms of cancer are essentially cured in a significant number of individuals, and other patients are significantly benefitted by the addition of chemotherapeutic agents to other forms of therapy.

    With continuing progress in cancer chemotherapy, there has been a concurrent change in the general category of physician who applies this treatment method. Cancer chemotherapy is no longer the domain of vir-

11

tually every practicing physician; instead, it is a treatment best employed or supervised by highly trained specialists in medical and pediatric oncology who must remain at the forefront of this rapidly changing field. The purpose of this chapter is to describe and define this general approach to cancer therapy in the broadest possible terms for those physicians who are not now focusing on this general method of treatment. Hopefully this will lead to an appreciation of the range of therapeutic possibilities now available and allow for a timely and appropriate search for knowledgeable consultation for cancer patients who may receive benefit from cancer chemotherapy. Specific details regarding the current chemotherapeutic approach to individual forms of cancer will be discussed in the other chapters in this volume. More detailed discussions of this approach are also available in larger texts.[2,8,11]

MECHANISM OF ACTION OF ANTICANCER AGENTS

The agents that have been found useful for clinical cancer therapy affect both normal cells and cancer cells, but they produce more damage to the cancer cell population than to normal tissues because of some quantitative difference in the alteration of the metabolic processes in these two cell populations. Although cytotoxic agents are not lethal to cancer cells selectively, the difference in the growth characteristics of cancerous and normal tissues as well as the minor unrecognized biochemical differences between these tissues probably combine to produce the selective effects. The "toxicities" observed with these agents are obviously the result of their concurrent effects on normal tissues.

Deoxyribonucleic acid (DNA), the genetic material of all cells, acts as the selective template for the production of specific forms of transfer, ribosomal, and messenger ribonucleic acid (RNA), and this determines which enzymes will be synthesized by the cell. These enzymes, in turn, are responsible for most of the continuing functions of cells, and interference with these processes will naturally affect continued function and proliferation of both normal and cancer cells. Most of the drugs used for cancer chemotherapy interfere in some way with these normal mechanisms of cell "business," and a better understanding of the normal cell cycle of preparation for mitosis and cellular division has lead to a clearer definition of mechanisms of drug action. To describe the mechanisms of action of cancer chemotherapeutic agents in these terms, it is important to define the normal cell cycle.

Cell Cycle of Dividing Cells[13,17]

The cell cycle of cells that divide, either for normal repair or as a part of uncontrolled proliferation (cancer), is shown in Figure 2-1. The time span of the individual phases of this cycle is variable, even in tissues that are proliferating in a controlled fashion, but the intracellular events in each phase are similar in all cells that divide. The cell is in one of the following phases: preparation for DNA synthesis by producing RNA precursors and protein (G1 phase); active DNA synthesis in preparation for complete and accurate duplication of nuclear material (S phase); preparation for actual cell division, a premitotic phase in which the cell is no longer synthesizing DNA (G2); and cell division by mitosis, a short period (M phase). Although all actively dividing cells are involved in one of these specific activities, most cell populations—normal or neoplastic—have a variable portion of cells in a resting phase (G0) in which there is no "reproductive" activity. Included in the resting phase are those cells that are in a permanently nondividing state as well as those cells that are capable of later recruitment into the active process of cell multiplication.

Both normal cell and cancer cell populations appear to divide more rapidly when their total volumes are small and more slowly when they are large. This leads to exponential growth producing short "doubling times" for tumors that are small. As the tumor mass increases, the "growth fraction" of the cancer population decreases and the doubling

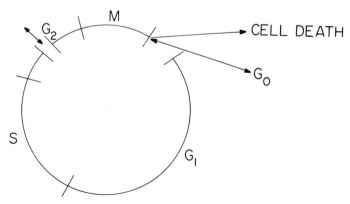

Fig. 2-1. The cell cycle. M, mitotic phase; G1, preparation preceding DNA synthesis; S, phase of DNA synthesis; G2, premitotic resting phase; G0, inactive resting phase from which cells may be recruited back into the cycle.

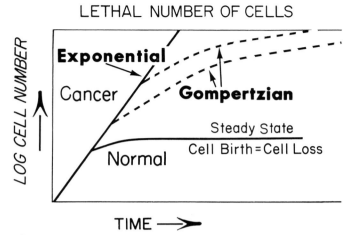

Fig. 2-2.   Diagram of growth of a typical cancer (Gomper-
zian growth curve). (Courtesy of Albert Munson, Ph.D.)

time lengthens.   Both normal tissues and cancers follow this biological
pattern described as "Gompertzian growth" (Fig. 2-2).   The implication
of this observation is that agents affecting the proliferating elements of the
cell cycle (the growth fraction) may be appropriate for small neoplastic
deposits, whereas agents that affect both the proliferating and the resting
compartments may be a necessary component of chemotherapy for larger
neoplastic masses.

Sites of Action of Chemotherapeutic Agents in Terms of the Cell Cycle

Information that has accumulated on the mechanism of action of the
various classes of agents has separated agents that are "S-phase specific"
in their action, those that are "S-phase specific and self-limited," those
that are "cycle nonspecific," and those that produce their effects by ar-
resting the cell during actual mitosis.   It is clear that some agents are effective only in inhibiting cells that are in the proliferative population compartment of a neoplasm and have no effect on the resting cells in G0.
These resting cells are injured by cycle nonspecific agents as these agents
exert their effect directly on the nuclear DNA, whether the cells are in the
"growth fraction" or not.   Thus the proportion of cells in a neoplasm in
the various compartments as defined in this fashion has a great deal to do
with the relative effectiveness of individual agents.

"Cell Kill" with Antitumor Cancer Chemotherapeutic Agents

Many of our clinical concepts and principles involved in the use of cancer chemotherapeutic agents are dependent on the "cell kill" hypothesis, which states that the survival of the host bearing the tumor is inversely related to the number of tumor cells that survive after administration of an agent.

Many of the data on which this hypothesis[22,23] is based were obtained from a leukemia animal model (L1210 system) in which it was shown that (a) the injection of a single cell can ultimately lead to the death of the host; (b) the larger the number of cells inoculated, the shorter the survival; (c) the interval between inoculation of the cells and death can be predicted by a knowledge of the number of the cells injected and the doubling time of the tumor cell population; and (d), survival is prolonged by destruction of a significant fraction of the cell population. Cell destruction by chemotherapeutic agents appears to follow first-order kinetics (e.g., a given dose will destroy a constant fraction of the existing cells and not a fixed number of cells). On this basis, the smaller the target to be affected, the smaller the residual volume of cells after a single treatment. Theoretically, the repeated use of an effective cytotoxic agent should eventually reduce the cell population to zero or to an insignificant number of cancer cells, which the host could dispose of by some other defense mechanism if the toxicity of the agent on normal tissues could be tolerated at the dose and frequency of drug administration required. Using this logic, it is clear that a small tumor mass would require less aggressive therapy than a larger tumor to produce a beneficial result.

One problem with this general concept of cell kill is that the tumor model on which this hypothesis is based differs from most human cancers by having almost a 100% growth fraction. The differences in the cell cycle characteristics of this model from those seen in human cancer may well give rise to misleading information regarding the appropriate choice and scheduling of chemotherapeutic agents for clinical use. Another discouraging feature of this cell kill hypothesis is that there are few demonstrations of the validity of this hypothesis in human cancer. This is partly because of differences between this animal model and human cancer in terms of the kinetics involved, but it is also because of the less potent drug-cancer combinations that are employed for clinical use. Nevertheless, the hypothesis is valid in a general sense if the agent or agents employed in patients have a significant anticancer affect.

USEFUL CHEMOTHERAPEUTIC AGENTS
FOR CANCER TREATMENT

The major categories of chemotherapeutic agents are the polyfunctional alkylating agents, antimetabolites, antitumor antibiotics, specific mitotic inhibitors, and a "miscellaneous" group of drugs. To this list should be added the various hormones that have been found so useful in the management of endocrine-responsive cancers, despite different concepts regarding their mechanisms of action. The clinical indications for all these agents are shown in Table 2-1. Although potentially useful new agents are constantly being developed by using newly acquired chemical and pharmacological knowledge as well as information obtained from experimental animal model systems, the general categories and the mechanisms of action of agents in each of these categories (Table 2-2) will follow the patterns outlined for these clinically useful agents.

Polyfunctional Alkylating Agents

Alkylating agents include those compounds that are capable of replacing a hydrogen atom in another molecule by an alkyl radical. They are thought to act by "binding" the DNA so as to prevent the separation of the two strands of DNA in the double-coiled helix that is necessary for cell replication. It has been suggested that there may be some differences in the modes of action of the various alkylating agents employed clinically, but the major differences between the various agents listed in Table 2-1 relate to the routes of administration, the metabolism of the individual agents, and the need or lack of need for metabolism of a carrier moiety to produce an "active" fraction. Agents in this category affect cells in all phases of the cell cycle in a nonspecific fashion. Although effective as single agents for many cancers, they rarely produce optimal clinical effect without being combined with other agents that affect a specific phase of the cell cycle.

Antimetabolites

Antimetabolites affect cells by inhibiting the biosynthesis of the nucleic acids that are essential components of both DNA and RNA. In this way they prevent both multiplication and normal function of cells. This inhibition of biosynthesis may relate to purines (6-mercaptopurine and 6-thioguanine), the production of thymidylic acid (fluorinated pyrimidines and methotrexate), and other similar interruptions in nucleic acid synthesis. These agents are particularly active against cells in the synthesis phase of the cell cycle (S phase) and usually affect cells only when they are in this portion of interphase (Fig. 2-1). For clinical use, antimetabolites are effective alone or in combination with other agents. The rate of destruction of susceptible cells in a tumor population is obviously determined by the life span of these cells that are prevented from undergoing mitosis by the effect of such agents on the S phase. One can easily see how differences in the cell kinetics of individual tumors may have considerable effect clinically on both the value and scheduling of these agents.

Antibiotics

The antitumor antibiotics are nonspecific in terms of their relationship to the cell cycle kinetics of a cancer, a property they hold in common with the alkylating agents, procarbazine, and the nitrosoureas. Their general mechanism of action is that of binding with DNA to block RNA production. The antimicrobial antibiotics specifically inhibit protein synthesis of bacterial ribosomes but have a substantially lesser effect on *mammalian* ribosomes. Thus these agents have a particular therapeutic value on microorganisms. The antitumor antibiotics that have been employed are less specific than this since they affect both normal and cancer cells, but a number of antibiotics have shown antitumor benefits in man.

Mitotic Inhibitors

Mitotic inhibitors can arrest mitosis in metaphase (Fig. 2-1). This function has been useful in "synchronization" of cell populations when mitotic inhibitors are combined with agents (the vinca alkaloids) specific for the S phase of the cycle. The specific mode of action of mitotic inhibitors makes treatment more effective when they are combined with agent(s) of other categories.

Miscellaneous Agents

Specific metabolic inhibition of normal metabolic processes by some agents has been useful in controlling some of the clinical manifestations of cancers that produce excessive amounts of hormone. Some drugs interfere with synthesis of proteins necessary for continued growth of cells. The steroid hormones inhibit the growth of cancer by mechanisms that are unclear at the present time, but these may well relate to interference at the cell membrane level.

The mechanisms of the anticancer effects of estrogens, progestational agents, androgens, and adrenocorticosteroids are assumed to be quite different from those of other pharmacologic agents under discussion. Actually, little information on mechanism of action is available.

Table 2-1
Effective Anticancer Agents with Major Toxicities and Current Clinical Indications

Class	Drug	Major Route of Administration	Usual Dose	Acute Toxic Signs	Major Toxic Manifestations	Disease for Which Agent is Commonly Employed (Single or Combination)
Alkylating agents	Mechlorethamine (nitrogen mustard)	IV	0.4 mg/kg (single or divided dose)	Nausea and vomiting	Bone marrow depression	Lymphomas, lung cancer
	Chlorambucil (Leukeran®)	Oral	0.1–0.2 mg/kg/day	None	Bone marrow depression	Lymphomas, chronic lymphatic leukemia, trophoblastic neoplasms
	Melphalan (L-PAM)	Oral	0.1 mg/kg/day × 7; 2–4 mg/day as maintenance	None	Bone marrow depression	Malignant melanoma, ovarian cancer, multiple myeloma, breast cancer, seminoma
	Cyclophosphamide (Cytoxan®)	IV	40 mg/kg single dose or 3.5–10 mg/kg/day × 10	Nausea and vomiting	Bone marrow depression, alopecia, hemorrhagic cystitis, oral ulceration	Lymphomas, multiple myeloma, lymphocytic and granulocytic leukemia, lung cancer, breast cancer, ovarian cancer, sarcomas
		Oral	50–200 mg/day (adjust for maintenance)	Nausea and vomiting		

	Route	Dose	Acute toxicity	Major or delayed toxicity	Indications
Triethylenethiophosphoramide (Thio-TEPA®)	IV	0.8–1.0 mg/kg or 0.2 mg/kg/day × 5	None	Bone marrow depression	Lymphomas, lung cancer, breast cancer
Busulfan (Myleran®)	Oral	2–6 mg/day	None	Bone marrow depression	Chronic granulocytic leukemia
Antimetabolites Methotrexate (amethopterin)	Oral	2.5–5 mg/day (15 mg/m²/week)	Nausea and vomiting	Oral and GI ulceration; bone marrow depression (toxicity increased by renal impairment); cirrhosis	Lymphomas and leukemias, multiple forms of squamous cancer, choriocarcinoma; breast cancer, sarcomas, histiocytosis X
	IV	20 mg/m² 2 × per week (rapid IV)	Nausea and vomiting		
Fluorouracil (5-FU)	IV (oral route less "dependable")	12.5 mg/kg/day × 3–5 days (intermittent); or weekly dose 10–15 mg/kg	Nausea (occasional)	Oral and GI ulceration, diarrhea, bone marrow depression	GI cancers, breast cancer, ovarian cancer
6-Mercaptopurine (6-MP)	Oral	2.5 mg/kg/day (90 mg/m²/day)	None	Bone marrow depression, liver dysfunction	Leukemias
6-Thioguanine (6-TG)	Oral	2 mg/kg/day	None	Bone marrow depression	Acute granulocytic leukemia
Arabinosyl cytosine (ARA-C)	IV	1.0–3.0 mg/kg/day × 10–20; 100 mg/m²/12 hr × 10 doses	Nausea and vomiting	Bone marrow depression, megaloblastosis, oral and GI ulceration	Acute granulocytic leukemia

Table 2-1 (continued)

Class	Drug	Major Route of Administration	Usual Dose	Acute Toxic Signs	Major Toxic Manifestations	Disease for Which Agent is Commonly Employed (Single or Combination)
Antibiotics	Adriamycin (Doxo- rubicin®)	IV	50–80 mg/m² in single or divided doses every 3 weeks	Nausea and vomit- ing	Stomatitis, GI disturb- ances, alopecia, bone marrow de- pression, cardiac toxicity	Sarcomas, breast cancer, lymphomas, lung cancer, thyroid cancer, Wilms' tumor
	Bleomycin (Blenoxane®)	IV	0.25 mg/kg/day × 5–7 days	Nausea, vomit- ing, chills, and fever	Stomatitis, alopecia, pulmonary fibrosis (5%)	Lymphomas, squamous cancers (head and neck), testis cancer
		IM	1.0–2.0 mg/day (maintenance)			
	Dactinomycin (actinomycin D)	IV	0.015 mg/kg/day × 5 every 6– 12 weeks	Nausea and vomit- ing	Stomatitis, oral ulcers, diarrhea, alopecia, bone marrow depression	Testis cancer, Wilms' tumor, sarcomas
	Mithramycin (mithracin®)	IV	0.025 mg/kg every other day × 3–4	Nausea and vomit- ing	Thrombocytopenia, hypocalcemia, hepatic toxicity	Testis cancer, tropho- blastic tumors (hyper- calcemia)

Category	Drug	Route	Dose	Acute toxicity	Delayed toxicity	Indications
	Mitomycin C (Mutamycin®)	IV	0.05 kg/day × 5	Nausea and vomiting	Bone marrow depression, skin lesions, pulmonary and renal toxicity (severe)	Multiple squamous carcinomas, GI cancer
Mitotic inhibitors	Vinblastine (Velban®)	IV	0.1–0.2 mg/kg/week	Nausea and vomiting	Alopecia, areflexia, bone marrow depression	Lymphomas, breast cancer, testis cancer, histiocytosis X
	Vincristine (Oncovin®)	IV	2 mg/m²/week	Joint pain	Areflexia, paresthesias, paralytic ileus, constipation, hypertension, hoarseness	Lymphomas and leukemias, breast cancer, sarcomas, Wilms' tumor
Nitrosoureas	BCNU	IV	100–200 mg/m² every 6 weeks	Nausea and vomiting	Bone marrow depression (delayed)	Lymphomas, melanoma, brain tumors
	Methyl-CCNU	Oral	200 mg/m² every 6–8 weeks	Nausea and vomiting	Bone marrow depression (delayed)	GI cancer, lung cancer, melanoma, brain tumors
	CCNU	Oral	80–100 mg/m²	Nausea and vomiting	Bone marrow depression (delayed)	Same as above
Miscellaneous cytotoxic agents	Imidazole, carboxamide (DTIC)	IV	4.5 mg/kg/day × 10 (repeat q. 4 weeks)	Nausea and vomiting	Mild bone marrow depression (delayed)	Melanoma, sarcomas

Table 2-1 (continued)

Class	Drug	Major Route of Administration	Usual Dose	Acute Toxic Signs	Major Toxic Manifestations	Disease for Which Agent is Commonly Employed (Single or Combination)
	Hydroxyurea (Hydrea®)	Oral	20–30 mg/day	Nausea (mild)	Bone marrow depression	Chronic granulocytic leukemia
	Mitotane (o,p'-DDD)	Oral	6–15 mg/kg/day	Nausea and vomiting	Mental depression, tremors, skin eruptions	Adrenocortical carcinoma (functioning)
	Procarbazine (Natulane®)	Oral	1–2 mg/kg/day	Nausea and vomiting	Depression of peripheral counts, bone marrow depression, mental depression	Lymphomas, lung cancer
	L-Asparaginase	IV	1000 units/kg/day × 10	Hypersensitivity reaction	Pancreatitis, liver dysfunction, coagulopathy	Acute lymphocytic leukemia
		IM	200 units/kg/day × 10			
Hormones Androgens	Testosterone propionate	IM	50–100 mg 3 × weekly	None	Masculinization, fluid retention	Breast cancer
	Fluoxymesterone (Halotestin®)	Oral	10–20 mg/day	None	Masculinization, fluid retention	Breast cancer

	Drug	Route	Dose		Side effects	Indications
	Testolactone (Teslac®)	IM	100 mg 3 ×/week	None	Masculinization, fluid retention	Breast cancer
Estrogens	Diethylstilbesterol	Oral	15 mg/day (1 mg for prostate cancer)	None	Fluid retention, uterine bleeding, feminization, hypercalcemia	Breast cancer, prostate cancer
	Ethinylestradiol (Estinyl®)	Oral	3 mg/day (0.1 mg/day for prostate cancer)	None	Fluid retention, uterine bleeding, feminization, hypercalcemia	Breast cancer, prostate cancer
Progestins	Hydroxyprogesterone caproate (Delalutin®)	IM	1 gm 2 ×/week	None	None	Endometrial cancer
	6-Methyl hydroxyprogesterone	Oral	100–200 mg/day	None	None	Endometrial cancer, renal cancer, breast cancer
	Provera®	IM	200–600 mg 2 ×/week	None		
Adrenocortical compounds	Cortisone acetate	Oral	20–100 mg/day	None	Fluid retention, hypertension, potassium depletion, susceptibility to infection	Lymphomas, leukemias, breast cancer
	Prednisone	Oral	10–100 mg/day	None		
	Dexamethasone (Decadron®)	Oral	0.5–4.0 mg/day	None		

Table 2-2
Mechanism of Action of Anticancer Chemotherapeutic Agents

Class	Mechanism of Action
Polyfunctional alkylating agents	Bind to DNA and prevent separation of the two strands of DNA (cross-link)
Antimetabolites	Inhibit biosynthesis of nucleic acids
Methotrexate	Blocks folic reductase, blocks purine ring biosynthesis, and inhibits methylation of deoxyuridylic to thymidylic acid
6-Mercaptopurine	Blocks purine ring biosynthesis and inhibits interconversion of purines
5-Fluorouracil	Blocks thymidylate synthesis and inhibits formation of thymidylic acid
Arabinosyl cytosine	Inhibits DNA polymerase and blocks reduction of cytidylic to deoxycytidylic acid
Antibiotics	Bind with DNA to block RNA production
Other	
Vinca alkaloids	Destroy "spindle" to produce mitotic arrest
L-Asparaginase	Hydrolyzes L-asparagine and prevents protein synthesis
Procarbazine	Depolymerizes DNA
Nitrosureas	Bind to DNA

The many clinical indications for this category of agents are shown on Table 2-1, but breast cancer, prostatic cancer, hypernephroma, and leukemia are the cancers for which they have been the most frequently employed (see Chaps. 7 and 11).

GENERAL CONSIDERATIONS IN CANCER CHEMOTHERAPY

Toxicity of Agents

Because the agents under discussion have relatively little specificity for cancer cells as opposed to normal cells, physicians are concerned about the toxicity experienced with each of the agents. The clinical evidence of toxicity of each of the agents is briefly listed in Table 2-1 Although there are individual differences among agents, the primary feature of toxicity of the agents in man is that they generally have a more pronounced effect on those normal cells that demonstrate rapid proliferation under normal circumstances. For this reason the gastrointestinal tract and the bone marrow are particularly sensitive tissues. It is important to distinguish reversible effects on normal cells between the intervals of drug administration from those effects that are irreversible. Anticancer effect may well be achieved by dosage and scheduling which allow repair in normal cell populations without dangerous sequelae during the period of "toxicity." This fine line between success and ineffectiveness is affected by small differences in the pharmacologic disposition of these agents in man for each drug and dosage schedule employed. It is also affected by the age and sex of the patient as well as by concurrent administration of other drugs. Therefore, careful investigations of absorption, distribution, and excretion are required with all agents before they are actually used. All agents are subjected to careful toxicologic studies in experimental animals before intensive efforts are made to test the anticancer usefulness of these agents in man. Metabolic studies of these agents are required in man at an early stage because of known differences in the metabolism and excretion of agents in different species. Dosage, optimal routes, and timing are all features of this investigation.

In the use of established chemotherapeutic regimes, it is usually necessary to accept some degree of "toxicity" if the optimal anticancer effect is to be achieved. The physician using these agents must be alert to the expected toxicities and be prepared to alter the regime as well as treat the effects of these agents on normal cells.

The bone marrow effects of most of the anticancer agents increase the risks of bleeding and infection, and this leads to the need for frequent monitoring of leukocyte and platelet counts and for judicious use of platelet and leukocyte infusions, antimicrobial antibiotics, and other mechanisms for reducing the likelihood of infection when the patient is in a susceptible state. Awareness of the more unusual infectious complications is important also so that these problems can be effectively diagnosed and treated. Gastrointestinal toxicity is almost universal because of the rapid cell turnover that occurs normally in the gastrointestinal tract. Alopecia is often a disturbing toxic effect that requires the use of a wig. Neurotoxicity occurs with several agents, particularly the vinca alkaloids. Pulmonary toxicity is infrequent but may be the limiting factor, especially with the antibiotic bleomycin, and cardiac toxicity is a specific limiting problem with adriamycin.

Appropriate monitoring procedures for identifying gastrointestinal and other toxicities must be built into the plan of therapy, along with judicious planning for alterations in the treatment schedule when toxicity is observed. Because of these assorted problems, most aggressive chemotherapeutic routines must be managed by physicians with considerable experience in the use of anticancer chemotherapy. A "brinksmanship" approach is probably required in most instances if the optimal anticancer effects are to be realized.

The teratogenic effects of many of the commonly used anticancer agents signal toxicity of more long-range significance. This is a concerning effect in children and adults in the reproductive years, particularly in those patients who experience long-term cancer control as a result of therapy. The later development of new cancers as a result of carcinogenic effect of these compounds is another late toxicity that will become more of a problem as the chemotherapeutic approach to cancer achieves more widespread acceptance.

Immunosuppression by Anticancer Chemotherapy

Several classes of chemotherapeutic agents originally used for cancer are now effectively employed for clinical immunosuppression for organ allografting. Although the host defense mechanisms are modified by many of the agents used to treat cancer, it is feasible to employ agents with maximum anticancer effects and minimal immunosuppressive features. It is also clear that any immunosuppression that is induced by anticancer agents depends on a complex interaction that includes dosage, drug scheduling, mode of action, and specific features of administration of the immunizing antigen used to monitor this effect. The general medical status of the patient receiving anticancer chemotherapy strongly influences the degree of immunosuppression experienced, since either the specific type of cancer or the patient's nutritional status may have produced a depression of the immunologic system before drug administration. The immunosuppressive effects of anticancer agents should be appreciated by the clinician who uses these drugs, but this property should not be a deterrent to the use of effective agents for cancer therapy.

Pharmacokinetics

Effective scheduling of agents for the treatment of cancers is dependent on the repair mechanisms for recovery of the normal tissues from the effects of these agents. The route of administration employed is often dictated by specific differences noted with the individual agents, but the route is dependent on the efficiency of gastrointestinal absorption, the metabolic fate, and the presence or absence of cell cycle specificities for individual agents. As more information accumulates on the detailed pharmacology and kinetics of anticancer agents and the kinetics of the cancers they affect, the scheduling of these agents is being placed on a more logical basis.

One of the major reasons for detailed research in the pharmacokinetics and the distribution of the anticancer agents is the known difference that does occur in the distribution of various agents within the body. The blood-brain barrier that exists for some agents is an excellent example of this problem as it may lead to a "sanctuary" for tumor cells in the central nervous system. This has been well demonstrated in the response of some patients with leukemia to systemic chemotherapy. In this instance appreciation of the capillary blocking factors in the brain and meninges has led to the effective use of agents by intrathecal administration and to the use of craniospinal irradiation to destroy cells isolated from the rest of the vascular system. The testes are another sanctuary for some cancer cells during systemic cancer chemotherapy.

More information is required to develop truly optimal schedules for therapy, but both new pharmacologic information and prospective clinical trials effectively comparing different treatment schedules are producing important data in this field where the margin between failure and success is so slim.

Drug Resistance

One of the major problems in the effective use of anticancer chemotherapy is the development of clinical resistance to these drugs. Repeated administration of agents to cancer patients over a long time interval has strong rationale from the standpoint of some of the concepts previously discussed, but resistant cell lines frequently develop with chronic therapy. An analogy to this problem is the development of resistant microorganisms in the therapy for infectious desease with antimicrobial agents. One theoretical solution to this problem is the therapeutic use of multiple drugs serially or in combination, but the success of any drug treatment program will be dependent on the number of resistant lines that develop in the tumor population as well as the number of drugs that can actually be used for treatment. Since the mechanisms leading to drug resistance are mainly speculative at the present time, the solutions to this problem are empirical rather than developed on substantial grounds.

"SPECIAL" APPROACHES TO ANTICANCER CHEMOTHERAPY

Regional Chemotherapy

Regional intra-arterial chemotherapy was first described in 1951 by Klopp et al.,[12] who used intermittent intra-arterial nitrogen mustard through external carotid artery catheters. Since that time a host of techniques have been developed for the intra-arterial infusion (fractionated or

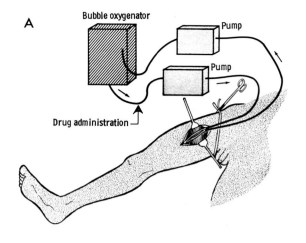

A

Bubble oxygenator

Pump

Pump

Drug administration

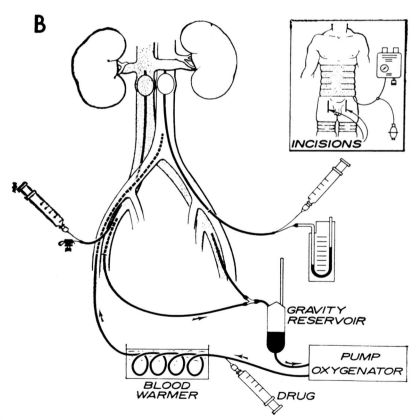

B

INCISIONS

GRAVITY
RESERVOIR

PUMP
OXYGENATOR

BLOOD
WARMER

DRUG

Fig. 2-3. Diagram of regional perfusion chemotherapy
with extracorporeal circut for (**A**) extremity and (**B**) pelvis.

continuous) and for isolated or semi-isolated regional perfusion of anatomic areas with extracorporeal equipment[3,14,24] (Figs. 2-3 and 2-4). This
approach had great appeal in the 1960s because of our relative disappoint-
ment with the results obtained from the systemic administration of available anticancer agents. Many ingenious refinements of regional arterial
techniques for chemotherapy were developed, and there is extensive literature describing attempts to employ this approach for virtually every anatomic site in the human body. Currently this approach is used for
treating only squamous carcinoma of the head and neck region, primary
and metastatic carcinoma in the liver, and recurrent and metastatic melanoma that is clinically confined to the extremities. The marginal benefit
that has resulted form this approach is demonstrated by the small number
of clinicians that still use it in clinical cancer chemotherapy.

In retrospect, the disappointing results following the regional arterial
approach to cancer chemotherapy are not surprising. Most advanced
cancers are not usually responsive to regional concentrations of chemotherapeutic agents that prove to be the maximum levels tolerated by the
normal tissues in the perfusion or infusion circuits. Although other
normal tissues (such as the bone marrow or the intestinal mucosa) are the
Achilles' heel with systemic anticancer chemotherapy, the local toxicity

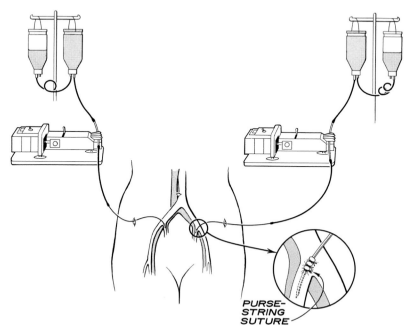

PURSE-
STRING
SUTURE

Fig. 2-4. Diagram of arterial infusion chemotherapy for prolonged continuous
regional administration to the pelvis.

limitation in these regional circuits is actually analogous to that associated with systemic drug administration. In addition, the regional localization of agents is often less striking than was imagined owing to other factors such as the systemic administration of the drug from the venous side of the anatomic circuit being infused; "leakage" from the regional perfusion circuit, which is usually less isolated than it would appear to be because of uncontrolled collateral vessels; and the later passage of the anticancer agent to the rest of the body by absorption and circulation from extracellular and intracellular fluid compartments after the regional perfusion has been clinically completed. For these reasons it appears unlikely that regional arterial chemotherapy will ever have a major impact on clinical cancer therapy except for those unusual circumstances where the agent is rapidly absorbed and "fixed" by the tissues being treated.

Although one might conclude from the above that there is no merit at the present time to any form of regional arterial chemotherapy for human cancer, a number of physicians still employ this approach with the conviction that the clinical results in selected situations are superior to those obtained with the systemic administration of chemotherapeutic agents now available to us. It is quite conceivable that there is some merit to the approach in selected circumstances, but the unfortunate fact is that no clinical trials have effectively compared this approach with less inconvenient alternatives. There may be a place for this type of therapy in the future, but this approach should be limited to those individuals and institutions equipped to answer these yet unanswered questions in a scientific fashion.

Combination Chemotherapy

There are a number of clear-cut examples of major therapeutic benefit from the simultaneous administration of two or more anticancer agents in the treatment of human cancer, but much of this progress has been achieved by the empirical trial of drug combinations without a truly sound basis for the choice of the individual agents. In some instances the combination employed includes so many agents that one might wonder if some disadvantages are produced by some of the components of the combination. There is a major need for development of combination protocols based on the knowledge that has developed regarding specific sites of action of drugs in the cell cycle, as well as for clinical trials to investigate these various drug combinations in a stepwise fashion. The optimal combination of anticancer agents would certainly be one in which synergy occurs, but most combination therapies employed thus far produce additive benefit at best.

Since toxicity is a major concern in the use of all anticancer agents, combination programs must be designed to minimize dangerous toxicity while exploiting the advantages of drugs that have anticancer mechanisms. A general rule of thumb that is useful in planning combination drug therapy is to use agents that have both different modes of action and different patterns of toxicity. Theoretically, this should reduce the possibility of drug resistance and, hopefully, achieve an additive effect from the individual components of the program.

The combination drug approach has been employed most effectively in the chemotherapeutic management of leukemia, but combination therapy for the management of "solid tumors" is much less advanced. In spite of the primitive nature of many clinical trials performed thus far, it is quite clear that acute lymphatic leukemia in childhood, Hodgkin's disease, carcinoma of the breast, and gastrointestinal cancer have been significantly benefitted by this general approach.[4,5,18] With the identification of few new individual agents with a major clinical effect on human cancer, the combination drug approach is one of great hope for the future.

Adjuvant Chemotherapy

The rationale for combining treatment modalities for better end results has a sound basis in experimental systems involving a number of animal models, and it is easy to understand the current enthusiasm for the clinical application of these findings. The combination of systemic chemotherapy with either surgical or x-ray treatment of a localized cancer has the appealing rationale that the systemic treatment may deal with the microscopic cancer (both within and without the local treatment field) that is not controlled completely by the strictly regional treatment. The key question is whether these experimental findings can actually be translated into the improved treatment of cancer in our human population.

Clinical data have now accumulated that demonstrate superior cancer control by adjuvant chemotherapy for Wilms' tumor,[25] embryonal rhabdomyosarcoma in children,[9] osteogenic sarcoma,[20] Ewing's sarcoma, and some testicular cancers.[1] One might logically conclude that the principle has been established that adjuvant chemotherapy is a worthwhile approach on the basis of these most impressive data. On the other hand, prospective clinical trials of this same approach for some of our major adult cancers, including gastric cancer,[16] lung cancer, and bladder cancer, have failed to show any benefit from the addition of chemotherapy to operative treatment. Adjuvant chemotherapy for colorectal cancer has produced either minimal or no benefit in all clinical trials performed thus far,[10,15] but recent trials of adjuvant chemotherapy for surgically treated breast cancer (in patients with lymph node metastases) strongly suggest the possibility of survival benefit from this surgery-drug treatment combination.[6,7] These data are probable justification for the routine application of adjuvant chemotherapy to patients with curable breast cancer at this time, but this statement cannot be made for most of the other common adult cancers that are currently being treated by surgery with hope of "cure."

It is clear that a common denominator in all clinical trials of adjuvant chemotherapy is the finding that adjuvant treatment has been of benefit only for those diseases for which the same systemic chemotherapeutic agents have been beneficial in the management of patients who have gross recurrent or metastatic disease. Many of our adjuvant chemotherapy programs have failed because of the relative weakness of the agents available for a specific cancer. These observations should be of benefit in the planning of future clinical trials as the hope that minimal residual disease would respond more effectively than gross disease has not been fulfilled. It is our belief that the adjuvant chemotherapy approach should be routinely applied only to those surgically resected or irradiated cancers for which reliable clinical data have established benefit from the combination of these two treatment methods.

CURRENT EFFECTIVENESS OF ANTICANCER CHEMOTHERAPY

There is no question regarding the positive accomplishments of anticancer chemotherapy for the treatment of human cancer. A number of patients with cancers now amenable to chemotherapeutic treatment can be expected to be rendered completely free of disease and, in some instances, to live a normal life span (Table 2-3). Another group of cancer patients have been demonstrated to have increased survival benefits as a result of chemotherapy. Even though the cancers in these groups benefitted by anticancer chemotherapy constitute only one-fourth of the cancers in this country (both from the standpoint of incidence and mortality), these findings conclusively establish the concept and capability of this treatment method.

The past accomplishments of cancer chemotherapy have led to some insights that should affect our future approach to this important field. First of all, the original concept that a "magic bullet" would be discovered and applied to human clinical cancer may be too simplistic and unrealistic. Future progress in the use of pharmacologic agents for the treatment of our more common cancers will certainly require intensive research in cancer cell biology and in basic and clinical pharmacology, extensive pharmacokinetic measurements, and carefully controlled therapeutic trials from which scientific answers can be obtained.

The future of cancer chemotherapy will not be determined by the physician who employs these agents without supervision by investigators

Table 2-3
Cancers Benefited by Chemotherapy

Resulting in Possible Normal Life Span	"Improved" Survival
Acute leukemia in children	Ovarian carcinoma
Hodgkin's disease	Breast carcinoma
Testicular cancer	Adult acute leukemia
Rhabdomyosarcoma	Acute granulocytic leukemia (children)
Ewing's sarcoma	Multiple myeloma
Wilms' tumor	Endometrial cancer
Burkitt's lymphoma	Prostatic cancer
Retinoblastoma	Lymphocytic lymphoma
Choriocarcinoma	Adrenocortical carcinoma
Osteogenic sarcoma	Malignant insulinoma
	Histiocytosis X
	Brain tumors

Modified from DeVita et al.[5]

who are on the forefront of this important field. Looking at the benefits achieved thus far, one could easily argue that all patients receiving cancer chemotherapy should be included in some form of carefully controlled clinical trial if we are to achieve progress at the rate we all desire. Possibly the interaction between the physicians in the community and the developing cancer center programs will be one route by which this objective can be achieved. Cancer chemotherapy has come of age, but we need to keep the ball rolling in clinical investigation if we are to exploit this treatment method effectively.

REFERENCES

1. Ansfield FJ, Korbitz BC, Davis HL, Ramirez G: Triple drug therapy in testicular tumors. Cancer 24:442–446, 1969
2. Cline MJ, Haskell CM: Cancer Chemotherapy. Philadelphia, WB Saunders Co, 1975
3. Creech O Jr, Krementz ET, Ryan RF, Winblad JN: Regional Perfusion utilizing an extra corporeal circuit. Ann Surg 148:616–632, 1958
4. DeVita VT Jr, Serpick AA, Carbone PP: Combination chemotherapy in the treatment of advanced Hodgkin's disease. Ann Intern Med 73:881–895, 1970
5. DeVita VT Jr, Young RC, Canellos GP: Combination versus single agent chemotherapy: A review of the basis for selection of drug treatment of cancer. Cancer 35:98–110, 1975

6. Fisher B, Carbone P, Ecomomou SG, Frelick R, Glass A, Lerner H, Redmond C, Zelen M, Band P, Katrych D, Wolmark N, Fisher ER, et al.: 1-Phenylalanine mustard(L-PAM) in the management of primary breast cancer. N Engl J Med 292:117–122, 1975

7. Fisher B, Slack N, Datrych D, Wolmark N: Ten year follow-up results of patients with carcinoma of the breast in a co-operative clinical trial evaluating surgical adjuvant chemotherapy. Surg Gynecol Obstet 140:528–534, 1975

8. Greenwald ES: Cancer Chemotherapy (medical outline series). Flushing, Medical Examination Publishing Co, 1973

9. Heyn RM: The role of chemotherapy in the management of soft tissue sarcomas. Cancer 35:921–924, 1975

10. Higgins GA, Dwight RW, Smith JV, and Keehn RJ: Fluorouracil as an adjuvant to surgery in carcinoma of the colon. Arch Surg 102:339–343, 1971

11. Holland JF, Frei E: Cancer Medicine. Philadelphia, Lea & Febiger, 1973

12. Klopp CT, Alford TC, Bateman J, Berry GN, Winship T: Fractionated intra-arterial cancer chemotherapy with methyl histamine hydrochloride: preliminary report. Ann Surg 132:811–832, 1950

13. Lamerton LF: Cell proliferation and the differential response of normal and malignant tissues. Br J Radiol 45:161–170, 1972

14. Lawrence W Jr: Regional cancer chemotherapy: An evaluation, in Ariel-IM (ed): Progress in Clinical Cancer, vol.1. New York, Grune & Stratton, 1965

15. Lawrence W Jr, Terz JJ, Horsley JS, Lovett WL, Brown PW, Ruffner BW, Regelson W: Chemotherapy as an adjunct to surgery for colorectal cancer. Ann Surg 181:616–623, 1975

16. Longmire WP, Kuzma JW, Dixon WJ: The use of thriethylene-thiophosphorami de as an adjunct to the surgical treatment of gastric carcinoma. Ann Surg 167:292–312, 1968

17. Mendelsohn ML: Cell cycle kinetics and mitotically linked chemotherapy. Cancer Res 29:2390–2393, 1969

18. Moertel CG: Clinical management of advanced gastrointestinal cancer. Cancer 36:675–682, 1975

19. Rhoads CP: Nitrogen mustards in the treatment of neoplastic disease. Official statement. JAMA 131:656–658, 1946

20. Rosen G, Suwansirikul S, Kwon C et al: High dose methotrexate with citrovorum factor rescue and adriamycin in childhood osteogenic sarcoma. Cancer 33:1151–1163, 1974

21. Rosen G, Wollner N, Tan C, Wu SJ, Haydu SI, Cham W, D'Angio GJ, Murphy ML: Disease—Free survival in children with Ewing's sarcoma treated with radiation therapy and adjuvant four-drug sequential chemotherapy. Cancer 33:384–393, 1974

22. Skipper HE, Schabel FM Jr, Wilcox WS: Experimental evaluation of potential anticancer agents. XII. On the criteria and kinetics associated with curability of experimental leukemia. Cancer Chemother Rep 35:1–111, 1964

23. Skipper H, Schabel F, Wilcox WS: Experimental evaluation of potential anticancer agents. XIV. Further studies of certain basic concepts underlying chemotherapy of leukemia. Cancer Chemother Rep 45:5–28, 1965
24. Sullivan RD, Miller E, Sikes MP: Antimetabolite–metabolite combination cancer chemotherapy. Cancer 12:1248–1262, 1969
25. Wolff JA: Advances in the treatment of Wilm's tumor. Cancer 35:901–904, 1975

3

Principles and Techniques of Immunotherapy for Cancer

The purpose of this volume is to summarize briefly the status of conventional clinical cancer management. For this reason some readers would submit that tumor immunology and clinical immunotherapy are still too investigational to warrant inclusion. Nevertheless, the widespread interest in the potential of this approach to human cancer requires review even though it has not been defined or refined enough to be ready for general use.

EXPERIMENTAL BASIS OF TUMOR IMMUNOLOGY

The mechanism of host resistance to neoplastic cells is dependent on recognition and response to specific tumor antigens that have been identified on cancer cells in many animal tumor models and in man. Although specific immunization of the host against these antigens may afford some protection against growth or continued survival of a small aliquot of cancer cells in these syngeneic (inbred) animal models, this immunity often is easily overcome by either the total mass of the tumor or its proliferative capacity. This disappointing feature of the relationship between cancer growth and immune mechanisms is best demonstrated by the observations that cancers do develop spontaneously and they do grow in immunologically competent hosts. This "weakness" of tumor-specific transplantation antigens and the host response to them is in contrast to the often stronger transplantation antigens that lead to the immunologic rejection of organ allografts between animals of differing strains. Nevertheless, the demonstration of both humoral and cell-mediated immunity in the tumor-bearing host has stimulated a great interest in exploiting these factors for either immunoprophylaxis or immunotherapy.

Convincing demonstration of tumor-specific transplantation antigens in man is a more difficult task than in laboratory animals for many reasons, not the least of which is the heterogeneity of our human population. Actually, there is no *direct* evidence to support the presence of tumor-specific antigens in man. Nevertheless, it would seem unlikely that man would not share these mechanisms with his fellow mammals, and indirect evidence of immunological reactions in man also supports their presence. Data of this type have been obtained by a variety of techniques including immunofluorescence, colony inhibition, complement fixation, immunodiffusion, lymphocyte blastogenesis, and lymphocyte-mediated cytotoxicity.

Clinical evidence of immune responses to cancer includes spontaneous regression of some cancers, occasional regression of metastases when the primary cancer is removed, the relationship between immunocompetence and cancer growth, and the difficulty experienced in attempts to autotransplant cancer cells in man. Serum or cell-mediated reactions against specific tumors in vitro yield additional evidence of the presence of tumor antigens, and tumor-associated antigens have been identified in this fashion for a large number of human cancers (Table 3-1). In general,

Table 3-1
Human Cancers for
Which There Is
Evidence for Tumor
Antigens

Burkitt's lymphoma
Nasopharyngeal cancer
Neuroblastoma
Malignant melanoma
Sarcomas
Leukemias
Urinary bladder cancer
Renal cancer
Wilms' tumor
Testicular tumor
CNS tumor
Breast cancer
Lung cancer
Gastrointestinal cancer
Endometrial cancer
Ovarian cancer

most human cancers of the same histologic type seem to share common antigens, a finding that has suggested, but certainly not established, a viral etiology for many of these cancers.

The immune response to a tumor antigen has the same two components that have been so thoroughly studied in organ transplantation systems. The cellular response has been accorded a major antitumor role, and the T-cell lymphocyte and the macrophage apparently corroborate in the recognition and killing of cancer cells. Another group of lymphoid cells that differentiate to cells that produce humoral antibody (B cells) may assist in the cell killing described or may actually serve to protect the cancer cell, probably by the formation of antigen-antibody complexes ("blocking factors")[12] (Fig. 3-1).

Cell-mediated responses to tumor cells have been demonstrated by a number of in vitro assays in animal model systems and in man,[7,23,27,35] as noted above, but the *in vivo* significance of these observations is not clear. The role of the serum antibodies that can be identified is even more difficult to define in view of the paradoxical effect of blocking serum described. Passive transfer of serum containing antibody does not usually suppress tumor growth in vivo and will actually enhance tumor growth under some experimental conditions. These findings emphasize both the complexity of the immune response to cancer growth and the reasons for problems in our attempts to harness these reactions for the immunotherapy for cancer.

Another series of important observations from both experimental systems and man relates to the capability of the immune systems of the tumor-bearing hosts to respond to antigenic stimuli. Although antibody formation is not usually impaired in the animal or the man harboring a

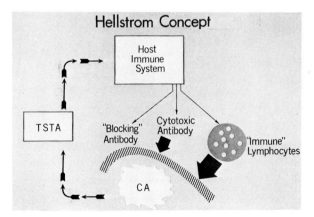

Fig. 3-1. Diagrammatic representation of "blocking" (from Hellstrom and Hellstrom[12]).

cancer (except for some lymphoproliferative disease), a large number of observations suggest a decrease in cellular immunity.[4–6] These range from the inability to sensitize the tumor-bearing host to chemical haptenes [such as dinitrochlorobenzene (DNCB)] to the suppression of delayed hypersensitivity responses to "recall" antigens to which the tumor host has previously been sensitized. The depression of blastogenic responses of lymphocytes to various mitogens [such as phytohemagglutinin (PHA)] by factors present in the serum of the tumor-bearing host is another expression of this immunosuppressive phenomenon.[2,6,20] These observations are probably a reflection of the deleterious effect of the neoplasm on the host immune system, rather than of carcinogenesis owing to a primary immune deficiency, but either explanation is tenable.

That the immunosuppressed renal transplant patients have a higher incidence of cancer than our "normal" population has been well established.[26] However, the preponderance of cancers of the lymphoreticular system in renal transplant patients, and the absence of an increased cancer incidence in immunosuppressed populations that do not have organ allografts, suggests that the phenomenon noted has more of a relationship to the host-versus-graft reaction than to the decrease in cellular immunity.[31] On the other hand, patients with some congenital immune deficiency syndromes have been shown to have a higher incidence of cancer than the normal population. Another clinical finding of interest is that some forms of cancer are associated with immunodeficiencies early in the clinical course (head and neck cancer and lymphomas), whereas in other forms (breast and colorectal cancer) these defects develop late in the disease course. All of these findings relate immunodeficiency (or suppression) to an increased growth capability of cancer in some way, but the phenomena have no simple explanation. Our hope, however, is to alter these immunosuppressive effects by various therapeutic approaches and thereby favor the host in his struggle against the invading neoplasm.

IMMUNOTHERAPY—EXPERIMENTAL TRIALS

As a background for trials of immunotherapy for cancer in man, it is important to review the results of attempts to alter neoplastic growth in animal model systems. The experimental methods employed thus far have not been very effective in modifying established tumor growth, and when an effect has been observed, it has usually been in an experimental system involving a small "tumor burden." The systemic approaches that have been employed have included nonspecific stimulation of the immune system by the so-called immunopotentiators [Bacillus Calmette Guerin (BCG), Corynebacterium Parvum (C. Parvum), Methanol extracted BCG residue (MER), Tilorone, Levamisole[3,7,32,38,39]], active immunization with some form of antigenic material obtained from the tumor itself,[1,33] passive immunization with serum or sensitized lymphoid cells,[16] and transfer of immune informational material such as transfer factor[17] or "immune RNA" from another animal.[27,28] Benefit, in terms of anticancer effect, has been observed with nonspecific systemic immunostimulation for immuno-prophylaxis, but this approach has been generally ineffective with estab-lished tumors unless it is combined with some form of anticancer chem-otherapy. Observations from successful laboratory trials of combined chemotherapy and nonspecific immunotherapy are encouraging also in view of the concern that the anticancer chemotherapeutic agents them-selves are often immunosuppressive.[34] When nonspecific immunopoten-tiators are brought into direct contact with the neoplasm by local injec-tion, they may be effective as the sole therapy (without chemotherapy) because of tumor destruction produced by the accompanying delayed hy-persensitivity reaction in the tumor itself.[39] These laboratory observa-tions have obvious implications for the clinical application of nonspecific immunotherapy to accessible lesions.

Passive immunization with serum or by adoptive transfer of sensi-tized lymphoid cells,[13,14,16] or RNA-rich fragments obtained therefrom,[28] has been effective under some circumstances, but this approach has been ineffective in suppressing the growth of established tumors in animal model systems. However, active immunization with tumor cells modi-fied by substances thought to "expose" antigenic determinants (such as neuraminidase)[33] has had intriguing antitumor effects in animal models with small established neoplasms. From all of these laboratory data it is apparent that immune mechanisms can be manipulated in favor of the host by various approaches, but these effects are "weak" at best and are better demonstrated in prophylaxis models rather than in animals with es-tablished neoplasms.

IMMUNOTHERAPY IN MAN

From the above brief summary of experimental data, it is not sur-prising that the immunologic approach to human cancer is still primitive and essentially undeveloped. One intriguing possibility in man is the exploitation of these immune mechanisms for immunoprophylaxis by immunization against etiologic agents (when they are identified), im-munization against tumor-specific antigens (when they can be isolated in a purified form), or nonspecific stimulation of the immune system. The last method would appear to be the most feasible approach for trial at the present time, for obvious reasons, but there are no truly con-vincing pilot data on prophylaxis that would encourage this approach.

The investigation of immunotherapy for established cancers in man has followed several lines. The cross-immunization of patients with similar neoplasms was carried out in several studies, after which cross-transfusions of lymphocytes or lymphocytes and plasma were carried out between these allogeneic pairs[13,14,25] (Fig. 3-2). The basis of these clinical trials was the hope that an effective subcellular immune fraction might be transferred from one individual to another since relatively rapid destruction of the allogeneic cells by the recipient was a foregone conclusion. Some objective clinical responses were observed in these studies, but evidence of the transfer of an immune response to the cancer patient was limited. Reinfusion of autologous lymphocytes after ex-vivo nonspecific stimulation by a mitogen (PHA) was attempted by several investigators with a few transient responses, but this approach was also disappointing.[9]

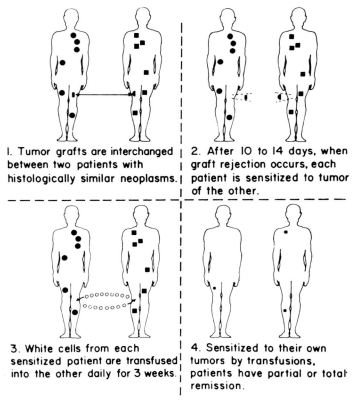

1. Tumor grafts are interchanged between two patients with histologically similar neoplasms.

2. After 10 to 14 days, when graft rejection occurs, each patient is sensitized to tumor of the other.

3. White cells from each sensitized patient are transfused into the other daily for 3 weeks.

4. Sensitized to their own tumors by transfusions, patients have partial or total remission.

Fig. 3-2. Immunotherapy: diagram of cross-immunization and subsequent cross-transfusion of white cells or white cells and plasma (from Nadler and Moore[25]).

Infusions of large amounts of unsensitized allogeneic lymphocytes ("fresh" or cultured), or spleen cells, produced similar infrequent tumor responses. All of these attempts at immunotherapy with lymphocytes of various types were disappointing despite some intriguing observations, and these studies confirm the laboratory observation regarding the importance of applying immunotherapy to subjects with a small tumor burden. These investigations generally failed to demonstrate a transfer of specific immune reactions to the recipient as a result of these cellular infusions, and they failed to produce enough benefit to justify this approach for clinical benefit.

Many investigators have attempted active immunization of patients with tumor vaccines of various types, but the results have generally been either ineffective or difficult to interpret because of the simultaneous administration of other therapies, or because of the absence of measurable tumor tissue when the approach was an adjuvant one after surgical resection.[13,14,18] The rationale of using this approach in patients with minimal residual disease after resection is certainly a good one, but objective evaluation of benefit is virtually impossible at this time. Other recent attempts to transfer specific immunologic reactivity with either transfer factor[37] or immune RNA[28] are also intriguing but highly experimental at the present time. It appears that the only immunotherapeutic approach with potential for successful application to man in the immediate future is the use of nonspecific immunostimulation.

One form of nonspecific immunotherapy that has clearly led to regression of cancer in man is the direct application or direct injection of superficial skin tumors with bacillus of Calmette and Guerin (BCG) or DNCB. This approach has been employed for both primary skin cancer[15] and for recurrent skin nodules after prior surgical treatment of malignant melanoma.[24] The delayed hypersensitivity reaction that subsequently develops destroys the injected lesion or nodule. In patients with multiple cutaneous lesions of melanoma, there is occasional regression of uninjected nodules as well. This approach for palliation of recurrent melanoma is limited in the clinical sense owing to the general observation that visceral lesions do not respond to the dermal injections of BCG.[24] The topical application of either BCG or DNCB to skin cancer has led to clinical regression, and the key mechanism of this response is also the hypersensitivity reaction produced. This has become a practical method of therapy for selected primary skin cancers as well as a palliative tool in some patients with recurrent melanoma in the skin.

There are much less convincing data on the use of BCG or other nonspecific immunostimulators as systemic treatment for established cancer. Although patients with leukemia,[11,19] colon cancer,[22] and malignant melanoma[10,21,30] may have been benefited by this approach in several trials, all patients in these studies also received other forms of therapy to reduce tumor volume. This combined approach certainly follows the dictum regarding tumor volume that was established in animal model systems, but it makes convincing evidence of benefit from the immunotherapy hard to develop. This is particularly true of use of nonspecific immunostimulation as an adjuvant to potentially curative treatment methods. Data from patients receiving BCG as an adjuvant after surgical therapy, compared with retrospective data on recurrence rate and survival after standard surgical treatment of stage 2 malignant melanoma, appear to show benefit from BCG[24] (Fig. 3-3). On the other hand, truly convincing evidence will require prospective clinical trials since the comparability of patients in these groups in these preliminary evaluations is far from definite.

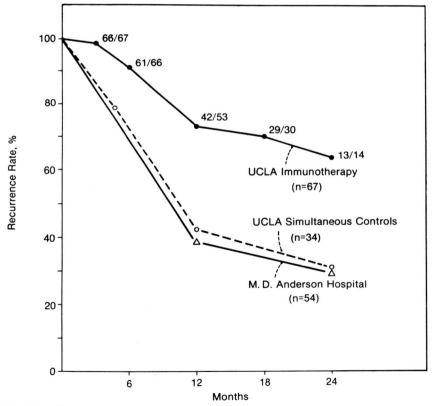

Fig. 3-3. Retrospective comparison of recurrence rates after surgical therapy for malignant melanoma (stage 2) with or without adjuvant BCG therapy (from Morton et al.[24]).

A factor of importance that should concern the clinician is that response of measurable disease occurs only in patients who initially have or subsequently develop a positive tuberculin reaction or a positive response to skin testing with DNCB.[24] It is also probable that the uncommon side effects of BCG, such as systemic BCG infection or inflammatory liver changes,[36] could be virtually eliminated by avoiding the administration of this form of therapy to patients who are immunosuppressed on either clinical or laboratory grounds.

The systemic use of BCG, C. Parvum, or MER as an adjunct to therapy certainly merits continued investigation, but the conflicting data from several studies, the variability of protocols owing to the different strains and dosages of live or dead organisms in the various preparations of BCG, and the multiple variations in the frequency of administration and duration of treatment make analysis extremely difficult. At this time the Food and Drug Administration still considers BCG to be an experimental agent, and it has not been cleared for general use. We believe it is safe to conclude that BCG, C Parvum, or similar agents should not be administered as "standard" therapy at this point in time unless given as part of a controlled clinical trial that is undertaken by physicians with appropriate experience.

In summary, we do not have enough clinical data to support the widespread use of any form of immunotherapy, with the possible exception of local application of agents to skin cancers or metastatic melanoma nodules in the dermis. Immunostimulation may well prove to be an effective systemic treatment or adjuvant to other forms of therapy in the future. However, well-planned clinical trials are required before this approach can be recommended for general use.

REFERENCES

1. Alexander P: Immunotherapy of cancer: Experiments with primary tumors and syngeneic tumor grafts. Prog Exp Tumor Res 10:22–71, 1968
2. Al-Sarraf M, Sardesal S, Vaitkevicius VK: Effect of syngeneic and allogeneic plasma on lymphocytes from cancer patients, patients with nonneoplastic disease, and normal subjects. Cancer 27:1426–1432, 1971
3. Bast RC Jr, Zbar B, Borsos T, Rapp HJ: BCG and cancer. N Engl J Med 290:1413–1458, 1974
4. Catalona WJ, Chretien PB: Abnormalities of quantitative dinitrochlorobenzene sensitization in cancer patients: correlation with tumor state and history. Cancer 31:353–356, 1973
5. Chakrovorty RC, Curutchet HP, Coppolla FS, Park CM, Blalock WK, Lawrence W Jr: The delayed hypersensitivity reaction in the cancer patient. Observations on sensitization to DNCB. Surgery 73:730–735, 1973

6. Chretien PB, Crowder WL, Gertner HR, Sample WF, Catalona WJ: Correlation of preoperative lymphocyte reactivity with the clinical course of cancer patients. Surg Gynecol Obstet 136:380–384, 1973

7. Crippen RG: Neoplasm Immunity: Theory and Application (Proceedings of a Chicago Symposium, 1974). Chicago, ITR, 1975

8. Falk RE, Mann P, Langer B: Cell-mediated immunity to human tumors. Arch Surg 107:261–265, 1973

9. Frenster JH, Rogoway WM: In-vitro activation and reinfusion of autologous human lymphocytes. Lancet 2:979, 1968

10. Gutterman J, Mavligit G, McBride C, Grei E, Hersh EM: BCG stimulation of immune responsiveness in patients with malignant melanoma. Cancer 32:321–327, 1973

11. Gutterman JV, Rodriguez V, Mavligit G et al: Chemoimmunotherapy of adult acute leukemia. Prolongation of remission in myeloblastic leukemia with BCG. Lancet 2:1405–1409, 1974

12. Hellstrom KE, Hellstrom I: Lymphocyte-mediated cytotoxicity in blocking serum activity to tumor antigens. Adv Immunol 18:209–277, 1974

13. Humphrey LJ, Boehm B, Jewell WR, Boehm OR: Immunologic response of cancer patients modified by immunization with tumor vaccine. Ann Surg 176:554–557, 1972

14. Humphrey LJ, Jewell WR, Murray DR, et al: Immunotherapy for the patient with cancer. Ann Surg 173:47–54, 1971

15. Klein E, Williams AC: Experiences with local chemotherapy and immunotherapy in premalignant and malignant skin lesions: Cancer 25:450–462, 1970

16. Krementz ET, Mansell PWA, Hornung MO, Samuels MS, Southerland CA, Benes EN: Immunotherapy of malignant disease; the use of viable sensitized lymphocytes or transfer factor prepared from sensitized lymphocytes. Cancer 33:394–401, 1974

17. Lawrence HS, Valentine FT: Transfer factor and other mediators of cellular immunity. Am J Pathol 60:437–452, 1970

18. Marcove RC, Mike V, Hurvos AG, Southam CM, Levin AG: Vaccine trials for osteogenic sarcoma. CA 23:74–80, 1973

19. Mathe G, Aniel JL, Schwarzenberg L, et al: Active immunotherapy for acute lymphoblastic leukemia. Lancet 1:697–699, 1969

20. Mavligit GM, Hersh EM, McBride CM: Lymphocyte blastogenesis induced by autochthonous human solid tumor cells: relationship to stage of disease and serum factors. Cancer 34:1712–1721, 1974

21. McCarthy WH, Cotton G, Carlon A, Milton GW, Kossard S: Immunotherapy of malignant melanoma—a clinical trial. Cancer 32:97–103, 1973

22. Moertel CG, Ritts RE, Schutt AJ, Hahn RG: Clinical studies of methanol extraction residue fraction of bacillus Calmette-Guerin as an immunostimulant in patients with advanced cancer. Cancer 35:3075–3083, 1975

23. Morton DL, Eilber FR, Joseph WL, et al: Immunological factors in human sarcomas and melanomas: a rational basis for immunotherapy. Ann Surg 172:740–749, 1970

24. Morton DL, Eilber FR, Holmes EC, Hunt JS, Ketcham AS, Silverstein MJ, Sparks FC: BCG immunotherapy of malignant melanoma (summary of a seven-year experience). Ann Surg 180:635–642, 1974

25. Nadler SH, Moore GE: Clinical immunologic study of malignant disease; response to tumor transplants and transfer of leukocytes. Ann Surg 164:482–490, 1966

26. Penn I, Starzl TE: Malignant tumors arising de novo in immunosuppressed organ transplant recipients. Transplantation 14:407–417, 1972

27. Pilch YH, Myers GH, Jr, Sparks FC, Golub SH: Prospects for the immunotherapy of cancer. Curr Prob Surg Jan/Feb, 1975

28. Pilch YH, Viltman LL, Kern DH: Immune cytolysis of human tumor cells mediated by xenogenic "Immune" RNA Implications for immunotherapy. Surgery 76:23–34, 1974

29. Rosato FE, Brown AS, Miller EE, Rosato EF, Mullis WF Johnson J, Moskovitz A: Neuraminidase immunotherapy of tumors in man. Surg Gynecol Obstet 139:675–682, 1974

30. Roth JA, Golub SH, Holmes EC, Morton DL: Effect of bacillus Calmette-Guerin immunotherapy on tumor antigen-induced lymphocyte-stimulated protein synthesis in melanoma patients. Surgery 78:66–75, 1975

31. Schwartz RS: Immunosuppressive chemotherapy and malignancy. Transplantation Proc [Suppl] 6:45–48, 1974

32. Sepsic HT, Rapp HJ: Systemic transfer of tumor immunity, delayed hypersensitivity and suppression of tumor growth. J Natl Cancer Inst 44:955–963, 1970

33. Simmons RL, Rios A: Cell surface modification in the treatment of experimental cancer: Neuraminidase or concanavalin A. Cancer 34:1541–1547, 1974

34. Sinkovics JG, Cabiness JR, Shullenberger CC: Disappearance after chemotherapy of blocking serum factors as measured in vitro with lymphocytes cytotoxic to tumor cells. Cancer 30:1428–1437, 1972

35. Smith RT: Possibilities and problems of immunologic intervention in cancer. N Engl J Med 287:439–450 1972

36. Sparks FC, Silverstein MJ, Hunt JS, et al: Complications of BCG immunotherapy in patients with cancer. N Engl J Med 289:827–830, 1973

37. Spitler LE, Levin AS, Blois MS, et al: Lymphocyte responses to tumor-specific antigens in patients with malignant melanoma and results of transfer factor therapy. J Clin Invest 51:92, 1972

38. Wampler, GL, Kuperminc, M, Regelson, W: Phase I study of Tilorone, a non-marrow depressing antitumor agent. Cancer Chemother Rep 57:209–217, 1973

39. Zbar B, Rapp HJ: Immunotherapy of guinea pig cancer with BCG. Cancer 34:1532–1540, 1974

Tapan A. Hazra, M.D.

4
Principles and Techniques of Radiotherapy

Radiotherapy is an important modality in the treatment of malignant disease as a curative procedure, as a palliative procedure, and as an adjunct to other forms of treatment.[21,22]   Radiotherapy selectively destroys or alters the growth potential of the neoplastic cells in situ without significantly compromising the normal tissues within which the tumor is located.   Exploitation of radiation in this fashion with a high degree of elegance is what must be understood when speaking of the radiotherapeutic method of neoplasm control.

The radiation used has been and is at present ionizing radiation.   Ionization is the result of knocking off electrons of stable atoms in the path of the radiation.   The atom then loses a unit of negative electrical charge (electron) and is left with an unbalanced surplus of positive charge.   The dislodged electron is usually captured by a neighboring atom, which thus acquires an extra unit of a negative charge (Fig. 4-1).   These abnormal fragments—one electrically positive because of the removal of electrons, the other electrically negative through the acquisition of extra ones—are called *ions,* and the process is called ionization.

The ionizing rays are of two types: waves and particles.

WAVES

Radiation is produced in a wide spectrum of wavelengths in nature (Fig. 4-2).   Differences in wavelengths give the rays their particular and characteristic physical properties.   Except for ordinary visible light, all

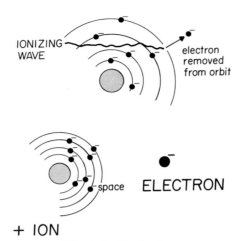

Fig. 4-1.   Ionization.

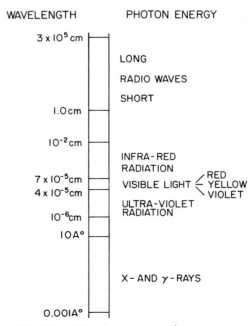

Fig. 4-2.   The electromagnetic spectrum.

the other radiation shown in the figure is invisible to us. Only the radiations in the x-ray range have the ability to ionize atoms. The others shown in the figure are of much longer wavelengths and are not ionizing in nature.

PARTICLES

The ionizing particles include alpha particles (rays), beta particles (rays), gamma rays, neutrons, protons,[30] and negative pi mesons.[1]

Alpha Rays

Alpha rays are the least penetrating of the particles and are easily absorbed. For example, they cannot penetrate even a thin layer of paper. They do not penetrate the skin and are as a consequence intensely ionizing over the short distance they travel. They are, therefore, very damaging to tissues. Even though they are heavily ionizing, alpha rays have little importance as tools in radiotherapy because of their inability to penetrate tissues.

Beta Rays

Beta rays are actually fast-moving electrons. Their penetrating power varies considerably according to the particular isotope emitting them (energy), but it is much greater than that of alpha rays. Beta rays can easily penetrate skin and in soft tissues they can travel distances ranging from small fractions of a millimeter up to approximately 2 cm, producing ionization all along their path. Beta-emitting isotopes may be used in several ways.

Surface therapy. Beta rays are often used as plaques for surface therapy. The most commonly used beta ray plaque today is the strontium 90 applicator,[6,12] which is particularly useful for treating the surface of the eye and such conditions as hemangiomas.

Intracavitary therapy.[15] A form of "internal surface" therapy, intracavitary therapy is commonly employed to control serous effusions. Colloidal gold 198 and phosphorus 32 are frequently used for this purpose.

Systemic therapy.[19,31] Common examples of systemic therapy are the use of radioactive phosphorus given IV for treatment of metastatic bone disease from prostatic cancer, and the use of radioactive iodine for thyroid disorders.

Interstitial therapy. Inserting radioactive sources in a tissue to treat local disease with high doses of radiation is known as interstitial therapy. The method is gaining importance in radiotherapy, especially in the treatment of prostatic cancer.[9]

Electrons

Electrons are physically identical to beta rays. Electron therapy is the term applied to use of these particles when they are produced by electron generators instead of being emitted by a radioisotope. Electron therapy has certain definite advantages over other types of treatment.[17] In electron therapy the dose distribution is more limited in depth, thus sparing the deeper tissues to a large extent. The range (depth) of electrons can be controlled and limited.

Neutrons[2,20]

Neutron beams are now available for clinical use. Clinical trials have begun, but it is still too early to assess properly the value of this form of treatment. Certain definite radiobiologic advantages accrue with neutron exposures. One advantage, which makes neutron therapy particularly useful in tumor treatment, is that the effect is not dependent on the presence of oxygen.

EQUIPMENT

To understand what goes on in a radiotherapy department, it is useful to have an acquaintance with the machines used by the radiotherapist. Detailed information can be found in many physics textbooks.[11]

The ordinary voltage in the electric mains in this country is approximately 120 V. In a typical diagnostic x-ray machine, voltage is about 80,000 V, or 80 kV. For therapy we use x-rays generated at widely different voltages, according to the degree of penetration required. A low-voltage machine produces rays of comparatively long wavelength, which are less penetrating than rays produced by high-voltage machines. The latter types of rays have shorter wavelengths and are more penetrating. Some of the commonly used machines are discussed below.

Superficial Therapy Units

Superficial therapy units (10–140 kV) are used mainly for skin lesions, both malignant and nonmalignant. The most widely used superficial x-ray unit delivers approximately 100 kV and can be used to treat skin lesions such as basal cell carcinoma, squamous cell carcinoma, and metastatic disease to the skin.

Deep Therapy Units

Before the development of supervoltage apparatus, deep therapy units (sometimes called orthovoltage therapy units; approximately 250 kV) were the standard machines (Fig. 4-3) in any radiotherapy department. Most of the clinical and biological experiences in radiotherapy have been acquired on this basis. These machines are now rarely used.

Megavoltage Units

There are several different types of megavoltage units (in excess of 1×10^6 kV) (Fig. 4-4) using different principles. The most important apparatus in this range is the linear accelerator, a high-energy electron accelerator that can be used as either an electron or an x-ray source. A much less common type of unit in this range, the Betatron, can also be used as both an x-ray and an electron source.

Gamma Ray Beam Units

The two radioisotopes most frequently used for teletherapy are cobalt 60 (Fig. 4-5) and cesium 137. Cobalt 60 beam units are also in the megavoltage range and are now universally used.

ADVANTAGES OF MEGAVOLTAGE

Depth dose. The obvious superiority of megavoltage therapy lies in its short wavelength x-rays and consequently greatly increased depth dose capability.

Build up (skin sparing effect). The maximum absorbed dose from megavoltage generators is not at the skin surface but a little below it. Just how far below depends on the voltage (Table 4-1) because the maximum ionization "builds up" to a peak below the surface being irradiated. This is important for the patient since skin reactions which once limited treatment are now much less troublesome with megavoltage therapy.

Definition. Megavoltage beams have sharper, better defined edges (Table 4-2) which results in more exact distribution of dosage to the tumor, sparing of adjacent organs, and less general body dosage (integral dose) to the patient. Thus a patient treated with megavoltage has less radiation-induced sickness than one treated with orthovoltage.

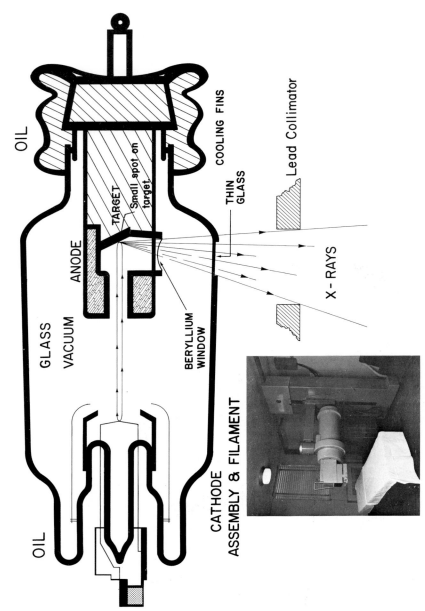

Fig. 4-3. Ortho-voltage therapy machine.

OIL

OIL

GLASS

VACUUM

ANODE

TARGET

Small spot on target

COOLING FINS

THIN GLASS

BERYLLIUM WINDOW

CATHODE ASSEMBLY & FILAMENT

Lead Collimator

X - RAYS

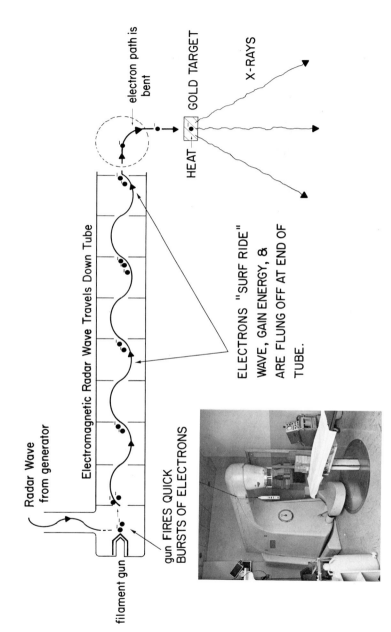

Fig. 4.4. **A.** A 6-MeV linear accelerator, megavoltage unit.

55

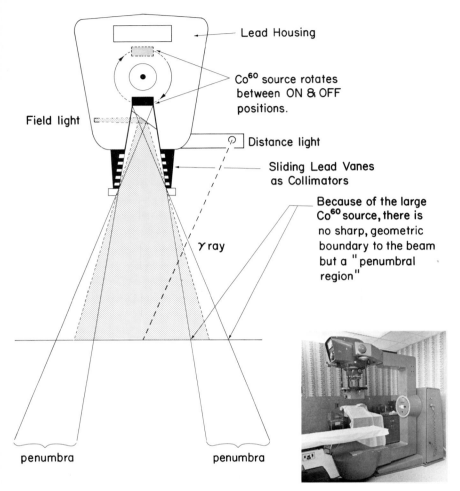

Lead Housing

Co⁶⁰ source rotates
between ON & OFF
positions.

Field light

Distance light

Sliding Lead Vanes
as Collimators

Because of the large
Co⁶⁰ source, there is
no sharp, geometric
boundary to the beam
but a "penumbral
region"

γ ray

penumbra   penumbra

Fig. 4-5.   Cobalt 60 unit.

Absence of differential absorption.   During the use of orthovoltage apparatus, the bones absorb approximately four to five times more radiation than soft tissues do.   With megavoltage units there is no differential absorption between bones and soft tissue so the risk of late bone necrosis is diminished.

Radiation Units

The roentgen (R) is the unit of measurement of the quantity of radiation from a beam as it emerges from the generating source or as it impinges on a surface being irradiated.   When the quantity of radiation a pa-

Table 4-1

Skin Dose Corresponding to 100 R in Air with
Different Field Size and Varying Beam Quality

Quality of Beam	Area of Field in sq cm		
	25	100	400
250 k V (HVL)			
2.0 mm) cu	109	126	136
Cobalt 60	20	30	40
6 MeV	11.5	17.0	27.0
18 MeV	10	15	10

tient is exposed to is measured over a period of time, one can calculate
the dose to which the patient is exposed. This is an *exposure dose.*
Roentgen (R) measurement applies only to air and only to x- or gamma
rays—amount of x- or gamma radiation which produces 1 esu (electro-
static unit of charge) of either sign in 0.001293 gm of air (1 cc of air at standard temperature and pressure).

What we need to know in radiation therapy is the amount of radiation
absorbed by the tissues and not by the air through which the beam passes.
The unit of *absorbed dose,* the rad, is the amount of energy absorbed in a
medium from the beam. One rad equals the absorption of 100 ergs/gm.
If the atoms of the absorbing material differ from those of air, the energy
absorption from the beam will differ from that calculated in air as
roentgens. The atoms of soft tissues in the body (muscle) are very similar
to those of air so that the exposure dose is almost equal to the absorbed
dose. But in bone, which is composed of different atoms, the energy absorbed may be significantly greater depending on the voltage of the radiation, although the energy absorption may actually be less than that of air.

Table 4-2

Showing Better Percentage Depth Dose and Lesser Scatter for
Megavoltage Machines

For 10 × 10 cm field	250 kV	Cobalt 60	6 MeV LA
At 4.0 width of			
20% isodose curve	13.1 cm	11.6 cm	10.7 cm
10% isodose curve	15.8 cm	13.4 cm	10.8 cm
Percent isodose curve			
on skin surface	100%	30%	20%
At depth of 5.0 cm	71%	79%	85%
At depth of 10.0 cm	40%	55%	66%

BIOLOGICAL EFFECTS OF
IONIZING RADIATIONS[5,8]

Although the various radiations are physically quite different, the biological effects they produce are similar. Once an atom is ionized, the molecule of which the atom is a part undergoes physicochemical changes. The evidence accumulated to date overwhelmingly supports the hypothesis that the critical target in radiation-induced cell death is the genetic material, DNA[16] (Figs. 4-6 and 4-7). Very rarely, the effects of the irradiation may be owing to a direct hit on the DNA molecule principally producing fission of the phosphate ester bonds between the sugars of one nuclide and the next. Usually the effect is indirect, resulting from the production of highly reactive short-lived free radicals (OH−) in the water that makes up so much of living material. These free radicals then react with DNA molecules.

When a cell absorbs radiation, two types of damage may be observed: (a) lethal damage which ends in the death of the cell, and (b) sublethal damage which can be repaired. When sublethal damage is adequately repaired, the cell will survive the initial insult.

Various factors modify the biological effects of ionizing radiations. Two of the important ones are linear energy transfer (LET) and oxygenation.[18,32]

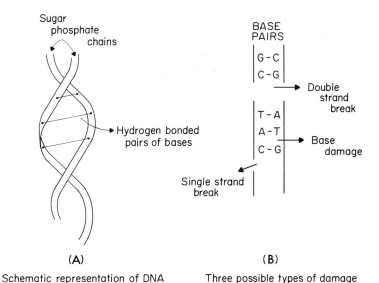

(A)

Schematic representation of DNA showing the double helix

(B)

Three possible types of damage in DNA due to ionizing radiation

Fig. 4-6. **A.** Schematic representation of DNA showing the double helix. **B.** Three possible types of damage in DNA owing to ionizing radiation.

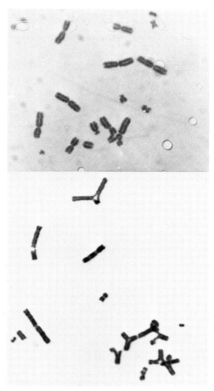

Fig. 4.7.   Radiation-induced chromosome aberrations in human lymphocytes.

LET

Ionizing radiation produces its biological effect by the deposition of energy in the nucleus of the cells irradiated. The probability of a lethal event occurring increases with the quantity of energy deposited in the tissues. The density of energy transfer (energy deposited) is known as the linear energy transfer of the particular radiation quality (Table 4-3).

Table 4-3
L.E.T (kev/μ) of Different Types of
Ionizing Radiation

Ionizing radiation	L.E.T.
200 kV x rays	0.4
Cobalt 60 x rays	0.2-2
Neutrons	3-30 (Peak at 7)
14.1 MeV	

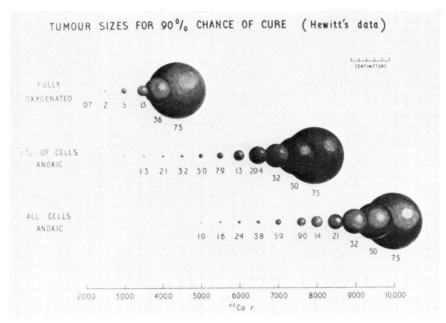

Fig. 4-8.   Oxygen effect.

Radiation with a high LET will be biologically more effective per rad than low-LET radiations.

In all instances the dose required to produce death (lethal dose) under hypoxic conditions is two or three times greater than the dose required under oxygenated conditions.   This oxygen effect (Fig. 4-8) has a far greater influence with low-LET radiation such as x-rays than with high-LET radiation such as alpha particles, and it has an intermediate value for fast neutrons.   For the oxygen affect to be observed, oxygen must be present during radiation exposure; just before or just after is not effective. Gray[7] was the first to postulate that the oxygen effect might be important in clinical radiation therapy because malignant tumors have hypoxic populations of cells.   The exact mechanism of the oxygen effect is not fully understood, although there is general agreement among various experts in the field that the effect concerns greater radical production in most cases.

FRACTIONATION[3,4]

It would, of course, be convenient to expose patients to single-shot radiation treatment.   This is, however, possible only for the very small superficial lesions, and even then the cosmetic results are liable to be inferior and the risk of necrosis high. Numerous treatment schedules have been developed exploiting the possibility of sparing normal tissues while obtaining the maximum lethal effect on the tumor as a result of splitting the total dose of radiation into a number of equal fractions over several days. Daily treatments Monday to Friday or Saturday to Wednesday (where Thursday and Friday are the weekends) are carried out as an administrative inconvenience, although there is no medical reason why it must remain as the only method or the best method. Many centers now are treating patients with different fractionation schemes (two or three times weekly) and obtaining equally good results with less strain on the patient.

Another variation of fractionation scheme is known as the split-course technique.[14,27] One or more radiation-free intervals of 2–3 weeks are interspersed between two fractionated treatment courses to allow time for normal tissue recovery. The splitting of the total dose of radiation into a number of equal fractions is now known to be associated with several complex factors. The important factors are intracellular repair of sublethal damage, reoxygenation of hypoxic cells, and cell division with repopulation and possibly synchronization of irradiated cell populations that subsequently divide.

These effects will vary for different tumors and normal tissues. The technical questions of dosage and time are of fundamental importance to the radiotherapist and are the subject of complex radiobiological experiments.

THE CELL CYCLE

Human cells multiply and divide by mitosis. It is now generally agreed that there is a variation of cellular radiosensitivity with cell age during the mitotic cycle.[28] The main characteristic of this radiosensitivity are (a) cells are most sensitive during mitosis (M) or close to mitosis; (b) G2, the time between DNA synthesis and M, is perhaps as sensitive as M; and (c) resistance is usually greatest in the S phase (DNA synthesis).

CLINICAL ASPECTS OF IONIZING RADIATION

Clinical radiotherapy is based on its capacity to destroy certain types of malignant growth in situ without damaging irreversibly normal tissues in which the tumor is growing. The therapeutic possibilities of using the killing action of radiation depend not on one factor but on the ratio between two factors, tumor lethal dose (TLD) and normal tissue tolerance

(NTT). This has been termed the *therapeutic ratio*. (NTT/TLD) This ratio determines if any lesion is clinically radiosensitive or radioresistant. Sensitive tumors are those in which the therapeutic ratio is high and normal tissues tolerate doses of several times the magnitude of the TLD. Resistant tumors are those in which the dose required to produce tumor lethality is almost as great or greater than the dose which destroys normal tissue.

Most human cancer cells are of limited sensitivity. Although cancer cells are generally more sensitive than normal tissues, the therapeutic ratio is low and the permissible dose exceeds the tumor lethal dose by only a small amount. It can, therefore, be said that radiosensitivity is not necessarily synonymous with radiocurability.

Once a diagnosis of malignancy has been reached, some crucial decisions must be made by joint consultation among surgeons, radiotherapist, and other oncologists (medical, pediatric, gynecologic, etc.).

For the patient with malignancy to receive optimum care, he or she should be referred to the radiotherapist for consultation and perhaps for treatment if it is indicated and if the recommendations are accepted. Before treatment is begun, all parties should agree on the total management policy to be followed.

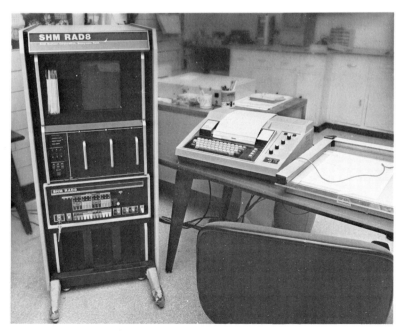

Fig. 4-9.   Computer planning unit.

The planning of radiotherapy[13] is extremely important, and special sophisticated equipment [simulators, computers (Fig. 4-9), devices to make molds or casts, and also devices to obtain the outline of the body] has been developed to help make radiotherapy more accurate and less strenuous on the patient.

The planning of radiation therapy consists of the following steps (Fig. 4-10): (a) delineating the treatment volume (the lesion and the surrounding area); (b) selecting the physical parameters of irradiation such as the machine, the fields, and the fractionation schedule (Fig. 4-10); and (c) adhering to established procedure. As a general rule, when established techniques produce good results there is little reason to alter them. This applies generally to the early, curable head and neck and gynecological cancers. It is equally true that when a tumor is known to be rarely curable by radiation therapy, such as in cancer of the esophagus or lung, the general treatment techniques used tend to be simple and rarely varied except in new clinical trials. As a result of the advantages of modern equipment and planning, particularly in the direction of greater patient tolerance to treatment, patients who previously might have been considered unsuitable for radiation can now be offered either definitive or palliative irradiation without too much strain or upset. This group includes pediatric patients and patients with Hodgkin's disease, prostatic cancer, as well as other cancers.

Quite often patients are seen at a stage of disease when it is obvious that neither surgery nor irradiation therapy alone is likely to achieve good results, and in order to give the patient a chance, the combination of two treatment methods is agreed on and carried out.[29] This combination may be affected two ways.

Postoperative irradiation.[24] This offers the patient the psychological advantage of ridding him of a diseased organ without undue delay. The surgeon also gains the technical advantage of being able to operate on nonirradiated tissue and is thus spared difficulties and complications otherwise encountered. Biologically, this combination is unsatisfactory since any extensive ablative procedure inevitably disturbs the vascularization of tissue, and hence any cancer cells growing under such conditions cannot be easily destroyed by irradiation. Recently, reports have been published that demonstrate that in certain sites, especially in the head and neck region, preoperative and postoperative irradiation yield the same results.

Preoperative irradiation.[23] Biologically, this combination is usually more satisfactory. It diminishes the tumor bulk and reduces the risk of dissemination of cancer cells during surgery. At the moment this combination is finding wide application in the treatment of advanced diseases of

64

VARYING TREATMENT TECHNIQUES FOR CARCINOMA OF BLADDER PLANNED WITH THE AID OF COMPUTER.

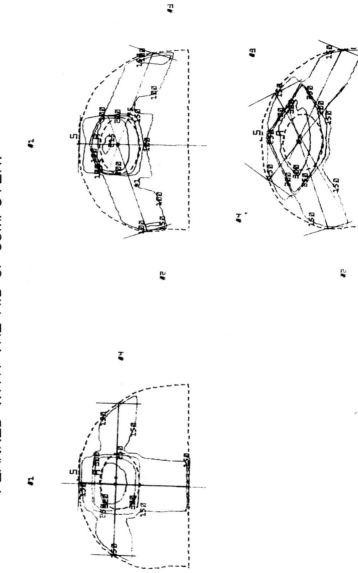

Fig. 4-10. Different treatment plans of carcinoma of the bladder.

the head and neck, bladder, and uterus. The problems presently unsolved are the optimum preoperative dose of radiation and the interval to be followed between radiation treatment and operation.

TREATMENT RESULTS

Malignant tumors curable by radiotherapy are in many instances quite the same as those curable by surgery, and the choice of method is often determined by local circumstances and experience. A considerable body of experience as to what can and cannot be achieved by radiotherapy has been gathered and is now available in the literature. It serves as an arbitrary guide subject to change as experience with new methodology grows. A summary of such a guide follows.

1. Neoplastic disease in which radiation therapy is used for curative purposes either alone or in combination with surgery and chemotherapy
   A. Carcinoma of the larynx
   B. Carcinoma of the skin (excluding melanoma)
   C. Early lesions of the mouth, including lip and tongue, in which the primary tumor must be treated by radiation therapy and the regional nodes by surgery
   D. Carcinoma of the uterine cervix
   E. Seminoma of the testes, in which the primary is treated surgically and the regional nodes by means of irradiation therapy
   F. Early lesions of the prostate
   G. Hodgkin's disease in stages 1, 2, and 3
   H. Most pediatric solid tumors, in which the primary is treated in conjunction with surgery and chemotherapy is used for micrometastases
2. Neoplasms for which the cure rates are rather low when treated by either surgery or radiation therapy alone, and for which combination treatment seems to produce better results
   A. Advanced lesions of the larynx and hypopharynx
   B. Carcinoma of esophagus
   C. Carcinoma of the tonsil and oropharyngeal region
   D. Carcinoma of the anorectal area in locally advanced stages.
3. Neoplasms rarely curable by any means (because of their aggressive nature and tendency for widespread dissemination at the time of first diagnosis) but often highly radiosensitive and, if localized, occasionally cured by irradiation alone or in combination with chemotherapy
   A. Non-Hodgkin's lymphoma
   B. Ewing's sarcoma of the bone
   C. Medulloblastoma
   D. Oat cell carcinoma of the lung

Large numbers of patients referred for radiation treatment are incurable by any means, and the treatment is often palliative. In all these cases the aims of the radiotherapist should be to make the patient more comfortable by relieving symptoms and prolonging an active and useful life if possible. The relief of pain owing to metastasis to bone is fairly simple and is usually accomplished with a relatively small dose of radiation. Similarly, palliative radiation therapy can be given to relieve obstruction of the luminal structures such as the superior vena cava, the ureters, and regional lymphatic channels. Radiation therapy as a palliative means is also used to control hematuria, hemoptysis, or vaginal bleeding owing to malignant disorders of the bladder, bronchus, and the uterus, respectively.

RADIATION EFFECT AND TOLERANCE OF NORMAL TISSUES[26,33]

It is generally assumed that the tolerance of normal tissue is the limiting factor in treating cancer by irradiation and that the normal tissue of general importance is connective tissue, probably the endothelium of the capillary blood vessels. There is a range of sensitivity stretching from the highly sensitive organs to the relatively insensitive organs. The former are regularly damaged by low doses of radiation, and the latter can tolerate much larger doses although not without sustaining some damage. As a general rule, the sensitive group includes the reproductive cells of the testis and ovary, the hematopoietic tissue, the epithelial lining of the alimentary tract, and the epithelium of the skin. The less sensitive group includes muscles, bones, fibrous tissue, and nerve tissue.

The limit of tolerance of various organs has been derived from clinical work. Dosage factors used in curing cancers of various sites are well documented in the literature. People vary in their sensitivity to ionization just as they do to ultraviolet rays (sunburn). As a general rule, the normal tissue reactions are worse if large volumes of tissue receive a large dose in a short time. Effects of radiation may be acute or late. Acute reactions occurring in patients undergoing treatment are usually reversible and are a function of "daily dose."

The late reactions include effects that occur months or years after completion of therapy, depending on the normal tissue in question. These are most definitely owing to endarteritis phenomena leading to impairment of the organ concerned. The late reactions are invariably irreversible and are a function of total dose. These sequalae include leukemia, carcinoma, other cancers, and genetic changes.

RADIATION AND IMMUNOLOGY[25]

That radiation is immunologically suppressive is generally agreed, but the precise effect of this immunological suppression on patients who undergo irradiation therapy for malignant disease is not clearly understood. There are conflicting reports, some of which suggest that the consequences of therapeutic irradiation may outweigh its benefits. On the other hand, some reports suggest that the adverse role of ionizing radiation on immune processes is probably more apparent than real and it is perhaps an expression of the method of investigation rather than the malfunction of the immune cells.

REFERENCES

1. Bond VP: Negative pions: their possible use in radiotherapy. Am J Roentgenol 111:9–26, 1971
2. Catterall M: Clinical experience with fast neutrons. Proc R Soc Med 65:839–843, 1972
3. Cohen L, Scott MJ: Fractionation procedures in radiation therapy: A computerized approach to evaluation. Br J Radiol 41:529–544, 1968
4. Ellis F: Fractionation in radiotherapy. Mod Trends Radiother 1:34–51, 1967
5. Fowler JF Current aspects of radiobiology as applied to radiotherapy. Clin Radiol 23:257–262, 1972
6. Friedell HL, Thomas CI, Krohmer JS: An evaluation of the clinical use of strontium 90 beta-ray applicator with a review of the underlying principles. Am J Roentgenol 71:25–39, 1954
7. Gray LH: Radiobiologic basis of oxygen as modifying factor in radiation therapy. Am J Roentgenol 85:803–815, 1961
8. Hall EJ Radiobiology for the radiologist. New York, Harper & Row Publishers, 1973
9. Hilaris BS, Whitmore W: Radiation therapy and pelvic node dissection in the management of cancer of the prostrate. Am J Roentgenol Radium Ther Nucl Med 121:832–838, 1974
10. International Commission on Radiation Units and Measurements: Radiation Quantities and Units, ICRU Report 19, ICRU Publications, Washington, D.C., 1971
11. Johns HE, Cunningham JR: The Physics of Radiology (ed 3). Springfield, Ill., Charles C Thomas Publisher, 1969
12. Krohmer JS: Physical measurements on various beta-ray applicators. Am J Roentgenol 66:791–796, 1951
13. Laughlin JS: Realistic treatment planning. Cancer 22:716–729, 1968
14. Levitt SH: The split-dose approach in radiation therapy. Radiol Clin North Am 7:293–299, 1969

15. Line D, Deeley TJ: Palliative therapy, in Deeley TJ (ed): Modern Radiotherapy—Carcinoma of the Bronchus. London, Buttersworths, pp 299–300
16. Little JB: Cellular effects of ioniaing radiation. N Engl J Med 278:308–315, 369–376, 1968
17. Loevinger R: Radiation therapy with high energy electrons, Parts I and II. Radiology 77:906–927, 1961
18. McEwan JB: Clinical trial of radiotherapy and high pressure oxygen. Ann R. Coll Surg 39:168–170, 1966
19. Maxfield JR Jr, Maxfield, JGS, Maxfield, WS: The use of radioactive phosphorus and testosterone in metastatic bone lesions from breast and prostate. South Med J 51:320–321, 1958
20. Morgan RL: Fast neutron therapy—clinical applications. Mod Trends Radiother 1:171–186, 1967
21. Moss WT, Brand WN, Battifora H: Radiation Oncology, Rationale, Technique Results (ed 4). St. Louis, CV Mosby Co, 1973
22. Murphy WT: Radiation Therapy (ed 2). Philadelphia, WB Saunders Co, 1967
23. Powers, WE: Preoperative and post-operative radiation therapy for cancer. Proceedings of the Sixth National Cancer Conference, New York, American Cancer Society, 1970, pp 33–38
24. Powers WE, Palmer LA: Biologic basis of preoperative radiation treatment. Am J Roentgenol 102:176–192, 1968
25. Radiation and Immune Defense Interaction in Interaction of Radiation and Host Immune Defense Mechanisms in Malignancy. Upton, NY, Brookhaven National Laboratory, 1974, pp 152–265
26. Rubin P, Casarett GW: Clinical Radiation Pathology. Philadelphia, WB Saunders Co, 1968
27. Scanlon PW: Initial experience with split-dose periodic radiation therapy. Am J Roentgenol 84:632–644, 1960
28. Sinclair WK: Cyclic x-ray responses in mammalian cells in vitro. Radiat Res 33:620–643, 1968
29. The Interrelationship of Surgery and Radiation Therapy. Vaeth JM (ed). Baltimore, University Park Press, 1970
30. Tobias CA, Todd PW: Heavy charged particles in cancer therapy. Conference on radiobiology and radiotherapy. Natl Cancer Inst Monogr 24:1–21, 1967
31. Tone ECK, Finkelstein P: Treatment of bone metastases with parathormone and radioactive phosphorus. J Urol 109:71–75, 1973
32. Wildermuth O: The present status of hybaroxic radiotherapy. Radiol Clin North Am 7:345–351, 1969
33. Zuckerman S: The sensitivity of the gonads to radiation. Clin Radiol 16:1–15, 1965

5

Management of Head and Neck Cancer

Neoplasms of the head and neck include a broad spectrum of fascinating lesions that present many diagnostic and therapeutic challenges to both the general physician and the oncologist. Although these tumors are relatively rare in incidence in our population in comparison to lung, breast, and gastrointestinal tract cancer, emphasis is indicated because of the frequent management questions that arise with this group of cancers. For the purpose of this discussion, neoplasms of the lining of the oral cavity, pharynx, larynx, and nasal passages will be considered separately from the glandular tumors (thyroid and salivary glands) and the more infrequent neoplasms.

SQUAMOUS CANCER OF THE LINING OF THE
UPPER ALIMENTARY AND RESPIRATORY PASSAGES

Lesions of these sites account for only approximately 3 percent of all cancers and 3 percent of all cancer deaths in the United States. There is even some hope for further reduction in incidence with improvement in oral hygiene, general nutrition, and curtailment of excessive tobacco and alcohol consumption. There is no factual evidence for the association between oral hygiene, nutrition, and chronic irritation of various types, but there are enough clinical correlations to establish some causal relationship between these factors and the development of squamous carcinoma of these sites. The associated socioeconomic, nutritional, hepatic, and pulmonary problems in many of these patients are also witness to the importance of these controllable factors in the genesis of head and neck cancer.

Diagnosis

Cancers in this group are readily accessible, at least in the oral cavity, and very easily and effectively treated when they are detected as small lesions. However, since there are many "hiding places" in this anatomic location, the examination must be carefully performed using both vision and palpation. The clinical problem is that pain or other symptoms are rare until the neoplastic process is relatively advanced and, correspondingly, difficult to treat. Special techniques such as oral cytology[42] and the topical application of toluidine blue[88] for identifying precancerous sites are intriguing possibilities for screening high-risk groups. However, a thorough oral examination as part of routine medical and dental examinations is probably our most valuable weapon in the control of these lesions.

Diagnosis of any lesion found in the nasal cavity, oral cavity, or oropharynx can be established by simple incisional, punch, or forceps biopsy of a small representative fragment of an ulcerated lesion of the mucosal surface. Topical or infiltration anesthesia may be employed, but ulcerating lesions are often insensitive and biopsy may be successfully employed without anesthesia in most instances. Biopsy of a mass lying beneath intact mucous membranes requires infiltration anesthesia, and the punch biopsy technique may be particularly useful here after incision of the mucosa. When biopsy of hypopharyngeal or laryngeal lesions is indicated because of symptoms or the presence of a palpable, clinically suspicious lymph node in the midcervical region, it is generally accomplished with appropriate biopsy forceps at the time of endoscopy. If lymph nodes are palpable, endoscopy should precede any consideration of obtaining histologic material from the enlarged lymph node other than the possibility of needle aspiration biopsy. This latter technique can be safely employed to establish the diagnosis of metastatic squamous carcinoma, but we generally defer aspiration biopsy until after a complete search, including endoscopy and nasopharyngeal examination, for the probable primary site. Diagnosis and management of the patient with a clinically positive cervical lymph node without a detectable primary lesion will be discussed subsequently.

DIFFERENTIAL DIAGNOSIS

Benign lesions. Examination of the lips, oral cavity, and pharynx may reveal the white plaquelike lesions of leukoplakia. Since this is a precancerous lesion, an excisional biopsy is worthwhile.[28] Many benign conditions may be found on careful examination of the mucosal surfaces of the head and neck, and some will require therapy, or at least a recognition of their presence.[89] These include mucoceles, papillomas, fibromas, hemangiomas, and benign mixed tumors of minor salivary glands. Gum lesions frequently confused with early neoplasms are denture fibromas, pyogenic granulomas, and giant cell reparative granulomas. The congenital lesions median rhomboid glossitis and palatine torus may also be concerning to the uninitiated, but no treatment is indicated in either case unless denture fitting problems are related to the latter lesion. An uncommon problem sometimes confused with cancer of the tongue is a lingual thyroid resulting from failure of the fetal thyroid tissue to descend into the neck. This presents as an elevated midline mass in the posterior tongue, and excision of the lesion may be required for mechanical reasons, even though thyroid tissue will usually be absent in the normal location.

Other malignant lesions. Glandular carcinoma (adenocarcinoma) may occur in any of the anatomic locations under discussion because of the presence of minor salivary gland tissue in association with all of these mucous membranes.[8] In general, these lesions should be evaluated and managed the same as squamous carcinoma. Another less frequent form of cancer is malignant melanoma arising from melanoblasts in the mucous membranes. The diagnosis may not be suspected until the biopsy of an ulcerated lesion is examined, but pigmentation of the lesion or the surrounding mucosa should suggest this diagnosis. In patients with primary malignant melanoma of the mucous membranes, the appropriate treatment is surgical resection of the type to be described subsequently for squamous carcinoma of the corresponding sites; but the poor prognosis and high incidence of distant metastases make a thorough search for distant disease mandatory before initiating treatment.

Malignant lymphoma arises in these same tissues, particularly in those areas rich in lymphoid tissue, such as Waldeyer's ring, the area encompassed by the nasopharynx, the tonsils, and the base of the tongue. The appropriate choice for local therapy for malignant lymphoma is radiation; therefore, it is imperative to confirm the diagnosis microscopically.

Staging

In all sites the stage of the neoplasm in an individual patient depends on the size and extent of the primary lesion, the clinical status of the regional (cervical) lymph nodes, and the presence or absence of distant metastasis. Both treatment planning and prognosis are dependent on appropriate staging of the neoplasm after the histologic diagnosis of cancer has been established, and the tumor-node-metastasis (TNM) system is a useful one.[90,91] There are specific minor differences in TNM staging for each anatomic site in the head and neck region and some continuing variations between the systems developed by the American Joint Committee and the Committee of the International Union Against Cancer, but these minor differences are on a common theme. Practically speaking, one needs to review TNM tables for each primary site at the time of staging for precise categorization. The general principles of the TNM system are outlined in Table 5-1.

Table 5-1
TNM Staging Scheme for Head and Neck Cancer

Stage	Description
T	
1	≤ 2 cm if measurable (as in oral cavity), or a small, noninfiltrating lesion limited to the site of origin as described specifically for each primary site
2	>2 cm but <4 cm (if in oral cavity), or limited infiltration or involvement of tissues adjacent to but within the organ of origin, as described for each primary site
3	>4 cm, or more infiltrative, or involving tissues outside the primary organ as specifically described for each primary site
N	
0	No suspicious lymph nodes palpable in the cervical region
1	Clinically palpable and suspicious lymph nodes in the ipsilateral cervical chain
2, 3	(N3 not used for some primary sites.) More advanced nodal disease such as contralateral or bilateral clinically suspicious lymph nodes, or "fixed" clinically positive nodes
M	
0	No clinical or radiographic evidence of metastasis (other than cervical lymph nodes)
1	Clinical or radiographic evidence of metastasis
Stage	
I	Small primary lesions (T1) without clinically suspicious cervical lymph nodes or distant metastases (NO, MO)
II	Slightly larger primary lesions (T2) without evidence of cervical lymph node or distant metastases (NO, MO)
III	More advanced primary lesions extending outside the organ of origin (T3), or primary lesion of any size (T1, T2, or T3) with clinically suspicious ipsilateral lymph nodes (N1)
IV	Neoplasms with contralateral cervical lymph node enlargement, bilateral cervical lymph node, or "fixed" lymph nodes (N2 or N3); patients with metastasis other than cervical lymph nodes (M1)

Treatment

The major treatment modalities available for potentially curable cancers of the head and neck are radiation therapy and surgical excision, but combinations of these two methods or a combination of either of these methods with systemic chemotherapy has also been proposed.

With the multiple alternatives available, the physician may be understandably confused regarding the preferable treatment for a specific patient. Unfortunately, treatment is often chosen on the basis of the limited perspective of an individual specialist, even though the diagnosis, evaluation of the extent of the disease, choice of primary treatment, and effective rehabilitation of the head and neck cancer patient all require special talents that cross our conventional disciplinary lines. Although the individual general surgeon, otorhinolaryngologist, plastic surgeon, oral surgeon, or radiotherapist may have special interest and training in the management of head and neck cancer problems, total care of high quality requires collaboration among these specialists as well as with medical oncologists, neurosurgeons, prosthodontists, speech therapists, and other allied health personnel. With no other group of neoplasms is the team approach more important to ideal patient care than with cancers of the head and neck.

CARCINOMA OF THE LIPS

Lip carcinomas are usually indolent and slow growing with an extremely low incidence of cervical lymph node metastasis. Small carcinomas of the lower lip are equally well treated by radiation therapy or simple surgical excision (V-lip excision). We prefer the latter approach because of its simplicity, convenience, and superb treatment results that are comparable to those achieved by radiation therapy.[10] The very large lip cancer seen frequently in the past seems to be a disappearing disease. The extent of reconstruction required for large lip cancers when treated by surgery often leads to a preference for primary radiation therapy for lesions of this extent.[25] The long-term results of radiation can be excellent and the cosmetic result unusually good. When resection is chosen for lesions involving the entire lower lip, reconstruction requires the use of a skin flap from the forehead or deltopectoral region. With all lip cancers, the cervical lymph nodes should be examined periodically for potential enlargement as subsequent neck dissection may be required in a few patients.[61]

Some patients are observed who have extensive leukoplakia on the lower lip—with or without a carcinoma. Because of the precancerous nature of this lesion, it is advisable to remove the mucosa of the entire lower lip as a prophylactic measure (lip shave). A satisfactory cosmetic result can be achieved by advancing the oral mucosa from the buccogingival sulcus, and this procedure can be combined with wedge (or V) excision of a carcinoma of the lip if it is also present. These findings are a specific indication for surgery, as opposed to radiation therapy, for treatment of the lip cancer despite the equal frequency of cancer control by these two methods.

ORAL CAVITY AND PHARYNX CANCERS

A major factor in the choice of therapy is the anatomic stage of the disease, but important additional factors are concurrent precancerous lesions, the possibility of other cancers, and the general debility and concurrent medical diseases often present (chronic pulmonary disease, hepatic cirrhosis, and cardiovascular disease). In addition to all of these factors, the reaction of the well-informed patient to the advantages and disadvantages of the alternatives requires careful assessment before developing a treatment plan. Our choice of therapy for cancers of these sites is based primarily on clinical staging, and our approach is presented with the realization that some features are necessarily arbitrary.

Small localized lesions of the oral cavity and pharynx, without clinical evidence of spread to cervical lymph nodes or other sites (stage I in TNM classification), are the most favorable lesions with any means of therapy. We prefer radiation therapy as primary treatment with close and prolonged follow-up for clinical signs of local recurrence or cervical lymph node metastasis. In some respects, radiation therapy may actually be more thorough or radical than surgical excision for these early lesions since the treatment field employed is larger than the field of surgical resection we are willing to employ. More radical excision, including contiguous structures and regional lymph nodes, does not seem justified for stage I lesions. Cryosurgery may be employed for selected stage I lesions on the basis of the favorable experience of others, but we have had no experience with this technique for early lesions.[36]

In contrast, the larger oral cavity and pharyngeal lesions with extensive involvement of adjacent anatomical structures, the mandible, or the cervical lymph nodes (an imprecise description of stage III or stage IV in the TNM classification) are treated with much less success using either radiation therapy or surgical excision. It is generally agreed, however, that the likelihood of success with surgical excision for these more-advanced lesions is greater than with primary radiation therapy, and we employ surgical resection by radical combined operations (including laryngectomy if required) for these distinctly less favorable lesions if the patient can accept medically and emotionally the increased immediate disability. In some centers a full course of radiation therapy is employed for lesions of this extent, and surgery is employed only subsequently if the clinical result is unsatisfactory.[31,49] This is based on the concept that surgery can salvage those patients who are considered ''radiation fail-

ures." However, the failure rate after radiation therapy for advanced lesions, the inability of this approach to reduce the extent of surgery eventually required in most instances, and the additional problems produced
by this maximal dosage of both treatment methods lead to our preference
for surgery as the initial approach to advanced-stage lesions of the oral
cavity and pharynx.

The major area of disagreement in choice of initial therapy for cancer
of the oral cavity and pharynx is in the intermediate stages from the standpoint of extent of disease (stages II and early III). We prefer surgical excision as primary treatment for lesions in these intermediate stages for the
same reasons given for the more advanced cases (stage IV). Our surgical
efforts are supplemented by an emphasis on the use of primary reconstructive procedures, which tend to offset both the cosmetic and functional disadvantages associated with radical surgery. With lesions in the
pharynx that require laryngectomy to achieve an adequate surgical
margin, the prognostic advantage of surgery seems to outweigh the advantage of retention of the larynx made possible by the use of radiation
therapy. This treatment decision is difficult, however, despite the post-
surgical possibility of esophageal speech. When choosing therapy for
intermediate stages, the physician must consider the patient's ability to
accept the treatment proposed.

PRIMARY CANCER OF THE LARYNX

In contrast to most of the lesions previously discussed, we individu-
alize the choice of therapy for patients with primary carcinoma of the
larynx with an inclination to favor radiation therapy whenever possible.[21,109,110] Our general approach for the smaller lesions of the supraglottic larynx and glottis (T1 and T2 lesions) has been radiation therapy for
the same reasons stated for stage I lesions of the oral cavity and pharynx,
but partial or supraglottic laryngectomy is undoubtedly an equally acceptable method for these lesions.[66] For glottic lesions with subglottic extension and for the larger lesions of the glottis and supraglottic region (T3 and
T4), we recommend total laryngectomy (often combined with radical neck
dissection) rather than radiation therapy in view of more adequate disease
control of lesions with these features. Social, medical, and psychological
factors may often temper the therapeutic decision for patients with primary carcinoma of the larynx, but laryngectomy appears to be the preferred approach for the more advanced lesions.[90,91]

CARCINOMA OF THE NASAL CAVITY
AND PARANASAL SINUSES

Carcinoma of the maxillary antrum, other paranasal sinuses, or nasal
cavity is generally associated with a poor prognosis when treated by
either radiation therapy or surgery, although radical resection of the max-

illa has generally been the preferred treatment.[34] Unfortunately, the disease usually is not diagnosed until it has extended into the soft tissues adjacent to the sinuses or into the ethmoid sinuses, and in either case the standard surgical procedure usually provides an inadequate margin because of the proximity of the disease to the base of the skull. With this background of essentially poor results by both of the primary treatment methods, Ketcham et al.[53] extended the procedure of maxillectomy to include en bloc excision of the ethmoid sinuses. This resection requires a combined craniofacial approach, which can be done with a reasonably low morbidity as well as effective rehabilitation. The anterior cranial fossa is approached through a frontal craniotomy as the initial part of the procedure (Fig. 5-1), and after it has been established that the disease has not extended into the sphenoid sinus at the base of the skull, the ethmoid complex can be resected in continuity with the facial portion of the dissection. The latter is carried out through a Weber-Ferguson incision, and the nasal bone, maxilla, pterygoid plate, and a portion of the nasopharynx are resected en bloc after the appropriate bony incisions are made in the floor of the frontal fossa. Although the orbital contents on the side of the lesion can be preserved in some patients, orbital exenteration is usually required. It is not possible at this time to state whether the end results will surpass those obtained in the past by primary radiation therapy or the standard surgical approaches, but we believe this is the procedure of choice in well-selected patients.

In some patients with advanced carcinoma of the maxillary antrum, the disease has extended into the soft tissues of the pterygomaxillary space. Involvement of this space is strongly suspected if there is trismus, pain in the ear or face, anesthesia in the area of distribution of the second and third division of the trigeminal nerve, or radiologic evidence of destruction of the posterior wall of the maxillary antrum and pterygoid plate. This extension of disease has previously prevented adequate surgical excision since the involved pterygoid fossa has the floor of the middle cranial fossa as one of its boundaries. For this problem, we have extended the procedure described by Ketcham et al.[53] to include an en bloc resection of the pterygomaxillary space by resection of the floor of the middle cranial fossa extradurally through a subtemporal craniectomy[100] (Fig. 5-1). The procedure is associated with acceptable morbidity, and it seems worthy of further trial in selected patients with cancers of the paranasal sinuses in view of the poor results with standard approaches. Technical problems in this combined craniofacial approach to head and neck cancer require attention, but our experience thus far has demonstrated that these can be overcome.[100,112,113]

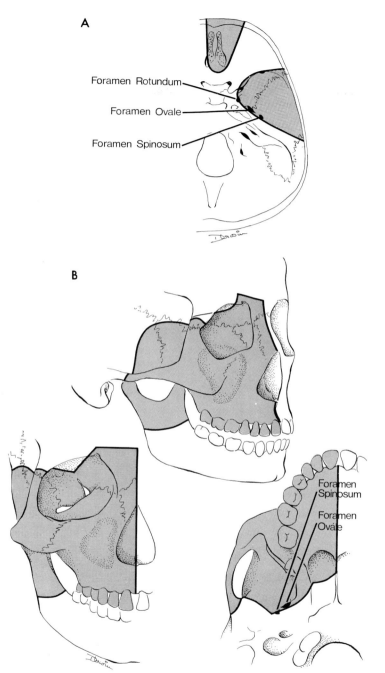

Fig. 5-1.   Diagram of anatomy of the combined craniofacial operative approach in patients with carcinoma involving the ethmoid sinuses and/or pterygoid fossa. **A.** Intracranial portion.   **B.** Maxillofacial portion.

NASOPHARYNGEAL CANCER

The anatomic location nasopharyngeal cancer precludes early diagnosis. Unfortunately, invasion of the base of the skull and cranial nerve involvement are frequent initial signs. The relationship of this primary site to the base of the skull makes adequate surgical resection impossible; therefore, appropriate treatment for all stages is radiation therapy. It should be added that patients with carcinoma of the pharynx extending into the nasopharynx are also treated with radiation therapy, rather than surgery, for the same anatomic reasons. Treatment planning should include both the primary site and the regional lymph nodes of the neck as the cancer in clinically involved lymph nodes from nasopharyngeal cancer is controlled by radiation therapy alone in a reasonable number of patients.[43,115]

Regional Lymph Node Metastases

A common denominator in the evaluation and staging, treatment planning, and prognosis of most squamous cancers of the head and neck region is the clinical and pathologic status of the regional (cervical) lymph nodes. The incidence of metastasis to these lymph nodes varies from a low incidence with lip cancer (5 percent) and paranasal sinus cancer (10 percent) to a higher level for oral cavity, pharyngeal, and laryngeal sites (greater than 50 percent). In addition to these variations, there is a direct relationship between local extent of the primary lesion and likelihood of metastasis. In the absence of clinically palpable lymph nodes in the cervical region, lymphatic metastasis may, obviously, be present. For these reasons, we include radical neck dissection in combination with resection of the primary lesion in all patients with primary cancer in whom the primary lesion of the oral cavity and pharynx is deemed advanced enough to warrant surgical therapy. There are no data to demonstrate a major advantage to such a combined operation (for patients with nonpalpable surgical lymph nodes) over later lymph node dissection when nodes do become palpable, but this combined type of operation allows some technical advantages relating to surgical access to the oral cavity and pharynx. In addition, it frequently saves the patient a subsequent operative procedure. This is particularly relevant to patients with stage III and IV lesions, for which the likelihood of metastasis in the cervical lymph nodes is high whether nodes are palpable at the time of initial evaluation or not.

Where one draws the line as to the practical advantage of performing an elective radical neck dissection is somewhat arbitrary. The incidence of histologic evidence of lymph node metastasis in patients with nonpalpable nodes with stage I oral cavity and pharyngeal lesions, lip cancer, nasal cavity and paranasal sinus cancer, and stage I and II primary laryngeal cancer is certainly low enough to lead the surgeon to omit neck dissection under these circumstances. In some of these sites, however, the relative midline nature of a more-advanced lesion does present a choice between omission of neck dissection and a simultaneous bilateral neck dissection. The increased morbidity from bilateral neck dissection makes this an unappealing choice in the absence of palpable or suspicious cervical lymph nodes or direct extension of the primary lesion into the cervical tissues.

If clinical evidence of cervical lymph node metastasis is present in patients with primary lesions at any of these sites and the primary lesion can be controlled, radical neck dissection is the preferred treatment except as previously noted with nasopharyngeal cancer. Radical neck dissection is indicated for this lesion if neck node metastasis persists after radiation therapy. Elective node therapy with radiation often controls metastastic disease in regional lymphatics, but this modality is less effective when the node disease has become advanced enough to be palpable.

The technique of radical neck dissection that we employ is that described by Hayes Martin.[64] This "standard" dissection is an en bloc dissection of the lymphatic tissues with no attempt to preserve the jugular vein, the sternocleidomastoid muscle, or the spinal accessory nerve. We usually prefer omitting or deferring neck dissection for a specific case of head and neck cancer to performing modified neck dissection, but the preservation of the spinal accessory nerve is a reasonable modification, particularly with elective neck dissection. The incisions for neck dissection that may be used are shown in Figure 5-2. We prefer the transverse incisions for cosmetic reasons, but incisions must be modified to fit specific problems.

A   B

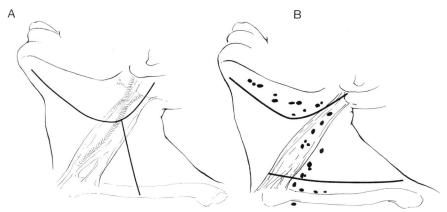

Fig. 5-2. Alternative incisions for unilateral radical neck dissection.

BILATERAL NECK DISSECTION[35,80]

Bilateral clinically positive lymph nodes and extensive bilateral soft tissue involvement are two indications for simultaneous bilateral neck dissection. The morbidity in terms of wound complications and facial edema is considerably greater than with unilateral neck dissection, which is the major reason for avoiding bilateral dissection in the absence of proof of bilateral disease. When the indications are present and there are no other signs of advanced disease, the procedure can be accomplished safely despite bilateral resection of the internal jugular veins. Postoperative facial edema is mild in some patients and severe in others, but the peak of edema may not be reached until 10–14 days postoperatively. Therefore, it is advisable to maintain a tracheostomy for this period as laryngeal edema may otherwise be a potential hazard. A useful incision for bilateral neck dissection is shown in Figure 5-3.

METASTASIS TO CERVICAL LYMPH NODES AS THE INITIAL SYMPTOM OF CANCER

A clinically silent primary cancer in the head and neck region (e.g., nasopharynx or pyriform sinus) or in some viscus below the clavicle may metastasize to the cervical lymph nodes, and the nodes may be the only clinical finding.[50,60] The anatomical location of the node mass may be of some help in directing the clinician's attention to the primary site since the supraclavicular (or scalene) lymph nodes usually contain metastases from cancers arising below the clavicle. The usual problem, however, is a metastatic mass in the midjugular lymph node chain, and this mass has multiple diagnostic possibilities. Although biopsy of the node mass may eventually be required for accurate diagnosis, it is preferable to carry out a thorough and accurate clinical and endoscopic examination of the oral cavity, nasopharynx, and larynx first because of the frequency of occult cancers in these sites. If the primary lesion is identified and biopsy obtained, there is no need to "violate" the planes of the neck by an inci-

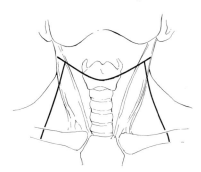

Fig. 5-3.   Incision for bilateral neck dissection.

sional biopsy as this may only complicate the subsequent surgical treatment.

If an occult primary lesion is not identified by the above examinations, chest radiograph, or esophagram, our next diagnostic maneuver is usually aspiration biopsy of the cervical mass. If metastatic squamous cancer is not detected by aspiration biopsy, histologic classification then requires open biopsy. Less-common primary cancers or lymphoma may be the cause of the enlargement, and on occasion the "clinically positive" node proves to be benign. If the aspiration biopsy does identify metastatic squamous cancer, sinus radiographs, direct laryngoscopy, and direct examination of the nasopharynx are required.

If a primary lesion is not yet identified, a "blind" biopsy of the nasopharynx is indicated. In addition, a bronchoscopy with bronchial washings may be helpful since a cryptic cancer can be detected by these procedures.

After a thorough workup has been completed, a few patients with histologically proven metastatic squamous cancer in the jugular chain will still not have an identifiable primary lesion. Under these circumstances treatment of the cervical metastases is appropriate and may be accomplished by either radiation therapy or surgery. Our preference is for radical neck dissection if the metastatic disease is centrally located and clinically limited to the jugular chain. In patients with more extensive lymphatic disease, radical neck dissection seems less appealing than radiation. Although repeated examinations often reveal the primary carcinoma at a later date, in some patients the primary lesion is never identified. Surprisingly enough, the results from treatment of patients with this unique situation have been reasonably satisfactory.

Planned Combination of Therapeutic Modalities for Head and Neck Cancer

The combination of a full therapeutic course of radiation therapy followed by surgical resection of the primary lesion and regional lymphatic bed has some rationale and is favored by a number of oncologists.[49] The absence of reliable data demonstrating benefit, and the added morbidity associated with this combination of two forms of therapy, has led us to avoid this approach at our own institution. Nevertheless, this approach has been used inadvertently when initial radiation therapy has failed to control the disease and surgery was required subsequently.

Many clinicians strongly believe that the combination of radiation and surgery has real hope for additional therapeutic benefits in head and neck cancer, particularly if the radiation dosage is below the full therapeutic range so as to reduce the complication rate.[68,98] Several reports

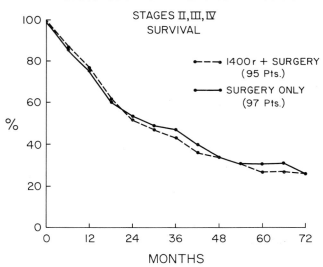

Fig. 5-4.   Data from prospective clinical trial of preoperative radiation therapy (1400 rads in 2 days) to the primary lesion and neck of patients with stages II, III, and IV squamous carcinoma of the oral cavity and pharynx (from Medical College of Virginia).

suggest benefit, but there are factors that obscure the data, especially the lack of randomized allocation of patients in such trials where benefit has been observed.   For this reason, we initiated a randomized clinical trial of low-dose preoperative radiation therapy (1400 rads in 2 days), stratified for primary site and stage, for patients undergoing primary surgical therapy for stage II, III, and IV cancers of the oral cavity and pharynx (Fig. 5-4).[57]   The increase in postoperative morbidity at this dosage level proved to be minimal, but no significant difference in recurrence rate or survival was demonstrated on longer follow-up in this study which included 192 patients.   A prospective clinical trial of preoperative radiation therapy at some other dose level conceivably might show some benefit, but we feel that available data fail to substantiate this approach at this time.

Other proposed combinations are primary radiation therapy with systemic chemotherapy and primary surgical therapy with systemic chemotherapy, but there are no data to support these approaches at this time. This will undoubtedly remain the case until more effective chemotherapeutic agents are developed for squamous carcinoma.

Prognosis

A summary of end results of treatment of epidermoid carcinoma of the head and neck using TNM staging is shown in Table 5-2.

**Special Considerations on the
Radiotherapeutic Management Squamous Carcinoma
of the Head and Neck**

With orthovoltage techniques used in the past, the major limitation of therapy for head and neck cancer was the tolerance of the overlying skin and the possibility of radionecrosis of bone included in the radiation portal. Adequate dosage for local control of the primary site often required interstitial therapy with radium needles or radon seeds in view of these limitations, but intraoral cones were applicable for some sites. Implantation of interstitial sources produced some problems in terms of even distribution of desired dosage, but this problem in treatment planning has now been largely obviated by present-day improvements in equipment for external beam radiotherapy. Nevertheless, interstitial irradiation is still appropriate for selected oral cavity lesions.

With cobalt and supervoltage therapy, the tolerance of skin and bone has increased and other considerations now become more significant. The cervical spinal cord is accessible to major damage at dosages that can now be achieved by external beam therapy. Although radiotherapy has an increased capability, treatment planning must be more precise to prevent grave complications. Present-day curative radiotherapy requires the skills and experience of a radiologist whose total effort is in the field of radiotherapy.

COMPLICATIONS[63]

The acute skin reaction of variable extent and the symptomatic mucosal changes in the treated field during therapy are particularly dis-

Table 5-2
End Results of Treatment of Epidermoid
Carcinoma of the Head and Neck

Site of Tumor	5-Yr Survival (%) According to Stage			
	I	II	III	IV
Oral cavity	75	65	35	15
Oropharynx	70	55	25	9
Glottis	95	85	60	10
Supraglottis	91	82	50	10
Hypopharynx	70	45	30	5
Lip	95	88	65	15

tressing to some patients, but these minor problems resolve with time. Permanent reduction in the amount of saliva secondary to a full course of well-administered radiation therapy (xerostomia) and permanent reduction in taste acuity are distressing problems for some but can be managed by topical medication. One extremely disabling complication, however, is the development of radionecrosis of bone within the radiated field.[24] The majority of patients with this problem have involvement of the mandible, but the process may involve the maxilla or other sites. Severe pain is the outstanding symptom of this complication, and the increased incidence in patients with infections associated with dental problems led radiotherapists in past years to advise total dental extraction before the initiation of therapy. With good dental care,[15,84] careful treatment of existing dental infections, and the use of supervoltage therapy, dentition can probably be maintained during radiation therapy, but dental status is still a major concern. If radionecrosis does occur, the only solution is wide removal of the affected bone and adequate coverage with healthy soft tissue. Pain is relieved soon after the procedure.

Special Considerations in the Surgical Management of Squamous Carcinoma of the Head and Neck

SURGICAL PROCEDURES

Tracheostomy. Airway management is a key factor in the treatment of patients with head and neck cancer. The patient may come to his physician with airway obstruction requiring relief if the patient is to tolerate subsequent evaluation and effective management. Most patients undergoing elective head and neck cancer surgery require tracheostomy as a prophylactic measure to allow the surgeon to proceed comfortably with the planned resection and reconstruction and to avoid or minimize respiratory complications in the postoperative period.

Tracheostomy is also routinely employed for patients undergoing bilateral radical neck dissection or a second contralateral radical neck dissection in view of the marked edema of mucous membranes that may occur with resulting airway problems.

Tracheostomy is performed under general anesthesia with an inlying endotracheal tube when this is feasible, but it is performed under local anesthesia under most emergency circumstances, if the patient has marked trismus, or if the tumor compromises the airway and prevents insertion of an endotracheal tube. We prefer the tracheostomy technique described by Bjork,[12] in which a flap or "trap-door" of the anterior tracheal wall is constructed. This minimizes the problems associated with the change of tracheostomy tubes (Fig. 5-5).

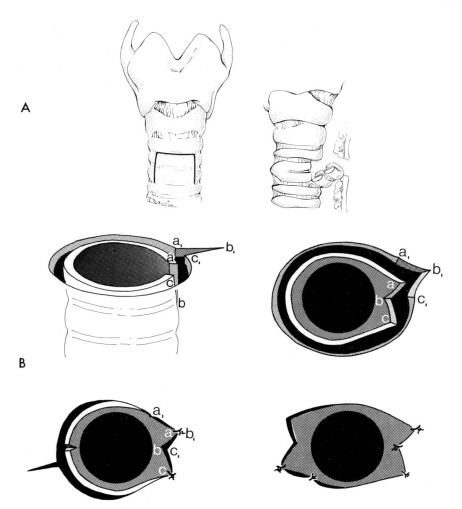

Fig. 5-5. **A:** Diagram of Bjork tracheostomy using an anterior flap of tracheal wall. **B:** Diagram of flaps developed for revision of a laryngectomy stoma that has become stenotic.

Two major complications to be avoided after tracheostomy are tube erosion of the major vessels in the upper mediastinum and muscosal necrosis (with subsequent stenosis) just below the tracheostomy stoma. These problems are prevented by selecting tracheostomy (or laryngostomy) tubes of proper configuration, size, and length for the individual patient; manipulating and changing tracheostomy tubes carefully; and avoiding prolonged high pressure in the external balloon that is often attached to the tube to prevent aspiration and facilitate use of respirators.

The stoma after laryngectomy is an end stoma that may develop stenosis at the skin level owing to a constricting circular scar. Revision can be effectively accomplished by transposition of small flaps of skin into bilateral incisions in the trachea (Fig. 5-5). This same procedure may be used as a primary method for stoma construction and may reduce the incidence of stoma stenosis.

Cervical esophagostomy. This technique for insertion of an esophageal feeding tube is convenient and has a wide range of uses in patients with cancer of the head and neck region. It has proven to be an alternative that is more acceptable than the nasal feeding tube when oral intake is not possible for more than a few weeks, and it may be used preoperatively, postoperatively, or as a means of sustenance during radiation therapy or palliative treatment. The procedure is accomplished simply by introducing a long clamp through the oral cavity and applying downward pressure with the tip of the clamp in the cervical esophagus well below the level of the cricoid cartilage.[79] The feeding tube is then grasped by the clamp exposed through a small "stab wound" in the neck, placed properly, and secured with a skin suture (Fig. 5-6).

Reconstruction of defects produced by surgical resection in the oral cavity and pharynx. After adequate surgical resection of cancer of the oral cavity or pharynx, primary closure of the operative defect is frequently possible, particularly if partial mandibular resection has been carried out. Unfortunately, primary closure after major resection leads to both cosmetic and functional disabilities that are often unacceptable. In more recent years, postsurgical disability has been reduced considerably by various skin flaps for providing new oral lining. These skin flaps also allow preservation of the mandible if it is not critically involved by tumor, and they allow mandibular replacement if resection of a segment of the mandible is required. This approach also reduces the fixation of the tongue and remaining oropharynx and reduces the disabling effects of surgery on swallowing and speech. Many methods have been employed to accomplish these objectives, including the flap constructed from the forehead[67,102] (Fig. 5-7), the deltopectoral flap based on the internal mammary vessels[4,6] (Fig. 5-8), the shoulder flap[22] (Fig. 5-9), and the nasolabial skin flap[18] constructed from the cheek (Fig. 5-10).

The nature of the blood supply of the forehead flap (temporal artery) and its location away from the field of possible prior radiation therapy make it an ideal source for new lining tissue at the time of the primary resection. We have found that it is usually possible to pass the flap into the oral cavity or pharynx through the channel created behind the zygomatic arch by resection of the coronoid process of the mandible and the accom-

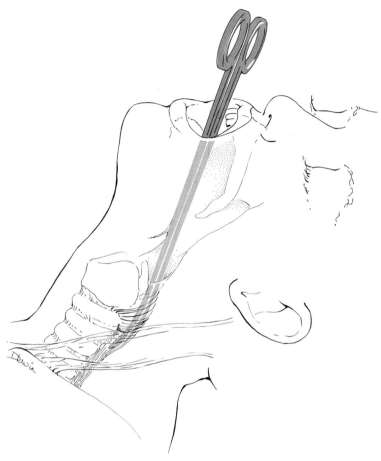

Fig. 5-6.   Diagram of technique of cervical esophagostomy using a "blind" approach.

panying temporal muscle attachment.   When an unusually wide flap is necessary for the reconstruction, the forehead flap is introduced into the oral cavity through an additional incision in the cheek.

The deltopectoral flap is also useful for primary reconstruction of large defects in the posterior oral cavity and pharynx, but the blood supply of this flap is not quite as ideal as that of the forehead flap. Although a split-thickness skin graft is employed to cover the bed of origin of either of these skin flaps, the fact that the skin graft used for the deltopectoral flap is concealed has certain advantages.

The shoulder flap has many potential applications as indicated in Figure 5-9, but the necessity of performing a "delay" in all cases makes it

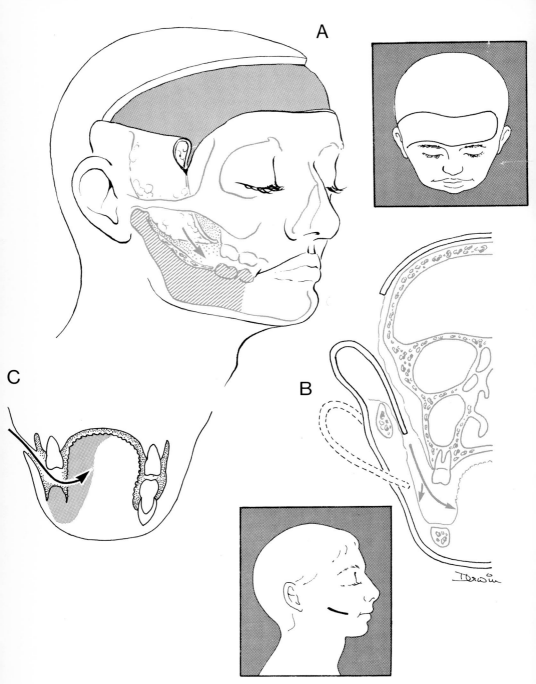

Fig. 5-7. **A:** Diagram of forehead skin flap for immediate reconstruction of oral cavity and/or pharynx. **B** and **C:** Flap is introduced through a tunnel behind the zygomatic arch after resection of the coronoid process of the mandible and temporalis muscle, or through a separate incision in the cheek.

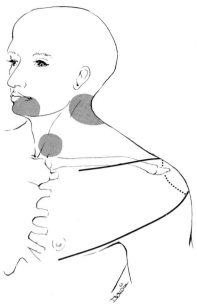

Fig. 5-8. Diagram of the deltopectoral skin flap used for primary or secondary reconstruction of the posterior oral cavity and pharynx, or providing skin coverage of the neck after extensive resection.

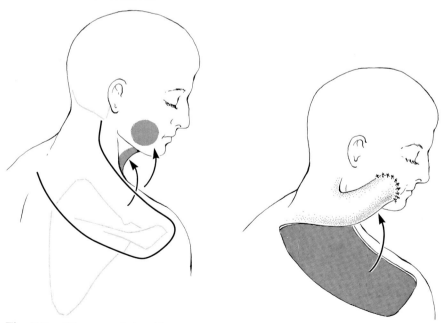

Fig. 5-9. Diagram of shoulder skin flap for various reconstructive purposes in patients undergoing major surgical resection procedures in the head and neck region.

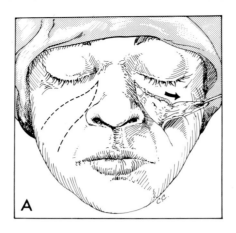

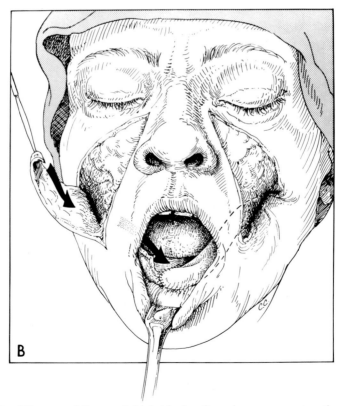

Fig. 5-10. Diagram of the nasolabial skin flap for primary reconstruction of small anterior oral cavity defects after surgical resection.

more appropriate for secondary reconstruction. Usually, we have considered the nasolabial flap for smaller defects in the anterior portion of the oral cavity as it has proven to be ideal for this purpose.

Although the general acceptance of primary reconstruction for early rehabilitation has proven to be a primary advance in surgery of head and neck cancer in recent years, it may still be preferable in some instances to create an external stoma at the time of resection. This has the disadvantage of a period of delay in physical and social rehabilitation, but the general condition of some patients or their local tissues may make the risk of a more extensive procedure to achieve reconstruction unwarranted.

Another functional advance after surgical resection for head and neck cancer is the development of improved methods for mandibular replacement. The primary reason for resection of a segment of mandible is direct invasion by disease or proximity of disease so that an adequate margin of resection cannot be accomplished without bone resection. Transfer of healthy lining tissue into the mouth and pharynx by the various skin flaps described above makes it possible to avoid mandibular resection for the simple purpose of achieving closure of the defect, and it also allows mandibular replacement with more likelihood of success in those patients in whom segmental resection of the mandible is required.

Mandibular replacement has been attempted in past years using a number of materials ranging from primary bone grafts to metal or acrylic splints.[51,82] Although provision of adequate soft tissue coverage of these replacements has solved one of the problems, the insertion of bone grafts or complex prostheses at the primary operative procedure has been associated with a high failure rate. For this reason, our preference is for the immediate insertion of a simple wire mesh segment to replace the resected mandible[101] (Fig. 5-11). The advantages of the immediate insertion of this prosthesis (with or without a condyle) over the later insertion of the more-refined prostheses by multiple secondary procedures include both an improved immediate cosmetic result and the reduction of problems produced by "shift" of the remaining mandible when no immediate replacement is employed.

Resection of carcinoma involving the ear or temporal bone. A combined intracranial facial approach is indicated for primary carcinoma involving the middle ear or for recurrent carcinoma of the skin or parotid gland involving the adjacent petrous portion of the temporal bone. Our early attempts to accomplish planned intracranial facial resection for lesions of this type were by a "piecemeal" approach and did not fulfill the accepted surgical principles of en bloc surgical excision for cancer.[111] With collaboration between neurosurgeons and surgical oncologists since that time, however, excellent techniques for en bloc excision of the pet-

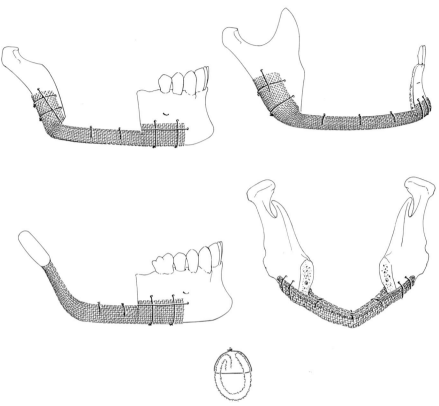

Fig. 5-11.   Diagram of stainless steel wire mesh prosthesis for mandibular replacement after surgical resection.

rous portion of the temporal bone have been developed by Lewis and
Page,[58] Conley and Novack,[20] and others.[40]   Major skin resection is also
frequently required, but coverage of the bone defect can be accomplished
by rotation of a suitable skin flap from the scalp with split-thickness skin
grafts applied to the area of origin of this flap (Fig. 5-12).

COMPLICATIONS OF SURGICAL TREATMENT

   Intraoperative complications.   A thoracic duct may be injured
during radical neck dissection, but ligation with fine suture material
solves this problem.   This is well tolerated as lymphatic collaterals are
numerous.   On rare occasions, an injured duct is not recognized until profuse drainage of lymphatic fluid is observed the first day after surgery.
Opening the operative wound and performing suture ligature of the open

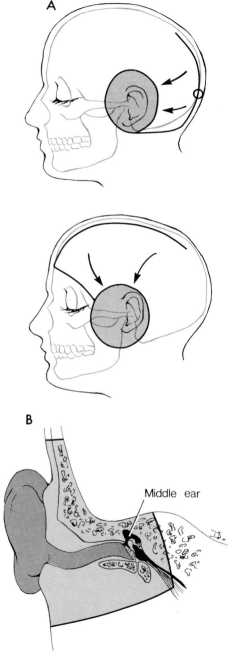

Fig. 5-12. **A:** Diagram of skin closure of operative defect after temporal bone resection using a rotation flap of scalp. **B:** Extent of bone resection.

Middle ear

duct is ideal management as the site of leak can be easily identified at this time. If the injury is not recognized until later or if the ligature is lost, elemental diet (to reduce lymph flow) and a pressure dressing on the lower neck are usually successful.

A vascular problem occurring during radical neck dissection is inadvertent damage to the subclavian vein, the subclavian artery, or one of the arterial branches of the thoracoacromial axis. Adequate exposure for controlling such hemorrhage often requires division or resection of the medial portion of the clavicle when the subclavian vein is injured, but arterial damage can often be managed by transverse division of the scalenus anticus muscle in the lower portion of the operative field. This approach gives excellent exposure of the subclavian artery for repair.

A rare, but potentially serious, intraoperative complication of surgery in the lower neck is development of ipsilateral, contralateral, or bilateral pneumothorax. Unexplained respiratory distress, cyanosis, or shock during neck dissection should always suggest the possibility of pneumothorax owing to mediastinal rupture with the escape of air trapped in this space as a result of partial respiratory obstruction. Although a portable chest radiograph in the operating room may be helpful, the emergency nature of pneumothorax may require immediate bilateral insertion of thoracostomy tubes.

Postoperative complications. The development of an external fistula between the oral cavity or pharynx and the wound in the neck is a distressing complication after surgical resection of head and neck cancer as it usually produces a major delay in the rehabilitation of the patient and may expose him to significant hazards. Initial management of the fistula is the establishment of adequate drainage by widely opening the external wound and instituting frequent wound sprays to cleanse the contaminated neck. The purpose of this approach is to allow protective granulation tissue to form in the wound and, hopefully, reduce the possibility of carotid artery exposure. Many fistulas close spontaneously after intensive wound care of this type, but secondary surgical procedures may be required.

Since exposure of the carotid artery with secondary hemorrhage is such a hazardous and serious postoperative complication of head and neck cancer surgery, it is appropriate in selected patients to plan methods for carotid artery protection, especially for those who require surgery after prior therapeutic doses of radiation therapy and for those who require bilateral neck dissection as a part of their surgical procedure.[69] Dermal graft coverage of the carotid artery has proven to be a reasonably effective method, and it is strongly recommended for those operative procedures in which the risk of subsequent exposure of the carotid artery is increased.[23,92]

REHABILITATION AFTER SURGICAL TREATMENT OF SQUAMOUS CARCINOMA OF HEAD AND NECK

Although the various primary reconstructive procedures can replace lost intraoral lining or bone, the use of removable prostheses and other intraoral devices can also be a practical and effective means of intraoral rehabilitation.[108] Prostheses are particularly useful in obturating defects of the hard or soft palate, but the prosthodontist must see the patient before resection if he is to participate effectively. He can then design and produce a temporary appliance that can actually be inserted at the time of the operative procedure. This has the advantage of allowing early speech and swallowing despite major bony loss, skin grafts, or intraoral packs. Individual problems, such as the surgical loss of the orbital floor, lead to special planning in terms of the prosthesis, but the prosthodontist is most effective if he is a member of the treatment team from the outset.

The external defects produced by major surgical resection in the region of the head and neck are probably best closed with living tissue, but this is often not feasible. Although the use of prosthetic materials to cover large external facial defects requires ingenuity, the available materials have been greatly improved and matching the color of the adjacent skin is less difficult now. The results of this cosmetic rehabilitation have often meant the difference between the patient's returning to work or self-isolation. Even if a staged reconstruction with living tissue is planned for a future date, prosthetic applicances may play a major role in rehabilitation.

The ability to use the esophagus as a source of useful speech after total laryngectomy is well established,[65] but the ability to create a useful voice varies from patient to patient. Patients requiring laryngopharyngectomy or resection of the cervical esophagus, and some with less radical resections, are sometimes impossible to train. Motivation is one major factor for success, and the assistance of an enthusiastic instructor for both speech and swallowing is another. A speech pathologist works closely with us in the follow-up care of our patients undergoing head and neck surgery, and this has been a major factor in effective rehabilitation. Some degree of success has been achieved with surgical procedures for producing an air bypass between the trachea and the cervical esophagus, with or without prosthetic tubes, and these have been recommended as either primary or secondary methods for facilitating esophageal speech after laryngectomy,[87,99] but we have no personal experience with these techniques.

Treatment of Recurrent Squamous Carcinoma
After Initial Treatment Failure

The patient with local recurrence after prior definitive therapy for epithelial carcinoma of the head and neck is a demonstration of improper choice of initial therapy, improper application of the method chosen, or lack of full recognition of the extent of the disease at initial evaluation. The low rate of salvage of patients with recurrent carcinoma emphasizes the need for extreme care in initial treatment planning and its execution. The best opportunity for permanent disease control is the initial treatment employed.

The patient with recurrent cancer of the head and neck usually has an infected, ulcerated mass in the oropharynx, larynx, face, or neck, and the increasing problems produced by this recurrence demand our attention. In addition to specific measures to be discussed, there is a need to reduce pain, reduce odor from infection and necrosis, and deal with disability from both breathing and swallowing problems. This management may range from general wound hygiene by mechanical sprays, dressings, and debridement of necrotic tissue to tracheostomy or tube esophagostomy when these are indicated. We have not found intra-arterial chemotherapy of particular benefit for this problem. Even if specific anticancer methods are not applicable to the individual patient, his symptom problems may be both complex and demanding for those responsible for this care.

RADIATION THERAPY FAILURE

The patient with residual or recurrent carcinoma after a primary effort to control the lesion by radiation therapy can be a difficult management problem, and surgery is often indicated.[17] Except for those patients manifesting lymph node metastases as their only disease, the extent of local resection required is difficult to define; and although wide resection of the previously involved area is accomplished under these circumstances, later recurrence is frequent when resection is employed as a secondary treatment method. A possible exception to this rule is recurrent glottic cancer after prior radiation therapy since total laryngectomy under these circumstances usually provides a good local margin.[21]

The extent of the resection of recurrent oropharymgeal lesions and the decreased vasculature of the irradiated tissues remaining after resection make primary closure difficult and fraught with wound complications. For this reason we often employ immediate skin flaps for new oral lining, as described earlier, and we are also more prone to resect nearby bone when surgery is employed after radiation therapy. Healthy skin coverage over mandibular replacement is also mandatory under these circumstances.

It is often preferable in debilitated patients with prior radiation to construct a pharyngostome superiorly and an esophagostome inferiorly if the resection is extensive. In many instances, a deltopectoral skin flap may be required to provide adequate skin coverage of the prevertebral fascia if the operative defect is large. Reconstruction of the cervical esophagus and pharynx in such patients is often not possible with previously radiated tissues, and primary reconstruction with skin flaps from other sites may be too ambitious. With these patients we have generally favored a secondary reconstruction with deltopectoral skin flaps, as described by Bakamijan and coworkers,[4-6] or by interposition of left colon[37] or stomach[52] between the pharyngostome and the gastrointestinal tract.

Colon interposition for esophageal replacement may be accomplished using either the right or the left colon after resection of the pharynx and cervical esophagus,[37] but the aditional length required for anastomosis to the proximal pharynx makes the left colon seem more suitable after laryngopharyngectomy. The procedure we have employed uses an antiperistaltic segment of transverse and left colon as outlined in Figure 8-1. Although both the substernal and subcutaneous routes have been satisfactory, the subcutaneous route has the advantage of increased safety.

SURGICAL FAILURE

The patient with recurrent carcinoma after primary surgery poses problems similar to those outlined for the patient who has recurrent carcinoma after radiation therapy. If the original surgery was only a local resection of the primary lesion, either radiation therapy or radical surgery may be employed for secondary treatment. Since the destruction of normal anatomic planes as a result of previous surgery necessitates a wider than usual resection, radiation therapy may be a more suitable choice for treatment.[30] However, the decreased blood supply to the anatomic area of the recurrence as a consequence of the prior surgery does decrease the effectiveness of radiation therapy.

If the recurrent cancer follows an initial attempt to control the primary lesion by resection and neck dissection, it is generally impossible to treat the recurrent disease effectively by additional surgery since the previous operative dissection field cannot be reexcised. Despite the restriction of blood supply to the area of tumor recurrence and the nearby host tissues, radiotherapy is probably the most effective choice of treatment, even though long-term control under these circumstances is infrequent. Experience with this type of patient leads to a fuller appreciation of the need for optimal therapy (surgery or radiotherapy) for patients with untreated primary cancer of the head and neck region.

Radiation therapists are understandably reluctant to offer a standard course of radiation therapy with its attendant acute radiation morbidity to patients with no real hope of long-term control and a suspicion that the side effects of the treatment may be as severe as the problems produced by the disease. One effective approach has been the technique of "split-dose therapy": Therapy is discontinued at the onset of initial radiomucositis, usually 12–14 days after the initiation of therapy, and is continued after 3 or 4 weeks when these initial reactions have abated. A total dosage of significance (5000–6000 rads) can be achieved by this route with some amelioration of patient distress from the treatment itself.

An unusual form of recurrence after surgical laryngectomy is recurrent carcinoma at the site of the tracheal stoma without clinical evidence of recurrence elsewhere in the operative field.[55] Various causes have been suggested for this pattern of recurrence, including implants from tumor cells floating in the subglottic area at the time of tracheostomy, preservation of the thyroid lobe on the side of the lesion, and possibly paratracheal lymph node metastases not resected at the time of the procedure. Radiation therapy is employed for this problem, but its effectiveness in palliation is limited by the location of the recurrence as well as the poor tolerance of the tracheal mucosa. In selected patients a surgical approach for this problem may be preferable, but the proximity of the cervical esophagus and the superior portion of the sternum requires their inclusion in the resection. For this circumstance, we have successfully employed the procedure described by Grillo[38,39] consisting of resection of the medial portions of the clavicles, the manubrium of the sternum, and the adjacent soft tissues and cervical esophagus with closure (and construction of a new mediastinal tracheostome) using a large, double-pedicle pectoral flap (Fig. 5-13). A gastrostomy is required after this procedure, and some patients may be candidates for the seconary colon interposition described previously.

CRYOSURGERY

Gage[36] and others[16] have shown that freezing some small intraoral cancers with a liquid nitrogen probe is an effective means of local disease control. In selected early cases, cryosurgery may be as effective as primary radiotherapy or local surgery; but there is inadequate experience for valid comparisons of this method with these established means of therapy. Whatever its role as primary therapy, this approach does have great potential as a palliative tool for patients with recurrent cancer after failure of primary treatment by radiation therapy or surgery. Some patients are clearly unsuitable for either radiation therapy or surgery under these circumstances, and we have found freezing to be a particularly useful palliative approach. The technique can be mastered with little experience, and it is an additional method suitable for the management of difficult problems.

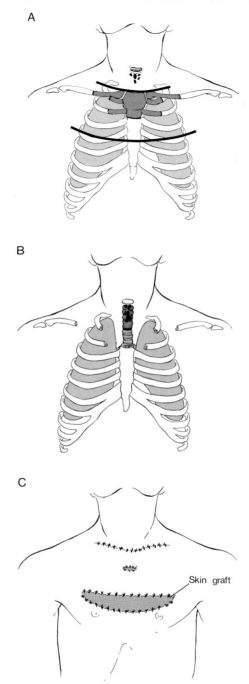

A

B

C

Skin graft

Fig. 5-13. Diagram of the creation of mediastinal tracheostomy after resection of stomal recurrence, manubrium of
sternum, and medial portions of clavicles (after Grillo).

99

CHEMOTHERAPY

Systemic chemotherapy for recurrent carcinoma of the head and neck has been disappointing with virtually all of the available anticancer agents.[27] This failure led to extensive trials of regional infusion chemotherapy using antimetabolites by continuous infusion or alkylating agents by intermittent infusion.[56,75] The lack of clearly defined arterial inflow sites after prior surgery is a serious drawback of this approach. The transient nature of the responses obtained in anatomically suitable patients, plus the technical problems and high complication rates, led most clinicians to abandon regional chemotherapy for head and neck cancer. At the present time, most chemotherapeutic attempts for the treatment of recurrent cancer of the head and neck employ systemic agents, and chemotherapy is generally used when no other treatment method is applicable for either the local or distant disease. Methotrexate has been a frequent choice, but some benefit has been achieved with multiple-drug combinations.

SYSTEMIC PROBLEMS

Since the local problems in patients with recurrent squamous cancer of the head and neck have been the most common cause of death in the past, the possibility of distant metastasis was not fully appreciated. Now that both surgery and radiotherapeutic methods have been improved, local control of head and neck cancer has been achieved more frequently. More treatment failures now demonstrate distant metastases in lung, liver, bone, or other sites. Before embarking on aggressive curative attempts in patients with recurrent head and neck cancer or advanced primary lesions, it is wise to explore fully the possibility of distant metastases. Survival times are usually quite short if distant disease is present.

One systemic problem in some patients with squamous carcinoma of the head and neck is the occurrence of hypercalcemia with either the primary lesion or its subsequent recurrence.[103] This is undoubtedly owing to a parathormonelike substance produced by some of these tumors. The significance of hypercalcemia is often ominous, but it does not necessarily establish the presence of distant metastases. All head and neck cancer patients we have observed with this finding have had large tumors, and the serum calcium has returned to normal with reduction of the gross disease by either surgical resection or effective radiotherapy. Subsequent recurrence of the disease is frequent in this group of patients, and it may be accompanied by return of hypercalcemia.

**OTHER NEOPLASMS OF THE HEAD
AND NECK REGION**

Thyroid Cancer

Even though it is an infrequent cause of death, thyroid cancer is one of the most controversial subjects in medicine. A unique feature of thyroid cancer is that it varies in severity from the very "benign" papillary cancer to the giant and spindle cell carcinoma, one of the most lethal cancers in man.

DIAGNOSIS

The majority of patients with thyroid cancer have no symptoms other than a palpable mass in the thyroid gland that has been observed by the patient or his physician, although systemic symptoms may arise from medullary carcinoma of the thyroid, a functioning tumor discussed in more detail in Chapter 12. There are also no reliable clinical characteristics to distinguish cancer of the thyroid from a benign thyroid nodule, even though specific signs—such as recurrent laryngeal nerve palsy or clinically enlarged cervical lymph nodes—may greatly increase suspicion of the malignant nature of the thyroid mass. Laboratory studies for thyroid function are usually not helpful in differential diagnosis since most patients with thyroid cancer are euthyroid, but a patient with a thyroid nodule that fails to take up radioiodine on scintiscan is generally considered a candidate for diagnostic surgery. It should be stressed, however, that less than 20 percent of such patients (13 percent in our institution) actually prove to have thyroid cancer, so other methods for diagnosis of the cause of a thyroid mass may prove particularly useful. For example, high titers of antithyroglobulin antibodies in the blood suggest autoimmune Hashimoto's thyroiditis. The classic triad of a low thyroid[131] I uptake and high serum PBI (protein-bound iodine) in association with a recent painful thyroid enlargement usually suggests thyroiditis, and this should be treated as such without diagnostic surgery. The patient should be followed carefully, however, as papillary carcinoma of the thyroid has been known to present as subacute thyroiditis; therefore, symptoms lasting over several months may require surgical intervention. Other scanning techniques (such as use of selenomethinone) may be helpful in the future in increasing our ability to restrict the number of patients subjected to diagnostic thyroid lobectomy. "Cold nodules" developing in children, particularly those with a previous history of radiation to the thymus or tonsil region, should always be treated promptly by surgical explortion because of the high incidence of thyroid cancer (75 percent) and the favorable prognosis in this age group.

CLASSIFICATION

A rational approach to planning therapy for thyroid cancer, as well as determining the prognosis, relates to pathologic classification.[118] The following classification is useful and affects therapeutic choice:

1. Papillary (including those mixed lesions with follicular components as well as occult sclerosing carcinoma[116])
2. Follicular (without any papillary components)
3. Hurtle cell
4. Medullary
5. Anaplastic (including giant and spindle cell carcinoma)

Since treatment planning depends on accurate histologic diagnosis, the method of surgical biopsy deserves comment. The biopsy procedure should consist of total unilateral thyroid lobectomy with resection of the isthmus because the pathologist cannot always give a definite dagnosis on frozen section of a nodule that is locally excised. A total lobectomy may well prove to be adequate therapy if the diagnosis is later found to be some form of thyroid cancer. Lobectomy with identification and preservation of the recurrent laryngeal nerve also avoids the likelihood of transecting and disseminating neoplastic tissue at the time of the surgical procedure. An attempt to achieve a histologic diagnosis by frozen section examination at the time of operation is worthwhile as this may affect the conduct of the operative procedure; however, it must be appreciated that the pathologist often has difficulty with frozen section diagnosis of thyroid cancer.

TREATMENT

Surgical Resection. Surgical resection (by lobectomy) of the primary lesion in the thyroid gland is indicated for all cancers of the thyroid except for those categorized as anaplastic carcinomas. These latter lesions are routinely found to be locally advanced at the time of diagnosis so that excision is not really feasible, and life expectancy is measured in months.[46,48,119] The major therapeutic approach to the anaplastic lesion is the palliative maintenance of an airway by tracheostomy for the comfort of the patient. We have generally employed postoperative external radiation therapy on the basis of an excellent response in a patient at our institution.

The treatment approach to the other categories of thyroid cancer listed is primarily surgical. This discussion will focus on the management of papillary,[14,32,33] follicular,[105] and Hurtle cell[106] carcinomas since the functioning medullary cancers are discussed more completely in Chapter 14.

Extent of thyroid resection. Total thyroidectomy for thyroid cancer of these histologic types has been proposed on the basis of the high incidence of microscopic involvement of the opposite lobe by multifocal cancer[47,81] (as high as 86 percent). This finding from whole-organ section studies is difficult to correlate with the clinical finding of only 4–12-percent incidence of subsequent clinical involvement of the opposite lobe in patients whose tumor was treated by unilateral lobectomy and isthmusectomy.[78,107] One disadvantage of routine bilateral thyroid lobectomy in various large surgical series is a 7–30-percent incidence of permanent hypoparathyroidism. In view of these considerations, our approach is total lobectomy on the side of the clinical thyroid mass including the isthmus. If the frozen section on this specimen demonstrates carcinoma, we proceed with subtotal thyroid lobectomy on the opposite side. Pains are taken to avoid disturbing the contralateral inferior thyroid artery and the thyroid tissue adjacent to the artery since this will protect the blood supply to the inferior parathyroid gland. The superior parathyroid may actually be included in the resection without the surgeon being aware of this because of its close relationship to the posterior capsule of the thyroid. It must be presumed that both parathyroids on the ipsilateral side have been resected or devascularized.

One not infrequent clinical problem is the subsequent report of papillary or follicular carcinoma several days after a unilateral thryoid lobectomy has been performed. It is not our practice to reoperate for the purpose of performing lobectomy or subtotal lobectomy of the grossly normal contralateral lobe under these circumstances, despite the reported pathologic data regarding multifocal disease. The data on clinical recurrence in the opposite lobe of patients so treated do not justify the disadvantage of secondary surgery.[78,107]

Management of regional lymph nodes. The regional lymph nodes may be enlarged in a patient with papillary, follicular, or mixed papillary and follicular thyroid cancer, and it is our policy to carry out radical neck dissection along with treatment of the primary cancer under these circumstances.[13] If node enlargement is contralateral or bilateral, it is appropriate to confirm histologic involvement by biopsy before bilateral neck dissection since the postoperative morbidity of bilateral dissection is considerably greater than that of unilateral dissection. Since metastatic thryoid cancer in nodes tends to remain within the capsule of lymph nodes, the true en bloc features of classic radical neck dissection are not quite as important as with metastatic squamous cancer. For this reason, we preserve the spinal accessory nerve during the dissection; but our procedure is otherwise the same as that used for squamous cancer of the head and neck. Some authors suggest that modified neck dissection (with preservation of the jugular vein and sternocleidomastoid muscle and omission of the submandibular gland dissection) is adequate for thyroid cancers of this type, and this is quite likely.[62] Whereas these restrictions of the procedure may have a sound rationale, it is important to include the paratracheal lymph nodes on the involved side. The surgical procedure can also be extended quite easily to include superior mediastinal node dissection if the lower paratracheal lymph nodes are involved.

The question of elective neck dissection for the patient with papillary or follicular thyroid cancer has been raised on the basis of finding histologically positive lymph nodes in 24–82 percent of clinically negative necks in various large series.[2,74,104] Despite these findings in most series, only 25–30 percent of patients will require subsequent therapeutic neck dissection if elective neck dissection is not performed.[44] This paradox is similar to that described for multifocal sites in the thyroid gland itself. Moreover, the end results of treatment are similar for patients with histologically positive nodes at time of elective dissection and for those treated by later therapeutic node dissection. In view of these factors, we do not perform elective neck dissection for papillary and follicular thyroid cancer under most circumstances. The poorer prognosis noted for thyroid cancer in men, particularly those over 40 years of age, and the uniformly good prognosis in young women are indications for some variations in this policy. Older men with thyroid cancer might be suitable candidates for elective node dissection, whereas young women certainly would not be. It is difficult to prove the value of elective node dissection for thyroid cancer under any circumstances, but these guidelines may be useful. Another indication for elective lymph node dissection is the finding of medullary carcinoma since this is a more aggressive lesion than papillary or follicular cancer (see Chap. 14).

Postoperative management. Thyroid feeding after thyroidectomy is mandatory to reduce the TSH stimulation of the thryoid tissue that remains in situ (and clinically confusing new thyroid "nodules"), to suppress the growth of any residual cancer that may be present, and to replace any hormonal deficiency produced by the thyroid resection. Our practice is to prescribe 2 grains of desiccated thyroid per day (or 0.2 mg of synthyroid) on a permanent basis, although other preparations (and dosage plans) are certainly acceptable.

Postoperative therapy with[131] I after thyroidectomy for thyroid cancer is probably not indicated because of the good life expectancy after surgery for this disease, the significant radiation dose required to complete the thyroidectomy, and the additional inconvenience and expense involved in using this treatment properly. However, the patient with residual or metastatic thyroid cancer is certainly a candidate for therapy of this type if the lesion is papillary or follicular.

Complications of surgical treatment. One complication of surgical treatment of thyroid cancer is a result of either deliberate or inadvertent resection or division of the recurrent laryngeal nerve. Although unilateral section may be associated with significant hoarseness in the early postoperative interval, this usually improves so that it is not very noticeable as the affected cord assumes a more midline position. Bilateral recurrent nerve injury is a catastrophic complication requiring permanent tracheostomy for airway purposes. Since palsy of one nerve may occur as a result of the disease process or surgery required for excision, every effort should be made to identify and preserve these nerves during thyroid cancer surgery.

Another less recognized nerve complication of surgery for thyroid cancer is injury to the motor branch of the superior laryngeal nerve resulting in palsy, which interferes with the ability to tense the vocal cord for singing and other activities. With care, this injury can be avoided at the time of dissection and ligation of the superior thyroid vessels without reducing the adequacy of the surgical resection. When radical neck dissection is combined with thyroid resection, the sensory portion of superior laryngeal nerve may be injured if care is not taken. The resulting problems with aspiration of secretions (from unilateral anesthesia of the larynx) can be severe. Although the patient can usually learn to swallow on the contralateral side, subsequent laryngectomy may be required to reduce aspiration and recurring pneumonia.

Hypoparathyroidism from bilateral excision or devascularization of all cervical parathyroid tissue may occur. For this reason we avoid total thyroidectomy unless there are specific local indications. Management of this complication is generally satisfactory with vitamin D and oral calcium preparations, but the problem is best avoided.

RADIOACTIVE THERAPY FOR RECURRENT OR METASTATIC DISEASE[11]

Patients with inoperable thyroid cancer or metastatic cancer outside the neck are candidates for a trial of[131] I therapy if the histologic type is papillary or follicular. Retention of significant amounts of ^{131}I in neoplastic thyroid tissue has been shown only for these two types. The procedure recommended is described below.

First, administer a thyroid ablation dose of [131]I (75–100 mCi) if routine scan shows residual thyroid tissue in the neck. Few carcinomas will take up significant ^{131}I under this circumstance. (Patients must not be receiving exogenous thyroid medication.)

Second, administer a tracer dose of [131]I (1.0 mCi) after myxedema has developed and determine uptake, if any, in known metastatic disease by scan and by measurement of urinary excretion of ^{131}I to quantitate retention.

Third, calculate the therapeutic dose of ^{131}I from excretion data if retention of the isotope can be confirmed by scan techniques. This treatment approach is repeated at yearly intervals following the same procedure, but lack of evidence of isotope localization in metastases is an indication for other therapy.

Results of this treatment vary with patient age and histologic type of neoplasm. A favorable response is more likely in the young patient with papillary cancer than in the older age group. Follicular cancer is much more likely than papillary cancer to be benefited in the older age group.

OTHER APPROACHES TO THYROID CANCER

An alternative to radioiodine therapy is TSH suppression with exogenous thyroid administration, although there are considerable disparity in opinion and few hard data on the efficacy of this approach to the control of established thyroid cancer in man. The rationale is good, some patients do clearly respond, and the side effects are minimal, so it must be considered a useful tool. Radiation therapy is also a treatment alternative that shows definite benefit in an occasional patient, but it has a relatively limited role in thyroid cancer management. Relief of pain from a bone metastasis is probably a specific indication for this method. Anticancer chemotherapy has not been beneficial for the management of recurrent and metastatic thyroid cancer, but recent data suggest possible benefit from actinomycin D in a few patients with anaplastic carcinoma of the thyroid.[77]

Some patients with papillary and follicular tumors develop locally recurrent cancer unresponsive to other palliative therapy. The slow growth and limited disability produced by the local disease make radical excision, particularly a disabling procedure such as laryngectomy, seem unwarranted. However, partial excision of the local disease may be useful if the gross disease disables or distresses the patient.

PROGNOSIS

A summary of the end results of treatment of the various categories of the thyroid cancers is shown in Table 5-3.

Table 5-3
End Results of Treatment of Thyroid Cancer

Type of Tumor	Survival (%)		
	5 Yr	10 Yr	20 Yr
Papillary	85	75	5
Follicular	80	70	40
Medullary	60	40	35
Anaplastic	5	—	—

Salivary Gland Tumors

Both benign and malignant salivary gland tumors occur eight to ten times more frequently in the parotid gland[95,96,116] than in the submandibular gland,[19] and the incidence of neoplasms occurring in the sublingual gland is neglibible. There is a greater frequency of benign tumors occurring in the parotid gland than in the submandibular gland (80 percent benign in the parotid, but only 60 percent benign in the submandibular gland). All of these factors affect our treatment approach to the major salivary glands. In most instances, the operation for diagnosis is the procedure employed for treatment if the lesion proves to be a benign mixed tumor, Warthin's tumor, Madelung's disease, or some form of inflammatory lesion.

DIAGNOSIS

With most benign-appearing masses in the parotid gland, the surgical biopsy consists of a superficial lobectomy after identification, preservation, and dissection of the facial nerve and its branches.[9] However, if the patient has a large parotid neoplasm, a facial nerve paresis or palsy, or other features that suggest cancer, an open incisional biopsy of the tumor may be the best course. Whatever the diagnosis proves to be, the entire biopsy wound must be removed at the time of definitive surgical resection if "seeding" of the subsequent surgical wound is to be avoided. In most clinical situations, however, pretreatment open biopsy has not been a useful approach, and aspiration biopsy is often inadequate from the standpoint of classification of the neoplasm.

The submandibular gland is anatomically close to the lingual and hypoglossal nerves, but this does not produce as disturbing a surgical problem as occurs with the facial nerve and the parotid gland. Biopsy of the submandibular gland is accomplished more easily than that of the parotid by total excision of the gland, and the subsequent treatment plan is dependent on the pathologic findings.

TREATMENT

The discussion thus far has centered on the surgical approach to diagnosis of salivary gland neoplasms, but surgical excision is also the preferred primary treatment method for salivary gland cancer as the malignant lesions are highly radioresistant.

Extent of Resection for Malignant Salivary Tumors. Total excision of the involved gland is indicated for most malignant tumors of the salivary glands. Total excision of the parotid usually includes a segment of the facial nerve and its major branches and, in some cases, adjacent muscles (masseter), bone (mandible, styloid process, ear canal), or a segment of skin. Total resection of the facial nerve may not prove necessary for low-grade mucoepidermoid cancers, but the other forms of parotid cancer require aggressive local resection as demonstrated by the alarmingly high local failure rates noted when surgical excision is accomplished with preservation of the facial nerve. Some return of facial nerve function has been observed in a few patients in whom no nerve graft is employed, but an immediate free nerve graft from the great auricular or lateral femoral cutaneous nerve has a high degree of success (approximately 70 percent) and is advisable. A satisfactory alternative has been the insertion of a fascial sling.

Cancer in the submandibular gland may be close to, or involving, the floor of the mouth or adjacent mandible. Under these circumstances, a preoperative biopsy may be useful since the subsequent resection should include these adjacent structures. In most instances, however, total excision of the gland and adjacent fat, nodes, and areolar tissue is the preferable approach to both diagnosis and treatment of the primary lesion.

Management of Regional Lymph Nodes. Malignant tumors of the salivary gland include malignant mixed tumor, mucoepidermoid cancer (high and low grade), adenoid cystic carcinoma (cylindroma), acinic cell carcinoma, adenocarcinoma, and squamous cell cancer. The advisability of neck dissection is determined on the basis of the histology of the neoplasm. For example, patients with adenoid cystic carcinoma, acinic cell carcinoma, or low-grade mucoepidermoid cancer rarely demonstrate regional lymph node involvement. Emphasis should be placed on adequate resection of the primary tumor for all of these lesions that are slow in their growth, prone to develop local recurrence, and extremely difficult to manage when they recur. Malignant mixed tumor, high-grade mucoepidermoid cancer, adenocarcinoma, and squamous carcinoma all merit consideration of elective neck dissection because of the high likelihood of occult lymphatic spread, but there is no strong evidence of therapeutic benefit from elective neck dissection in previously untreated cases. In patients with moderate extension of the primary lesion into the cervical region, those with clinically involved cervical nodes, or patients being treated surgically for recurrent cancer, there is a strong argument for inclusion of neck dissection with the operative procedure.

Complications of Treatment of Salivary Tumors. Facial nerve palsy or other nerve palsies may occur as a result of the disease process or as a result of the extent of resection required to encompass the disease. A transient paralysis or paresis of the facial nerve may occur also as a result of trauma during dissection, but function returns in 6–8 weeks in most instances.

Incomplete resection of the parotid gland may be associated with a small salivary fistula, particularly after partial excision of the gland for a benign neoplasm. Although radiation therapy has been employed for management, the fistula is virtually always temporary and heals without difficulty. The gustatory sweating complex[72,97] after parotid resection (Frey's syndrome) is sometimes mistaken for a fistula because of localized sweating from the cheek that is associated with eating. When particularly troublesome, this symptom can be treated with section of the auriculotemporal nerve at the level of the tympanic membrane by an endaural approach; but symptoms frequently return after this procedure.

Management of Recurrent Cancer of the Salivary Glands. Local failure of surgical treatment is a distressingly frequent problem in the management of these cancers, and the prognosis is clearly related to the histological type as defined earlier. Neither radiation therapy nor anticancer chemotherapy has been particularly useful in management, but radiation has produced some success in control of relatively undifferentiated salivary gland cancers. Secondary surgical resection is usually employed for recurrence to control symptoms when it is feasible. If it is possible to encompass the disease by secondary surgery, resection of the adjacent temporal bone by a combined craniofacial approach (as described earlier) may be indicated.

PROGNOSIS

A summary of end results of treatment of malignant salivary gland tumors is shown in Table 5-4.

Table 5-4
End Results of Treatment of
Malignant Salivary Gland Tumors

Type of Tumor	Survival (%)	
	5 Yr	10 Yr
Mucoepidermoid (low grade)	86	86
Mucoepidermoid (high grade)	22	10
Adenoid cystic	45	28
Malignant mixed	63	39
Acinic cell	66	27
Epidermoid	30	15

LESS-COMMON NEOPLASMS OF THE
HEAD AND NECK REGION

Nasopharyngeal Angiofibromas

These lesions are seen almost exclusively in male adolescents, are locally invasive, do not metastasize, and usually regress as the patient enters adulthood.[29,73] The clinical manifestations are related to the anatomical location of the lesion in the posterior nasal cavity or nasopharynx and may include nasal obstruction, epistaxis, edema of the face, and exophthalmos. These tumors are extremely vascular, and biopsy may result in massive hemorrhage.

Resection of the tumor is the treatment of choice despite the inconvenient anatomic location and the usual inability of the surgeon to accomplish total excision. A transpalatine approach or the transnasal route through a lateral rhinotomy is employed, but some lesions may actually require a craniofacial approach. When resecting this lesion, the surgeon must be prepared to cope with the massive bleeding that often occurs. Repeated cryosurgery is an attractive alternative for management since the sole purpose of therapy is to deal with the local problem until the tumor regresses (at or about the age of 25). Radiation therapy and hormone therapy have not been particularly helpful means of management.

Esthesioneuroblastoma

Esthesioneuroblastoma is an unusual tumor that arises from the olfactory membrane in the nasal cavity.[3,45] The clinical manifestations are nasal obstruction, epistaxis, and symptoms and signs resulting from invasion of the surrounding structures (edema of the nose, exophthalmos, diplopia, etc.). This neoplasm is locally aggressive in its growth but has a low incidence of distant metastasis. The only really valuable form of treatment is a well-planned craniofacial resection to eradicate the esthesioneuroblastoma. Radiation therapy has not controlled this neoplasm in the experience of others.

Neoplasms of the Lacrimal Gland

Lacrimal gland neoplasm is an uncommon cancer that usually presents as a progressive swelling arising from the medial aspect of the orbit.[1,83] It has a histological pattern similar to that seen in salivary glands. Approximately half of these rare lesions are benign mixed tumors, and the remaining tumors represent a wide variety of adenocarcinomas. Once the histologic diagnosis is established, treatment must be aggressive to avoid local recurrence. In dealing with benign mixed tumors, the entire gland must be removed including the capsule. In the management of malignant tumors, an orbital exenteration is usually mandatory to accomplish adequate resection. The surgeon should not hesitate to proceed with resection of the bony orbit through a combined craniofacial approach if this is necessary for adequate local resection of the disease. Radiation therapy may be employed in order to preserve the eye in patients with small lesions of the lacrimal gland, but surgical resection must be employed for treatment failure in this circumstance.

Chemodectomas

Chemodectomas are uncommon benign neoplasms that arise from nonchromaffin tissue in the region of the carotid body at the bifurcation of the carotid artery,[86] the cervical portion of the vagus nerve,[71] or the glomus jugulare in the middle ear.[41,93] The overwhelming majority of chemodectomas occur in the neck and present either as an asymptomatic pulsatile neck mass near the angle of the mandible or as a cervical mass that bulges into the pharynx. Although the location of the neoplasm is essentially the same if the lesion originates from the vagus nerve or the carotid body, it is of interest that the lesions originating from the vagus nerve generally bulge into the pharynx, whereas those originating from the carotid body are felt more easily by external palpation. The differential diagnosis includes other possible causes of the neck mass, as well as the possibility of a carotid artery aneurysm. Carotid angiography demonstrates a characteristic radiographic picture that can establish the diagnosis with confidence.

In view of the benign nature of the lesion (less than 5 percent ever develop malignant change), its site of origin with associated technical problems and the essential absence of symptoms other than the presence of a mass lead one to consider the treatment plan with great care. Dissection of the carotid body lesion from the carotid artery itself may be difficult, and resection of a tumor originating from the vagus nerve usually produces a greater nerve deficit than is present preoperatively. For these reasons our general policy is to carry out a surgical resection only in younger patients and avoid a surgical approach in patients who are more than 60 years of age. If there is progressive enlargement of the mass or some aditional symptomatology produced by the physical presence of the mass, surgery can be considered for the older patient.

At the time of operation, the tumor should be dissected from the carotid bifurcation with care. It is probably preferable to settle for partial removal than to proceed with carotid artery resection or ligation if the tumor adheres to the vessel. Under some circumstances a "patch graft" might be considered, but this should rarely be necessary. For those lesions originating from the vagus nerve, it is virtually impossible to separate the tumor from the nerve with preservation of the vagus, which explains why resection usually results in additional nerve palsy not present before the procedure. The vagal nerve neoplasm usually is high in the neck so that both superior laryngeal palsy and recurrent laryngeal nerve palsy are produced after total resection.

The similar neoplasm originating from the glomus jugulare is even more uncommon than the two lesions discussed above. It usually causes symptoms related to the middle ear involvement (tinnitus, vertigo, or bleeding from the external ear). The surgical approach is similar to that for radical mastoidectomy.

Neoplasms of the Mesodermal Tissues of the Head and Neck

Both benign and malignant soft part tumors and bone neoplasms occur in the head and neck region as in other sites of the body. These soft part and bony lesions are described in more detail in the chapter describing sarcomas (Chap. 10) and in the chapter on pediatric neoplasms (Chap. 13). The diagnosis and management are identical to those of these same lesions in other locations. The compact anatomy of the head and neck region makes adequate surgical resection of these lesions more difficult than in other anatomic areas, but the principles are the same. Some lesions characteristically occur in the jaws because of the unique feature of the presence of teeth. There are a number of cysts of various kinds, and odontoblastoma is the most common odontogenic neoplasm. Management of all these lesions is surgical for both diagnosis and therapy.

Carcinoma in a Branchiogenic Cyst

This lesion of the neck is quite rare, and histologically it is a squamous carcinoma indistinguishable from other squamous cancers of the head and neck region. Many patients so designated initially prove subsequently to have metastatic disease from malignant occult primary lesions somewhere in the head and neck. Radical neck dissection is the appropriate treatment for this cancer after adequate pretreatment evaluation has established the diagnosis.

REFERENCES

1. Adam YG, Farr HW: Primary orbital tumors. Am J Surg. 122:726–731, 1971
2. Attie JN, Khafif RA, Steckler RM: Elective neck dissection in papillary carcinoma of the thyroid. Am J Surg 122:464–471, 1971

3. Bailey BJ, Barton S: Olfactory neuroblastoma. Arch Otolaryngol 101:1–5, 1975

4. Bakamijan VY: A two stage method for pharyngoesophageal reconstruction with a primary pectoral skin flap. Plast Reconstr Surg 36:173–184, 1965

5. Bakamijan VY, Holbrook LA: Prefabrication technics in cervical pharyngoesophageal reconstruction. Br J Plast Surg 26:214–222, 1973

6. Bakamijan VY, Long M, Rigg B: Experience with medially based delto-pectoral flap in reconstructive surgery of the head and neck. Br J Plast Surg 24:174–183, 1971

7. Ballantyne AJ, Fletcher GH: Surgical management of irradiation failures of non-fixed cancers of the glottic region. Am J Roentgenol Radium Ther Nucl Med 120:164–168, 1974

8. Batsakis JG: Neoplasms of the minor and lesser major salivary glands (collective review). Surg Gynecol Obstet 135:289–298, 1972

9. Beahrs OH, Chong GC: Management of the facial nerve in parotid gland surgery. Am J Surg 124:473–476, 1972

10. Beckman JS, Westbrook KC, Thompson BW: Lip cancer: Surgical management. Am J Surg 128:732–734, 1974

11. Benua RS, Cicale NR, Sonenberg M, Rawson RW: The relation of radioiodine dosimetery to results and complications in the treatment of metastatic thyroid cancer. Am J Roentegenol 87:171–182, 1962

12. Bjork VO: Partial resection of the only remaining lung with the aid of respirator treatment. J Thorac Cardiovasc Surg 39:179–188, 1960

13. Block MA, Miller JM, Horn RC Jr: Thyroid carcinoma with cervical lymph node metastasis. Am J Surg 122:458–463, 1971

14. Buckwalter JA, Thomas CG Jr: Selection of surgical treatment for Well-differentiated thryoid carcinomas. Ann Surg 176:565–578, 1972

15. Carl W, Schaaf NG, Chen TY: Oral care of patients irradiated for cancer of the head and neck. Cancer 30:448–453, 1972

16. Chandler JR: Cryosurgery for recurrent carcinoma of the oral cavity. Arch Otolaryngol 97:319–321, 1973

17. Chu A, Fletcher GH: Incidence and causes of failure to control by irradiation the primary lesions in squamous cell carcinomas of the anterior two-thirds of the tongue and floor of mouth. Am J Roentgenol Radium Ther Nucl Med 117:502–508, 1973

18. Cohen IK, Theogaraj SD: Nasolabial flap reconstruction of the floor of the mouth after extirpation of oral cancer. Am J Surg 130:479–480, 1975

19. Conley J, Myers E, Cole R: Analysis of 115 patients with tumors of the submandibular gland. Ann Otol Rhinol Laryngol 81:323–330, 1972

20. Conley J, Novack AJ: The surgical treatment of malignant tumors of the ear and temporal bone. Arch Otolaryngol 71:635–652, 1960

21. Constable WC, Marks RD, Robbins JP et al: High dose preoperative radiotherapy and surgery for cancer of the larynx. Laryngoscope 82:1861–1869, 1972

22. Corso PF, Gerold FP, Frazell EL: The rapid closure of large salivary fistulas by an accelerated shoulder flap technique. Am J Surg 106:691–695, 1963

23. Curutchet HP, Terz JJ, Lawrence WL Jr: The value of the autogenous dermal graft for carotid artery protection. Surgery 71:876–880, 1972

24. Daly TE, Drane JB: Osteoradionecorsis of the jaws. Cancer Bull 24:86–89, 1972

25. Del Regato JA, Sala JM: The treatment of carcinoma of the lower lip. Radiology 73:839–844, 1959

26. Doberneck RC, Antoine JE: Deglutition after resection of oral, laryngeal, and pharyngeal cancers. Surgery 75:87–90, 1974

27. Dowell KE, Armstrong DM, Aust JB, Cruz AB Jr: Systemic chemotherapy of advanced head and neck malignancies. Cancer 35:116–1120, 1975

28. Einhorn J, Wersall J: Oral carcinoma in cases of leukoplakia of the oral mucosa. Acta. Otolaryngol 224:20–22, 1967

29. Fitzpatrick PJ, Rider WD: Radiotherapy of nasopharyngeal angiofibroma. Radiology 109:171–178, 1973

30. Fletcher GH, Evers W Th: Radiotherapeutic management of surgical recurrences and postoperative residuals in tumors of the head and neck. Radiology 95:185–188, 1970

31. Fletcher GH, Jesse RH, Lindberg RD, Koons CR: The place of radiotherapy in the management of squamous cell carcinoma of the supraglottic larynx. Am J Roentgenol. 108:19–26, 1970

32. Franssila KO: Is the differentiation between papillary and follicular thyroid carcinoma valid? Cancer 32:853–864, 1973

33. Frazell EL, Foote FW Jr: Papillary cancer of the thyroid: A review of 25 years of experience. Cancer 11:895–922, 1958

34. Frazell EL, Lewis JS: Cancer of the nasal cavity and accessory sinuses. A report of the management of 416 patients. Cancer 16:1293–1301, 1963

35. Frazell EL, Moore OS: Bilateral radical neck dissection performed in stages. Experience with 467 patients. Am J Surg 102:809–814, 1961

36. Gage AA: Cryotherapy for oral cancer. JAMA 204:565–569, 1968

37. Gregorie HB, Jr: Esophagocoloplasty. Ann Surg 175:740–749, 1972

38. Grillo HC: Obstructive lesions of the trachea. Ann Otol Rhinol Laryngol 82:770–777, 1973

39. Grillo HC: Terminal or mural tracheostomy in the anterior mediastinum. J Thorac Cardiovasc Surg 51:422, 1966

40. Hanna DC, Richardson GS, Gaisford JC: Suggested technic for resection of the temporal bone. Am J Surg 114:553–558, 1967

41. Hatefield PM, James AE, Schulz MD: Chemodectomas of the glomus jugulare. Cancer 30:1164–1168, 1972

42. Helsper, JT, Sharp GS, Bullock WK: The mouth wash technique: A method for screening for intra-oral carcinoma. Am J Surg 106:802–806, 1963

43. Henderson BE: Nasopharyngeal carcinoma: Present status of knowledge. Cancer Res 34:1187–1188, 1974

44. Hutter RV, Frazell EL, Foote FW Jr: Elective radical neck dissection: An assessment of its' use in the management of papillary thyroid cancer. Cancer 20:87–93, 1970

45. Hutter RV, Lewis JS, Foote FW Jr, Tollefsen HR: Esthesioneuroblastoma. Am J Surg 106:748–753, 1963
46. Hutter RV, Tollefsen HR, DeCosse JJ et al: Spindle and giant cell metaplasia in papillary carcinoma of the thyroid. Am J Surg 110:660–668, 1965
47. Iida F, Yonekura M, Miyakawa M: Study of intraglandular dissemination of thyroid cancer. Cancer 24:764–771, 1969
48. Jereb B, Stjernsward J, Lowhagan T: Anaplastic giant-cell carcinoma of the thyroid. (a study of treatment and prognosis.) Cancer 35:1293–1295, 1975
49. Jesse RH, Lindberg RD: The efficacy of combining radiation therapy with a surgical procedure to patients with cervical metastases from squamous cancer of the oropharynx and hypopharynx. Cancer 35:1163–1166, 1975
50. Jesse RH, Perez CA, Fletcher GH: Cervical lymph node metastases; unknown primary cancer. Cancer 31:854–859, 1973
51. Joel Jose: Mandibular reconstruction with inert materials. Plast Reconstr Surg 2:322–327, 1972
52. Kakegawa, T, Tsuzuki T, Sasaki T: Primary pharyngogastrostomy for carcinoma of the esophagus situated in the cervicothoracic segment. Surgery 73:226–229, 1973
53. Ketcham KS, Chretien PB, Van Buren JM, Hoye RC, Beazley RM, Herdt JR: The ethmoid sinuses; a re-evaluation of surgical resection. Am J Surg 126:469–476, 1973
54. Kissin B, Kaley MM, Su WH, Lerner R: Head and neck cancer in alcoholics: The relationship to drinking, smoking, and dietary patterns. JAMA 224:1174–1175, 1973
55. Kuehn PG, Tennant R: Surgical treatment of stomal recurrences in cancer of the larynx. Am J Surg 122:445–450, 1971
56. Lawrence W Jr: Regional cancer chemotherapy: An evaluation. Prog Clin Cancer 1:341–393, 1965
57. Lawrence W Jr, Terz JJ, Rogers C et al: Preoperative irradiation for head and neck cancer: A prospective study. Cancer 33:318–323, 1974
58. Lewis JS, Page R: Radical surgery for malignant tumors of the ear. Arch. Otolaryngol 83:114–117, 1966
59. Lore JM Jr: An Atlas of Head and Neck Surgery, vol. 2. Philadelphia, WB Saunders Co, 1973
60. MacComb WS: Diagnosis and treatment of metastatic cervical cancerous nodes from unknown primary sites. Am J Surg 124:441–449, 1972
61. Mahoney LJ: Resection of cervical lymph nodes in cancer of the lip: Results in 123 patients. Can J Surg 12:40–43, 1969
62. Marchetta FC, Sake K, Matsuura H: Modified neck dissection for carcinoma of the thyroid gland. Am J Surg 120:452–455, 1970
63. Marchetta FC, Sako K, Maxwell W: Complications after radical head and neck surgery performed through previously irradiated tissues. Am J Surg 114:835–838, 1967
64. Martin H, Del Valle B, Ehrlich H, Cahan WG: Neck dissection. Cancer 4:441–499, 1951

65. Martin Hayes: Rehabilitation of the laryngectome. Cancer 16:823–841, 1963

66. Martin Hayes: Surgery of Head and Neck Tumors. New York, Paul B Hoeber, 1957

67. McGregor IA: The temporal flap in intra-oral cancer: Its use in repairing the post-excisional defect. Br J Plast Surg 16:318–335, 1963

68. Moore C, Mullins F, Scott M: Preoperative irradiation in cancer of the head and neck. Am J Surg 124:555–558, 1972

69. Moore OS, Karlan M, Sigler L: Factors influencing the safety of carotid ligation. Am J Surg 118:666–668, 1969

70. Morrison R: Review article—Radiation therapy in diseases of the larynx. Br J Radiol 44:489–504, 1971

71. Murphy TE, Huvos AF, Frazell EL: Chemodectomas of the glomus intra-vagale: Vagal body tumors, nonchromaffin paragangliomas of the nodose ganglion of the vagus nerve. Ann Surg 172:246–255, 1970

72. Myers EN, Conley J: Gustatory sweating after radical neck dissection. Arch Otolaryngol 91:534–542, 1970

73. Neel HB, Whicker JA, Devine KD, Weiland LH: Juvenile angiofibroma (review of 120 cases). Am J Surg 126:547–556, 1973

74. Noguchi S, Noguchi A, Murakami N: Papillary carcinoma of the thyroid. II. Value of prophylactic lymph node excision. Cancer 26:1061–1064, 1970

75. Oberfield RA, Cady B, Booth JC: Regional arterial chemotherapy for advanced carcinoma of the head and neck. (A ten year review.) Cancer 32:82–88, 1973

76. Pollack RS: Tumor Surgery of the Head and Neck. Basel, S Karger, 1975

77. Rogers JD, Lindberg RD, Hill CS, Jr, Gehan E: Spindle and giant cell carcinoma of the thyroid; a different therapeutic approach. Cancer 34:1328–1332, 1974

78. Rose RG, Kelsy MP, Russell WO, et al: Follow-up study of thyroid cancer treated by unilateral lobectomy. Am J Surg 106:494–500, 1963

79. Royster HP, Noone BR, Graham WP III, Theogaraj SD: Cervical pharyngostomy for feeding after maxillofacial surgery. Am J Surg 116:610–614, 1968

80. Rufino CD, MacComb WS: Bilateral neck dissections. Analysis of 180 cases. Cancer 19:1503–1508, 1966

81. Russell WO, Ibanez ML, Clark RL, White EC: Thyroid carcinoma: Classification, Intraglandular dissemination, and clinicopathological study based upon whole organ sections of 80 glands. Cancer 16:1425–1460, 1963

82. Sako K, Marchetta FC: The use of metal protheses following anterior mandibulectomyand neck dissection for carcinoma of the oral cavity. Am J Surg 104:715–720, 1962

83. Sanders TE, Ackerman LV, and Zimmerman LE: Epithelial tumors of the lacrimal gland. A comparison of the pathologic and clinical behavior with those of the salivary glands. Am J Surg 110:592–655, 1962

84. Scannell JB: The function of the dental specialist in the treatment of cancer of the head and neck. Am J Surg 110:592–594, 1965

85. Shah JP, Tollefsen HR: Epidermoid carcinoma of the supraglottic larynx. Role of neck dissection in initial surgical treatment. Am J Surg 128:494–499, 1974

86. Shamblin WR, ReMine WH, Sheps GS, Harrison EG Jr: Carotid body tumor (chemodectoma): Clinicopathological analysis of 90 cases. Am J Surg 124:510–514, 1971

87. Shedd D, Dakamjian V, Sako K, Mann M, Barba S, Schaaf N: Reed-Fistula method of speech rehabilitation after laryngectomy. Am J Surg 124:510–514, 1972

88. Shedd DB, Hukill PB, Bahn S: In vivo staining properties of oral cancer. Am J Surg 110:631–634, 1965

89. Silverman S Jr, Griffith M: Studies on oral lichen planus: II. Follow-up on 200 patients, clinical characteristics, and associated malignanay. Oral Surg 37:705–710, 1974

90. Smith RR, Caulk R, Frazell E, Holinger et al: Revision of the clinical staging system for cancer of the larynx. Cancer 31:72–80, 1973

91. Smith RR, Frazell EL, Caulk R, Holinger PH, Russell WO: The American Joint Committee's proposed method of stage classification and end-result reporting applied to 1,320 pharynx cancers. Cancer 16:1505–1520, 1963

92. Smithdeal CD, Corso PF, Strong EW: Dermis graft for carotid artery protection; yes or no? (A ten year experience.) Am J Surg 128:484–489, 1974

93. Spector GJ, Maisel RH, Ogura JH: Glomus tumors in the middle ear; I. An analysis of 46 patients. Laryngoscope 83:1652–1672, 1973

94. Spiro RH, Alfonso AE, Farr HW, Strong EW: Cervical node metastasis from epidermoid carcinoma of the oral cavity and oropharynx. Am J Surg 128:562–567, 1974

95. Spiro RH, Hubos AG, Strong EW: Adenoid cystic carcinoma of salivary origin. (A clinico-pathological study of 242 cases.) Am J Surg 128:512–520, 1974

96. Spiro, RH, Huvos AG, Strong EW: Cancer of the parotid gland. A clinico-pathologic study of 288 primary cases. Am J Surg 130:452–459, 1975

97. Spiro RH, Martin H: Gustatory sweating following parotid surgery and radical neck dissection. Ann Surg 165:118–127, 1967

98. Strong EW: Preoperative radiation and radical neck dissection. Surg Clin North Am 49:271–276, 1969

99. Taub S, Bergner LH: Air bypass voice prosthesis for vocal rehabilitation of laryngectomees. Am J Surg 127:748–756, 1973

100. Terz JJ, Alksne JF, Lawrence W Jr: En bloc resection of the pterygoid region in the management of advanced oropharyngeal carcinoma. Surg Gynecol Obstet 130:349–352, 1970

101. Terz JJ, Bear ES, King RE, Lawrence W Jr: Primary reconstruction of the mandible with a wire mesh prosthesis. Surg Gynecol Obstet 139:198–200, 1974

102. Terz JJ, Lawrence W Jr: Primary reconstruction of oropharyngeal surgical defects with a forehead flap. Surg Gynecol Obstet 129:1–5, 1969

103. Terz JJ, Estep H, Bright R, Lawrence W Jr, Curutchet HP, Kay S: Primary oropharyngeal cancer and hypercalcemia. Cancer 33:334–339, 1974

104. Tollefsen HR, Decosse JJ: Papillary carcinoma of the thyroid. The case for radical neck dissection. Am J Surg 108:547–551, 1964

105. Tollefsen HR, Shah JP, Huvos AG: Follicular carcinoma of the thyroid. Am J Surg 126:523–528, 1973

106. Tollefsen HR, Shah JP, Huvos AG: Hurthle cell carcinoma of the thyroid. Am J Surg 130:390–394, 1975

107. Tollefsen HR, Shah JP, Huvos AG: Papillary carcinoma of the thyroid. Recurrence in the thyroid gland after initial surgical treatment. Am J Surg 124:468–472, 1972

108. van Slooten EA, Horree WA, Kruisbrink JJ: Some principles of surgical and prosthodontic treatment of patients with malignant tumors of maxilla. Arch Chir Neerl 21:1–15, 1969

109. Wang CC: Megavoltage radiation therapy for supraglottic carcinoma. Results of treatment. Radiology 109:183–186, 1973

110. Wang CC: Treatment of glottic carcinoma by megavoltage radiation therapy and results. Am J Roentgenol Radium Ther Nucl Med 120:157–163, 1974

111. Ward GE, Loch WE, Lawrence W Jr: Radical operation for carcinoma of the external auditiry canal and middle ear. Am J Surg 82:169–178, 1951

112. Westbury G, Wilson JSP, Richardson A: Combined craniofacial resection for malignant disease. Am J Surg 130:463–469, 1975

113. Wilson JS, Blake GB, Richardson AE, Westbury G: Malignant tumors of the ear and their treatment. Br J Plast Surg 27:77–91, 1974

114. Wise RA, Baker HW: Surgery of the Head and Neck. Chicago, Year Book Medical Publishers, 1962

115. Wizenberg MJ, Bloedorn FG, Weiner S, Gracia J: Treatment of lymph node metastases in head and neck cancer: A radiotherapeutic approach. Cancer 29:1455–1462, 1972

116. Woods JE, Chong GC, Beahrs OH: Experience with 1360 primary parotid tumors. Am J Surg 130:460–462, 1975

117. Woolner LB, Lemmon ML, Beahrs HO et al: Occult papillary carcinoma of the thyroid gland: a study of 140 cases observed in a 30-year period. J Clin Endocrinol 20:89–105, 1960

118. Woolner LB, Beahrs OH, Black BM, et al: Classification and prognosis of thyroid carcinoma: A study of 885 cases observed in a 30 year period. Am J Surg 102:354–387, 1961

119. Wychulis AR, Beahrs OH, Woolner LB: Papillary carcinoma with associated anaplastic carcinoma in the thyroid gland. Surg Gynecol Obstet 120:28–34, 1965

Paul C. Adkins, M.D.
and L. Thompson Bowles, M.D.

6

Management of Cancer of the Lung and Mediastinum

LUNG CANCER

Carcinoma of the lung is by far the most common thoracic neoplasm encountered in practice. Although this entity was uncommon and rarely recognized before the twentieth century, the incidence of bronchogenic carcinoma has increased considerably in the past 65 years, accounting for an estimated 83,800 deaths in the United States in 1976. It is the most common visceral cancer in men in this country at the present time.

Even though routine chest films have become a standard procedure in annual physical examinations of adults, it is unfortunate that nearly half the patients with bronchogenic carcinoma have reached a stage of inoperability when first seen by the surgeon. This may be in part because of procrastination on the part of the patient, who fails to detect obvious symptoms through fear or ignorance, or because of undue delays on the part of the physician managing the patient with an undiagnosed abnormality on chest x-ray. Studies are currently underway to evaluate techniques in the early diagnosis of lung cancer, particularly for high-risk segments of the population, but the rate of resectability of this tumor remains low.

Cell Type

Numerous classifications of bronchogenic carcinoma have been proposed, but the most widely accepted classification identifies the following cell types: epidermoid carcinoma, adenocarcinoma, large cell undifferentiated carcinoma, small cell undifferentiated (oat cell) carcinoma, and bronchiolar-alveolar carcinoma. Precise differentiation is important from a histological standpoint; moreover, the differences in the biological behavior of each of the cell types are of prognostic significance. Occasionally, there may be an admixture of different cell types within the same tumor mass. The most common of these is a mixture of adenocarcinoma and epidermoid carcinoma, the so-called adenosquamous carcinoma.

EPIDERMOID CARCINOMA

The most common form of bronchogenic carcinoma, epidermoid carcinoma, accounts for approximately 40 percent of all cases. It is found more frequently in men than in women in a ratio of approximately 9 to 1. The neoplasm tends to originate in the mainstem or lobar bronchi, frequently resulting in obstruction of the distal portions of the bronchial tree and secondary infection or atelectasis. In addition, ulceration and bleeding are not infrequent and may be the initial manifestation of this tumor. Metastasis tends to occur early by travel to regional lymphatics and direct invasion of adjacent structures. Some epidermoid carcinomas are exceedingly well differentiated and tend to grow slowly over a period of months or years.

ADENOCARCINOMA

Adenocarcinoma accounts for approximately 20 percent of pulmonary malignancies and is likely to originate in a secondary bronchus or peripherally within the lung. It is seen slightly more frequently in men than in women in a ratio of approximately 2 to 1. In women alone it is the most common cell type. Adenocarcinoma tends to spread by way of the bloodstream to distant sites, although lymphatic invasion may occur. Additionally, adenocarcinoma may develop at the site of a previous scar within the lung as a result of old disease or injury. The tumor may occur within the scar or immediately adjacent to it and is termed "scar carcinoma." The fact that this form of adenocarcinoma originates in association with a scar does not appear to alter the behavior or prognosis.[8]

In view of the peripheral location, many adenocarcinomas are silent and are detected on routine chest films. In other instances, clinical manifestations may be present only after metastases have occurred.

UNDIFFERENTIATED CARCINOMAS

Various forms of undifferentiated carcinomas account for approximately 35 percent of all bronchogenic neoplasms. These include a number of anaplastic or poorly differentiated malignancies arising either peripherally or centrally. These carcinomas tend to grow rapidly and spread by both lymphatic and vascular involvement. Distant metastases may occur early. These tumors may be divided into the large cell undif-

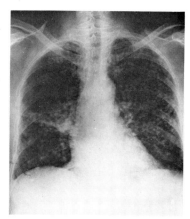

Fig. 6-1. Multiple nodular densities in both lungs. Open lung biopsy proved this to be a multicentric bronchiolar-alveolar carcinoma.

ferentiated and small cell undifferentiated (oat cell), the latter being more malignant in terms of both growth and spread. Extension may occur to mediastinal structures resulting in compression and obstruction of the superior vena cava or occasionally the pulmonary artery.

BRONCHIOLAR-ALVEOLAR CARCINOMA

The least frequent of all bronchogenic carcinomas, bronchiolar-alveolar carcinoma, is found in approximately 5 percent of cases. Bronchiolar-alveolar carcinoma tends to occur in the terminal bronchi or alveoli. Not infrequently, the tumor is multicentric and its histologic features resemble those seen in a contagious disease of sheep known as Jagziekte. In its multicentric form (Fig. 6-1), bronchiolar-alveolar carcinoma causes a significant amount of bronchial irritation resulting in large amounts of foamy or "soap suds" sputum. The unicentric form tends to present as a solitary peripheral nodular density. Spread occurs by way of the lymphatics and bloodstream.

Symptoms

Bronchogenic carcinoma may cause a variety of symptoms depending on the location of the neoplasm and the degree of obstruction or invasion of adjacent structures. A relatively small percentage of patients have no symptoms at all, and their tumor is detected on a routine chest roentgenogram. In most instances, this is a peripheral well-localized carcinoma.

The most common presenting symptom in a patient with carcinoma of the lung is a cough. Many of these people are heavy smokers, and a chronic cough is relatively common. Nevertheless, change in the character of the cough should alert the physician to the possibility of something other than the chronic tracheobronchitis of the smoker. Other frequently encountered presenting symptoms are hemoptysis, dyspnea, and manifestations of a pulmonary infection secondary to bronchial obstruction. The type and extent of symptoms are primarily dependent on the location and size of the neoplasm. Hemoptysis is usually associated with a centrally located ulcerating neoplasm. Dyspnea or infection may be the result of atelectasis or pneumonitis distal to the point of obstruction of a lobar or mainstem bronchus by tumor. Occasionally, one may see a lung abscess as a result of either lobar obstruction and infection or, less commonly, a cavitation within a carcinoma.

Extension of the neoplasm outside the lung may cause symptoms such as pain as a result of chest wall involvement, dyspnea associated with phrenic nerve paralysis, or hoarseness as a result of recurrent laryngeal nerve involvement by the tumor. A carcinoma of the lung occurring in the superior pulmonary sulcus may cause arm and shoulder pain because of brachial plexus involvement, or it may cause a Horner's syndrome from extension to the stellate ganglion.

In recent years, a group of symptoms associated with bronchogenic carcinoma has been classified as extrapulmonary manifestations not associated with metastases.[22] These symptoms include the carcinomatous neuromyopathies and may be detected in as many as 15 percent of patients with bronchogenic carcinoma. Symptoms are most frequently associated with oat cell carcinoma, but they are seen occasionally with other cell types. These symptoms include polymyositis or a myasthenia-like picture, peripheral neuropathy, and subacute cerebellar degeneration. Another group of metabolic manifestations associated with oat cell carcinoma includes Cushing's syndrome, inappropriate antidiuretic hormone production, hypercalcemia, hypoglycemia, gynecomastia, and the carcinoid syndrome. Extraction of the primary tumor occasionally results in regression of these metabolic manifestations, but in general the prognosis is extremely poor since the symptoms are associated with small cell or undifferentiated oat cell carcinoma.

Clubbing and generalized hypertrophic pulmonary osteoarthropathy are other systemic manifestations of bronchogenic carcinoma. This entity is not generally associated with oat cell carcinoma but with more differentiated forms of the neoplasm, and it may or may not regress after removal of the primary carcinoma.

Radiographic Patterns

The appearance of bronchogenic carcinoma on chest roentgenogram may be extremely varied depending on the size and location of the neoplasm. In general, it is wise to pursue a policy of suspecting bronchogenic carcinoma in any patient over the age of 35 with an unexplained pulmonary density on the chest roentgenogram. Unnecessary delays in pursuing diagnostic studies or procrastination on the part of the physician too often leads to a stage of inoperability while the patient is under observation.

One of the common roentgenographic manifestations of bronchogenic carcinoma is a solitary peripheral nodule, the so-called coin lesion (Fig. 6-2). Our policy is to advise surgical excision of any solitary peripheral nodule that contains no central core of calcification or concen-

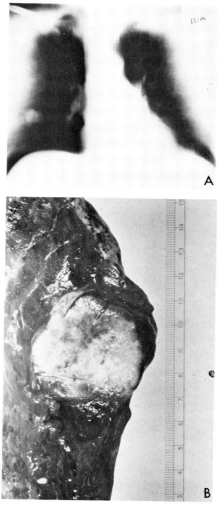

Fig. 6-2. **A:** Tomogram of midlung field demonstrating solitary nodule without calcification. **B:** At operation this proved to be a peripheral adenocarcinoma without lymph node involvement.

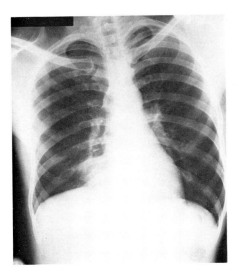

Fig. 6-3.   Peripheral epidermoid carcinoma of right lower lobe.

tric rings of calcium.   The appearance of calcium flecks adjacent to a solitary nodule does not exclude the possibility of bronchogenic carcinoma or
the so-called scar carcinoma.   When a solitary nodule is detected on a
chest film, tomography may be helpful in ascertaining whether or not calcium is present within the lesion.   If calcium is detected, it is then reasonably safe to assume that this represents a granuloma and not carcinoma.
Other peripherally occurring bronchogenic carcinomas may not appear as
a discrete nodules but as irregular infiltrating densities of varying sizes
(Fig. 6-3).

When the neoplasm occurs centrally, it may cause segmental, lobar,
or even total lung atelectasis.   If infection occurs in the lung distal to the
tumor, the radiographic appearance may simulate that of pneumonia or a
lung abscess (Fig. 6-4).   Since the common sites for a postaspiration
pyogenic lung abscess are the posterior segments of the upper lobes and
the superior segments of the lower lobes, the appearance of a lung abscess
in other areas of the lung should strongly suggest that one is dealing with a
malignancy.   Direct extension of a tumor to the hilum of the lung or
involvement of hilar lymph nodes may cause hilar enlargement on the
chest roentgenogram.

A carcinoma of the lung occurring in the apex may extend directly to
the chest wall, presenting the classic appearance of the superior sulcus or
Pancoast tumor.   The classic roentgenographic appearance of this tumor
is that of a density at the apex of the lung with evidence of destruction of
portions of the first, second, or third ribs immediately adjacent to the
tumor (Fig. 6-5).

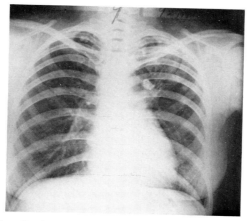

Fig. 6-4.   Cavitary carcinoma in left upper lobe in patient
with history of tuberculosis.   Note calcified left hilar nodes.

Diagnosis and Evaluation

In any patient whose chest roentgenogram discloses an abnormality
suspected of being carcinoma of the lung, an orderly series of studies
should be undertaken in order to confirm the diagnosis and assess the degree of spread (staging) of the neoplasm.   Using currently available techniques, physicians can obtain a histological diagnosis in the vast majority
of patients before thoracotomy, and they can ascertain the degree of

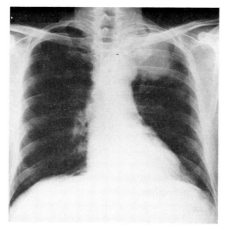

Fig. 6-5.   Superior sulcus tumor at apex of left lung.   No
destruction of first rib. This patient also had arm and
shoulder pain and a Horner's syndrome.

operability by proper evaluation techniques, thus avoiding an unnecessary or fruitless thoracotomy.

Staging of bronchogenic carcinoma consists of evaluating: the size of the primary tumor, the presence or absence of ipsilateral and contralateral mediastinal node involvement, and the presence or absence of distant metastases. Thus the surgeon can select those patients for whom resection of the tumor and adjacent lung carries a reasonably favorable prognosis and exclude those for whom surgical resection is of little or no value.

BRONCHOSCOPY

The introduction of fiberoptic bronchoscopy as a diagnostic technique has greatly enhanced the surgeon's ability to obtain a preoperative diagnosis of peripherally located carcinomas. Before the availability of this instrument, the standard rigid bronchoscope afforded visualization of the mainstem and lobar bronchi and the orifices of the segmental bronchi. Since more than half of the bronchogenic neoplasms occur distal to these points, preoperative biopsy was frequently impossible. However, with the fiberoptic bronchoscope, one can visualize the segmental and subsegmental bronchi and obtain biopsy material. An additional technique that has provided further accessibility to peripheral lesions is bronchial brushing, which may be carried out in conjunction with fiberoptic bronchoscopy. A small catheter with a brush at the top is passed into subsegmental bronchi and a tissue sample is obtained.

A variation of the brushing technique is that performed without bronchoscopy through a percutaneous puncture of the cervical trachea. Under fluoroscopic guidance, the brush is advanced to the area of the suspected carcinoma of the lung and a specimen is obtained for histological examination (Fig. 6-6). Using these techniques, a positive histological diagnosis can be obtained in over three-fourths of the patients with pulmonary lesions. During bronchial brushing, contrast material can be injected and a bronchogram of the involved segment obtained. This may be helpful in demonstrating bronchial obstruction and further assessing the degree of involvement of the specific area of the lung.

A practical approach is the employment of all of these techniques at one time. A rigid bronchoscope can be introduced to visualize the trachea and main bronchi. If a diagnosis is not readily apparent, the fiberoptic bronchoscope can be passed through the rigid bronchoscope and be used for exploring the more distal portions of the tracheobronchial tree. Finally, brushing can be carried out with the fiberoptic bronchoscope in place and bronchography can be performed. For all except small peripheral lesions, a histological diagnosis should be achieved in the vast majority of instances using this technique.

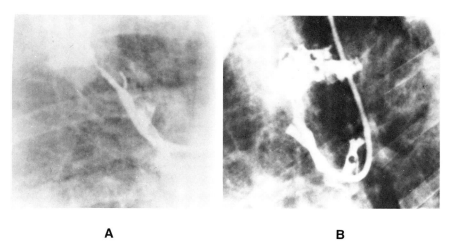

A   **B**

Fig. 6-6.   Spot films of bronchial brushing of peripheral lesions.   Bronchography is performed in conjunction with this procedure.   Note narrowing of segmental bronchus on left and obstruction of bronchus on right.

MEDIASTINOSCOPY AND MEDIASTINOTOMY

A knowledge of the lymphatic drainage patterns of each of the lobes of the lung is extremely important in preoperative evaluation of the patient with bronchogenic carcinoma.   The nodes draining the three lobes of the right lung are located in a lymphatic "sump" located inferior and posterior to the right upper lobe bronchus, but above the takeoff of the right middle lobe and superior segmental bronchus of the right lower lobe (Fig. 6-7).   All three lobes of the right lung drain into this sump.   This knowledge is of some practical importance to the surgeon deciding on the extent of resection.   Since carcinomas located in the right lower lobe may drain to this group of nodes, in order to achieve an adequate resection, it may be necessary to remove the right lower and middle lobes with their accompanying nodes.   On the other hand, the right upper lobe lymphatics drain to this sump occurring above the bronchi to the middle lobe and superior segment so that right upper lobectomy alone is adequate to achieve exposure and removal of the nodes draining that lobe.   From this lymphatic sump, the drainage goes to the right superior tracheobronchial nodes, then to the peritracheal nodes and the right supraclavicular nodes. Spread to the contralateral mediastinal nodes from the right lung is uncommon and occurs in only approximately 5 percent of the cases. Spread of tumor from the right upper lobe to the carina or contralateral lymphatic chain is exceedingly rare.

The drainage of the left lung is somewhat different. The lymphatic

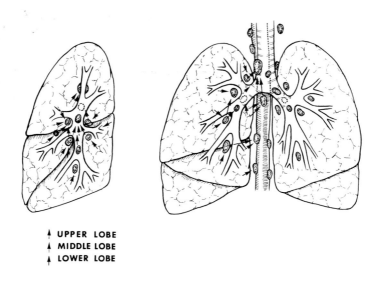

↑ UPPER LOBE
↟ MIDDLE LOBE
↑ LOWER LOBE

Fig. 6-7.   Lymphatic drainage of right lung.

sump consists of a group of nodes lying in the fissure between the upper
and the lower lobes (Fig. 6-8).   One of these nodes lies immediately posterior to the main pulmonary artery before it enters the fissure.   Consequently, the performance of a lobectomy alone on the left does not assure
exposure and removal of all the lymphatic nodes draining either the upper
or the lower lobes.   In addition, the mediastinal node drainage from the
left lung is somewhat different in that spread to the carinal nodes and to
the contralateral peritracheal nodes from the left lung occurs with equal
frequency as drainage to the ipsilateral peritracheal and supraclavicular
nodes.   Carcinomas of both lower lobes may spread as well to the nodes
of the interior pulmonary ligament and periesophageal chain.

       With this knowledge of lymphatic drainage, it is obvious that biopsy
of the appropriate hilar and mediastinal nodes is extremely helpful in assessing the degree of spread of a given carcinoma.   With carcinomas of
the left lung, evaluation of not only the ipsilateral but also the carinal and
contralateral mediastinal nodes is extremely important in evaluating resectability.   Until recent years scalene node biopsy was considered the
standard procedure in evaluation of the patient with bronchogenic carcinoma; however, from a practical standpoint, it has been found that in
the absence of palpable supraclavicular nodes, the yield of positive diagnosis by scalene node biopsy was relatively uncommon.   With the introduction of mediastinoscopy by Carlens[6] in 1959, a technique of biopsying

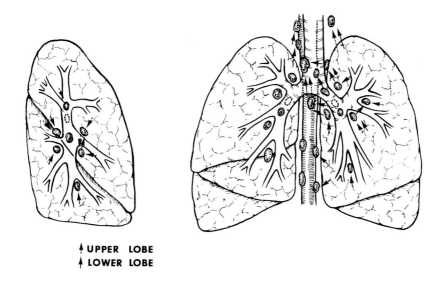

↑ UPPER LOBE
↑ LOWER LOBE

Fig. 6-8.   Lymphatic drainage of left lung.

mediastinal nodes has proven to be extremely helpful.   At our institution, mediastinoscopy has supplanted scalene node biopsy as a method of evaluation in all patients except those who have definite palpable supraclavicular nodes.

The indications for mediastinoscopy are a patient with any central pulmonary density suspected of being carcinoma or a peripheral density with any suggestion of hilar or mediastinal adenopathy.   In those individuals with peripheral lesions and no evidence of mediastinal adenopathy on tomograms of the mediastinum, the yield from mediastinoscopy is extremely small and this study is not routinely employed.

Technique of mediastinoscopy.   In our institution, mediastinoscopy is performed under general endotracheal anesthesia.   It is frequently combined with bronchoscopy and bronchial brushing.   The patient is placed in the supine position with the head and neck slightly hyperextended (Fig. 6-9).   After routine preparation and draping of the skin, a 4-cm transverse incision is made two finger breadths above the suprasternal notch.   The incision is carried down to the peritracheal fascia which is incised.   Using blunt dissection with the finger, a plane is developed down into the mediastinum staying close to the trachea.   This

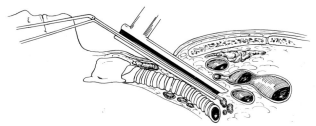

Fig. 6-9. Technique of carinal node biopsy at mediastinoscopy (see text).

should place the finger dorsal to the great vessels. Once the plane has
been developed as far as the operator's index finger will reach, the mediastinoscope is introduced into this incision. With continued blunt dissection, the mediastinoscope can be passed sufficiently far to visualize
the lymph nodes in the superior portion of the right hilum, the carina, and
the superior portion of the left hilum. Once the lymphatics in these areas
are visualized, they are aspirated with a 6-inch #20 needle and a small
syringe to make sure they are not blood vessels. Once this has been as-
certained, a special biopsy forceps is passed and biopsies of representative nodes are carried out. We have found a special combination suction and cautery device to be extremely helpful in controlling small
amounts of bleeding which may occur in the mediastinum in association
with this procedure. Using the above techniques, mediastinoscopy can
be carried out with minimal risk.

Mediastinoscopy has proved to be very helpful, especially in evaluating lesions of the right lung, which do not tend to drain to the contralateral nodes. On the other hand, mediastinoscopy does not afford access
to the lymph nodes of the left lung located anterior to the arch of the aorta
or between the aorta and the pulmonary artery. Access to these lymphatics may be gained by another technique, anterior mediastinotomy.[21] This
technique affords access to the lymphatics of the hilum located anteriorly
and out of reach of the mediastinoscope and is particularly helpful for
neoplasms in the left lung.

Technique of mediastinotomy. With the patient under general anesthesia, the anterior thorax is prepared and draped in the usual fashion. A
4-cm incision is made in the second or third intercostal space beginning
approximately 1 cm lateral to the border of the sternum. Dissection is
carried down to the intercostal muscles which are split, exposing the
medial reflection of the parietal pleura. Care is taken to avoid the internal mammary vessels at the most medial aspect of the incision. Using
blunt dissection, the mediastinal pleura is reflected laterally without en-

tering the pleural space and the anterior mediastinal nodes are encountered. These can be biopsied either under direct vision or by the introduction of a mediastinoscope through the incision. If further exposure is necessary, a segment of one of the costal cartilages can be resected. When further evaluation of the extent of a carcinoma is necessary, mediastinotomy can be combined with mediastinoscopy, and the hilum of the left lung can be palpated bimanually introducing the index finger of the right hand through the mediastinoscopy incision in the neck and the index finger of the left hand through the anterior mediastinotomy incision. If further evaluation is necessary, the mediastinal pleura can be incised and the hilum of the lung palpated and biopsied through this approach.

In addition to the above methods of evaluation, we frequently employ bone and liver scans in patients with signs or symptoms of distant metastases. Thus patients with extension of tumor beyond the limits of resectability are defined before thoracotomy, and it is uncommon to perform a thoracotomy and be unable to perform a definitive resection.

Contraindication to Exploratory Thoracotomy

Certain clinical manifestations indicate spread of the neoplasm to an extent that precludes definitive resection of a bronchogenic carcinoma. When these are present and a histologic diagnosis of cancer can be obtained, thoracotomy is not justified. Absolute contraindications include dissemination of the malignancy to distant sites, such as the brain, liver, and bone. Extension to contralateral mediastinal lymph nodes or to the supraclavicular node is also a sign of inoperability. The presence of a sanguineous pleural effusion in which malignant cells can be demonstrated indicates that the neoplasm has spread to the parietal pleura and is considered a sign of inoperability. Paralysis of the ipsilateral vocal cord in the presence of a lung cancer invariably means the neoplasm has invaded the mediastinum, generally around the arch of the aorta, and is not resectable. This manifestation is almost invariably associated with left-sided malignancies because of the course of the left recurrent laryngeal nerve.

In addition to the above, there are certain relative contraindications to exploration. Under these circumstances, the majority of tumors with these manifestations are not resectable, but occasionally resection can be carried out. Relative contraindications include paralysis of the ipsilateral diaphragm, chest wall involvement, and extension across the carina. Occasionally, the phrenic nerve is involved in the tumor mass as it descends the pericardium, and it may be possible to resect a portion of the pericardium including the phrenic nerve and the adjacent neoplasm. However, phrenic nerve paralysis associated with a neoplasm in the upper part of the lung rarely proves to be resectable. Involvement of the chest wall by direct extension of the carcinoma is not infrequent and is often associated with severe chest wall pain. Provided the tumor has not extended to other areas, it is possible to resect the involved segment of the chest wall in continuity with the lung or lobe with gratifying results.[13] In unusual circumstances a carcinoma of the mainstem bronchus extends to or just beyond the carina. Provided the trachea itself is not involved, it is technically possible to perform a pneumonectomy on the involved side, resect the proximal portion of the contralateral mainstem bronchus, and reanastomose the distal end of that bronchus to the trachea. The use of prosthetic materials to replace the trachea or carina is currently undergoing clinical investigation, but its application is extremely limited.[10]

Thoracic surgeons generally believe that if a histological diagnosis of oat cell carcinoma can be obtained operation is contraindicated. The results of surgical resection of this form of bronchogenic carcinoma are so poor that radiation alone or combined with chemotherapy is considered the most appropriate method of treatment.

Surgical Management

Before operation, it is common practice to perform pulmonary function studies on patients who are candidates for a pulmonary resection. In the normal individual the right lung carries approximately 55 percent of the total pulmonary function and the left lung 45 percent. A left pneumonectomy is tolerated better than a right pneumonectomy in most instances. However, if a neoplasm totally obstructs a mainstem bronchus or involves a major portion of the lung, the involved lung is probably contributing little to the total pulmonary function and its removal will not seriously reduce the patient's ventilation.

Generally, if the neoplasm and involved nodes, if any, are limited to one lobe, lobectomy yields approximately the same results as pneumonectomy.[15] In rare instances small localized carcinomas have been treated by localized resections such as segmentectomy or wedge resection with good results. However, lobectomy or pneumonectomy is the more widely accepted procedure, primarily depending on the location and extent of the neoplasm. If a carcinoma involves the mediastinal nodes but has not extended past this point, radical pneumonectomy can be performed. This involves removal of all mediastinal nodes and intrapericardial division of the pulmonary artery and pulmonary veins along with the lung.

It is beyond the scope of this chapter to describe the technical aspects of performing the above operative procedures. All are performed through a posterolateral thoracotomy, which gives the surgeon the option of performing lobectomy, pneumonectomy, or radical pneumonectomy as the situation dictates. If there is some question regarding the patient's ability to tolerate pneumonectomy, intraoperative occlusion of the main pulmonary artery for 5 minutes has proved to be helpful. If the patient tolerates this without significant change in blood pressure, pulse rate, or electrocardiographic pattern, it is usually safe to go ahead with the resection. If, however, occlusion of the pulmonary artery produces significant and persisting change in any of these parameters, a resection of that magnitude will probably not be well tolerated.

The use of preoperative radiation in the management of patients with bronchogenic carcinoma has not proven to be of significant benefit.[4] Extensive trials with this combined therapy during the 1960s did increase the resectability rate but failed to increase longevity and were associated with a significant increase in the number of postoperative complications. Exception to this is the patient with the superior sulcus or Pancoast tumor. This form of bronchogenic carcinoma is usually an epidermoid carcinoma occurring at the apex of the lung and usually involving the adjacent portions of the brachial plexus, the first or second rib, and not infrequently the stellate ganglion producing a Horner's syndrome. Before 1956 this form of bronchogenic carcinoma was generally considered inoperable and carried an extremely poor prognosis. The work of Shaw and Paulson and subsequent reports by Paulson[23] have demonstrated that using a preoperative irradiation dose of 3000–3500 rads followed by radical resection of the upper lobe, adjacent chest wall, and segments of the brachial plexus has yielded gratifying results with 35 percent 5-year survival rates. More recent reports from investigators at the University of Michigan[17] indicate that in their hands radiation alone yielded an equally satisfactory 5-year survival rate.

Results of Surgical Treatment of Bronchogenic Carcinoma

In assessing the results of surgical resection in the treatment of this tumor, it appears that the most important prognostic factor is the extent of nodal involvement. If one excludes the oat cell carcinomas, histologic type seems to be a less important prognostic factor than extent of nodes involved. Most recent reports indicate that in the absence of nodal metastases 5-year survival rates are between 34 and 48 percent. On the other hand, if lobar of hilar nodes are involved (stage II), the 5-year survival rates are between 17 and 30 percent. Small differences have been noted in survival rates of patients with various cell types. Slightly improved results are likely for those individuals with epidermoid carcinoma, and slightly less satisfactory results occur in patients with adenocarcinoma and undifferentiated carcinoma. However, these results do not appear to be as significant to survival as the relationship of nodal involvement.[18,23,24]

Chemotherapy for Lung Cancer

Although none of the currently available chemotherapeutic agents produce major benefits in the treatment of lung cancer, there are a number of agents that are associated with measurable regressions. These include alkylating agents, antimetabolites (particularly methotrexate), nitrosoureas, procarbazine, hydroxyurea, vinca alkaloids, hexamethylmelamine, and others. The alkylating agents, particularly nitrogen mustard and cyclophosphamide, produce useful benefit in approximately one-third of lung cancer patients who can be evaluated. Responders to the other agents range from 15 to 30 percent, but there is little if any prolongation of survival in responders to therapy with any of these drugs when they are used as single agents.

The future of chemotherapy for lung cancer is undoubtedly in the area of combination chemotherapy, but this field has been slow to develop. Some of the combinations that have been employed are shown in Table 6-1. It is of interest that the objective response observed with combination drug therapy is higher than with single agent therapy, particularly with the small cell (oat cell) carcinomas. Objective responses as high as 60% have been reported and responders do appear to live longer than non-responders.

Table 6-1
Drug Combinations Employed for Treatment of Lung Cancer

Drugs	References
Cyclophosphamide, Methotrexate, Actinomycin D, and Vincristine	Hansen et al. (Cancer 30:315, 1972)
Cyclophosphamide, Vincristine, and Procarbazine	Eagen et al. (Cancer 33:527, 1974)
Hexamethyl melamine and Methotrexate	Weiss and Wilson (Ca. Chemo. Rep. 55:299, 1971)
Nitrogen mustard, Vinblastine, Procarbazine, and prednisolone	Laing et al. (Lancet 1:129, 1975)

TUMORS OF THE MEDIASTINUM

Tumors occurring in the mediastinum are generally anatomically accessible and surgical removal is frequently possible. A knowledge of the mediastinal anatomy and pathology is essential for effective diagnosis and proper management. The mediastinum may be regarded as that segment of thoracic anatomy bounded cephalad by the thoracic outlet and caudad by the diaphragm, laterally by the pleura, anteriorly by the sternum, and posteriorly by the vertebral column. The subcompartments of the mediastinum are the anterior, superior, middle, and posterior. Consideration of mediastinal tumors is conveniently organized by these anatomic compartments (Fig. 6-10).

Specific neoplasms of the mediastinum characteristically occur in one or more of these anatomic subcompartments, allowing the physician to make a reasonable preoperative diagnosis based on the location and radiographic appearance of the mass.

MEDIASTINUM

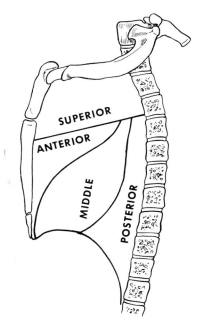

Fig. 6-10.   Diagram of mediastinal compartments.

Anterior-Superior Compartment of the Mediastinum

The anterior-superior space may be considered that area which extends from the thoracic outlet above down to a line between the inferior border of the manubrium and the fourth thoracic vertebra with lateral borders at the mediastinal pleura. Structures contained in this compartment are the proximal trachea and esophagus, the thymus, and the aortic arch with its brachiocephalic branches. Downward extensions of the thyroid gland may be in this area, and embryonic rests may also persist in the anterior-superior mediastinum. The tumors most commonly encountered here are teratodermoids, thymonas, and substernal or intrathoracic goiters. Parathyroid tumors, lymphomas, and epidermoid carcinomas occur less commonly in this space.

CLINICAL CONSIDERATIONS

Common signs and symptoms of tumors in the anterior-superior compartment are cough, dyspnea, dysphagia, and manifestations of superior vena caval obstruction. Less frequent involvement of the phrenic or laryngeal nerves may occur with resultant diaphragmatic paralysis or vocal cord palsy. Gradual enlargement of a mass in this area may cause compression of the trachea or the esophagus, resulting in stridor or dysphagia. Systemic manifestations may include myasthenia gravis associated with thymoma, hyperthyroidism associated with an active thyroid adenoma occurring in the mediastinum, and hyperparathyroidism associated with the parathyroid adenoma.

Teratodermoid tumors compose a spectrum of dysgenetic tumors ranging from the relatively simple dermoid cyst to the potential and frequently malignant teratoma. These lesions represent the development of endodermal, ectodermal, and/or mesodermal tissue which is abnormal to the anatomic location. Although this kind of tumor is usually present at birth, it is rarely observed until the patient is older and the tumor has grown and developed to a size sufficient to be seen on x-ray or to cause symptoms. Not infrequently, teratodermoids are asymptomatic. Histologically, a wide spectrum of cellular patterns may be seen in this group, ranging from mature cellular elements representing teeth, hair, cartilage, and other classic components of a dermoid cyst, to a highly anaplastic cell seen with the malignant teratoma. Malignancy and invasiveness are generally a function of the degree of maturity of the cellular elements of this tumor. Radiographically, a teratodermoid most commonly presents as a rounded density in the anterior-superior mediastinum, but occasionally it may be lobulated. In the more mature forms of the tumor, calcification in teeth or bone or a calcific rim may be visible and serve to establish a diagnosis. Gross appearance of the lesion at surgery may vary from a well-encapsulated, thin-walled cystic lesion to a lobulated firm tumor mass. The tumor itself may contain components of skin, including hair, sebaceous glands, and sebaceous material, as well as teeth, cartilage, or muscle. Solid tumors must be regarded as potentially malignant teratomas and every effort should be made to achieve complete removal.

Thymoma is another type of relatively common anterior-superior mediastinal tumor. Approximately one-third of these tumors cause signs and symptoms.[25] The most common of these are cough, dyspnea, dysphagia, and superior caval obstruction. Another third are asymptomatic.[19] The remaining third are associated with systemic conditions in which the relationship to the thymus is poorly understood. Some of the more prominent diseases of this last category include myasthenia gravis, anemia, pancytopenia, thrombocytopenia, hypogammaglobulinemia, and some forms of autoimmune disease.

The four common cell types encountered in thymomas are lymphoid, spindle cell, epithelial, and rosette forming. Most thymomas contain more than one of these cell types, but only one is likely to predominate. Predicting the biological behavior of the tumor on the basis of its histology is notoriously difficult; however, the gross appearance is considerably more helpful. Tumors that remain within the thymic capsule are completely resectable, and postoperative recurrence is most unusual.[29] If the thymoma reveals gross invasion of the capsule and local extension, postoperative radiation therapy should be employed, but the probability of 5-year survival is significantly diminished.[16] These tumors have a characteristic appearance at the time of surgery: they are yellowish gray, lobulated, and variable in size up to several centimeters in diameter. In approximately 80 percent of patients with this tumor, the lesion is encapsulated. The other 20 percent infiltrate the capsule and invade local structures.[1]

The relationship of thymic abnormality and systemic diseases is poorly understood. Approximately about 75 percent of patients with myasthenia gravis have some thymic disease. It is of interest that myasthenia gravis also occurs in patients with a normal thymus. The histologic abnormalities most common in myasthenia patients are thymoma, which occurs in approximately one-third of myasthenia cases, and thymic hyperplasia.[26]

Radiologic studies may be useful in assessing resectability of the thymus lesion, but a tissue diagnosis is essential to plan proper treatment. Mediastinoscopy may be helpful, as may anterior mediastinotomy, but most of these patients come to thoracotomy with or without a tissue diagnosis. Complete removal of a thymoma may or may not significantly alter the course of associated myasthenia gravis. Reports are variable in their findings, although there is general agreement that young women with thymic hyperplasia are likely to have the most successful outcome after surgery. Thomas[26] reviewed a number of series and reported that the presence of myasthenia gravis was associated with a poorer prognosis for patients who had a thymoma. Weissberg et al.[28] reported that 15 patients had myasthenia gravis in their series of 35 thymomas, and 5 of the 11 managed by surgery had significant remission postoperatively. One of their surgically treated patients actually got worse postoperatively. Alpert and coworkers[2] suggest that remission of myasthenia after thymectomy is in part a variant of time, and they report 7 percent remission after 1 year and 60 percent by 8 years. Response after thymectomy has been variable for other systemic conditions as well, and it is difficult to predict the postthymectomy course in patients who also have anemia, pancytopenia, or other hematologic or immunologic disease. Wolfe et al.[30] emphasized the importance of the operative management of the patient's respiratory status after surgery for myasthenia gravis. Anticholinasterase drug management is facilitated by a nasotracheal tube preoperatively, intraoperatively, and for a period of time postoperatively. Respiratory failure can be lethal in the postoperative period. Radiation of the thymus yields variable results in myasthenia gravis, and steroid therapy has been used to treat thymoma with occasional success.[11]

Substernal thyroid is a relatively rare condition. Retrosternal extension of thyroid disease is not uncommon but should be considered a primary problem of the neck rather than the mediastinum. Substernal thyroid tumors are usually asymptomatic, but they may on occasion present as thyroid adenomas associated with hyperthyroid conditions. In these patients, radioactive iodine uptake studies may be helpful in making the diagnosis, and surgical therapy must be weighed against radioactive iodine therapy. The possibility of malignancy in a substernal adenoma must be considered but is extremely rare.

Parathyroid adenomas are usually small and cause no mechanical compression symptoms. These lesions may be embedded in the thymus gland and can be enormously difficult to locate in the mediastinum even with the best possible exposure. The precise location of these tumors is usually unknown preoperatively, and surgery is frequently indicated after cervical exploration has failed to reveal either adenoma or hyperplasia in the hyperparathyroid patient. Occasionally, mediastinal parathyroid tumors may reach sufficient size to cause cough or dysphagia, and they can be identified by chest x-ray or barium swallow.[20] Although the parathyroid adenoma commonly occurs in the anterior or superior mediastinum, it has been found rarely in the posterior mediastinum. The systemic signs and symptoms in these patients are those of hyperparathyroidism with hypercalcemia and abnormal phosphorus excretion.

A group of rare tumors may also occur in the anterior-superior compartment of the mediastinum. These are lymphangioma, hemangioma, paraganglioma including chemodectoma, lipoma, hemangiopericytoma, liposarcoma, fibrosarcoma, leiomyosarcoma, mesothelioma, and seminoma. Primary epidermoid carcinoma may arise in the mediastinum. Although all these tumors are uncommon, they must be remembered in the differential diagnosis. The mesenchymal tumors are often malignant and surgically curable.[3] The signs and symptoms that can result from their presence are those of other tumors of this area—namely, cough, dyspnea, or dysphagia. Chemodectomas rarely secrete catechol or its metabolites and cause systemic symptoms.

Tissue diagnosis is essential in all patients with tumors identified in the anterior-superior mediastinum. Although mediastinoscopy or anterior mediastinotomy may often be useful in obtaining cells for diagnosis, surgical exploration of the mediastinum is nearly always indicated for a mediastinal tumor once the presence of the tumor is known and unless compelling surgical contraindications exist. Median sternotomy is the most advantageous surgical approach to the anterior-superior mediastinum. On the rare occasion in which lateral extension is pronounced, anterolateral thoracotomy may be preferable. If bilateral growth is considerable, bilateral anterior thoracotomy transecting the sternum may be necessary.

Middle Compartment of the Mediastinum

The middle compartment of the mediastinum is that space which is anatomically located from the level of the fourth thoracic vertebra inferiorly to the diaphragm and bounded anteriorly by the manubrium and posteriorly by the esophagus. Within this space is contained the heart, the ascending aorta, the tracheal bifurcation and mainstem bronchi, and the lymph nodes surrounding the tracheal bifurcation.

The middle mediastinum tumor that is most often malignant is the lymphoma.[1] Lymphoma occurs rarely in the anterior-superior section. In the middle mediastinum, lesions that can cause symptoms and be radiologically similar to neoplasms are pericardial cysts and bronchogenic cysts (Fig. 6-11, 6-12, and 6-13). Prominent adenopathy from tuberculosis, sarcoidosis, and chronic fungal infections can cause compression symptoms and appear radiologically as rounded densities. Lymph nodes bearing metastatic tumor from lung, esophagus, and organs below the diaphragm may also resemble tumors of the middle mediastinum on x-ray.

Lymphomas may present as a diffuse disease, but confinement to the mediastinum also occurs. Van Heerden et al.[27] reported 97 cases of lymphoma localized to the mediastinum. Lymphosarcoma, reticulum cell sarcoma, and Hodgkin's disease may be localized in the midmediastinum and surgical excision may be possible. Radiologically, these tumors may

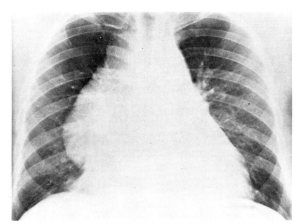

Fig. 6-11.   Lymphoma of the middle mediastinum.

be bilateral lobulated masses.   There may be compression of the trachea, and occasionally extension into the posterior mediastinum may result in esophageal compression.   These tumors are frequently asymptomatic if confined to the mediastinum and may be detected only on a routine chest film (Fig. 6-14).   Some patients have systemic symptoms of low-grade fever, anorexia, weight loss, or a vague feeling of discomfort in the chest.

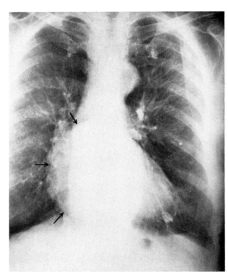

Fig. 6-12.   Anteroposterior view of bronchogenic cyst.

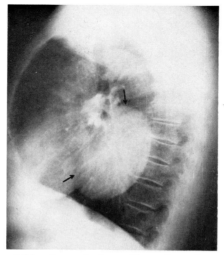

Fig. 6-13.   Lateral view of bronchogenic cyst.

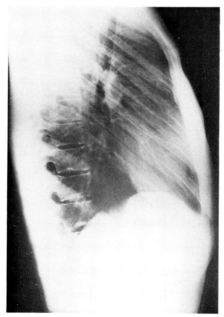

Fig. 6-14.   Lateral view of Hodgkin's disease of medias-tinum.

In the absence of palpable supraclavicular nodes, mediastinoscopy is frequently useful in establishing a tissue diagnosis of lymphoma. If the supraclavicular nodes are palpable, however, biopsy of one of these is usually sufficient to establish the diagnosis. In the event that mediastinoscopy or supraclavicular node biopsy is not diagnostic, an anterior mediastinotomy may be performed for biopsy of the involved nodes. Occasionally it is not possible to identify the lymphoma preoperatively, and the area can be explored through a posterolateral thoracotomy. If possible, the tumor mass should be completely resected. In any event, the surgeon's attempt to remove the entire tumor should be tempered by the knowledge that postoperative irradiation is very effective in controlling residual tumor and will increase the probability of a successful outcome even if total resection is not feasible.

Once the diagnosis of lymphoma of the mediastinum is established, staging should be carried out and appropriate therapy employed—irradiation, chemotherapy, or both. The cell type of the lymphoma is important in predicting its biological behavior. Patients with Hodgkin's disease have a rather good 5-year prognosis, whereas those with a lymphocytic type of lymphoma have a much poorer outlook.[5]

Posterior Mediastinum

The posterior compartment is that portion of the mediastinum adjacent to the vertebral column and containing the esophagus, the descending thoracic aorta, and the sympathetic nerve chains. Tumors of the posterior mediastinum are predominately neurogenic in origin. Duplication cysts of the esophagus and esophageal tumors, benign and malignant, as well as aneurysms of the descending thoracic aorta, must be considered initially in the differential diagnosis. The neurogenic lesions are usually asymptomatic and are discovered in a routine chest x-ray or chest x-ray taken for another condition. When signs or symptoms do occur, pain in the back or posterior chest wall is most common. In extreme cases, local invasion can cause paralysis, dysphagia, and cough.

Neurofibromas are the most common neurogenic tumors. These lesions are solid, arise from nerve sheaths in the posterior mediastinum, and may be seen in patients with von Recklinghausen's disease. Neurilemomas, malignant schwannomas, and neuroblastomas all occur in the posterior mediastinum. These neurogenic lesions are most likely to be malignant in children, but malignancies may be encountered in adults. Paragangliomas commonly occur in the posterior mediastinum but may grow in the anterior compartment. Paragangliomas are sometimes hormonally active and cause the signs and symptoms related to excess blood levels of catecholamines. Sweating and episodic hypertension may be the presenting complaints in these patients. With the exception of patients who have malignant schwannomas, patients with nerve sheath tumors generally have quite a good prognosis.

Neuroblastomas arise from the sympathetic nervous system and occur most frequently in children.[12] In fact, neuroblastomas are the most common soft tissue tumors in children, and 20 percent of all these lesions are mediastinal.[9] These posterior lesions are often high in the mediastinum, nonencapsulated, and locally invading. They are quite sensitive to radiation, and 5-year cures are rather common even for those patients who have had surgical procedures that failed to remove all the tumor. Preferred treatment is surgical resection of all or as much tumor as possible followed by radiation. Grosfeld et al.[14] reported an 88-percent survival rate (8 of 9 patients) in patients under 1 year of age.

Ganglioneuromas are the most common of the sympathetic nerve tumors. These tumors are well encapsulated and frequently are histologically well differentiated. In some patients with ganglioneuromas, vanillylmandelic acid (VMA) level may be elevated in the urine. Postoperative return to normal VMA urine levels generally heralds an excellent prognosis. Ganglioneuroblastomas may appear encapsulated and lobulated, and such tumors can be completely removed. In general, however, these tumors are poorly differentiated, tend to metastasize rapidly, and carry a poor prognosis.

Pheochromocytomas may be encountered in other parts of the mediastinum but are usually seen in the posterior compartment. They resemble pheochromocytomas in other locations and give rise to the same kinds of signs and symptoms. Paroxysmal hypertension may suggest the presence of this tumor, and palpitations, perspiration, chest pain, and headaches are the signs and symptoms associated with increased blood levels of catecholamines. Pheochromocytomas are sometimes malignant and present as brown, soft, highly vascular tumors. Surgical excision offers a complete cure in benign growths.

Chordomas, rare lesions arising from embryonic remnants of the notochord, present as tumors attached to the vertebral bodies. Surgical attempts to remove these tumors are often frustrating, and local recurrence postoperatively is common even though distant metastases are rare.

Tumors of the posterior mediastinum are difficult to assess preoperatively. Vena cavagram, barium swallow, and aortography may all be useful in establishing gross anatomic characteristics of the lesion; however, posterolateral thoracotomy with attempt at surgical removal offers the highest probability of diagnosis and cure. Tumors demonstrating preoperative evidence of vena caval compression or esophageal or tracheal invasion, of course, offer the poorest prognosis. Tissue diagnosis is necessary to plan therapy, but thoracotomy is indicated whenever the tumor is identified unless there are reasons to avoid surgery. A high percentage of these benign lesions are completely resectable, and many of the malignant lesions can be resected and cured.

REFERENCES

1. Ackerman LV, Rosai J: Surgical Pathology. St. Louis, CV, Mosby Co, 1974
2. Alpert LK, Papatestes A, Karle A, Osserman RS, Osserman K: A histologic reappraisal of the thymus in myasthenia gravis. Arch Pathol 91:55, 1971
3. Benjamin SP, McCormack LM, Effler DB, Groves LK: Primary tumors of the mediastinum. Chest 62:297–303, 1972
4. Bloedorn FG, Cowley RA: Irradiation and surgery in the treatment of bronchogenic carcinoma. Surg Gynecol Obstet 111:141, 1960
5. Burke WA, Burford JH, Dorfman RF: Hodgkin's disease in the mediastinum. J Thorac Cardiovasc Surg 3:287, 1967
6. Carlens E: Mediastinoscopy. Dis Chest 36:343, 1959
7. Enquist RW, Tormey DC, Jenis EH, Warkel RL: Malignant chemodectoma of the superior mediastinum with elevated urinary homovanillic acid. Chest 66:209, 1974
8. Freant LJ, Joseph WL, Adkins PC: Scar carcinoma of the lung. Fact or fantasy? Ann Thorac Surg 17:531, 1974
9. Gale AW, Jelihovsky T, Grant AF, Leekie BD, Nicks R: Neurogenic tumors of the mediastinum. Ann Thorac Surg 16:141, 1973
10. Graziano JL, Spinazzola A, Neville WE. Prosthetic replacement of the tracheal carina. Ann Thorac Surg 4:1, 1967
11. Green J, Forman WH: Response of thymoma to steroids. Chest 65:114, 1974
12. Greenfield LJ, Shelley WM: The spectrum of neurogenic tumors of the sympathetic nervous system: maturation and adrenergic function. J Natl Cancer Inst 35:215, 1965
13. Grillo HC, Greenberg JJ, Wilkins EW: Resection of bronchogenic carcinoma involving the thoracic wall. J Thorac Cardiovasc Surg 64:400, 1972
14. Grosfeld JL, Weinberger M, Kilman JW, Clatworthy HW: Primary mediastinal neoplasms in infants and children. Ann Thorac Surg 12:179, 1971
15. Jones JC, Kern WH, Chapman ND, Meyer BW, Lindesmith GG: Long-term survival after surgical resection for bronchogenic carcinoma. J Thorac Cardiovasc Surg 54:383, 1967
16. Kilman JW, Kassen KP: Thymoma. Am J Surg 121:170, 1971
17. Kirsh MM, Dickerman R, Fayos J, Lampe I, Pellegrini R, Gago O, Sloan H: The value of chest wall resection in the treatment of superior sulcus tumors of the lung. Ann Thorac Surg 15:339, 1973
18. Kirsh MM, Kahn DR, Gago O, Lampe I, Fayos JV, Prior M, Moores WY, Haight C, Sloan H: Treatment of bronchogenic carcinoma with mediastinal metastases. Ann Thorac Surg 12:11, 1971

19. Lattes R: Thymomas and other tumors of the thymus: analysis of 107 cases. Cancer 15:1224, 1962

20. Lee YT, Hutcheson: Mediastinal parathyroid carcinoma detected on routine chest films. Chest 65:354, 1974

21. McNeill TM, Chamberlain IM: Diagnostic anterior mediastinotomy. Ann Thorac Surg 2:532, 1966

22. Morton DL, Itabashi HH, Grimes OF: Nonmetastatic neurological complications of bronchogenic carcinoma. J Thorac Cardiovasc Surg 51:14, 1966

23. Paulson DL: Carcinoma of the lung. Curr Probl Surg Nov, 1967

24. Shields TW, Yee J, Conn JH, Robinette CD: Relationship of cell type and lymph node metastasis to survival after resection of bronchial carcinoma. Ann Thorac Surg 20:501–510, 1975

25. Takita H, Mongoya RB: Thymoma: clinical pathological observation. NYJ Med 70:2667, 1970

26. Thomas TV: Thymus and myasthenia gravis. Ann Thorac. Surg 13:499, 1972

27. Van Heerden JA, Harrison EG Jr, Bernatz PE, Kiely JM: Mediastinal malignant lymphoma. Chest 57:518, 1970

28. Weissberg D, Goldberg M, Pearson FG: Thymoma. Ann Thorac Surg 16:141, 1973

29. Wilkens EW Jr, Edmunds LH, Cast Ceman B: Cases of thymoma at the Massachusetts General Hospital. J Thorac Cardiovasc Surg 52:322, 1966

30. Wolfe WG, Sealy WC, Young, WG: Surgical management of myasthenia gravis. Ann Thorac Surg 14:645, 1972

7

Management of Breast Cancer

Breast cancer is the most prevalent cancer in women in the United States today. Of the major cancers we attempt to modify by management, it is also the cancer that appears to be the most amenable to diagnostic and therapeutic efforts. Nevertheless, we still can expect approximately half of the women with the diagnosis of breast cancer to die of this disease within 10 years of diagnosis. The death rate from breast cancer (approximately 25/100,000 female population) has remained relatively stable in the United States over the last 40 years.

The pathologic categories of breast cancer include a large number of histologic types of epithelial neoplasms (infiltrating duct carcinoma, lobular carcinoma, colloid carcinoma, medullary carcinoma, comedocarcinoma, and papillary carcinoma) as well as malignant neoplasms of mesenchymal origin (sarcomas), but the predominant cell type is infiltrating duct carcinoma or "scirrhous" cancer.

DIAGNOSIS

Although various technical advances have contributed to the earlier detection of breast cancer, a systematic and thorough clinical examination is required whenever there is a suggestion of breast disease. Since more than 90 percent of breast cancers are still discovered by the patients themselves, it is also essential that women be taught breast self-examination. This is a key aspect of our diagnostic effort. Excellent descriptions of self breast examination and medical examination are available[50] and will not be repeated here.

The diagnosis of the primary cancer in the breast is effectively established by aspiration or open surgical biopsy when a mass or some other physical irregularity is identified in the breast. The major differential diagnostic problem is produced by the hormonally induced variations in the breast that we have termed cystic "disease," but various benign neoplasms also require biopsy confirmation for differentiation. The decision regarding the need or appropriate site for biopsy is sometimes difficult in patients with large breasts, and xeromammography has proven to be a useful adjunct to this decision process in equivocal situations. It has also proven to be a useful technique for delineating additional sites appropriate for biopsy if a specific clinical finding in the breast leads to the need for an open biopsy. It should be stressed, however, that radiologic examination cannot eliminate the need for additional diagnostic investigation if there is any clinical suspicion of breast disease.

Our approach to the patient with a physical finding suspected of being cystic disease is to obtain xeromammograms. When the physical and radiologic examinations suggest the diagnosis of macrocysts or cystic disease, we aspirate or attempt to aspirate these "masses." We are then satisfied regarding the diagnosis if nonbloody fluid is obtained and there is complete disappearance of the concerning physical finding. If the clinical or radiologic diagnosis is in doubt, or if the attempt to aspirate the presumed cyst does not match the above requirements, open surgical biopsy is necessary unless aspiration biopsy has revealed cancer. Open biopsy can be accomplished under local or general anesthesia, but our preference in patients with cystic disease is for general anesthesia. This allows precise and adequate resection of the anatomic area of concern and also facilitates reconstruction of the defect produced.

Aspiration biopsy is a convenient technique for establishing the diagnosis of breast cancer in a patient with a suspicious mass, and it has become a more "respectable" procedure that it once was in the eyes of many surgeons. The technique is that of staining and examining a smear of a small quantity of tissue obtained from a mass by negative pressure produced in an appropriate syringe. This approach definitely requires close collaboration with the pathologist, who must be experienced in diagnosing cancer from cytologic examination of individual cells. In a patient with clinical findings diagnostic for or indicative of breast cancer, it is a simple office procedure that may confirm the clinical diagnosis histologically. If findings are "positive," aspiration biopsy allows for an efficient "staging" approach to the patient before developing a specific treatment plan. This type of biopsy may be readily employed during an attempted aspiration of a suspected breast cyst if the characteristic fluid is not obtained. However, the absence of cancer cells on this examination does not establish a benign diagnosis, and the patient then requires a more formal biopsy for diagnostic confirmation.

It was formerly believed that treatment by operation should be performed immediately upon obtaining histologic proof of breast cancer by open surgical biopsy. It has become obvious, however, that this concept was without basis, and many clinicians now prefer to perform breast biopsy before a thorough workup of the patient for metastatic disease. They then plan the appropriate laboratory investigations for staging if and when the diagnosis of cancer is established. Although this approach is optimal in some patients, we usually prefer to obtain the chest x-ray, standard biochemical determinations, and isotope bone scans before open surgical biopsy (if an attempted aspiration biopsy has not been diagnostic) in all patients with breast lesions truly suspicious of breast cancer. Since operation is still our primary treatment of localized breast cancer, it does allow the patient the convenience of having one combined operative procedure rather than two trips to the operating room.

Early Diagnosis

Our lack of progress in improving treatment results for clinically apparent breast cancer has led to a great interest in screening asymptomatic women for the presence of occult nonpalpable breast cancer. However, the role of xeromammography for the diagnosis of breast cancer in the absence of any physical findings is an entirely different situation than described earlier for a patient with a palpable breast mass. The specific role of this technique for screening asymptomatic patients without physical findings still requires clarification. Xeromammography can certainly detect cancers not clinically apparent to the patient or physician, but the yield of significant lesions in unselected populations is low,[47,76] and the cost of the examination in terms of equipment and manpower is considerable. Therefore, this examination, which also involves exposure to radiation, should be used selectively rather than universally in our female population. For example, women over 35 with positive family history of breast cancer, with abnormal thermograms, or with questionable physical findings might be realistic candidates for this complex radiologic screening examination. These and other criteria being studied currently may lead to use of xeromammography for a fraction of the asymptomatic women entering an organized screening process, and they may also bring the yield from this examination into a higher and more rewarding range.

The radiologic finding of an "occult" breast cancer that eventually proves to be *infiltrating* breast cancer should lead to the same staging approach and treatment plan as used for patients who have palpable breast cancer since this minimal lesion will have behavioral characteristics similar to those of the more obvious breast cancers, even with the favorable feature of being small. A real reward of screening, however, is the detection of an occult *noninfiltrating* cancer. This is probably a situation in which clinical cancer can be prevented by appropriate treatment.

Other diagnostic approaches for screening asymptomatic female populations for breast cancer have included serum assays for carcinoembryonic antigen[105] and urinary assays for polyamines.[72,108] Neither of these assays appears to be of value for detecting subclinical disease as each assay shows a low frequency of abnormal evaluations even in populations of women with established breast cancer. Breast thermography is being more thoroughly evaluated for screening purposes, but it has the opposite disadvantage: that of finding frequent temperature variations between the breasts in patients without clinically significant breast disease. This lack of specificity clearly reduces the value of thermography. This screening technique may have usefulness in our attempt to identify the "high-risk" populations suitable for xeromammography, but the breast screening projects have not shown it to be of particular benefit thus far.

STAGING OF BREAST CANCER

The choice of therapy for breast cancer, as with all cancers, depends on appropriate staging of the cancer in individual patients. The staging classifications of breast cancer extend from the most primitive (inoperable versus operable) to the more precise attempts to develop staging criteria with more reliable prognostic significance (TNM classification). Certain problems are inherent in any clinical staging system, but staging does provide both a common language among clinicians and a means for making logical decisions in treatment planning.

A number of systems have been used including the Manchester system, the "Columbia" system, and the TNM system (both American Joint Committee and the UICC).[50] Although these systems appear different on superficial examination, an attempt to classify hypothetical clinical findings by all these staging methods reveals few real discrepancies among them (Table 7-1). Clinicians are frustrated by the inherent inaccuracy in the clinical assessment of the disease that is present and the uncertainty contained in the use of descriptive terms such as "fixation to pectoral muscles," "fixation to the chest wall," and "fixed axillary lymph nodes." These staging systems also fail to take the dynamic growth characteristics of the cancer into consideration.[17] From a review of these systems it appears that the most significant aspects of these classifications are the actual size of the primary cancer in the breast,[28,40] the presence and extent of axillary lymph node enlargement, and the observed presence or absence of distant metastasis. These prognostic factors do affect our treatment planning and they must be defined using an accepted language.

In the past the term "inoperable" was synonymous with incurable, but the imprecision of this concept has been demonstrated by long-term cancer control following radiation therapy in some patients considered to be "inoperable."[49,113] However, identification of a status of incurability on clinical evaluation is important so that the patient can be spared some of the local disadvantages of treatment (particularly mastectomy) if this is the case. Progress has been achieved in this important aspect of classification or staging by means of bone scintiscanning, which can demonstrate bone metastases in an asymptomatic stage in patients who have breast cancer.[68,90] Bone scintiscanning is not truly specific; there are occasional "false positives," but these can be minimized if the clinician obtains biopsy confirmation of metastasis in any patient who has a *solitary* abnormality on bone scan. The other major sites for distant spread from breast cancer (lung, liver, and distant lymph nodes) are less amenable to laboratory detection, but chest x-ray and liver function tests fulfill this role reasonably well.

The following clinical findings indicate advanced "inoperable" disease, and their presence allows categorization of the patient for palliative therapy:

1. distant metastases of any kind,
2. metastatic involvement of supraclavicular lymph nodes,
3. fixed involved axillary lymph nodes,
4. arm edema secondary to axillary metastases,
5. chest wall fixation by neoplasm,
6. involvement of the entire breast by neoplasm,
7. "inflammatory" cancer of the breast.

Although some of the more subtle regional findings on physical examination of the breast may be disputed by various clinicians and staging systems (in regard to "operability"), the key concern—the presence of occult metastatic disease—will be clarified by the appropriate pretreatment studies described.

The ultimate prognosis of the breast cancer patient treated by surgery or irradiation is clearly related to the stage of disease at the time of diagnosis.[50] For stage I (or A) the 5-year and 10-year survival figures are 83 percent and 68 percent, respectively. For patients in stage II (or B),

Table 7-1
Comparison of Clinical Staging Systems for Breast Cancer

"Manchester" Staging System		Columbia Classification		TNM Staging System (American Joint Committee, 1973)	
Primary	*A. Nodes*	*Primary*	*A. Nodes*	*Primary*	*A. Nodes*
I Operable	Not palpable	(A) no edema, ulceration, or fixation	Not palpable	T1: <2 cm without (1a) or with (1b) pectoral muscle or fascia fixation	N0: not palpable; N1a: palpable but not considered to contain growth
II Operable	Mobile and palpable	(B) no edema, ulceration, or fixation	Mobile and palpable (<2.5 cm)	T0: no tumor; T1: <2 cm; T2a: 2–5 cm; or T2b: 2–5 cm with pectoral fixation	N1b: palpable, clinically "positive"; N0, N1a, or N2

III	Borderline operable	Mobile and palpable or not palpable	(C) any one of the following: 1. edema (<1/3 breast skin) 2. ulceration 3. fixation to chest wall	Mobile and palpable 1. nodes >2.5 cm 2. "fixed" nodes	T3: >5 cm without (3a) or with (3b) pectoral fixation; T4: fixation, ulceration, edema, or satellite nodules; and T1 or T2	N0; N1; N2: fixed; or N3: supraclavicular, infra-clavicular, or arm edema
IV	Inoperable	"Fixed" and/or distant metastasis	(D) more advanced lesions in-cluding: 1. combination of 2 signs listed under C 2. edema of skin (>1/3 breast) 3. satellite skin nodules 4. inflammatory cancer 5. palpable supraclavicular nodes 6. parasternal "tumor" 7. arm edema 8. distant metastases	Any T with distant metastases (M1)	Any N with distant metastases (M1)

153

these figures are 57 percent and 39 percent. The 5-year survival figures for stage III (C), 34 percent, and for stage IV (D), 18 percent, are considerably lower, as might be expected.

CHOICE OF TREATMENT OF
PRIMARY BREAST CANCER

If a patient has localized breast cancer without grave signs suggesting or establishing incurability by regional means of therapy, many treatment alternatives are available. From these a choice must be made. At this time there are data suggesting no particular advantage from some of these approaches over others, but there are few reliable data for establishing the truly optimal treatment. The treatment alternatives are listed in Table 7-2. Data at this time appear to have reliably answered some of the questions raised by a consideration of these treatment alternatives. There is essentially general agreement that: (a) no benefit from surgical removal of the internal mammary lymph nodes (as a routine operative approach) has been demonstrated;[14,58,66] (b) no benefit has been demonstrated from the administration of postoperative radiation therapy or prophylactic castration after radical mastectomy;[41,62,86,92] (c) radiation therapy can control breast cancer effectively, but its relative effectiveness, in comparison to that of surgical methods, has not been completely clarified.[88,113]

Some questions are being answered by recently completed studies of primary surgical treatment of breast cancer (but with inadequate follow-up time for full confidence in the answers): Should axillary lymph nodes be treated as part of the initial treatment effort if they are not clinically palable?* Is radiation therapy equal (or superior) to axillary dissection if

Table 7-2
Primary Treatment Alternatives for
Localized Breast Cancer

1. Radical mastectomy[2,50,51]	
2. Extended radical mastectomy[112] (internal mammary lymph nodes)	With or without radiation therapy
3. Modified radical mastectomy[75] (preservation of pectoral muscles)	
4. Total (simple) mastectomy[24,79]	
5. Segmental mastectomy[25]	
6. Primary radiation therapy[49,88] (after biopsy)	

* NSABP Protocol #4.

treatment for nonpalpable axillary lymph nodes proves to be beneficial?* If the axillary lymph nodes are clinically involved, is radiation therapy equal (or superior) to axillary dissection?*   Are the results of local or regional treatment of breast cancer improved by adjuvant therapy with systemic methods (chemotherapy or immunotherapy)?

The answers obtained thus far to the above questions *suggest* that the treatment results are no different whether axillary nodes are treated initially or not if they are not palpable, and the end results of treatment of clinically involved nodes are similar whether treated by surgery or radiation therapy.   After years of "negative" results, adjuvant systemic chemotherapy has now been shown to reduce the incidence of recurrence and metastasis in the early period after primary surgical treatment of breast cancer.[11,34,39,42,64]   These answers are considered inconclusive at present, but confidence in these findings will certainly develop from the long-term follow-up of the clinical trials concerned.   Treatment planning should cautiously exploit this available information, and we believe all patients with lymphatic metastases should receive adjuvant chemotherapy.

Important questions regarding the regional treatment of breast cancer remain unanswered: Is there a demonstrable therapeutic advantage to the surgical removal of the pectoral muscles over their preservation (radical mastectomy versus modified radical mastectomy) in terms of end results?   Is partial mastectomy equal to more aggressive methods of resection for breast cancer when the cancer is *clinically* well localized?   Is radiation therapy after partial mastectomy (or incisional biopsy) equal in treatment result to methods relying on surgical removal of the breast with or without regional lymph nodes?

The answer to the first question is probably "no," in view of the early answers obtained in the clinical trials mentioned in the previous category of questions.   However, a specific clinical trial addressed to this point would be indicated if long-term results from the earlier trials did eventually demonstrate a need for the initial treatment of nonpalpable axillary lymph nodes.   The frequency of other microscopic cancerous foci in the breast with established cancer makes partial mastectomy appear to be a poor choice for the treatment of curable breast cancer at this time, but some patients (although it is impossible to define which ones) could conceivably be treated on a local basis with this approach.

The answer to the last question must await results of ongoing clinical trials.   Data from clinical trials in Great Britain[6] appear to demonstrate that partial mastectomy combined with postoperative radiation therapy equals radical mastectomy in terms of end results if the nodes are *not* clinically involved at the time of initial evaluation *and* if "salvage" surgery is considered acceptable for some patients in the radiation therapy group. These results may be modified, however, by alterations in radiation therapy dosage used in subsequent clinical trials in this country.

Choice of Surgical Treatment

Despite these unanswered and partially answered questions about available treatment strategies, the clinician must decide on the primary therapy for his patient with breast cancer. In this regard it seems fair to make the following statements about therapy for breast cancer patients with clinically localized disease: First, partial mastectomy, with or without radiation therapy, should not be employed on a general basis until clinial trials establish that this is equal (or superior) to methods employing removal of the entire breast.[23,95,101] Second, mastectomy, with or without axillary dissection, is indicated if no clinically involved axillary lymph nodes are present. Third, mastectomy with axillary lymph node dissection (radical mastectomy or "modified" radical mastectomy)[75] or mastectomy combined with adequate postoperative x-ray therapy should be performed if axillary lymph nodes are clinically palapable. Finally, adjuvant systemic chemotherapy should be employed in addition to mastectomy in patients who have histologically demonstrated axillary lymph node metastases.[39]

These conclusions regarding our current information are not entirely compatible since knowledge of axillary lymph node status for the purpose of chemotherapy decisions will not be available in patients who do not undergo axillary dissection. Nevertheless, these premises are helpful in developing a logical treatment plan and our clinical approach is as follows.

Careful clinical and laboratory evaluation of the patient is first accomplished to eliminate those patients from a mastectomy group who will not ultimately benefit in terms of long-term survival.

Mastectomy with axillary dissection is performed in patients with "localized" or "operable" cancer (despite lack of proof of need for lymph node dissection in patients with clinically negative axillae) because of our interest in axillary node staging and its helpful role in selecting patients for adjuvant chemotherapy.[97] We believe either radical mastectomy or "modified" radical mastectomy is acceptable for this purpose, and we see little real difference between these procedures in most situations.

Adjuvant systemic chemotherapy is administered postoperatively to patients with pathologic evidence of axillary lymph node metastases. If the initial reported clinical results are substantiated, this is more likely to improve overall results than any of the modifications of regional treatment that have been discussed. Our own patients are entered into cooperative clinical trials comparing the currently standard adjuvant chemotherapy with potentially superior modifications of this regime.

A reasonable alternative to the above plan is elimination of axillary dissection in patients with clinically negative axillae, but logic in this circumstance would dictate adjuvant chemotherapy for all patients since there would be no way to determine which patients had lymphatic metastasis. It also should be stressed that the extent of the regional treatment of breast cancer must be modified on occasion by age and concurrent medical problems.

Management of Patients with Breast Cancer Unsuitable for Surgical Therapy

If a patient with breast cancer has advanced local disease that will not be satisfactorily encompassed by a surgical procedure, we favor radiation therapy to the breast and regional lymphatics if there is no clinical evidence of distant metastatic disease. Radiation therapy is our most effective palliative tool for breast cancer; long-term control of some "inoperable" patients is accomplished by a course of radiation therapy to the breast, supraclavicular region, axilla, and internal mammary chain,[49,113] using cobalt or supervoltage therapy. Many surgeons stress the value of palliative "toilet" mastectomy for some of these patients before or sometime during radiation therapy. There are major disadvantages to this approach, particularly in the patient with bulky regional disease, and it may complicate rather than expedite the radiation plan. Local regrowth of cancer in the operative wound is not unexpected in such patients, and local tolerance to radiation may be reduced. In our experience "palliative" simple (or total) mastectomy is rarely indicated in the patient who is considered a suitable candidate for primary radiation therapy.

In some patients with "inoperable" breast cancer this characterization is primarily owing to the presence of distant metastasis, whereas the local manifestations of the disease are more limited. Under these circumstances radiation therapy to the breast may be omitted from the initial treatment plan. Reliance for local control can then be placed on systemic means of palliative therapy. The systemic treatment plan and our priorities for choice of therapy are discussed in the section on recurrent and metastatic disease.

"Borderline Operable" Breast Cancer

A small group of patients have no evidence of distant metastases but have physical findings in the region of the breast that lead to concern about the advisability of using an operation as the primary therapy. It is conceivable that such patients might enjoy long-term control by regional treatment methods, but the volume of disease may be excessive for complete reliance on radiation therapy for local control. Although the classification, is arbitrary we have placed such patients in a category of "borderline operable" in our clinic. These patients are thoroughly evaluated because we suspect that the disease may be inoperable. For this group we add ipsilateral supraclavicular (or scalene) lymph node biopsy to the pretreatment evaluation, despite the absence of palpable cervical nodes, on the supposition that these patients have a high risk of demonstrating microscopic lymphatic disease outside the field of potential surgical resection. We supplement our systemic workup and bone scintiscan with a complete radiologic bone survey on the same basis. Bone marrow aspiration for cancer cells is performed also in selected cases.

If this thorough pretreatment evaluation reveals occult, previously unrecognized metastatic disease, the patient is then properly classified as "inoperable" and treated in the fashion outlined previously. If no occult metastatic spread is detected on this pretreatment evaluation, we manage this select group of patients by a full course of radiotherapy to the breast, axilla, and supraclavicular region on the assumption that occult disease may become manifest at an early time on subsequent follow-up examinations. One month after completing radiation therapy, the patient is again fully evaluated by clinical and laboratory investigation; if no distant disease can be detected, radical mastectomy is performed.

The above approach is essentially that described earlier by Fletcher.[43] Our criteria for treating selected patients in this fashion are (a) a primary breast lesion larger than 10 cm in diameter, (b) clinically involved axillary lymph nodes larger than 2 cm but not "fixed," (c) absence of distant metastases, and (d) patients who are neither elderly nor suffering from concurrent medical disease. The value of this approach for this select group of "questionable" breast cancers has not been determined; but it is of interest that all but 2 of 32 patients treated in this fashion have demonstrated residual cancer in the surgical specimen (either the breast or regional lymph nodes), a factor partially confirming the inability of radiation therapy to control cancer when it is in a relatively advanced stage. Of additional interest, only 2 of these 32 patients manifested local recurrence on short-term follow-up examination ranging up to 8 years. However, of the 32 patients entering this treatment program, 24 have manifested distant metastases during the period of follow-up. This approach requires continued cautious evaluation in this selected group.

SPECIAL PROBLEMS IN MANAGEMENT OF LOCALIZED BREAST CANCER

Management of Noninfiltrating (in situ) Cancer

The noninfiltrating form of breast carcinoma may be discovered by a biopsy of either a clinically benign breast mass or a nonpalpable lesion discovered by xeromammography. Carcinoma may be of duct origin (intraductal) or lobular origin (lobular carcinoma in situ).

Careful follow-up studies by McDivitt et al.,[78] Hutter and Foote,[56] and others[116] demonstrate the finding of in situ lobular cancer is of great prognostic significance. This preinvasive form of breast cancer is associated in most series with a high incidence of multiplicity of lesions and a significant incidence of subsequent invasive breast cancer in the same breast, and to a lesser extent in the opposite breast. On this basis it is our current conviction that the pathologic finding of in situ lobular cancer merits mastectomy of some type with an appropriate biopsy examination of the opposite breast.[111] Our preference is for total (simple) mastectomy on the side of the histologic finding, and management of the opposite breast is dependent on the biopsy findings from that breast. The choice of site for biopsy in the opposite breast will be benefited by preoperative xeromammography. In the absence of xeromammographic findings, a generous segment for biopsy should be obtained from the upper outer quadrant and/or the mirror image site in the "normal" breast.

If the noninfiltrative breast lesion in question is an intraductal lesion, the question of appropriate therapy is much more difficult to determine in view of the lack of sufficient data on the multifocal nature of this process in the same or the opposite breast and the lack of information regarding the capability of xeromammography to detect additional lesions that may be present. It is tempting to consider adequate resection of the involved area in the breast by segmental mastectomy and then carry out frequent follow-up evaluations, both clinical and radiologic. However, we prefer total (simple) mastectomy in view of inadequate data to substantiate a more-limited approach. Contralateral breast biopsy is performed if xeromammographic findings indicate an appropriate site for this, but routine "blind biopsy" seems less rewarding in these patients.[65] A detailed radiologic and pathologic study of these totally resected breasts is clearly indicated as the findings might substantiate a less-aggressive approach to this clinical problem in the future and thereby demonstrate some positive evidence of value to the patient from this type of "early diagnosis."

Contralateral Breast Biopsy in Patients with Unilateral Infiltrating Carcinoma of the Breast

Patients with infiltrating lobular carcinoma of the breast constitute a particularly "high-risk" group for the development of carcinoma of the opposite breast, this risk being even greater than that stated for patients with cancer of the breast as a whole. This fact is substantiated by the data referred to for in situ lobular carcinoma of the breast in the previous section. For this reason we carry out elective biopsy of the clinically normal contralateral breast during initial treatment of infiltrating lobular carcinoma in all patients, even if xeromammograms fail to reveal a suspicious area.[37,65] It has been proposed that such a biopsy be repeated at intervals in this population of patients, and the clinical data tend to substantiate this idea.

Patients with the more frequent form of infiltrating duct cancer represent a somewhat different situation than described for lobular carcinoma. Urban[111] has advised routine generous contralateral "blind" biopsy of the opposite breast as standard procedure for patients with infiltrating duct carcinoma, as well as for those with lobular carcinoma, on the basis of the "yield" he has observed, as well as the ever-present concern regarding the known risk of carcinoma in the opposite breast. In our series of routine contralateral "blind" breast biopsies, we discovered one infiltrating and four noninfiltrating cancers in a consecutive series of 109 patients.[65] In view of this relatively low yield from "routine" contralateral breast biopsy and the concomitant improvement in xeroradiographic techniques for discovery of occult lesions, we have shifted our emphasis to selective rather than routine biopsy of the opposite breast. Selection of patients and the site for biopsy is based on preoperative xeromammographic findings since all of our patients undergo this examination before the operation for breast cancer.

Operative Management of Patients with Suspicious Radiologic Findings in the Absence of a Palpable Breast Mass

The frequency of this clinical problem has closely followed the development of sophisticated radiologic techniques (xeromammography).[47,76] The major problem for the surgeon is to be certain that he has excised the area in question for adequate pathologic examination. Close coordination and consultation with the radiologist regarding the location of the process in question are obviously mandatory before surgical biopsy, but other techniques have been suggested for more accurate localization of the lesion seen on the xeromammograms.[94,96] Some techniques are of particular importance in patients in whom the suspicious lesion does not have tiny focal calcifications since their absence makes radiologic confirmation of the removal of the suspicious lesion difficult by specimen radiology (Fig. 7-1). A simple and effective method we have employed is the preoperative placement of a needle into the suspicious area using xeromammographic control.[11] Then 0.5 cc of methylene blue is instilled into the breast tissue after there is confidence that the needle tip is adjacent to the area of concern. During surgery the area of the involved quadrant is opened and the segment containing the dye is resected (Fig. 7-2). We prefer to avoid additional surgery at the time of biopsy of this type of lesion as the pathologist usually requires extensive sections and careful study before rendering a final diagnosis.

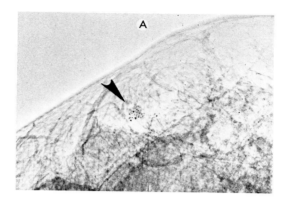

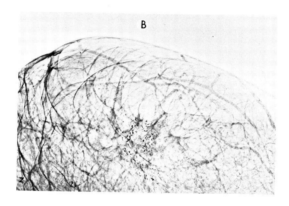

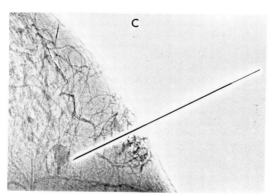

Fig. 7-1. **A&B:** Xeromammograms with "suspicious" calcification. **C:** Xeromammogram without calcification with
needle adjacent to the nonpalpable mass detected by radiologic examination. (Courtesy of Harold Goodman, M.D.)

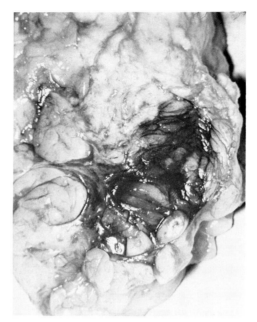

Fig. 7-2.   Photograph of breast specimen injected with dye preoperatively to identify the nonpalpable breast lesion detected by xeromammography.

Bilateral Infiltrating Cancer of the Breast

The increased incidence of infiltrating breast cancer in patients who have already had breast cancer is well known, and it is not surprising that an occasional patient may have synchronous bilateral infiltrating cancers of the breast.[93,117]   The principal problem in this situation is the differentiation of an independent primary lesion in the contralateral breast. Although a patient with breast cancer has an increased likelihood of developing a simultaneous or subsequent contralateral primary breast cancer, metastasis to the opposite breast is actually a more common occurrence.   This difficult differential diagnosis is aided by the histologic demonstration of in situ carcinoma within the duct system of the breast in question, a comparison of the histologic types of the two cancers thought to be independent primaries, and determination of the presence or absence of other metastatic lesions in the patient.   If the clinical presentation of the breast mass in the contralateral breast occurs some time after the original breast cancer has been treated (metachronous) and the investigations described indicate that the lesion is probably not a metastasis,

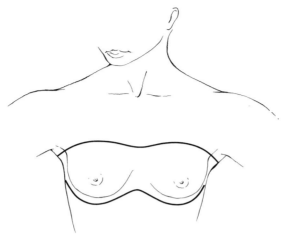

Fig. 7-3.   Incision for simultaneous bilateral mastectomy.

mastectomy is certainly indicated if the clinical findings are compatible with the definition of "operability" discussed previously.

If the bilateral breast lesions occur synchronously, bilateral mastectomy can be accomplished in suitable cases by using a transverse incision extending from one axilla to another.   Generous resection of skin in the region of both breasts is essential, but the butterfly design of the incision prevents necrosis of central skin overlying the sternum (Fig. 7-3).   This operative incision can also be employed for patients with infiltrating cancer in one breast and noninfiltrating cancer in the other.   If a radiologically suspicious lesion is detected in the contralateral breast of a patient with unilateral breast cancer, we prefer to complete the pathologic diagnosis on this apparently less significant lesion before embarking on the primary operation for the proven cancer.

Paget's Disease of the Breast

Paget's disease, an uncommon clinical presentation of intraductal carcinoma of the breast, can be diagnosed by biopsy of the characteristic eczematous lesion of the nipple.   If no mass is present in the breast, the incidence of infiltrating cancer on microscopic study of the resected breast is less and axillary lymph node metastases are quite rare (Table 7-3).[4,83]   Most surgeons believe that total mastectomy, with or without removal of the lower axillary nodes, is appropriate treatment for Paget's disease when there is no palpable breast mass, and this is our preference. Patients with Paget's disease of the nipple and a palpable breast mass

Table 7-3

Frequency of Infiltration of Breast Cancer and Lymphatic
Metastases in Relation to Presence or Absence of a Mass
in Patients with Paget's Disease

		Pathologic Findings	
	No.	Infiltrative Cancer	Lymphatic Metastases
Paget's disease without breast mass	96	33(34%)	13(14%)
Paget's disease with palpable breast mass	113	106(94%)	74(65%)

Data from Ashikari et al.[4]

share all of the clinical features of patients with breast cancer without
Paget's disease, and they should be treated accordingly.

The presence of nipple discharge without a nipple lesion has a significance totally different from that of Paget's disease. In women under
the age of 40, nipple discharge is virtually always owing to benign disease
(duct ectasia or intraductal papilloma). Moreover, nipple discharge is
rarely owing to cancer in the older age group, except in a few patients
with blood or blood-tinged fluid in the discharge. Excision of the entire
subareolar duct system is the most practical approach for both diagnosis
and control of the discharge (clear or blood-tinged) if no breast mass is
palpable. Virtually all of these operative procedures primarily benefit the
patient's peace of mind since the usual finding is a benign process.

Metastatic Cancer in the Axilla
Without a Breast Mass

If the histologic diagnosis from an excised axillary lymph node in a
patient without breast mass is compatible with the diagnosis of breast
cancer, and if there are no clinical or laboratory findings to suggest another primary cancer or distant metastasis, the classic approach has been
radical mastectomy on the basis that an occult breast primary with lymphatic metastases is the most likely explanation for the findings. The
technique of xeroradiography and the techniques available for searching
for distant metastasis have refined the management of this problem in
many instances. Nevertheless, in some cases uncertainty remains after
these more sophisticated examinations. In this instance we still perform
radical mastectomy if our pathologist believes the lesion in the axillary

lymph node is probably metastatic breast cancer and if we are unable to detect other metastases by laboratory means (including ipsilateral scalene node biopsy).

Carcinoma of the Breast During Pregnancy and Lactation

The diagnosis of breast cancer during pregnancy and lactation is often delayed and is certainly more difficult than at other times. This association is infrequent, but it has developed the deserved reputation of being a grave problem. This is primarily because the disease is usually locally advanced at the time of initial treatment and the incidence of lymphatic metastases is high. Patients who have no lymph node metastases in their surgical specimen have control rates comparable to those of patients who are not pregnant, but those who have positive nodes have an unusually poor prognosis. Even in the larger series studied, the data are too scanty to draw positive conclusions regarding the potential theoretical benefits of therapeutic abortion and/or castration of these patients.[54,74] In view of this we believe that pregnant or postpartum patients with breast cancer should be treated solely on the basis of the extent of their breast disease.

"Inflammatory" Breast Cancer

This rare (1 percent) clinical presentation of primary breast cancer is characterized by local physical signs of acute inflammation similar to erysipelas, but there is no fever, tenderness, or leukocytosis.[38] In pregnant or lactating women this form of breast cancer is often mistaken for cellulitis or mastitis. These unique physical findings are owing to extensive neoplastic infiltration of the subepidermal lymphatics, and the diffuse growth pattern in this type of patient may not even produce a clearly defined breast mass. If a biopsy of the skin of the breast confirms this diagnosis, the patient is not suitable for surgical therapy since total removal of disease of this type is not really feasible. Radiation therapy is recommended for local management, but long-term control is usually not possible if the process fulfills the pathologic criteria for inflammatory carcinoma.

Carcinoma of the Male Breast

Although breast cancer in the male is rare and represents less than 1 percent of all breast cancers, the presence of a mass in the older adult male breast warrants suspicion of a malignant tumor.[22,36,85] This suspicion should be increased if nipple discharge is also present. Clinical assessment and therapeutic choice are analogous to those described for women, but adequate skin resection in men undergoing mastectomy always requires graft coverage. The overall survival rate is slightly lower than that in women, and this difference is observed primarily in patients with lymph node metastases. It is of interest that orchiectomy, as a palliative method of therapy, has a higher response rate in patients with metastatic disease than that achieved by oophorectomy for a similar-stage female breast cancer. Data on other endocrine ablative procedures and nonsurgical palliative methods are too limited for such comparisons.

Malignant Mesenchymal Tumors of the Breast

The major forms of sarcoma of the breast are the malignant form of cystosarcoma phyllodes,[109] primary lymphoma of the breast,[32] angiosarcoma of the breast,[104] and a variety of assorted stromal sarcomas.[10] The last includes categories from malignant mesenchymoma to fibrosarcoma, but all of these sarcomatous lesions are extremely rare in a population of patients with breast masses. Most surgeons feel that adequate local resection, usually by total mastectomy, is appropriate therapy for most of these mesodermal lesions because the prime cause of treatment failure is either local recurrence or hematogenous spread. Metastasis to the regional lymph nodes is not a pathologic feature of most of these lesions. Radical mastectomy has been recommended for the rare highly malignant angiosarcoma of the breast, but none of the reported cases has demonstrated axillary node mestatasis despite a small but definite incidence of lymphatic metastasis with this type of sarcoma in other sites.

"Local Recurrence" After Primary Therapy for Breast Cancer

In a clinical trial of segmental mastectomy combined with radiation therapy (Atkins et al.[6]), there were patients with local recurrence following this therapy who were subsequently managed successfully by radical mastectomy. On this basis one could assume that secondary surgical resection is a reasonable choice for recurrence after limited surgery, but the preeminence of primary surgery by mastectomy in this country makes this problem an infrequent occurrence. The subsequent appearance of clinically involved lymph nodes after prior mastectomy without axillary dissection is another situation where secondary surgery is indicated with some hope of ultimate "success."

The fact that local "recurrence" in the operative wound area after radical mastectomy and distant metastatic disease appear simultaneously

Table 7-4
Treatment of "Local" Recurrence After Mastectomy

Clinical Factors	Type of Treatment
Local recurrence only and no prior chest wall irradiation	Local irradiation only
Local recurrence only, prior chest wall irradiation, and "free interval" >3 years since mastectomy	Chest wall resection
Local recurrence only, prior chest wall irradiation, and "free interval" <3 years	"Systemic" therapy
Symptomatic local recurrence plus other recurrent disease; no prior chest wall irradiation	Local irradiation plus "systemic" therapy

in many patients has led to the conclusion that this form of local "recurrence" is usually just one manifestation of disseminated incurable breast cancer. However, data from the Mayo Clinic tend to refute this concept for patients with a significant interval between primary treatment and the appearance of the local recurrence.[103] In this study patients developing recurrent disease in the operative area more than 4 years after mastectomy had a reasonable chance of long-term control by means of secondary local measures if there were no clinical or laboratory manifestations of generalized disease when the local problem appeared. The long-term study of chest wall resection for chest wall "recurrence" reported by Shah and Urban[102] supports this contention. On the other hand, most patients who developed local recurrence less than 4 years after mastectomy rapidly developed evidence of disseminated disease regardless of the treatment employed for the local recurrence. Thus treatment of local recurrence after mastectomy varies with these time factors and the nature of the prior treatment.

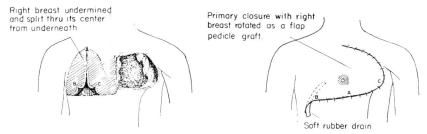

Fig. 7-4. Diagram showing use of the opposite breast to cover the operative defect at time of chest wall resection (from Urban and Baker[112]).

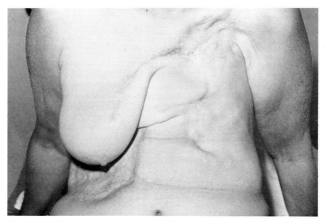

Fig. 7-5. Postoperative view of postmastectomy patient requiring chest wall (including sternum) resection for radionecrosis. Chest wall defect closed by large previously delayed
flap from contralateral breast and anterior thorax.

Our approach is summarized in Table 7-4. In those rare patients
with recurrence who are suitable candidates for resection of the chest
wall, we have employed either fascia lata or Marlex mesh for the chest
wall defect. Satisfactory skin coverage after resection has been achieved
by mobilization and splitting of the undersurface of the opposite breast as
described by Urban and Baker[112] (Fig. 7-4). It may be necessary in some
instances to delay a skin flap prior to resection, as was done in another patient requiring resection of the central portion of the sternum for radionecrosis (Fig. 7-5). Solutions to these problems must be individualized for
obvious reasons, but adequate skin coverage of the chest wall defect is
mandatory.

METASTATIC BREAST CANCER

Disseminated breast cancer is often responsive to our palliative tools,
be they endocrinologic or chemotherapeutic, but there are currently no
absolute guides for determining which patients will respond to various
treatments. Some clinical responses are quite dramatic; the response
rate with most treatments is reasonably high, and the predictability of
response to any one treatment is far from clear-cut despite recent advances in development of predictive assays. For these reasons, patients

with recurrent and/or metastatic breast cancer should probably receive the benefit of continued trials of palliative therapy as long as these can be reasonably tolerated.

The major clinical variables affecting probability of response to any palliative therapy include the anatomic sites of metastasis, the free interval between the initial treatment and the appearance of recurrent or metastatic disease, and the age and menopausal status of the patient. Prior clinical experience with these variables in the treatment of patients with hormonal and chemotherapeutic agents has led to guidelines for priority of treatment choices under various clinical circumstances. The relatively recent development of various tissue assays, particularly estrogen receptor activity, has further refined our approach to clinical management in spite of the paucity of information on the mechanisms by which any of these palliative methods work.

Metastatic disease from breast cancer usually develops in one or more of the following sites: soft tissues of adjacent or distant sites, distant lymphatics, bones, lungs, pleura, peritoneum, liver, and central nervous system. Analysis of the course of patients with disseminated carcinoma of the breast reveals that patients with metastasis to the central nervous system, the liver, and possibly the peritoneum fall into a "dire prognosis group."[27] Patients with metastasis to these sites have been shown to have a median survival period of only 6 months, and they are generally less responsive to palliative measures than patients in whom the pattern of metastatic disease involves other sites. Analysis of the pattern of recurrent disease also reveals that patients with a large number of sites of recurrent and metastatic disease have a shorter survival than those in whom the pattern of metastatic disease is more limited. On the other hand, patients with soft tissue or bone disease as the major or only manifestation of metastatic breast cancer usually have a longer survival and are more responsive to most therapies than patients in the dire prognosis group. The objective in managing patients in all categories is to improve the quality of life at the least "cost" for each individual circumstance, and these variations in the ultimate outcome may affect the magnitude of the treatment effort.

Another finding apparent in all studies of patients treated for recurrent and metastatic breast cancer is that there is a direct relationship between the length of the disease "free interval" and the duration of response to palliative treatment. This is not surprising since the length of this interval implies some correlation with the degree of aggressiveness of the individual cancer. Age and menopausal status also play a significant but unexplained role in choice of therapy. This is best exemplified by the definite response of some premenopausal patients to castration and the significant response to estrogen administration in many patients who are well beyond the menopause.

"Local" Therapy for Metastatic Disease

Although a relatively localized area of bone metastasis, a bulky lymph node or soft tissue mass, a mediastinal node mass producing esophageal or superior vena caval narrowing, or a pleural effusion represents just one manifestation of disseminated disease in a patient with metastatic breast cancer, it may be the only symptomatic finding. The ideal palliative therapy for this problem is often regional rather than systemic. Radiation therapy is particularly useful for localized manifestations of metastatic disease as the likelihood of effective response (approximately 75 percent) surpasses that with any systemic means at our disposal. This is certainly true for the palliative therapy for symptomatic bone metastasis or radiologic evidence of bone metastasis that may be a potential future site for pathologic fracture, but localized soft tissue disease is also responsive. We find it useful in many instances to defer systemic approaches to therapy in such patients until additional metastatic disease becomes manifest. This allows a more accurate assessment of the response to the systemic therapy chosen. On the other hand, patients already receiving a systemic treatment approach may benefit significantly from localized radiation to a particularly symptomatic or concerning site of metastatic disease.

Although radiation therapy is our most frequently employed regional technique, chemotherapy may play a similar regional treatment role for recurring pleural effusions. Intrapleural administration of an alkylating agent, such as nitrogen mustard (0.2 mg/kg) or, preferably, thio-TEPA (30–50 mg/kg), is frequently quite effective in control of this local problem. The amount of agent absorbed does not severely interfere with ongoing systemic chemotherapy.

Surgery is rarely indicated for localized metastatic disease, but there are some notable exceptions to this general rule. Pathologic fracture of a long bone (such as femur or humerus) or radiologic or clinical findings suggesting impending fracture are effectively managed by the operative insertion of appropriate skeletal fixation devices, after which radiotherapy can be employed.[100] Laminectomy for cord decompression is also indicated on an emergency basis when this acute neurologic problem arises, and radiation therapy and chemotherapy are used subsequently.

At some point patients requiring various forms of local palliative therapy will need a systemic approach. It is often useful at that time to have other sites of metastatic disease for objective evaluation of the response to the systemic approach employed, but this is obviously not mandatory.

Choice of Systemic Method of Palliative Therapy for Disseminated Breast Cancer

The methods of systemic therapy frequently employed are listed in Table 7-5 along with an estimate of the frequency of objective remission of breast cancer that has been experienced with each of these methods in the past. Two practical factors must be considered in the choice of systemic therapy: (a) the statistical likelihood of significant benefit from a therapy in a specific clinical setting, and (b) the disadvantages and difficulties produced by the treatment itself. Our policy for choice of palliative systemic treatment is generally based on the clinical factors shown in Table 7-6, but this choice will obviously be modified by any predictive information obtained from biochemical assays. The priority of treatment for each group is based on the concept that it is generally advisable to choose the therapy most likely, statistically, to produce benefit of some duration if the "inconvenience" of the approach does not outweigh the lower response expected from the next best choice. If estrogen receptor assays or related determinations are "positive," endocrine ablation tends to have the top priority within these ground rules, except for those patients who are well past the menopause (> 10 years). Combination chemotherapy has initial response rates similar to those of endocrine manipulation, but the benefit tends to persist for a longer time when the response is obtained from hormonal methods (ablative or additive). It should be stressed that the choices outlined are still quite arbitrary and may be modified by other factors such as the patient's willingness to accept the recommendations made, the patient's ability to follow necessary requirements of the treatment (e.g., maintenance therapy after adrenalectomy or

Table 7-5

Systemic Treatment Alternatives and Estimates of Expected Objective Response to Palliation of Breast Cancer

Treatment	Premenopause (%)	Menopause 0–10 (%)	Menopause 10+ (%)
Androgens	15–20	15–20	15–20
Estrogens		0–10	30
Corticoids	< 10	< 10	< 10
Bilateral oophorectomy	35	<3.5	—
Bilateral adrenalectomy	30	40–50	40–50
Hypophysectomy	30	40–50	40–50
5-Fluorouracil	20	20	20
Combination chemotherapy*	40–50	40–50	40–50

* Responses of shorter duration than with endocrine measures.

hypophysectomy), and the general medical status of the patient in regard to ability to tolerate the therapy planned.

The special problems listed at the bottom of Table 7-6 require additional comment. As noted earlier, central nervous system metastases are generally associated with a poor response to palliative therapy as well as a short survival time. Experience has shown that radiation therapy is the most effective treatment method for palliation of symptomatic CNS metastasis,[18] but the overall survival time is still quite limited. Steroid therapy is usually employed to reduce cerebral edema during radiation rather than for any anticancer effect, but not all radiotherapists are convinced of its value.

Liver metastases are often present in patients with other patterns of metastatic disease, but they may not be a major clinical feature and may become known only at time of celiotomy for oophorectomy and adrenalectomy. Other patients have significant hepatomegaly and alterations in liver function. In these situations the liver is often the major focus of metastatic disease. Although this latter disease pattern is associated with a more limited response to all palliative therapy, combination chemotherapy is the optimal treatment in view of the limited response to hormonal methods.[12,84]

Table 7-6
Treatment Plan for Palliation of Recurrent or Metastatic
Breast Cancer

Systemic Treatment of Bone, Lung, Pleura, and Soft Tissue Metastases			
	First Rx	Second Rx	Third Rx
Premenopausal	Oophorectomy or	→ Adrenalectomy* → Combination chemotherapy	
		→ Combination chemotherapy → New agents	
Menopause to 10 years post-menopausal	Adrenalectomy* →	Combination chemotherapy → New agents	
>10 years post-menopausal	Estrogen	→ Combination → chemotherapy	New agents
		→ Adrenalectomy* → Combination chemotherapy	

Treatment of Other Metastatic Sites	
CNS	Radiation therapy, steroids, and combination chemotherapy
Liver	Combination chemotherapy

* "Negative" estrophilin or failure to respond to oophorectomy discourages this choice.

CRITERIA FOR EVALUATION OF RESPONSE

Guidelines for evaluation of response differ somewhat for the different palliative modalities, but objective regression of measurable disease (usually 50 percent or more) without progression of other sites or appearance of new lesions is the measure generally used. For endocrine ablation by adrenalectomy or hypophysectomy, a duration of response of 6 months is usually appended for a patient classification to be a "response."

ENDOCRINE METHODS OF MANAGEMENT

Hormones

The various hormones that have been commonly employed for the management of breast cancer and estimates of expected response are seen in Table 7-5. Although androgens are widely used, we give them a low priority in our choice of treatments because of the relatively low objective response rates obtained.[20,21,48] The primary role of estrogen therapy in the management of metastatic breast cancer is in the patient who is well past menopause (usually 10 or more years), but this is arbitrary and based on the possibility of disease stimulation (rather than regression) in younger groups.[21,61] One feature of hormonal administration that must be appreciated is the phenomenon of "rebound regression."[7,59] Cessation of estrogen therapy after relapse of disease may lead to a second response in approximately 10 percent of patients. This response may occur whether or not estrogen initially produced a response, but it is less likely when the hormonal program has been unsuccessful. In view of this phenomenon, it is important when estrogens are discontinued to have an interval of several weeks without therapy before instituting a new treatment plan. This type of clinical response has been observed in a few patients after androgen withdrawal, but not after withdrawal of corticosteriods or progesterone. The phenomenon of "rebound regression" only highlights our lack of understanding of the mechanisms of the various hormonal alterations we exploit. In addition to the considerations discussed above, both estrogens and androgens have been thought to initiate or aggravate hypercalcemia in some patients with bony metastasis.[9,63] For this reason these hormones are contraindicated in patients demonstrating an elevated serum calcium on initial evaluation. Corticosteriods have been useful in lowering elevated serum calcium, but the presence of hypercalcemia is usually an index of rapidly progressive metastatic disease and subsequent treatments are usually less effective. High water intake (oral or parenteral), steroids, and low dosage of mithramycin (0.8–1.5 mg) are effective methods for the acute management of hypercalcemia. Nonhormonal systemic chemotherapy is subsequently employed for overall disease management.

Corticosteroids have been used extensively as single agents for the palliative treatment of breast cancer, but they produce a very low incidence of response.[115] There are also some effective combination drug protocols of chemotherapeutic agents that include steroids without evidence that they actually affect the response rate. Progesterones have been of some benefit, particularly in combination with estrogens,[22,67] but we have had no experience with these agents and do not consider them a primary choice in the management of patients with recurrent and metastatic breast cancer. Nevertheless, some oncologists prefer these and other hormonal trials before offering surgical endocrine ablation because of the obvious disadvantages associated with surgical procedures for palliation. Another hormone approach shown to be of value recently is the use of antiestrogens that are thought to compete with estrogen for binding sites on neoplastic tissue.

Endocrine Ablation

OOPHORECTOMY

Surgical castration of the premenopausal patient is well established as a simple, effective means of management of metastatic breast cancer, despite the relatively low rate of response.[44,62] It produces its effects much more rapidly than radiation castration, which may require 6–8 weeks for complete suppression of ovarian function. When the patient has reached menopausal status or is immediately premenopausal, the likelihood of response is markedly diminished. Our general approach is to carry out both oophorectomy and bilateral adrenalectomy on such patients if an endocrine ablative procedure appears a suitable choice for palliative treatment.

CLINICAL FACTORS AFFECTING RESPONSE
TO ADRENALECTOMY OR HYPOPHYSECTOMY

The following clinical trends have been observed, but often they are not precise enough to satisfy the clinician regarding the choice of palliative treatment for the individual patient.[12,16,29,46,55,82]

Age. Patients under 45 years of age have low response rates in most series (approximately 30 percent), and the duration of response is frequently short. Patients over 45 have objective response rates of 50–60 percent with a longer duration of response.

Menopausal status. Actively menstruating women have a response rate to combined adrenalectomy and oophorectomy that is in the same range as that for oophorectomy alone (approximately 30 percent), a finding demonstrating no significant benefit from the addition of adrenalectomy or the use of hypophysectomy in this group of patients. Postmenopausal patients generally have objective response rates to adrenalectomy or hypophysectomy in the range of 50 percent.

"Free interval." Response to these ablative therapies in patients with "no interval" or up to a 2-year interval is in the 40-percent range. Response is in the 60-percent range if recurrence free interval is more than 2 years. Free interval may have been overemphasized as a determinant for treatment choice in the past, but the longer interval is certainly preferable.

Prior response to palliative oophorectomy. If objective response to prior oophorectomy definitely occurs, most investigators have observed a higher than usual response rate to a subsequent adrenalectomy or hypophysectomy. Some consider this the most significant clinical factor affecting the results of these ablative methods, but it is a less clear-cut determinant in other series.

Effect of pattern of disease on response. As previously noted, patients with CNS metastasis, clinical liver metastasis, peritoneal metastasis, hypercalcemia, and lymphangitic pulmonary spread have a short survival time and limited palliative benefit after all methods of therapy. Response to endocrine ablation with any of these patterns is uniformly poor in comparison to response to treatment in patients with other clinical presentations. Soft tissue disease and/or bone metastases have responded well to endocrine ablation (over 60-percent response in postmenopausal patients, with a mean duration of 18 months).

BENEFIT OF LABORATORY METHODS FOR
PREDICTING RESPONSE TO
ADRENALECTOMY AND OTHER APPROACHES

The effect of the various hormonal balances that encourage or discourage growth of established tumor are far from understood. It was once hoped that the maturation index from the vaginal smear would be a useful guide for identifying potential responders to adrenalectomy or hypophysectomy, but this has not proved to be the case. Extensive metabolic data have been accumulated, beginning with the work of Atkins and his coworkers,[5] using analysis of various urinary steroids as a guide to response to the endocrine ablative procedures for metastatic breast cancer. Discriminate functions calculated from their data seemed to demonstrate some correlation between the ratio of androgenic and corticosteroid metabolites in the urine and the clinical response to adrenalectomy or hypophysectomy.[1,13,52] However, others have had great difficulty confirming this work. There was also an extensive cooperative study in the United States measuring a wide range of steroid metabolites in the urine of patients undergoing adrenalectomy or hypophysectomy in an attempt to develop a similar predictive method for more clear-cut separation of patients who would or would not respond to these methods.[77] Although there were some differences in urinary steroid metabolites in the responding and nonresponding group, variations were too imprecise to serve the purpose of prediction.

More recently, other predictive methods for selecting patients responsive or unresponsive to hormonal therapy have been developed. These include measurement of tissue estrogen receptor protein (estrophilin)[57] or tissue sulfokinase activity,[30] therapeutic trial of levodopa,[80] and therapeutic trial of "chemical adrenalectomy" with aminoglutethimide and ACTH suppression.[71,98]

All the above methods have shown some degree of benefit in early trials for predicting response to hormonal therapies but each must still be considered investigative at this time. The most applicable to clinical usage at present is the determination of estrogen receptor protein in breast cancer tissue. This indicates the presence or absence of cytoplasmic or membrane receptor sites in tissue for a hormone (estradiol) that trigger the chain of events that characterize the effect of the hormone on the tissue in question. Such sites are present on various hormonally responsive normal tissues (e.g., the breast), but they are apparently lost with the neoplastic transformation in some patients and this loss seems to be associated with the loss of hormonal "control." However, despite potential clinical usefulness, adequate tissue for this assay may not be available at the time needed for a therapeutic decision. Using the current (and changing) criteria for a "positive" or "negative" assay, approximately 50–60 percent of patients fall into the positive group. The negative estrogen receptor status does appear to separate those patients who will not respond to hormonal methods.[7,9,70,73,87] The response rate to all hormonal approaches in the estrogen receptor positive group is higher than in "unselected" patients in all studies of this method, but other receptor measurements (for progesterone and other pertinent hormones) will clearly be needed to refine this selection process. As this general selection approach is further refined and as the mechanisms are better understood, it may even be possible to reinduce the ability of a cancer to bind estrogen or other hormones and make hormonal treatment approaches effective in patients in whom they are now ineffective.

From the practical standpoint, estrogen receptor assays appear to be a useful means of analysis of patients with metastatic cancer to complement clinical criteria for the choice between hormone treatment and chemotherapy. Results of these assays are often not available due to absence of suitable tissue for assay or lack of appropriate laboratory services. Under these circumstances, treatment planning is reasonably effective using only the clinical data listed. When this general approach to the assay of breast cancer tissue is further developed and better understood, it will become a necessary part of the initial evaluation of the diagnostic biopsy and may well be used as a guide for choice of effective adjuvant therapy after "curative" treatment.

The other predictive methods listed are less well described, but they may eventually supplement estrogen receptor assays in the assessment of breast cancer patients. Dao and Libby[29,30] report favorable experience with determination of sulfokinase activity on breast cancer tissue, but other investigators are less enthusiastic.[69,82] Our own experience with this approach has been less-precise in the predictive sense, but various methods for refining this assay are possible and it may prove to be useful in the future. Minton[80] has reported the relief of bone pain with a relatively demanding regime of levodopa administration (with concurrent alteration in serum prolactin levels) as a predictor of subsequent response to endocrine ablative therapy, and this may prove also to be a useful clinical tool. "Chemical" adrenalectomy by pharmacologic means (aminoglutethimide and dexamethasone),[71,98] although reversible, has some procedural disadvantages. We have recently shown an excellent correlation between response to this "chemical" adrenalectomy and subsequent response to surgical adrenalectomy. These current investigations may lead to the use of this approach as either a standard predictive method for endocrine ablation therapy or as a nonoperative substitute for surgical adrenalectomy.

Management of Patients Undergoing Adrenalectomy and Hypophysectomy for Breast Cancer

BILATERAL ADRENALECTOMY

Since bilateral adrenalectomy requires general anesthesia, potential candidates for this approach must have sufficient "reserve" to tolerate the operation without significant risk. In addition to standard means of assessment, we usually perform pulmonary function tests and evaluate the "blood gases," particularly in patients with pulmonary or pleural involvement. Asymptomatic pulmonary metastases frequently respond to adrenalectomy, but patients with pulmonary symptoms or the lymphangitic form of pulmonary spread have too high a risk for this form of palliative treatment. Bilateral adrenalectomy can be easily included in the armamentarium of the general surgeon in the many communities where skilled neurosurgeons with special interest in the pituitary are not available.

TECHNIQUE AND POSTOPERATIVE
MANAGEMENT OF PATIENTS
UNDERGOING ADRENALECTOMY

Our choice of operative approach varies with the habitus of the patient and the presence or absence of the ovaries. Even if the patient is postmenopausal, the possible role of the ovaries in the steroid alteration to be achieved makes their removal advisable even though some data seem to discount this. If the patient has not had bilateral oophorectomy performed at some time before adrenalectomy, the abdominal route may be chosen unless obesity is a major problem. This allows both oophorectomy and adrenalectomy to be performed through a single incision. If only bilateral adrenalectomy is required, we prefer the flank approach with bilateral incisions through the bed of each of the 12th ribs, using either the lateral or the prone position (Fig. 7-6). This approach has less morbidity than the abdominal approach, and we now prefer it even if oophorectomy is also planned. Under this circumstance, the ovaries are removed through a small lower abdominal incision.[12]

Because there are no practical means for determining the increased quantity of corticosteroids required in the postoperative period owing to the stress caused by the operative procedure itself, our routine for maintenance "overtreats" these patients during this period. We find intramuscular cortisone acetate useful during the first few postoperative days as it allows scheduled administration of cortisone replacement without dependence on a continuously functioning intravenous system. Since absorption occurs at a slow rate, the intramuscular schedule may be begun the night before surgery on the assumption that effective serum levels from these depots will be achieved by the evening after surgery. For the operative period itself, the patient is maintained on intravenous hydrocortisone (100 mg), and an additional 100 mg is given in a liter of intravenous solution in the immediate postoperative period. Intramuscular cortisone acetate is reinitiated immediately on return to the recovery room, and, except for the intravenous dosage listed above, all subsequent parenteral cortisone is given by this route or the oral route with arbitrary reduction of dosage every 1–2 days until the maintenance dosage is reached. Since oral cortisone is absorbed more rapidly than the intramuscular form, parenteral cortisone can be discontinued as soon as oral medications are tolerated by the patient. In unusually obese patients we prefer intravenous hydrocortisone rather than the intramuscular preparation while parenteral replacement is required because of uncertain rates of absorption from intramuscular depots.

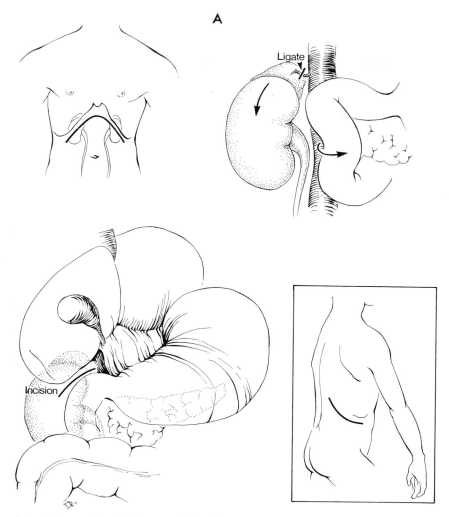

Fig. 7-6 A.   Abdominal approach for bilateral adrenalectomy: Right adrenal.   Insert shows incision for flank approach.

In view of the "excess" dosage administered during the immediate
postoperative period and the sodium conservation and postassium excretion associated with this, all intravenous fluid replacement should be in
terms of 5 percent glucose in water with 40 mEq of potassium chloride in
each liter.   Intravenous saline is avoided unless there is significant gastrointestinal fluid loss requiring replacement.
Our standard maintenance dosage of 37.5 mg of cortisone acetate

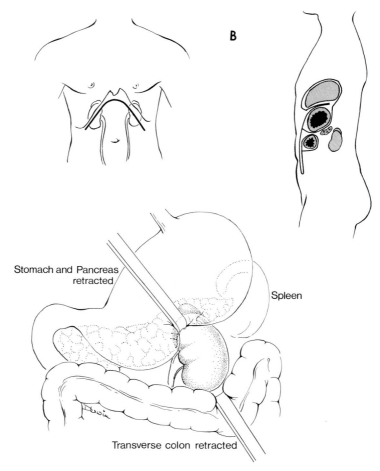

Fig. 7-6**B**.   Operative approach for bilateral adrenalectomy: Left adrenal.

orally per day (12.5 mg t.i.d.) with 0.1 mg of fludrocortisone acetate (Florinef®) daily has been quite satisfactory in all patients.   Cortisone replacement must be increased whenever there is unusual stress from intercurrent injury or illness.   Each patient is given a card with appropriate instructions regarding this for herself and her physician.

HYPOPHYSECTOMY

Hypophysectomy as a means of endocrine ablation for metastatic breast cancer has appealing aspects of both a theoretical and practical nature.   In addition to altering the trophic stimulation of other endocrine glands, pituitary destruction might conceivably eliminate tumor stimulation by removing prolactin or pituitary growth hormone. However, the actual mechanism of benefit from pituitary destruction in patients with breast cancer is still not defined, and the similarity of the response rates to that following adrenalectomy[45,118] suggests that the major mechanisms involved in response are also similar. Furthermore, patients in relapse after treatment by one of these methods uniformly fail to respond to the other. The choice between hypophysectomy and bilateral adrenalectomy must be made on the basis of factors other than response rates.

Technique and management of patients undergoing hypophysectomy. Pituitary destruction has been carried out by several methods including transcranial resection[89,91] and transphenoidal resection[107]—the latter method having gained popularity in recent years. Selective destruction of the pituitary by a radioactive implant (yttrium 90) or cryosurgery techniques has also produced results comparable to that achieved by resection. The latter method (cryohypophysectomy) can be performed by skilled hands under local anesthesia using stereotactic placement of the freezing probes. Hypophysectomy by any of the approaches has a distinct advantage over adrenalectomy from the standpoint of immediate postoperative recovery.[91,114] However, confidence in regard to total destruction of the pituitary with some techniques, the increased complexity of maintenance therapy, the low but definite possibility of a cerebrospinal fluid fistula, and the occasional problem of diabetes insipidus balance these postoperative differences between the procedures. Widespread use of methods to resect or destroy the pituitary is also limited by the special skills required to accomplish these procedures effectively.

The replacement plan after hypophysectomy is the same as that described for postadrenalectomy patients, but thyroid hormone replacement is necessary in the former. Diabetes insipidus is an uncommon complication that requires appropriate additional replacement therapy in some patients.

CHEMOTHERAPEUTIC MANAGEMENT

Although the various clinical features described, such as pattern of disease and disease "free interval," have a general effect on response to all palliative treatment methods, the clinical response to systemic chemotherapy has no clear-cut relationship to age or menopausal status and a less-striking relationship to the prior history of response to various hormonal treatments. Some clinical features of breast cancer that are uniformly bad omens for endocrine approaches have been associated with real benefit from systemic chemotherapy. For these reasons chemotherapeutic agents are a particularly attractive choice for therapy when patients fail to respond or relapse after response to endocrine ablation or exogenous hormone administration, when the clinical presentation makes endocrine approaches unadvisable, or when predictive assays suggest a low likelihood of response to endocrine methods. In addition to these considerations, the improvement in response rates noted with combinations of agents over that generally achieved with single agents in the past has made systemic chemotherapy more appealing under many clinical circumstances when it would not have had a real priority on the basis of the single-agent therapy results.

Single Agents

The alkylating agents were the first nonhormonal agents employed for metastatic breast cancer, and cyclophosphamide is generally acknowledged to be the most effective of this class for this disease. Of the antimetabolities, 5-fluorouracil has been the most extensively studied and used single agent, but methotrexate is another antimetabolite shown to have a definite effect on breast cancer. Many data on response rates to these agents, ranging from 15–35 percent in various series,[3,15] have been accumulated using a wide range of dosage schedules. Of the antibiotics, adriamycin has been the most impressive single agent in the therapy for breast cancer, with a reported response rate of 35 percent. In addition, the effectiveness of this agent was established at this level in a population of patients with breast cancer many of whom had failed to respond to other single agents or combinations that are known to be effective. There has been less intensive evaluation of a number of other agents in all classes, but adriamycin is currently the only single agent that effectively "competes" with combination chemotherapy.[15] An intensive study of new agents may lead to a rapid change in this situation.

Combination Chemotherapy

The rationale of combining drugs was first exploited in the treatment of leukemia, but the impetus to this approach in breast cancer was the initial experience with the "Cooper regime."[19] This combination chemotherapy for breast cancer did not develop in a stepwise experimental manner since proof of the importance of some agents in the combinations is not established. Nevertheless, the use of combination chemotherapy is a major step forward in the palliative management of breast cancer, and it is also the basis for current and future clinical trials of adjuvant chemotherapy.

Some of the logical prerequisites for choice of agents for a successful combination for treating any cancer are that the drugs have some evidence of activity against the disease as single agents, the drugs have some differences in their mechanisms of action, and the toxicities should be somewhat different to avoid major dosage reductions owing to overlapping toxicity (see Chap. 2). These conditions are difficult to achieve, but most have been met by the regimes currently in use. Clinical trials have tested various combinations ranging from three to five agents, and although the results are impressive, they do fall short of the additive response for each of the agents in the combination when used optimally alone.[8,15,33,60] No specific drug combination can be considered truly optimal at present, but currently effective combinations are shown in Table 7-7. Although more investigation is required to determine the optimum combinations, dosages, and scheduling, standard therapy at any one point

Table 7-7
Chemotherapy Combinations Employed for Metastatic
Breast Cancer[15]

Combination	Originator
5-Drug combinations	
5-Fluorouracil Methotrexate Cyclophosphamide Prednisone Testosterone	Greenspan, 1966
5-Fluorouracil Methotrexate Cyclophosphamide Vincristine Prednisone	Cooper, 1969
4-Drug combinations	
5-Fluorouracil Methotrexate Cyclophosphamide Vincristine	Central Oncology Group, 1973
3-Drug combinations	
5-Fluorouracil Vincristine Prednisone	Acute Leukemia Group B, 1973
5-Fluorouracil Cyclophosphamide Prednisone	Mayo Clinic, 1974
5-Fluorouracil Methotrexate Cyclophosphamide	Eastern Cooperative Oncology Group, 1974

in time must depend on the results of well-planned prospective clinical trials. This is a general treatment approach that should yield improved clinical results over the next few years.

Combining Systemic Chemotherapy with Endocrine Ablation Procedures

In an attempt to achieve palliation for metastatic breast cancer, it is probably unwise to employ more than one systemic treatment method simultaneously. The disadvantages of the differing therapies are additive, and the response or lack of response from each therapy chosen will soon become evident. Management approach can then be altered logically. Actually the serial use of the two major different systemic methods (endocrine and chemotherapeutic) may produce a longer period of benefit in some patients than the combination of the two approaches.

The combination of bilateral adrenalectomy and 5-fluorouracil has been recommended on the basis of a reportedly higher overall response rate from the combination.[81] However, the alternative approach, that of using chemotherapy at the time of adrenalectomy failure or relapse, yields similar overall response rates from the statistical point of view.[12] This observation demonstrates an additive (not synergistic) benefit which is essentially equal by either approach. Serial treatment makes the procedures less complex for the patient and could conceivably produce some extension of survival.

EPILOGUE

Breast cancer is one of our few common cancers for which there is understandable optimism for significant improvement in treatment results in the near future. This opinion is based on what appear to be new clues in diagnosis, possible benefit from new adjuvant programs, better laboratory methods of assessing and possibly understanding the response of metastatic disease to palliative therapy, and significant improvements in our approach to chemotherapy.

REFERENCES

1. Ahlquist KA, Jackson AW, Stewart JG: Urinary steroid values as a guide to prognosis in breast cancer. Br Med J 1:217–221, 1968
2. Anglem TJ, Leber RE: The dubious case for conservative operation in operable cancer of the breast. Ann Surg 176:625–632, 1972

3. Ansfield FJ, Ramirez F, Mackman S, Bryan GT, Curreri AR: A 10 year study of 5-fluorouracil in disseminated breast cancer with clinical results and survival times.   Cancer Res 29:1062–1066, 1969

4. Ashikari R, Park K, Huvos AG, Urban JA: Paget's disease of the breast. Cancer 26:680–685, 1970

5. Atkins HJB, Bulbrook RD, Falconer MA, Hayward JL, MacLean KC, Schurr PH: Ten years' experience of steroid assays in the Management of breast cancer.   Lancet 2:1255–1260, 1968

6. Atkins SH, Hayward JL, Klugman DJ, Wayte AB: Treatment of early breast cancer: A report after ten years of clinical trial.   Br Med J 2:423–429, 1972

7. Baker LH, Vaitkevicius VK: Reevaluation of rebound regression in dis-seminated carcinoma of the breast.   Cancer 29:1268–1271, 1972

8. Baker LH, Vaugh CB, al-Sarraf M, Reed ML, Valtkevicious VK: Pro-ceedings: Evaluation of combined vs. sequential cytotoxic chemotherapy in the treatment of advanced breast cancer.   Cancer 3:513–518, 1974

9. Beckett VL: Hypercalcemia associated with estrogen administration in patients with breast carcinoma.   Cancer 24:610–616, 1969

10. Berg JW, DeCosse JJ, Francchia AA, Farrow J: Stromal sarcomas of the breast (a unified approach to connective tissue sarcomas other than cysto-sarcoma phyllodes).   Cancer 15:418–424, 1962

11. Bonadonna G, Brusamolino E, Valagussa P, et al: Combination chemo-therapy as an adjuvant treatment in operable breast cancer.   N Engl J Med 294:405–410, 1976

12. Brown PW, Terz JJ, King RE, Lawrence W Jr: Bilateral adrenalectomy for metastatic breast carcinoma.   Arch Surg 110:77–82, 1975

13. Bulbrook RD, Greenwood FC, Hayward JL: Selection of breast cancer patients for adrenalectomy or hypophysectomy by determination of urinary 17-hydroxy corticosteroids and aeticholanolone.   Lancet 1:1154–1157, 1960

14. Caceres E: An evaluation of radical mastectomy and extended radical mastectomy for cancer of the breast.   Surg Gynecol Obstet 125:337–341, 1967

15. Carter SK: The chemical therapy of breast cancer.   Semin Oncol 1:131–144, 1974

16. Chamberlain A, Dao TL, Bross IDJ, Nemoto T, Slack NH: Efficacy of adrenalectomy in treatment of patients with metastatic cancer of the breast. Surg Gynecol Obstet 138:891–895, 1974

17. Charlson ME, Feinstein AR: An analytic critique of existing systems of staging for breast cancer.   Surgery 73:479–498, 1973

18. Chu FC, Hilaris BB: Value of radiation therapy in the management of in-tracranial metastases.   Cancer 14:577–581, 1961

19. Cooper RG: Combination chemotherapy in hormone resistant breast cancer.   Proc Am Assoc Cancer Res 10:15, 1969

20. Cooperative Breast Cancer Group: Testosterone propinate therapy in breast cancer.   JAMA 188:1069–1072, 1964

21. Council on Drugs, Subcommittee on Breast and Genital Cancer, Committee on Research, American Medical Association: Androgens and estrogens in

the treatment of disseminated mammary carcinoma; Retrospective study of 944 patients. JAMA 172:1271–1283, 1960

22. Crichlow RW: Carcinoma of the male breast. Surg Gynecol Obstet 134:1011–1019, 1972

23. Crile G JR: Multicentric breast cancer—the incidence of new cancers in the homolateral breast after partial mastectomy. Cancer 35:475–477, 1975

24. Crile G Jr: Results of simple mastectomy without irradiation in the treatment of operative stage I cancer of the breast. Ann Surg 168:330–336, 1968

25. Crile G Jr, Esselstyn CB Jr, Hermann RE, Hoerr SO: Partial mastectomy for carcinoma of the breast. Surg Gynecol Obstet 136:929–933, 1973

26. Crowley LG, Macdonald I: Delalutin and estrogens for the treatment of advanced mammary carcinoma in the postmenopausal woman. Cancer 18:436–446, 1965

27. Cutler SJ, Asire AJ, Taylor SG: Classification of patients with disseminated cancer of the breast. Cancer 24:861–869, 1969

28. Cutler SJ, Black MM, Mork T, Harvei S, Freeman C: Further observations on prognostic factors in cancer of the female breast. Cancer 24:653–667, 1969

29. Dao TL: Ablation therapy for hormone-dependent tumors. Annu Rev Med 23:1–18, 1972

30. Dao TL, Libby PR: Conjugation of steroid hormones by breast cancer tissue and selection of patients of adrenalectomy. Surgery 66:162–166, 1969

31. Dao T., Nemoto T, Chamberlain A, Bross I: Adrenalectomy with radical mastectomy in the treatment of high-risk breast cancer. Cancer 35:478–482, 1975

32. Decosse JJ, Berg JW, Fracchia AA, Farrow JH: Primary lymphosarcoma of breasts; A review of 14 cases. Cancer 15:1264–1268, 1962

33. DeLena M, Brambilla C, Morabito A, Bonadonna G: Adriamycin plus vincristine compared to and combined with cyclophosphamide, methotrexate, and 5-fluorouracil for advanced breast cancer. Cancer 35:1108–1115, 1975

34. Donegan WL: Extended surgical adjuvant thiotepa for mammary carcinoma. Arch Surg 109:187–192, 1974

35. Donegan WL: Mastectomy in the primary management of invasive mammary carcinoma. Adv Surg 6:1–101, 1972

36. Donegan WL, Perez-Mesa CM: Carcinoma of the male breast: A 30 year review of 28 cases. Arch Surg 106:273–279, 1973

37. Donegan WL, Perez-Mesa CM: Lobular carcinoma—an indication for elective biopsy of the second breast. Ann Surg 176:178–187, 1972

38. Ellis DL, Teitelbaum SL: Inflammatory carcinoma of the breast. Cancer 33:1045–1047, 1974

39. Fisher B, Carbone P, Economou SG, et al: 1-Phenylalanine mustard (L-PAM) in the management of primary breast cancer. N Engl J Med 292:117–122, 1975

40. Fisher B, Slack NH, Bross IDJ, et al: Cancer of the breasts: Size of neoplasm and prognosis. Cancer 34:1071–1080, 1969.

41. Fisher B, Slack NH, Cavanaugh PJ, Gardner B, Ravdin RG, et al: Post-

operative radiotherapy in treatment of breast cancer: Results of the NSABP clinical trial. Ann Surg 172:711–732, 1970

42. Fisher B, Slack N, Katrych D, Wolmark N: Ten year follow-up results of patients with carcinoma of the breast in a co-operative clinical trial evaluating surgical adjuvant chemotherapy. Surg Gynecol Obstet 140:528–534, 1975

43. Fletcher JH: The advantages of preoperative irradiation. JAMA 200:140–143, 1967

44. Fracchia AA, Farrow JH, DePalo AJ, Connolly DP, Huvos AG: Castration for primary inoperable or recurrent breast carcinoma. Surg Gynecol Obstet 128:1226–1234, 1969

45. Fracchia AA, Farrow JH, Miller TR, Tollefsen RH, Greenberg EG, Knapper WH: Hypophysectomy as compared with adrenalectomy in the treatment of advanced carcinoma of the breast. Surg Gynecol Obstet 133:241–246, 1971

46. Fracchia AA, Randall HT, Farrow JH: The results of adrenalectomy in advanced breast cancer in 500 consecutive patients. Surg Gynecol Obstet 125:747–756, 1967

47. Frankl G, Fosenfeld DD: Xeroradiographic detection of occult breast cancer. Cancer 35:542–548, 1975

48. Goldenberg IS, Waters MN, Ravdin RS, Ansfield FJ, Segaloff A: Androgenic therapy for advanced breast cancer in women: A report of the Cooperative breast cancer group. JAMA 223:1267–1268, 1973

49. Guttman RJ: Survival and results after 2 million volt irradiation in the treatment in primary operable carcinoma of the breast with proved positive internal mammary and/or highest axillary nodes. Cancer 15:383–386, 1962

50. Haagensen CD: Diseases of the Breast. Philadelphia, WB Saunders Co, 1971

51. Haagensen CD: The choice of treatment for operable carcinoma of the breast. Surgery 76:685–714, 1974

52. Hayward JL, Bulbrook RD: The value of urinary steroid estimations in the prediction of response to adrenalectomy or hypophysectomy. Cancer Res 25:1129–1134, 1965

53. Herrmann JB: Management of the contralateral breast after mastectomy for unilateral carcinoma. Surg Gynecol Obstet 132:777–779, 1973

54. Holleb AI, Farrow J: The relation of carcinoma of the breast and pregnancy in 283 patients. Surg Gynecol Obstet 115:65–71, 1962

55. Horsley JS III, Alrich EM, Sears HF, et al: Adrenalectomy for metastatic mammary cancer. Ann Surg 173:906–912, 1971

56. Hutter RVP, Foote FW Jr: Lobular carcinoma in situ (long term follow-up). Cancer 24:1081–1085, 1969

57. Jensen EV, Block GE, Smith S, Kiper K, DeSombre ER: Estrogen receptors and breast cancer response to adrenalectomy. Natl Cancer Monogr 55–70, 1971

58. Kaae S, Johnson H: Five year results: Two random series of simple mastectomy with postoperative irradiation vs. extended radical mastectomy. Am J Roentgenol 87:82–88, 1962

59. Kaufman RJ, Escher GC: Rebound regression in advanced mammary carcinoma. Surg Gynecol Obstet 113:635–640, 1961
60. Kaufman S, Goldstein M: Combination chemotherapy in disseminated carcinoma of the breast. Surg Gynecol Obstet 137:83–86, 1973
61. Kennedy BJ: Hormonal therapies in breast cancer. Semin Oncol 1:119–130, 1974
62. Kennedy BJ, Mielke PW, Fortuny IE: Therapeutic castration vs. prophylactic castration in breast cancer. Surg Gynecol Obstet 118:524–540, 1964
63. Kennedy BJ, Tibbetts DM, Nathanson IT, et al: Hypercalcemia, complication of hormone therapy of advanced breast cancer. Cancer Res 13:445–459, 1953
64. Kholdin SA, Deemarsky LY, Bavly JL: Adjuvant long term chemotherapy in complex treatment of operable breast cancer. Cancer 33:903–906, 1974
65. King RE, Terz JJ, Lawrence W Jr: Experience with opposite breast biopsy in patients with operable breast cancer. Cancer 37:43–45, 1976
66. LaCour J, Bucalosi P, Caceres E, Jasobelli G, et al: Radical mastectomy versus radical mastectomy plus internal mammary node dissection. Cancer 37:206–214, 1976
67. Landau RL, Ehrlich EN, Hughes C: Estradiol Benzoate and progesterone in advanced human breast cancer: A combination found effective in advanced cases. JAMA 182:632–636, 1962
68. Lentle BC, Burns PE, Dierich H, Jackson FI: Bone scintiscanning in the initial assessment of carcinoma of the breast. Surg Gynecol Obstet 141:43–47, 1975
69. Leung BS, Fletcher WS, Lindell TD, et al: Predictability of response to endocrine ablation in advanced breast carcinoma: A correlation to estrogen receptor and steroid sulfurylation. Arch Surg 106:515–519, 1973
70. Leung BS, Krippaehne WW, Fletcher WS: Prognostic value of estrogen receptor to endocrine ablation in cancer of the breast. Surg Gynecol Obstet 139:525–528, 1974
71. Lipton A, Santen RJ: Proceedings: Medical adrenalectomy using aminoglutethimide and dexamethasone in advanced breast cancer. Cancer 33:503–512, 1974
72. Lipton A, Sheehan LM, Keesler GF: Urinary polyamine levels in human cancer. Cancer 35:464–468, 1975
73. Maass H, Engel B, Homeister H, et al: Estrogen receptors in human breast cancer tissue. Am J Obstet Gynecol 113:377–382, 1972
74. MacDonald I: Carcinoma of the breast in pregnancy and lactation. JAMA 201:529, 1967
75. Madden JL: Modified radical mastectomy. Surg Gynecol Obstet 121:1221–1230, 1965
76. Malone LJ, Frankl G, Dorazio RA, Winkley JH: Occult breast carcinomas detected by xeroradiography. Ann Surg 181:133–136, 1975
77. Masnyk IJ, collaborating investigators: Unpublished data.
78. McDivitt RW, Hutter RVP, Foote FW Jr, Stewart FW: In situ lobular car-

cinoma: A prospective follow-up study indicating cumulative patient risks. JAMA 201:82–86, 1967

79. McWhirter R: Simple mastectomy and radiotherapy in the treatment of breast cancer. Br J Radiol 28:128–139, 1955

80. Minton JP: The response of breast cancer patients with bone pain to L-DOPA. Cancer 33:358–363, 1974

81. Moore FD, Van Devanter SB, Boyden CM, Lokich Jacob, Wilson RE: Adrenalectomy with chemotherapy in the treatment of advanced breast cancer; objective and subjective response rates; duration and quality of life. Surgery 76:376–388, 1974

82. Moseley HS, Fletcher WS, Leung BS, Krippaehne WW: Predictive criteria for the selection of breast cancer patients for adrenalectomy. Am J Surg 128:143–150, 1974

83. Nance FC, DeLoach DH, Welsh RA, Becker WF: Paget's disease of the breast. Ann Surg 171:864–874, 1970

84. Nemoto T, Dao TL: Significance of liver metastasis in women with disseminated breast cancer undergoing endocrine ablative surgery. Cancer 19:421–427, 1966

85. Paterson R, Russel MH: Clinical trials in malignant disease. II. Clin. Radiol. 10:130–133, 1959

86. Paterson R, Russel MH: Clinical trials of malignant disease. III. Breast cancer: Evaluation of postoperative radiotherapy. Clin Radiol 10:175–180, 1959

87. Pearson OH, McGuire WL, Bodkey J, Marshall J: Estrogen receptors and prediction of the response of metastatic breast cancer to hypophysectomy, in Estrogen Receptors in Human Breast Cancer. New York, Raven Press, 1975

88. Pearson OH, Ray BS: Hypophysectomy in the treatment of metastatic mammary cancer. Am J Surg 99:544–552, 1960

89. Peters V: Wedge resection and irradiation in early breast cancers. JAMA 200:134–135, 1967

90. Pistenma DA, McDougal R, Kriss JP: Screening for bone metastases (are only scans necessary?). JAMA 231:46–50, 1975

91. Ray B: Hypophysectomy as palliative treatment. JAMA 200:974–975, 1967

92. Robbins GF, Lucas JC, Fracchia AA, et al: An evaluation of postoperative prophylactic radiation therapy in breast cancer. Surg Gynecol Obstet 122:979–982, 1966

93. Robbins GF, Berg JW: Bilateral breast cancers (a prospective clinical pathologic study). Cancer 17:1501–1527, 1964

94. Rosato FE, Thomas J, Rosato EF: Operative management of nonpalpable lesions detected by mammography. Surg Gynecol Obstet 137:491–493, 1973

95. Rosen PP, Fracchia AA, Urban JA, Schottenfeld D, Robbins GF: "Residual" mammary carcinoma following simulated partial mastectomy. Cancer 35:739–747, 1975

96. Rosen PP, Snyder RE, Robbins G: Specimen radiography for nonpalpable breast lesions founded by mammography: procedures and results. Cancer 34:2028–2033, 1974

97. Rush BFJ: Axillary dissection in Breast Cancer: A staging procedure. Surgery 77:478, 1975

98. Santen RJ, Lipton A, Kendall J: Successful medical adrenalectomy with amino-glutethimide: Role of altered drug metabolism. JAMA 230:1661–1665, 1974

99. Savlov ED, Wittliff JL, Hilf R, Hall TC: Correlations between certain biochemical properties of breast cancer and response to therapy: A preliminary report. Cancer 33:303–309, 1974

100. Schurman DJ, Amstutz HC: Orthopedic management of patients with metastatic carcinoma of the breast. Surg Gynecol Obstet 137:831–836, 1973

101. Shah JP, Rosen PP, Robbins GF: Pitfalls of local excision in the treatment of carcinoma of the breast. Surg Gynecol Obstet 136:721–725, 1973

102. Shah JP, Urban JA: Full thickness chest wall resection for recurrent breast carcinoma involving the bony chest wall. Cancer 35:567–573, 1975

103. Snyder AF, Farrow GM, Masson JK, Payne WS: Chest wall resection for locally recurrent breast cancer. Arch Surg 97:246–253, 1968

104. Steingaszner LC, Enzinzer FM, Taylor HB: Hemangiosarcoma of the breast. Cancer 18:352–361, 1965

105. Steward AM, Nixon D, Zamcheck N, Aisenberg A: Carcinoembryonic antigen in breast cancer patients: serum levels and disease progress. Cancer 33:1246–1252, 1974

106. Terenius L, Johansson H, Rimsten A, Thoren L: Malignant and benign human mammary disease: Estrogen binding in relation to clinical data. Cancer 33:1364–1368, 1974

107. Tollefsen HR, Miller TR, Gerold FP: Transantral sphenoidal hypophysectomy. Am J Surg 112:569–576, 1966

108. Tormey DC, Waalkes TP, Ahmann D, Behrke CW, et al: Biological markers in breast carcinoma. I. Incidence of abnormalities of CEA, HCG, three polyamines, and three minor nucleosides. Cancer 35:1095–1100, 1975

109. Treves N, Sunderland DA: Cystosarcoma phyllodes of breasts: malignant and benign tumor, clinico-pathological study of 77 cases. Cancer 4:1286–1322, 1951

110. Urban JA: Radical excision of the chest wall for mammary cancer. Cancer 4:1263–1285, 1951

111. Urban JA: Bilaterality of breast cancer—biopsy of the opposite breast. Cancer 20:1867–1870, 1967

112. Urban JA, Baker HW: Radical mastectomy with en bloc resection of the internal mammary lymph node chain. Cancer 5:992–1008, 1952

113. Vaeth JM, Clark JC, Green JP, Schroeder AF, Lowy RO: Radiotherapeutic management of locally advanced carcinoma of the breast. Cancer 30:107–112, 1972

114. VanGilder JC, Goldenberg IS: Hypophysectomy in metastatic breast cancer. Arch Surg 110:293–295, 1975

115. West CD, Li MD, McLean JP, Escher GC, Pearson OH: Cortisone in-
     duced remissions in women with metastatic mammary cancer. Proc Am
     Assoc Cancer Res 1:51, 1954
116. Wheeler JE, Enterline HT, Roseman JM, et al: Lobular carcinoma in situ
     of the breast. Cancer 34:554–563, 1974
117. Wilson ND, Alberty RE: Bilateral carcinoma of the breast. Am J Surg
     126:244–248, 1973
118. Wilson RE, Piro AJ, Aliapoulios MA, Moore SD: Evaluation of adrenalec-
     tomy and hypophysectomy in the treatment of metastatic cancer of the
     breast. Cancer 24:1322–1330, 1969

8

Management of Gastrointestinal Cancer

The neoplasms to be covered in this chapter range from those in the cervical esophagus to those arising from the anus, anatomic territory that is the domain of the surgeon for the most part. There have been few recent technical advances in the therapeutic approach to this group of neoplasms, but their diagnosis and management have seen some improvement, due mainly to more active participation of the gastroenterologist, the endoscopist, and the cytologist. Esophageal cancer is still an almost overwhelming challenge; gastric cancer is steadily decreasing in incidence in the United States but is still a reasonably frequent killer; small bowel cancer remains a rare lesion; whereas colorectal cancer has become the most prevalent cancer in our population. Cancers of the accessory organs of the gastrointestinal tract (liver, biliary tract, and pancreas) are less frequent than colorectal cancer, but their diagnosis and differentiation from benign diseases are still a frequent clinical problem. Progress in both diagnostic measures and therapy for this entire group of neoplasms is sorely needed.

ESOPHAGEAL CANCER

Carcinoma of the cervical and thoracic esophagus, like cancer of the oral cavity, pharynx, and larynx, is clearly associated with mucosal injury (primarily by tobacco, chemicals, and other irritants) and nutritional deficiencies of various sorts (excess alcohol consumption, vitamin deficiency, and general malnutrition). These are probably our most impor-

193

tant leads in view of our poor diagnostic and therapeutic abilities at the present time.

Diagnosis

Esophageal cancer is usually diagnosed after the major symptom, dysphagia, has already produced some degree of weight loss, dehydration, and general malnutrition. Unfortunately, the distensibility of the esophagus allows adequate deglutition until the primary lesion has progressed to a significant size or has involved other local or distant structures. The concept of early diagnosis is really not feasible for carcinoma of the esophagus at this time.

The procedures employed for establishing a diagnosis of esophageal cancer are the barium esophagogram and endoscopy with either the rigid or flexible instrument. Histologic confirmation is achieved by forceps biopsy or brush cytology from the distal lumen at the time of endoscopy.[165] The overwhelming majority of these lesions are squamous carcinomas (as in the oral cavity and pharynx), but sarcoma (leiomyosarcoma), carcinosarcoma, or malignant melanoma may occur. Lower esophageal cancer is the most common (43 percent), midthoracic esophageal cancer is next in incidence (37 percent), and the cervical esophageal cancer is the least common of the three types of esophageal cancer. The last lesion is rarely seen in comparison to the frequency of squamous carcinoma of the oral cavity, pharynx, or larynx.

Interestingly enough, the prominent sites for squamous carcinoma of the esophagus are those areas of esophageal narrowing in the cricopharyngeal region, the region of the bifurcation of the trachea and arch of the aorta, and the esophagogastric junction. In this same regard, chronic esophageal obstruction from peptic esophagitis, stricture, or achalasia also seems to have some causal relationship to cancer of the esophagus. From the clinical standpoint, the differential diagnosis of esophageal cancer includes various benign conditions (benign neoplasms, achalasia, hiatus hernia, Plummer-Vinson syndrome, and scleroderma) as well as other malignant processes producing extrinsic compression of the organ (lung cancer, mediastinal neoplasm, and metastatic carcinoma in the mediastinum).

Staging

In contrast to that of more accessible cancers, clinical staging of esophageal cancer is difficult. The full extent of infiltration of the tumor (T) cannot often by fully appreciated by either radiography or endoscopy, and the regional node status (N) cannot be evaluated except with the cervical esophageal lesions. Unfortunately, metastases (M) (primarily to dis-

tant lymph nodes, liver, lungs, and bone) are frequent by the time the diagnosis of esophageal cancer is established, and pretreatment evaluation fo-
cuses primarily on this pessimistic aspect of the staging process. It is
probably wise to carry out a "staging celiotomy" before deciding the specific treatment plan directed to intrathoracic primary lesions if the standard clinical and laboratory investigations fail to reveal metastatic disease.[54] The aggressiveness of the subsequent therapeutic approach may
be affected in many instances, and the possibility of finding signs of incurability is great.

Treatment

Both local and distant treatment usually fail after radiation therapy or
surgical resection for esophageal cancer, and we must accept that most of
the benefits we may produce relate to palliation, even in what appear clinically to be favorable settings. Actually, the problems of dysphagia, aspiration, and malnutrition produced by the local disease are severe, and
they do require a therapeutic effort despite the grave ultimate prognosis
for most patients with esophageal cancer. Unfortunately, there has been
no success thus far with anticancer chemotherapy for esophageal cancer,
and the subsequent discussion relates to the other available methods.

CARCINOMA OF THE CERVICAL ESOPHAGUS

The choice of treatment between radiation therapy and surgical excision can be accomplished for cancer of the cervical esophagus using criteria similar to those described for squamous carcinoma of the head and
neck region (see Chap. 5). Since a truly early lesion in this anatomic location is rarely found by the physician, most patients seem better suited
for surgical resection with reconstruction to allow reasonably normal deglutition. However, it must be admitted that the reported late end results
of the surgical approach are actually no better than those achieved by
radiation therapy, and the latter treatment method does allow retention of
the larynx. This is probably why patients with carcinoma of the cervical
esophagus are treated with radiation therapy at most institutions and also
why our clinical experience is limited primarily to the surgical treatment
of radiation treatment "failures." Our preference for surgical resection
is based on the frequency of failure of radiation therapy to control the
local disease (Table 8-1).

When surgical resection of the cervical esophagus and larynx is accomplished for primary lesions of this site, we prefer reconstruction of the
cervical esophagus by colon interposition[50,134] since the distal line of esophageal resection is usually too low after adequate resection to create the
cervical esophagostomy required for later reconstruction by local or distant skin flaps (Fig. 8-1). We believe it is preferable to carry out this re-

Table 8-1
Squamous Cell Carcinoma of the Esophagus: 5-Yr Treatment
Results for Patients with Localized Disease

Site	Surgery*		Radiation†	
	Patients	%	Patients	%
Cervical	2/10	20	14/46	30
Upper and midthoracic	6/56	11	12/73	16
Lower thoracic	29/91	32	6/50	12
Total	37/157	24	32/169	19

   * Based on data from "curative" resection only at Mayo Clinic (Gunnlaugsson GH, Wychulus AR, Roland C, Ellis FH Jr: Surg Gynecol Obstet 130:997–1005, 1970).
   † Based on report by Pearson.[122]

construction as a secondary procedure in view of the magnitude of the initial operative procedure, which may also require resection of the adjacent trachea and manubrium, and the general medical and nutritional state of most of these patients. In all fairness, it is difficult to compare realistically the effectiveness of radiation therapy and surgery for carcinoma of the cervical esophagus since the long-term results have been poor by both approaches. It is our conviction, however, as in analogous situations in the head and neck region, that it is preferable to proceed with a surgical approach, rather than the alternative method of radiation therapy, if surgery will ultimately be required in most instances for local control. The basis for this is the increase in morbidity and the less-desirable immediate results after surgery in heavily irradiated fields.

CARCINOMA OF THE THORACIC ESOPHAGUS

Midthoracic esophageal cancers pose particularly difficult therapeutic problems. There are multiple alternatives using either surgical resection or radiation therapy, but poor long-term results as well as major early complications occur with both general treatment methods (Table 8-1). It is difficult to make a strong argument for either approach, but it is important to stress the need for therapeutic efforts to maintain the patient's ability to swallow if at all possible. Esophageal obstruction is the most distressing aspect of this type of cancer in this anatomic location. The various therapeutic alternatives that have been proposed are listed below:

1. esophageal resection and immediate reconstruction with stomach, colon, or small intestine;
2. resection of the entire thoracic esophagus with later reconstruction, usually by a segment of right or left colon;

3. surgical bypass of the esophageal obstruction, usually by a segment of colon, with later total thoracic esophagectomy;
4. surgical bypass as described in (3) with subsequent radiation therapy to the primary lesion in the esophagus;
5. alternative (4) with surgical resection after completion of radiation therapy;
6. preoperative radiation therapy (low or high dose) with later surgical resection of the esophagus and primary or secondary reconstruction;
7. primary radiation therapy to the esophageal lesion with bougienage and/or insertion of a prosthetic tube (intraluminal prosthetic tube).

A strong argument cannot be made for any of the alternatives listed (and preferred by one or more authors),[50,53,101,109,119,121,122,134] but it should be stressed that (a) the patient with esophageal cancer is best served if he continues to swallow during his remaining life; (b) surgical gastrostomy alone has not given this type of patient adequate relief of the local symptoms from esophageal obstruction; and (c) the presence or absence of extrathoracic metastatic disease should make a difference in the degree of treatment effort that the patient is asked to accept. In our institution patients in reasonably good general condition without extrathoracic metastasis (usually confirmed by celiotomy) are treated by surgical resection of midthoracic esophageal cancer, whereas radiation therapy is employed for those patients whose condition is less satisfactory than this. Secondary reconstruction with left colon is preferred. In many institutions radiation therapy is considered the treatment of choice for carcinoma of the midthoracic esophagus because of the relatively high postoperative mortality and the poor long-term results achieved by surgical resection. In view the factors discussed, it is difficult to find fault with this approach. It should be stressed, however, that the treatment plan should effectively deal with the major symptom problem, dysphagia, since palliation is the primary accomplishment that we can hope for at this time.

CARCINOMA OF THE DISTAL ESOPHAGUS

Some of the same problems and considerations described for carcinoma of the midthoracic esophagus apply to patients with distal esophageal lesions, but some features of cancer in the distal esophagus makes surgery a more appealing choice than radiation therapy. First of all, the distal location of these lesions makes surgical resection with primary restoration of alimentary tract continuity more feasible since the stomach can often be brought into the lower thorax for esophagogastric anastomosis at the time of resection (Fig. 8-2). In one stage, this effectively relieves esophageal obstruction, the primary management problem. Some patients who have lesions in this location are successfully treated by surgery from the long-term standpoint (Table 8-1). This is far from an

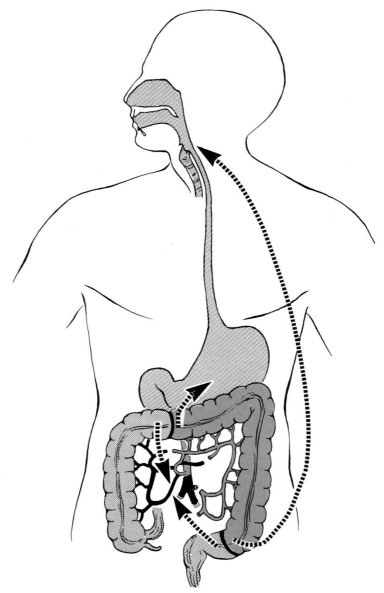

Fig. 8-1.   Antiperistaltic left colon transposition for esophageal reconstruction

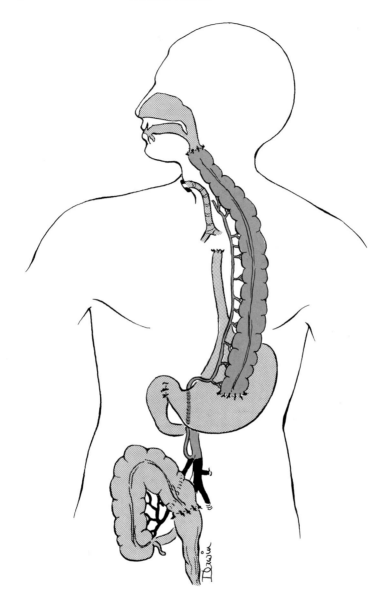

after cervical or total thoracic esophagectomy.

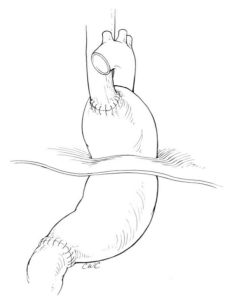

Fig. 8-2. Primary reconstruction of esophagogastric anastomosis after resection of distal third of esophagus.

ideal long-term result and little different from what can be achieved by radiation therapy, but the improvement in operative morbidity and mortality from this procedure in recent years makes this a much more acceptable approach than it once was.

ENDOSCOPIC AND NONOPERATIVE APPROACHES TO ESOPHAGEAL OBSTRUCTION FROM CANCER

Although results of the surgical introduction of prosthetic devices to maintain the esophageal lumen have been disappointing in the past because of operative morbidity and mortality, subsequent displacement, obstruction of the prosthesis, or other complications, Boyce[19] and Palmer[116] have developed a simple method of bougienage and peroral esophageal tube placement for patients who have some lumen still present. This approach is adaptable to most patients with carcinoma of the esophagus and particularly to those patients with carcinoma in the midthoracic esophagus. Peroral placement of an indwelling prosthesis is much safer and more easily accomplished than operative placement and may even be used effectively when a small tracheoesophageal fistula is present. The prosthesis can be inserted in the awake patient with an anesthetic gargle, using fluoroscopy to permit examination of the postintubation tube position (Fig. 8-3). The patient has no sensation of a foreign body in his

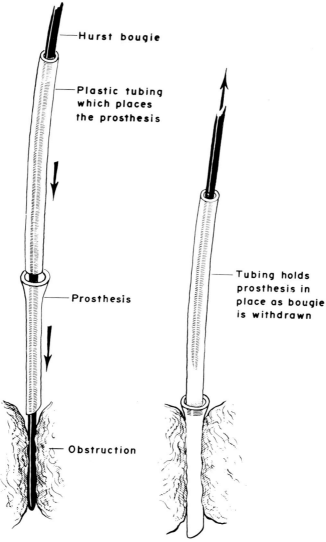

—Hurst bougie

—Plastic tubing
which places
the prosthesis

—Prosthesis

—Obstruction

—Tubing holds
prosthesis in
place as bougie
is withdrawn

Fig. 8-3. Insertion of a plastic prosthesis into the esophagus (from Palmer[116]).

esophagus after introduction of such a tube by this method and is able to
take a relatively normal diet with a tube of 0.5-inch inside diameter. This
technique does not alter the progression of the carcinoma, but it improves
the quality of life of most esophageal cancer patients whether or not radiation therapy is also used. This approach combined with primary radiation therapy for cancers of the midthoracic esophagus is a worthwhile
consideration for selected patients.

Complications of Treatment

SURGICAL RESECTION

There are many potential complications following surgery for carcinoma of the esophagus. This is not surprising since both the abdominal and thoracic cavities are entered, and the patients are quite debilitated in most instances. This is a major reason for staging the operative procedures in many instances in which a surgical approach has been chosen. The cardiopulmonary complications are often the most difficult ones to deal with, and careful pretreatment evaluation is required before selection of therapy if the frequency of this complication is to be maintained in a reasonable range.

RADIATION THERAPY

One of the major problems associated with radiation therapy for carcinoma of the esophagus is that relief of the esophageal obstruction cannot be instantly achieved by radiation therapy alone. Therefore, many physicians consider other methods—such as bougienage, peroral insertion of a prosthetic tube, or both—in conjunction with radiation therapy. The major fear of the radiation therapist treating a midthoracic esophageal cancer is the possibility of development of a tracheoesophageal fistula since the trachea is so close to the esophageal lesion in this type of patient. This complication may be a result of the treatment itself or actually a result of the regression of the carcinoma involving the adjacent trachea, but the results are usually catastrophic from the standpoint of the patient's course. The insertion of a peroral prosthesis as previously described is a useful method of management for this problem in selected cases.

GASTRIC CANCER

For unknown reasons the incidence of carcinoma of the stomach in both men and women in the United States has continued to decline over the past 30 years. This is not a worldwide phenomenon as certain countries, particularly Japan, Chile, Iceland, and Finland, have a higher incidence of gastric carcinoma than the United States. More than half of the male cancer deaths in Japan are owing to gastric cancer, and the disease occurs at a much younger age than generally seen in this country.

Diagnosis

The history and physical examination of patients with potentially "curable" gastric cancer often reveal nonspecific findings that do not even suggest the specific diagnosis. We found vague symptoms of "indigestion" in over 80 percent of patients in our series, and the typical "ulcer syndrome," or periodic pain relieved by food intake, was discovered in only approximately 10–15 percent.[98,99] Nausea and vomiting, fullness after meals, weight loss, hematemesis, melena, or even free perforation on occasion are other symptoms of gastric cancer. Dysphagia may also be a presenting complaint in patients with lesions of the cardia. Only 5–6 percent of patients in our own series had no gastrointestinal symptoms; unexplained weight loss or anemia from blood loss prompted the gastrointestinal workup. Physical findings are usually absent in potentially resectable cases, but an abdominal mass may be present.

Findings are rather characteristic in patients who have metastatic disease from gastric cancer. The most frequent sites of metastasis are the supraclavicular lymph nodes, the peritoneum (manifested by ascites or "rectal shelf"), and the liver. Ovarian metastases can be large and, occasionally, a pelvic mass is the initial physical finding. Lung, brain, skin, bone, or bone marrow metastases can occur, but the clinical evidence of metastatic disease in these sites generally leads one to suspect the validity of the clinical diagnosis of gastric cancer.

Since the history and physical examination are rarely rewarding unless the patient had advanced disease, the classic method for diagnosing gastric cancer has been radiologic. Radiologic techniques for identifying small inconspicuous lesions of the stomach have been improved, a factor that may lead to "earlier" diagnosis of gastric cancer, or premalignant lesions, and might improve the high mortality. No concerted effort has been made in this country to accomplish earlier radiologic identification of potential cancers, but both radiologic and endoscopic techniques for the diagnosis of asymptomic gastric lesions have been refined in Japan. The use of double contrast methods by the introduction of air through a nasogastric tube or by air-producing tablets allows better definition of very small superficial lesions. Hopefully, these radiologic inprovements will have a favorable influence on gastric diagnosis in the United States.[136]

Another major advance in the diagnosis of gastric carcinoma is the fiberoptic gastroscope, an instrument that has revolutionized gastric endoscopy by making it easier on both the patient and the operator. The added value of easily visualizing (and photographing) gross pathology in the stomach had led to the use of endoscopy in patients with symptoms and radiographic findings in the past considered too insignificant to merit the rigor of endoscopy with the then available equipment. Thorough endoscopic evaluation with biopsy of a possible gastric lesion seen on radiographic examination does increase diagnostic accuracy. Endoscopy is now easy and effective enough to be considered in the evaluation of any patient with gastric symptoms despite absence of radiographic findings. The Japanese experience has demonstrated an increasing proportion of

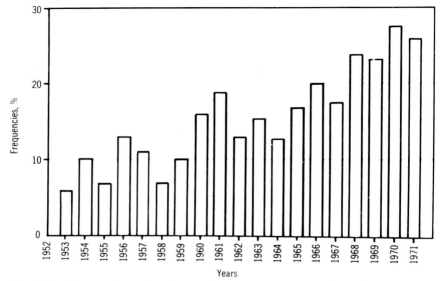

Fig. 8-4. Frequencies of early gastric cancers among total gastric cancers resected (from Nagayo T, Yokoyama H: JAMA 228:889, 1974).

superficial cancers as a result of aggressive diagnostic efforts, including endoscopy, and this has resulted in higher resectability and surgical control rates for gastric cancer (Fig. 8-4). We have seen no such improvement in the United States, where mass survey approaches are not really practical, but the Japanese experience should prompt a vigorous combined diagnostic approach to all patients who have any suggestion of gastric disease as well as to asymptomatic "high-risk" populations. This includes patients with achlorhydria, atrophic gastritis, or stools positive for occult blood in the absence of an obvious cause.

The increase in use of gastric cytology is also a favorable trend from the standpoint of diagnosis of more favorable lesions. There are many techniques for obtaining specimens for cytologic studies, ranging from various brushes to differing methods of lavage, but all have been helpful if an experienced cytologist and cytology laboratory are involved. In some studies gastric cytology has increased the diagnostic yield by as much as 20 percent, particularly when the cytologic specimen was obtained with a direct brush technique at the time of endoscopy.

In addition to advances in radiology, endoscopy, and cytology, there has been considerable interest in tumor markers, particularly serum studies of the tumor-associated antigen (carcinoembryonic antigen) that was initially found in the serum of patients with carcinoma of the colon.

It has become evident that this particular assay has no usefulness for early diagnosis of gastric cancer (or other neoplasms in man), but this general approach may have some merit for diagnosis in the future.

The differential diagnosis of gastric cancer includes peptic ulcer, benign neoplasms, unusual inflammatory problems such as syphilis or tuberculosis, and various functional prepyloric abnormalities that may be difficult to differentiate from carcinoma on radiologic study. The diagnostic measures described thus far are helpful in clarifying the diagnosis, but surgical exploration may be required for definitive diagnosis in a number of clinical situations.

Treatment of Gastric Cancer

At the present time, surgery provides the only satisfactory curative treatment for gastric cancer. However, the end results of treatment of "resectable" lesions are affected more by the pathologic findings than by the surgeon's skill. Many clinicopathologic reviews have clearly shown that the salvage of patients with anaplastic, infiltrative lesions (which progress to a "leather bottle" stomach) is extremely low, whereas patients with polypoid carcinomas or "ulcerocancers" have a reasonable prognosis after surgical resection (Fig. 8-5).[98,99] It is also clear that the presence or absence of regional lymph node metastasis is the most significant prognostic feature in patients with "curable" lesions at the time of surgical exploration: 45–50-percent 5-year survival if regional lymph nodes do not contain metastasis; 15 percent if they do.

CHOICE OF OPERATION

All patients with gastric cancer, except those with definite evidence of peritoneal metastasis (ascites containing malignant cells or "rectal shelf"), documented liver metastases, or proven distant metastases should be subjected to exploratory celiotomy in order to select potentially "curable" patients. If a regionally localized process is found at the time of exploration, adequate resection of the primary neoplasm, as well as the actual and potential lymphatic extensions, is required. Unfortunately, signs of incurability are revealed at the time of exploratory celiotomy in the majority of patients, but approximately 40 percent of patients who are explored are candidates for a "curative" attempt.

What is "adequate" resection? At one time the use of total gastrectomy for patients with small gastric cancers was advanced on the theoretical basis that removal of the entire organ of origin and the regional lymphatic bed would increase cure rates. Retrospective evaluation of our clinical experience has not supported this approach for cancer of the distal half of the stomach;[78] these lesions can usually be adequately re-

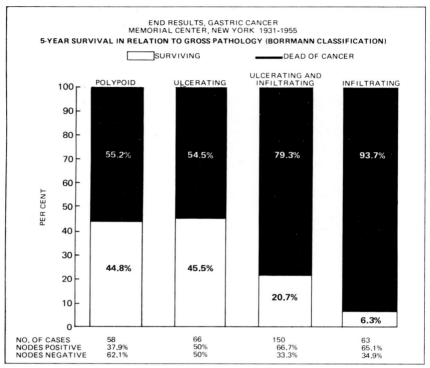

Fig. 8-5.   Prognosis after ''curative'' resection according to gross pathologic type.

sected, including potential lymphatic extensions, by distal radical subtotal
resection.   In addition, liberal use of total gastrectomy for distal-half lesions did not favorably affect survival rates.   Larger lesions of pars media
of the stomach and lesions of the proximal stomach usually close to the
esophagogastric junction require the proximal line of resection to be
through the distal esophagus.   Since esophageal anastomosis is the major
added hazard of either proximal or total gastrectomy, we prefer total gastrectomy rather than subtotal resection of the stomach for lesions requiring resection of the cardia.   The established risk of an esophageal anastomosis is not avoided by retaining the distal portion of the stomach,
and the functional value of the small, distal gastric remnant after adequate
proximal gastrectomy is often inferior to that afforded by other possible
means of ''reservoir'' construction.

    Although a careful exploration is intended to prevent a radical opera-
tion when cure is not possible, it is also important to confirm the diagnosis
of cancer under certain circumstances.   For instance, if a typical gastric
cancer is observed grossly, it may not always seem essential to obtain a

positive biopsy before resection, particularly if the procedure is less radical than total gastrectomy. However, a gastric ulcer with an associated mass may mimic a malignant process, and a total gastric resection may be overly aggressive treatment from the standpoint of both morbidity and potential increase in mortality. Therefore, gastrotomy and biopsy are often indicated to diagnose gastric cancer in questionable cases before performing radical resections, particularly total gastrectomy. Every effort should be made to avoid the spillage of gastric content and tumor cells during these operative biopsy procedures.

Since microscopic spread beyond the gross margins of the tumor is commonly found, the removal of a generous margin of normal stomach around the carcinoma is the major principle of gastric resection for malignant lesions of all sites. In distal gastric lesions, generous resection of the first portion of the duodenum is required; in proximal lesions, a generous margin of distal esophagus must be removed. Failure to control a potentially curable cancer by not achieving adequate gross margins around the primary neoplasm is a serious, avoidable error.

LYMPHATIC SPREAD

In designing a radical gastrectomy for patients with "curable" gastric cancer, one must consider the removal of potential regional lymphatic extensions. Although the incidence of regional lymphatic spread varies with different gross and histologic types of cancer, the overall incidence of lymphatic spread from carcinoma of the stomach is high, approximately 60 percent. In addition, gross observations do not reveal whether or not regional metastases are present. Frozen section examination of isolated nodes is not of real benefit except in the evaluation of nodes outside the anatomic boundary of a feasible "en bloc" resection. Potential areas of lymphatic spread must always be considered in the design of radical gastrectomy since the true status of the regional lymphatics can be determined only after treatment has been completed.

Since regional lymphatics accompany the blood vessels on both the lesser and greater curvatures of the stomach, lymphatic spread of gastric cancer to these sites always warrants consideration. Detailed autopsy studies, and studies of cleared surgical specimens after total gastrectomy and distal pancreatectomy, have also demonstrated many instances of regional spread to the pancreatic group of lymph nodes (Fig. 8-6).[97,99] Since metastasis to lymph nodes in the splenic hilum is always accompanied by metastasis to the more proximal nodes along the body and tail of the pancreas, it is reasonable to assume that these hilar nodes are an extension of lymphatic metastases occurring initially in the retrogastric portion of the splenic artery chain (pancreatolienal nodes). That this area of spread is still within the limits of "curative" resection is shown by the long-term survival of several of our patients after resection of involved

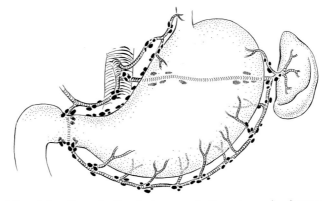

Fig. 8-6. Lymphatic drainage of the stomach demonstrating the pancreatolienal lymph nodes.

pancreatolienal nodes. However, routine clinical trial of this approach led
to no clear-cut increase in the overall salvage of gastric cancer patients,
but rather to a definite increase in both morbidity and mortality.[78]

SPECIFIC OPERATIONS

The extent of resection of the "gastric bed" of lymphatic-bearing
tissues obviously varies with the location and size of the lesion and the
general status of the patient. Radical distal subtotal gastrectomy (Fig.
8-7) does not include resection of the nodes adjacent to the cardia of the

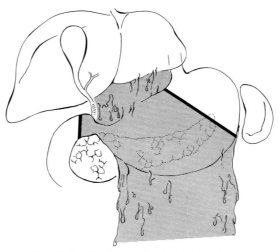

Fig. 8-7. Radical subtotal gastrectomy.

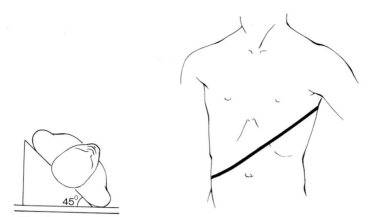

Fig. 8-8. Thoracoabdominal incision for radical gastrectomy.

stomach, the pancreatolienal nodes along the splenic artery, or the lymph nodes in the splenic hilum. However, both logic and prior studies of operative specimens have shown that these lymph node groups are not involved in patients with cancers of the distal third of the stomach, except when nonresectable areas of lymphatic spread in the region of the head of the pancreas have already developed. Regional lymphatic spread of these sites has been demonstrated in potentially curable cancers of the pars media and proximal stomach—a major theoretical reason for considering total gastrectomy or even extended total gastrectomy (distal pancreas and spleen) for such cancers (Figs. 8-8 and 8-9). Nevertheless, high

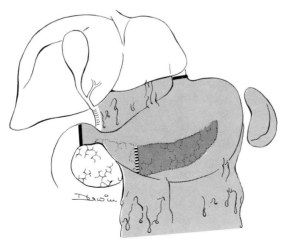

Fig. 8-9. Extended total gastrectomy.

subtotal gastrectomy appears to be a reasonable approach to the treatment of a small lesion in the pars media, particularly if a generous margin around the gross tumor can be removed. Because of the relatively limited gains with the extended procedures, the patient's age and medical disability must also be carefully weighed before deciding on the extent of resection. See Nora's *Operative Surgery*[74] for a description of the technical details of all of these operative procedures.

COMBINED ORGAN RESECTIONS

Some otherwise resectable gastric cancers are adherent not only to the pancreas or spleen, but also to the transverse mesocolon and the midcolic vessels. There should be no hesitation about the division of the mesocolon, leaving adherent tissue attached to the surgical specimen. Adequate collateral blood supply of the transverse colon may allow sacrifice of the midcolic vessels without colon resection, but any question of the adequacy of the blood supply should prompt colon resection along with gastric resection. The left lobe of the liver, which is occasionally adherent to a more proximal gastric cancer, can also be resected in continuity with the gastrectomy under these circumstances. Resection of adjacent adherent organs prevents "violation" of the surgical margins, but local invasion of adherent structures may be difficult to demonstrate later histologically. Invasion of adjacent organs or structures causes concern, but it is probably associated with a better prognosis than is lymphatic spread.

Resection of a segment of transverse colon, the body and tail of the pancreas, the spleen, or a portion of the liver combined with resection for gastric carcinoma can provide benefits; however, whether combined organ resection is applicable to the head of the pancreas is difficult to answer. Pancreatoduodenectomy is a truly major extension of gastrectomy, and vital structures in this area, particularly the superior mesenteric artery and portal vein, reduce the anatomic possibility of an en bloc resection. In addition, most gastric cancers involving the head of the pancreas to this extent also involve other structures in the porta hepatis or elsewhere, rendering the patient "incurable." The data of Berry and Rottschafer[14] give no support for this approach. It is conceivable that pancreatoduodenectomy could be advisable as a "curative operation," but there are no reported clinical data demonstrating benefits from this approach. Personal experience is limited to 3 patients in whom pancreatoduodenectomy seemed the logical approach: 2 developed recurrent carcinoma within 12 months, and the third patient is alive and well more than 4 years after resection.

ALIMENTARY TRACT RECONSTRUCTION

After distal subtotal gastrectomy, continuity should always be restored by gastrojejunostomy rather than gastroduodenostomy. The former procedure avoids the problem of gastric outlet obstruction in patients who develop recurrent carcinoma following attempted "curative" resection. Gastric cancer recurs in the region of the pancreas ("gastric bed"); therefore, a gastroduodenostomy would be more likely to be involved in this regrowth of cancer than a gastrojejunostomy.

The weakest point in the reconstruction after total gastrectomy is the esophageal anastomosis, and this should be carried out as precisely as possible with interrupted sutures through all layers (Fig. 8-10). Continuity is best restored by end-to-side esophagojejunostomy using some form of jejunal reservoir pouch distal to this anastomosis. Our preference is a double-lumen jejunal pouch with a distal Roux-y anastomosis, which creates a reservoir to substitute for the resected stomach.[76,120,135]

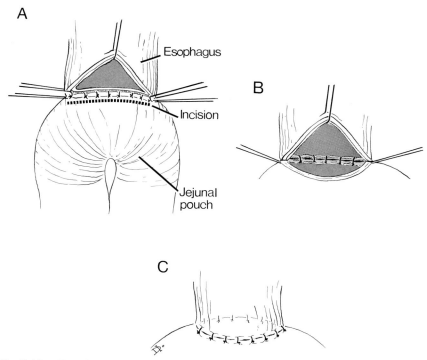

Fig. 8-10. Esophagojejunostomy is accomplished by interrupted sutures through all layers of the esophagus and the jejunum. An outer row of sutures buttresses this anastomosis, but this inner layer is the key portion of the anastomosis.

The details of the jejunal reservoir construction we prefer are shown in Figure 8-11.[74] The reservoir is partially constructed by carrying out a long side-to-side jejunojejunostomy (approximately 6–8 inches) after folding the jejunum on itself. Care is taken to avoid connecting the jejunal incisions to the apex of the bowel loop as the blood supply of the portion of bowel for esophageal anastomosis must be preserved. The jejunum of the afferent loop is divided several centimeters proximal to the long jejunojejunostomy, and the distal (or pouch) lumen is closed. The proximal lumen of the limb is brought to the efferent limb for anastomosis 6–8 inches distal to the pouch itself. Actually, all portions of this part of the reconstructive procedure can be effectively accomplished with gastrointestinal stapling instruments if desired, but we have felt more confident using a suture technique on the esophageal anastomosis.

This specific form of reservoir reconstruction is designed to prevent reflux of duodenal secretions into the esophagus, and the Roux-y anastomosis tends to reduce the rate of outflow of foodstuff from the reservoir area. This type of reconstruction definitely seems to reduce the postgastrectomy symptoms and nutritional problems previously associated with simple esophagojejunal anastomosis as a means for restoring continuity. Other methods of reconstruction after total gastrectomy that attempt to

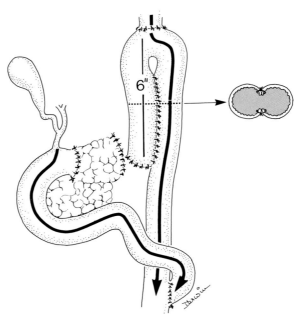

Fig. 8-11. A useful method for reconstruction after total gastrectomy.

achieve some form of reservoir-substitute for the stomach may well be equal to this one, but none of these techniques is more simply accomplished.

PALLIATIVE SURGERY

A significant number of patients have unfavorable operative findings, such as tiny serosal implants, a solitary liver metastasis, an ovarian metastasis, or metastatic disease in lymph nodes outside the range of "en bloc" dissection. This is the case in approximately 60 percent of those patients with gastric cancer who are subjected to operation with the hope that a "curative" procedure can be accomplished. A palliative procedure is then planned or the abdomen is then closed without further surgery, except for biopsy confirmation of these findings.

We prefer palliative resection (without major attention to regional node areas) if the procedure can be accomplished without total gastrectomy, without transection of gross tumor at the site of the planned anastomosis, and without major hazard to the patient. If these conditions are met, palliative resection can give significant relief of symptoms in the majority of patients and also prolongs survival.[77] If these conditions cannot be met in the incurable patient, we prefer to close the abdomen without performing gastrojejunostomy, gastrostomy or jejunostomy, which rarely relieves symptoms or prolongs life expectancy (Table 8-2). In carefully selected patients, total gastrectomy can be employed, but this procedure is rarely indicated for palliation because of the longer recovery and adjustment period required after this type of operation compared to

Table 8-2
Duration of Life After Noncurative Operations for
Gastric Cancer

Treatment	No. of Patients		Average Duration (Mo)
Laparotomy only	239		4.6
Bypass operations	86		4.2
Gastrostomy		32	6.9
Jejunostomy		27	3.3
Gastroenterostomy		27	3.9
Palliative resection	108		9.0
Subtotal gastrectomy		67	9.5
Total gastrectomy		41	8.2

* From Lawrence and McNeer.[77]

the course after partial gastrectomy. Total gastrectomy might be seriously considered for palliation in the patient with virtually complete obstruction and a limited quantity of nonresectable disease.

NONSURGICAL TREATMENT OF GASTRIC CANCER

Radiation therapy and systemic drug therapy are the nonsurgical methods available for treatment of gastric cancer, but they are both inappropriate for primary treatment of potentially curable disease. There is no evidence at present that either of these methods is of value as an adjuvant to surgical resection in favorable cases, although our only hope for future improvement in end results will obviously depend on some form of adjuvant therapy preceding or following surgical resection.[88]

For palliative treatment of patients who have lesions unsuitable for gastric resection, systemic chemotherapy can be employed with some benefit; but radiation therapy is effective in few instances because the disease is not localized in most patients. On the other hand, radiation therapy has been useful in relieving localized areas of obstruction, particularly in the region of the cardia, and patients with chronically bleeding gastric cancers have also been said to be benefited by radiation. The nature of the pattern of spread of gastric cancer in the patient who is not amenable to surgical therapy usually makes systemic chemotherapy seem more appropriate as a palliative tool.

Systemic cancer chemotherapy generally has been less effective for gastric cancer than for colorectal cancer, probably because of the relatively rapid clinical course of most patients who are not effectively treated by gastric resection. Many chemotherapeutic agents have been employed as single agents with generally disappointing results, and the antimetabolite 5-fluorouracil (5-FU) was the most effective of these agents until combination drug regimes were developed.[29] Approximately 15–20 percent of patients treated with 5-FU demonstrated transient evidence of improvement of a limited degree with no increase in survival time. In contrast, various combinations of agents studied in advanced gastric cancer patients in prospective clinical trials have produced somewhat higher rates of objective response to therapy with apparent increase in patient survival. Response rates in the 30–50-percent range have been recorded with the combination of 5-FU and nitrosourea compounds (BCNU and methyl-CCNU). Hopefully, this investigation is a first step toward more effective anticancer chemotherapy for gastric cancer after years of general dissatisfaction with single-agent therapy. As these data are more firmly established, and more effective combination regimes are developed, it is hoped that effective adjuvant chemotherapy will be developed for patients undergoing surgery for gastric cancer.

Survival Data

Until some major improvement in therapy for gastric cancer is established, treatment decisions will be assisted by an appreciation of survival curves after therapy for patients in various "stages" of disease (see Fig. 8-12). These curves are from an old study from Memorial Sloan-Kettering Cancer Center, but there have been no change in treatment methods and no evidence of a major change in prognosis of patients with gastric cancer.[44] These curves demonstrate quite clearly that the 5-year period is an excellent "yardstick" for evaluating treatment methods since the majority of patients who develop further difficulty do so within 3 years of the primary surgical treatment. After resection, 90 percent of those patients in our series surviving 5 years without evidence of residual cancer have remained free of disease.

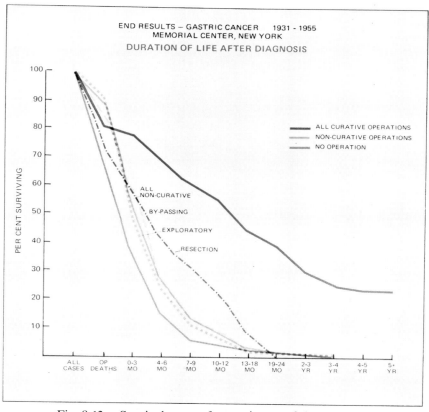

Fig. 8-12. Survival curves for carcinoma of the stomach.

Since approximately two-thirds of patients seen with gastric cancer have either physical examination or operative findings at the time of diagnosis that eliminate the possibility of surgical "cure," and since no more than one-third of those patients considered candidates for curative resection are well 5 or more years after treatment, only 10 percent of all patients with the diagnosis of carcinoma of the stomach enjoy long-term survival. It is quite apparent, then that we will continue to have a significant number of patients with gastric carcinoma who require thoughtful palliative management.

Special Management Problems

PEPTIC ULCER VERSUS CANCER

Ulcerocancer of the stomach appears to be a discrete gross pathologic type of gastric cancer with some favorable clinical features (higher resectability and curability rates). For this reason it is particularly important to differentiate this lesion from benign gastric ulcer as early as possible in the clinical course.[133] The vagaries of the radiologic diagnosis of gastric ulcer versus ulcerocancer were great enough in the past for many clinicians to recommend surgery for most gastric ulcers. Others took the opposite attitude that medical therapy should be pursued in all patients for an extended period. They argued that the overall prognosis for gastric cancer was so poor that the inconvenience and disability experienced by the group requiring gastrectomy for benign lesions outweighed any potential salvage in the cancer group. Since the prognosis for ulcerocancer is clearly better than that for most other gross types, this latter approach is not well founded. However, the other extreme, surgery for all gastric ulcers, also seems unwise with the diagnostic precision now available.

Our approach to these questionable ulcerating lesions is to recommend exploration and resection of the gastric ulcer if there has been a significant prior bleeding episode, if the prior history of peptic ulcer disease and the present symptoms are disabling, or if cytologic, radiologic, or endoscopic findings are suspicious in any way. If all tests suggest benign gastric ulcer, a therapeutic trial seems quite justified as diagnostic accuracy with these criteria exceeds 95 percent. Follow-up radiographic and gastroscopic examination should show some evidence of healing in 3–4 weeks if this regime is to be continued, and eventual complete healing is required or operation will be indicated at a later date.

For those patients with gastric ulcers that require surgery, the operative approach to the lesion varies somewhat with the location in the stomach, the size of the lesion, and the relationship of other organs to the process in question. Biopsy of several sites on the edge of the ulcer through a gastrotomy has several disadvantages, including potential tumor cell spillage in the peritoneal cavity and the possibility of an erroneus frozen section diagnosis. Nevertheless, gross examination of the ulcerating lesion and generous biopsies through the gastrotomy are indicated if the diagnosis of cancer would lead to a radical procedure such as total gastrectomy or an extended combined organ resection. Gross inspection and frozen section examination of a gastric ulcer are certainly not foolproof, but the accuracy of this approach is considerably greater than that of external palpation through the wall of the unopened stomach.

For distal gastric ulcers it is often easy to carry out a radical distal subtotal gastrectomy for any lesion with a suspicion of cancer without opening the stomach for biopsy evaluation. The lymph node–bearing tissues are resected as if the lesion is an ulcerocancer so as to avoid the gastrotomy, but the actual gastric resection is carried to the same extent for benign or malignant lesions.

GASTRIC POLYPS

A "polyp" of the stomach may be an adenomatous polyp, a cancer appearing as a "polyp" in terms of gross configuration, an inflammatory polyp, or a benign or malignant neoplasm of mesodermal origin. The relative rarity of gastric polyps tends to eliminate consideration of the adenomatous polyp as a significant precancerous lesion, but the management of polypoid lesions of the stomach is still confused by differing concepts of their neoplastic potential.[12,99,149]

Two features suggesting a relationship between the adenomatous polyp and cancer of the stomach are (a) the high incidence of adenomatous polyps in a stomach with established cancer (25–35 percent), and (b) the high incidence of achlorhydria and the presence of atrophic gastric mucous membrane in patients with adenomatous polyps and in those with cancer. Although 10–15 percent of adenomatous polyps do develop cytologic atypism (carcinoma in situ),[12] there is little evidence on long-term follow-up examination that this lesion proceeds to clinical cancer. Fortunately, these cytologic changes have not been observed frequently in polyps less than 2 cm in diameter, a factor that allows us to develop a reasonable and logical treatment plan for polypoid lesions.

If single or multiple polypoid lesions of the stomach cause symptoms, such as bleeding or obstruction, surgical intervention is certainly indicated. The solitary polyp, or multiple lesions of limited extent, can be treated by limited gastric resection. If there are no symptoms, the polypoid lesion less than 2 cm in diameter can be safely observed by serial radiographic and gastroscopic examinations on the basis of data from a number of series. However, if a single lesion is larger than 2 cm in diameter, exploratory celiotomy is indicated for excision of the entire lesion in question. If there is diffuse polyposis, gastrectomy may be required to eliminate the abnormality, but there is no evidence for a relationship comparable to that of familial polyposis and colon cancer.

BENIGN NEOPLASMS OF THE STOMACH

There are a number of potential benign neoplasms and pseudoneoplasms of the stomach, but these are rare in proportion to the malignant lesions. After the adenomatous polyp discussed previously, the next most common benign gastric neoplasm is the leiomyoma. These may become quite large before producing symptoms, and one of the most frequent symptoms heralding their presence is gastric bleeding from a small ulcer in the overlying mucosa. Other mesodermal tumors—lipomas, neurogenic tumors, glomus tumors, accessory pancreas and inflammatory tumors (eosinophilic granuloma or inflammatory polyps)—are all extremely rare and require only local resection of the lesion with repair of the stomach. Carcinoid of the stomach is a rare lesion and is usually thought to be a carcinoma from its gross features at time of operation. Actually, this neoplasm is usually treated as a carcinoma, and this seems reasonable since some of these lesions are capable of metastasis. Carcinoids are discussed in more detail in the section on small intestinal neoplasms.

OTHER MALIGNANT TUMORS
OF THE STOMACH

The overwhelming majority of malignant gastric tumors are glandular carcinomas (adenocarcinomas). Leiomyosarcoma and primary lymphoma of the stomach are so rarely encountered that these diagnoses frequently lead to confusion regarding appropriate treatment. Actually, the neoplastic lesion is often resected on the assumption that it is a carcinoma on the basis of gross evaluation, and the unsuspected diagnosis of sarcoma is revealed later. In each instance the general plan of resection is identical to that for carcinoma. One major difference, however, is that the prognosis for both leiomyosarcoma of the stomach and primary lymphoma of the stomach is considerably better than that for primary adenocarcinoma (approximately twice as high 5-year survival rates).

Although the primary objective of surgery for these uncommon lesions is identical to that for carcinoma, the relative radiosensitivity of lymphoma has led to the recommendation that all patients with primary lymphoma of the stomach be given radiation therapy after the surgical resection.[30,96] Cases of lymphosarcoma or reticulum cell sarcoma of the stomach are too infrequent to establish the value of radiation therapy conclusively, but the dogma has a reasonable basis particularly for those with lymphatic metastases.

One related gastric lesion that may confuse both the surgeon and his surgical pathologist is "pseudolymphoma."[13] This diffuse or discrete lesion accompanies some benign gastric ulcers and undoubtedly represents an atypical inflammatory response in the region of the ulcer. Differentiating this lesion from true lymphoma at the time of operation is frequently a difficult problem for the surgical pathologist since some lymphomas also develop ulceration. The extent of resection obviously depends on the eventual pathologic decision.

RECURRENT GASTRIC CARCINOMA

It is not too surprising that a few patients who survive for a considerable period after partial gastrectomy for cancer do develop cancer in the gastric remnant. Since an inadequate margin around the primary lesion is rare at the site of proximal transection of the stomach, the likelihood of this "late recurrence" being a second primary gastric cancer is somewhat higher than the likelihood of a "recurrence" of the original cancer. Whatever mechanism for the presence of neoplasm in the gastric remnant of the individual patient, some lesions are amenable to a second resection with hope for cure. Secondary operation under these circumstances usually entails resection of the remaining stomach, along with the spleen and body and tail of the pancreas, but the procedure does seem justified in rare selected cases. In virtually all patients with regrowth of gastric cancer after prior resection, the appropriate therapy is multiple-drug chemotherapy as described previously.

**CANCER OF THE PANCREAS AND
EXTRAHEPATIC BILIARY TREE**

In contrast to gastric cancer, cancer of the pancreas in the United States is increasing in frequency for both men and women. The majority of pancreatic cancers occur in the head of the gland, and the diagnostic difficulties are well known. It is doubtful that there is a significant etiologic relationship between this cancer and chronic pancreatitis, but there is a weak association in some series. The only etiologic clue we have at present for cancer in the extrahepatic biliary tree is the frequent association of gallbladder cancer with cholelithiasis.

In the pancreas the pathology of malignant lesions includes adenocarcinoma arising from the ducts or acini, cyst adenocarcinoma, islet cell carcinoma (functioning or nonfunctioning), lymphoma, and other forms of sarcoma. The first lesion listed accounts for more than 95 percent of these lesions. There are also various common benign neoplasms and a fascinating group of functioning neoplasms (discussed in Chapter 14). In the extrahepatic biliary tree virtually all malignant lesions are variations of adenocarcinoma. For the purpose of this discussion cancer of the pancreas and extrahepatic biliary tree will be considered together as the presentation, diagnosis, and management have many common features.

Clinical Diagnosis

Jaundice is a common sign of most of these neoplasms, and most symptoms—other than the pain of advanced disease—are relatively nonspecific. Actually, the initial management problem with this group of neoplasms is establishing a diagnosis since benign inflammatory disease of the pancreas or the biliary tree can readily simulate cancer of these structures. Standard upper gastrointestinal radiographic study rarely helps much in this differentiation because of wide variation in the shape of the duodenal sweep. In addition, gross involvement of the duodenum by cancer of the pancreas is usually a sign of advanced disease. Primary carcinoma of the duodenum leads to a clinical presentation that is indistinguishable from these pancreatic and biliary tree cancers, and barium studies (particularly hypotonic duodenography) are helpful in this differentiation.[40]

Some investigators use pancreatic scans with selenomethionine to aid in diagnosis of pancreatic lesions, but these scans have not been particularly useful and have not been at all helpful in achieving "early" diagnosis. Ultrasound for diagnosis and evaluation of pancreatic disease has been described,[81] but, although useful for demonstrating bile duct obstruction and following the course of inflammatory disease and pseudocysts, ultrasound provides no specific diagnostic information needed for these cancers. Selective angiography may demonstrate abnormal tumor vessels or ominous encasement of major arteries in the region of the pancreas,[46] but this method has had little practical application in our own experience since it usually only confirms our impression that disease is present and does not delineate the anatomic and pathologic features. Duodenal aspiration after administration of a pancreatic secretogogue (secretin) produces data on qualitative and quantitative variations in pancreatic juice,[37] as well as material for cytologic study, but this too provides little practical help. All of these examinations have failed to provide either early diagnosis or clear delineation of the established cancer, and virtually all of these lesions are now detected at operation at an incurable stage.

The major tests required by the clinician for evaluation of the patient with apparent obstructive jaundice are studies confirming the mechanical nature of the obstruction as well as localizing the specific site since surgical resection or biopsy is usually required to obtain the histologic diagnosis. Percutaneous transhepatic cholangiography has been a useful diagnostic method for these purposes, particularly if the patient is prepared for definitive surgery soon after the study. A more direct approach to the same technique has been described using "mini-lap," or laparoscopy, with needle aspiration and injection of the biliary tree, but these variations on transhepatic cholangiography require special preparation and coordination not feasible for routine performance in most institutions.[11] A practical and rewarding diagnostic approach to this type of clinical problem is duodenoscopy with retrograde cannulation and radiographic study of the biliary and pancreatic duct systems.[17,130] With this approach one can confirm the diagnosis of biliary obstruction, localize the anatomic site of obstruction, and possibly obtain material for histologic diagnosis. At the present time this appears in experienced hands to be a useful diagnostic approach to the patient with apparent obstructive jaundice being prepared for surgical exploration. The specific information obtained may greatly facilitate conduct of the subsequent operative procedure in such a patient, but this approach has not been useful for early diagnosis of pancreatic cancer.

DIAGNOSTIC PROBLEMS AT TIME OF SURGICAL EXPLORATION OF THE JAUNDICED PATIENT

Since the neoplasms under consideration (carcinoma of the pancreas, carcinoma of the extrahepatic biliary tree, carcinoma of the ampulla of Vater, and carcinoma of the duodenum) are all best treated by operation if there is a curative possibility, the next step in the differential diagnosis of obstructive jaundice is exploratory celiotomy. The diagnostic questions at the time of surgical exploration of the jaundiced patient include (a) Is the extrahepatic biliary tree really obstructed? (b) Is the obstruction of the biliary tree owing to a benign process or a neoplasm? (c) If there is a mass in the pancreas, is it a form of chronic pancreatitis or a cancer obstructing the pancreatic duct and producing pancreatitis, or is the mass itself a primary pancreatic neoplasm? (d) If there is biliary obstruction owing to neoplasm, what is its primary site?

The validity of the diagnosis of biliary tract obstruction is usually well established before surgery on the basis of the liver function tests and the other preoperative diagnostic tests discussed. The primary site may also be delineated preoperatively, but the second diagnostic question listed above, that of determining the presence or absence of neoplasm, is often difficult. An operative cholangiogram may be useful, particularly in those patients who have not had "successful" preoperative cholangiography by the transduodenal or transhepatic route. The last two questions are sometimes difficult to answer at the time of exploration, and biopsy must be considered. In most instances we believe it is preferable to proceed with resection if there is a resectable mass in the head of the pancreas without metastasis since "benign" biopsy reports on pancreatic masses have been so unreliable.

Treatment

Surgery is the only "curative" treatment for periampullary neoplasm but the ultimate prognosis is so poor after surgical resection of carcinoma of the head of the pancreas that many clinicians logically question the value of resection for this lesion. A philosophic argument continues unresolved with most surgeons favoring pancreatic resection, despite significant morbidity and mortality, because of rare instances of long-term survival after this operation when it is performed for carcinoma of the head of the pancreas. Crile[32] states that the average patient with carcinoma of the head of the pancreas large enough to be palpable may live longer and more comfortably if no attempt to resect the lesion, but there is certainly no general agreement on this point. However, the adoption of this conservative philosophic approach to all patients with a firm mass in the head of the pancreas would eliminate the possibility of curative resection of the more favorable lesions in the duodenum, distal common duct, and the ampulla of Vater that may also present grossly as masses in the head of the pancreas. The pancreatic mass in these instances represents pancreatitis on the basis of the obstructing neoplasm. Since the final pathologic classification of the underlying lesion is often not made until after the resection has been completed and the specimen studied carefully in the pathology laboratory, we contend that pancreatoduodenectomy should be accomplished without biopsy in all such patients of reasonable age and physical condition if all of the gross neoplasm can be resected. Patients with primary cancers of the ampulla, distal common duct, and duodenum have a reasonable chance for long-term survival after resection;[31] (Table 8-3) and those lesions originating in the pancreas itself and treated by resection have palliation as good as, and possibly better than that achieved with "bypass." Such lesions also have a remote chance for "cure."[6,36,67,156,164]

Determining resectability of pancreatobiliary cancers is one of the most tedious aspects of surgery for these sites once it has been determined that no distant peritoneal or liver metastases are present. Mobilization and careful palpation of the duodenum are required since biopsy proof of a benign neoplasm in the ampulla of Vater or duodenum may lead to a more limited resection.[160] The duodenum can be reconstructed by a

Table 8-3
Carcinoma of the Biliary Tree and
Pancreas: End Results of Treatment

Site	5-Yr Survival (%)
Head of the pancreas	0–10
Body and tail of the pancreas	0
Ampulla of Vater	35
Bile duct	25
Gallbladder	5

number of techniques after partial resection (see Fig. 8-18), and the papilla can even be reimplanted if necessary.[70]

The next step is dissection of the major vessels (portal vein and superior mesenteric artery) juxtaposed to the head of the pancreas as their involvement precludes resection in our view (see Fig. 8-13). Many surgeons have proposed resection of the portal vein with graft replacement, portocaval shunt, or even more extensive vascular resection with graft and replacements.[41,111] However, vascular involvement is generally associated with neoplastic extension to other extrapancreatic sites as well as to the specific vascular attachment, and we do not believe it is realistic to resect the pancreas when this type of "local extension" is apparent. We consider this an indication for palliative "bypass" operation.

Before embarking on a major pancreatoduodenal resection, it is also important for the surgeon to assess regional lymph node areas that will not be included in the surgical specimen. The nodes to be evaluated most carefully are in the region of the celiac axis, the hepatoduodenal ligament in and around the major structures of the porta hepatis, and in the base of the mesentery of the small bowel near the superior mesenteric artery. One might even consider metastases in the immediately adjacent regional lymph nodes of the head of the pancreas a contraindication for pancreatoduodenectomy, since this anatomic site is not as suitable for an "en bloc" resection of regional nodes as is the stomach or colon. We prefer to consider these regional nodes potentially resectable on the basis that lymphatic metastasis from primary sites other than the head of the pancreas may be controlled by resection. For this reason we carry out no biopsies of lymph nodes that would ordinarily be included in the surgical specimen of a standard pancreatoduodenectomy.

The value of biopsy of the head of the pancreas is often discussed. Many surgeons feel impelled to justify a major procedure of the type required for periampullary cancer by first obtaining a biopsy. This is a solution to treatment decisions for many surgical diseases, but this situation is different. Biopsy of a mass in the head of the pancreas may produce complications without assisting in resolving the problems for which it was intended. For this reason we prefer to determine the resectability of a mass on clinical grounds at the operating table. We feel that pancreatic biopsies should be reserved to document cancer in those patients in whom the dissection demonstrates nonresectability of the neoplasm.

RESECTION

By the time thorough exploration and dissection have been accomplished to determine resectability, the resection of distal stomach, duodenum, and head of the pancreas is easily accomplished. A major question that remains unresolved is the advisability of total pancreatectomy versus the classic Whipple procedure, which retains the grossly uninvolved portion of the distal pancreas when the primary lesion appears to arise from the head of the pancreas. It is conceivable that invasive cancer may be left in the pancreatic remnant after pancreatoduodenectomy despite the appearance of a grossly free margin beyond the tumor, and cutting across the pancreatic duct in the region of the neck of the pancreas may allow contamination of the peripancreatic area by viable tumor cells in the pancreatic juice. A third, but unlikely, cause for failure of pancreatoduodenectomy to control this lesion is in situ cancer in the remaining pancreas. In view of these possibilities, however, and the generally poor end results from standard surgical resection for cancer of the head of the pancreas, Hicks and Brooks[59] and ReMine et al.[128] have suggested that total pancreatectomy may be a preferable procedure. Total pancreatectomy adds little to the technical problems of pancreatectomy, it obviates one of the anastomoses associated with alimentary tract reconstruction, and patients are controlled relatively well with pancreatic enzymes and insulin after initial recovery from the operation. The results reported by ReMine after total pancreatectomy suggest that this technique may have merit, but we currently use this procedure only in selected instances and suspect that it will not have a major impact on results.

Reconstruction after pancreatic resection for cancer. Truncal vagotomy is routinely performed as a reasonable precaution against development of a marginal ulcer at the gastrojejunostomy site. The anatomic method of reconstruction we prefer is shown in Figure 8-13, although other variations, including simple ligature of the duct in the pancreatic remnant, have been described. Ligation of the duct does reduce the number of anastomoses by one, but our limited experience with this approach in 2 patients was associated with a subsequent pancreatic fistula in both.

BYPASS OPERATIONS FOR CARCINOMA OF THE PERIAMPULLARY AREA

A patient with nonresectable periampullary cancer is most easily treated by a cholecystojejunostomy and routine gastrojejunostomy. We use a loop of proximal jejunum for anastomosis to the enlarged thick-walled gallbladder, unless the neoplasm extends as far as the cystic duct, and perform the gastrojejunostomy distal to this anastomosis to reduce the possibility of marginal ulcer. The use of an enteroenterostomy between the two limbs of jejunum on either side of the gallbladder anastomosis or the use of a Roux-en-y loop of jejunum for the cholecystojejunostomy are "optional" variations. Some surgeons favor choledocho-duodenostomy, choledochojejunostomy, cholecystoduodenostomy, or cholecystogastrostomy as alternative means of bypassing the biliary obstruction. Further growth of the nonresectable neoplasm is more likely to occlude any anastomoses to the duodenum because of proximity, and anastomosis of the gallbladder to the stomach has both this disadvantage and that of total diversion of alkaline bile into the gastrin-producing antrum. The need for gastrojejunostomy is often questioned in such patients who have no gastroduodenal obstruction. Nothing is more frustrating, however, than the development of partial or complete duodenal obstruction at a later date in a patient known to have a nonresectable periampullary cancer.

Surgical Treatment of Lesions of Sites Other Than the Periampullary Area

CARCINOMA OF THE BODY OF THE PANCREAS

The body is a "silent" area of the pancreas, and the first symptoms are usually those secondary to invasion of surrounding structures, intra-abdominal metastases with ascites, or other distant metastases. Surgery accomplishes little more than establishing a diagnosis under these circumstances. One exception to this rule is the relatively rare cystic lesion, cystadenocarcinoma, and its benign counterpart and precursor lesion, cystadenoma.[9,157] Resection of the appropriate portion of pancreas is frequently curative with this uncommon lesion, and fortunately the dominant location for this lesion is in the distal portion of the gland. This is also the most common site for the functioning neoplasms of the pancreatic islets, which are discussed in Chapter 14.

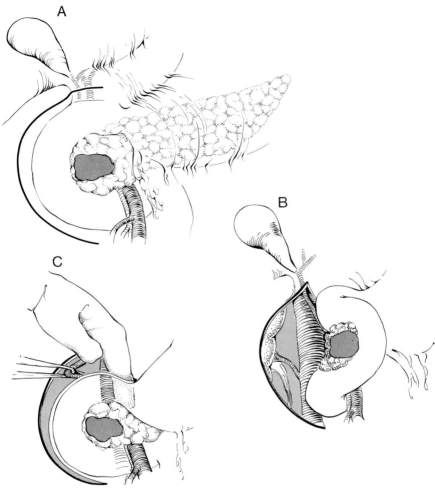

Fig. 8-13. **A, B,** and **C:** Operative steps in determining resectability and performing pancreatoduodenectomy for periampullary cancer. **D** and **E:** Resection and reconstruction.

CARCINOMA OF THE GALLBLADDER

Gallbladder cancer tends to occur in elderly patients, is frequently advanced in terms of local growth by the time it is clinically apparent, and is rarely cured except for the occasional patient with the chance finding of a gallbladder cancer detected as a result of elective cholecystectomy for stones.[10,105,158] In our own experience, and that of others, gallbladder cancers involving only the mucosa (in situ) or the adjacent muscularis are routinely cured by simple cholecystectomy and no further treatment is indicated.[110] At the other extreme, patients with direct gross invasion of

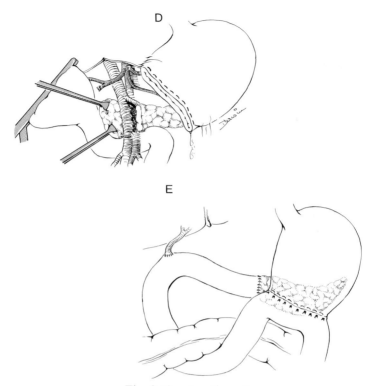

Fig. 8-13. (continued)

the liver bed and/or metastases will not be benefited by aggressive surgical resection (including hepatectomy), and invasion of the porta hepatis in these patients is sufficient to make resection impossible without leaving residual cancer. Patients with gallbladder cancers intermediate between these two extremes have been treated unsuccessfully by cholecystectomy (or extended cholecystectomy) in the past. Right hepatic lobectomy with cholecystectomy and dissection of the regional lymph nodes is probably worthwhile in this setting if the age and medical status of the patient will allow it. Unfortunately, no convincing data are available to support this approach, particularly with neoplastic involvement of the cystic duct lymph node, and cases suitable for this approach are very uncommon.

CARCINOMA OF THE PROXIMAL EXTRAHEPATIC DUCTS

From the standpoint of the surgeon, cancers of these sites have most of the disadvantages demonstrated by cancer of the gallbladder owing to the close proximity of other anatomic structures in the porta hepatis. This prevents adequate local resection of the lesion unless it is in the distal portion of common duct. However, the rather chronic nature of some extrahepatic bile duct cancers (often leading to misdiagnosis as chronic sclerosing cholangitis) has often allowed significant benefit from palliative surgery directed to the biliary obstruction.[152]

Proximal lesions in the bile duct near the bifurcation may require curettage both to establish diagnosis and to drain the obstructed biliary tree. It is probably unrealistic to consider this type of lesion for total curative resection because of the immediate proximity of arterial and venous structures supplying both lobes of the liver, but resection has been successful and may be seriously considered in conjunction with hepatic lobectomy if the primary site is localized to only one of the major ducts. Insertion of a stent with limbs extending into both the right and left hepatic ducts is advisable under most circumstances, and the distal limb of the tube can be inserted into a loop of jejunum brought to the liver for the purpose of relieving the jaundice.[15,25]

Nonsurgical Treatment of Cancers of Pancreatic and Periampullary Areas, Bile Ducts, and Gallbladder

Since the primary curative treatment of cancers of all of these sites is surgical, radiation therapy and anticancer chemotherapy are reserved for patients not suitable for total resection or for those with recurrent lesions after unsuccessful surgical treatment. The limited effectiveness of resectional therapy for most of these lesions has led to considerable interest in these nonsurgical approaches, but the results have generally been disappointing. There are also no data to support the use of either radiation or chemotherapy as an adjuvant to surgical resection.

Radiation therapy has been employed for palliation of unresectable cancers in these sites, but the results have been inconclusive and many therapists feel the disadvantages far outweigh any potential benefit. Nonresectable and recurrent pancreatic cancers have also been resistant to all tested drug approaches. Although the standard gastrointestinal chemotherapeutic agent 5-fluoruracil has produced little patient benefit, some benefit and prolongation of survival time have been demonstrated for patients with localized disease after combined therapy with 5-FU and radiation therapy.[58,104] New drug combinations need to be developed and tested for this aggressive group of cancers.

Prognosis

A summary of the end results of treatment of pancreatobiliary cancers is shown in Table 8-3.

PRIMARY LIVER CANCER

Primary malignant tumors of the liver are relatively uncommon in the United States, whereas they are a major cause of death from cancer in some other parts of the world, particularly Southeast Asia and Africa. The reasons for this geographic and racial difference in incidence are unclear at the present time, although dietary contamination with aflatoxin and other carcinogens may play a role. The association of primary liver cancer with cirrhosis is variable but definite, and postnecrotic cirrhosis is the type most commonly found. In our own series[34] concomitant cirrhosis was present in 60 percent of the patients in whom sufficient pathologic material was available to make this judgment. The histologic forms of primary liver cancer include hepatic cell (hepatocellular), ductal origin (cholangiocellular), a mixture of these, and sarcomas of mesenchymal origin.

Clinical Diagnosis

Clinical diagnosis of primary liver cancer is complicated by the fact that the symptoms, physical findings, and many laboratory abnormalities are frequently the same as in patients with cirrhosis. One specific diagnostic approach is the serum alpha-fetoprotein determination.[83,124,153] The specificity of this test for liver cancer appears to be very high, with embryonal or tetratomatous tumors being virtually the only other conditions in which this fetal protein is significantly elevated, but elevations do occur with various forms of hepatitis.[16] Despite certain geographic, sex, and age differences that have been noted in regard to results obtained with this test, it is a useful adjunct to diagnosis and may have screening possibilities in some parts of the world. Hepatomegaly is a specific enough finding, however, to initiate other diagnostic studies, the most useful being the liver scan and selective arteriography (Fig. 8-14), even if alpha-fetoprotein values are not diagnostic.[4,68] Radioisotope scanning is simple, safe, and reasonably accurate for detecting liver abnormalities measuring at least 2 cm in diameter, but it is nonspecific and imprecise in estimating extent of disease. It has the advantage of being noninvasive, like ultrasound, an untried technique of potential usefulness for diagnosis of liver neoplasms. Selective celiac axis angiography is important for both refinement of diagnosis and classification of the extent of disease. If

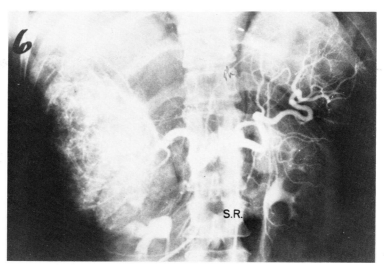

Fig. 8-14. Arteriogram demonstrating abnormal vasculature in primary liver cancer involving right lobe.

the patient undergoes exploration for possible hepatic resection, the angiographic findings are also useful since many variations in vascular anatomy do occur.

Needle biopsy of the liver has proved to be an effective means of establishing the diagnosis of hepatoma, particularly if the selective angiogram demonstrates bilateral lobar involvement. On the other hand, in most instances we prefer surgical exploration for biopsy, rather than needle biopsy, to reveal those patients that may be suitable candidates for resection, as well as to avoid peritoneal spillage of cancer cells in potentially curable cases.

Treatment

According to the microscopic classification of Eggal, primary liver cancer is solitary (massive), nodular (actually multinodular), or diffuse. Even in the absence of extrahepatic metastases (which usually occur in lymph nodes, peritoneum, or lung), only the solitary-type lesion is amenable to surgical resection for obvious reasons. Ultimate staging usually requires exploratory celiotomy (or laparoscopy), but selective arteriography may demonstrate bilobar disease and palliative treatment can then be planned.

In our series only 20 percent of the hepatic cancers were localized in one lobe of the liver, and only 18 percent of patients who underwent exploratory laparotomy for resection were actually suitable for hepatic lobectomy.[34] This figure differs from those reported by some authors in other parts of the world. Cohen and Tan[27] reported a resectability rate of 36 percent and Wang and Li[155] found 38 percent resectable cancers (130 of 336) in a collective study in China.

The presence of cirrhosis is not a contraindication for hepatic resection, but the possibility of postoperative liver failure is increased. Lin and Chen[82] performed seven hepatic lobectomies for primary liver cancer in patients with cirrhosis; 3 of the patients died within 2 months of surgery. Of the 2 patients with cirrhosis in our own series of liver resections, 1 died (with ascending cholangitis) after 2 months and the other patient lived for 64 months.

SURGICAL RESECTION

Before 1950 there were only 8 published cases of long-term survival after surgical resection of primary liver cancer, and all were patients suitable for extremely limited hepatic resections. The feasibility of elective hepatic lobectomy involving the right lobe was then established in the early 1950s, and this extended the possibility of surgical resection to patients considered incurable. There are no reliable data regarding the results and prognosis of liver cancer treated by hepatic lobectomy, but there are enough reported patients with long-term survival after resection to warrant continued application of this method in anatomically suitable cases.[1,7,20,35,42,66,89,93]

Elective resection of the right lobe (or "extended" right lobe) of the liver is clearly of greater magnitude than resection of the smaller left hepatic lobe, but the operation is commonly performed with acceptable morbidity. The key features of liver surgery relate to control of hemorrhage at the time of operation and appropriate supportive care during the postoperative period.

Pack and Baker[115] and others have stressed the importance of controlling the vascular inflow to the hepatic lobe undergoing resection as well as controlling the hepatic veins draining the lobe (Fig. 8-15). One precaution, of course, is to avoid injury to hepatic venous drainage from the remaining liver. Another precaution is to be certain that the malignant lesion is clearly resectable from the standpoint of liver tissue near the vena cava; as an error in judgment regarding this could also lead to serious hepatic vein or vena caval injury.

Methods of major liver resection have been refined in recent years, particularly the "finger fracture" technique for transecting hepatic parenchyma (Fig. 8-16). This has obviated any need for complex clamps or massive sutures to control bleeding from the divided parenchyma. To accomplish this simple and convenient method of hemostasis, the liver cap-

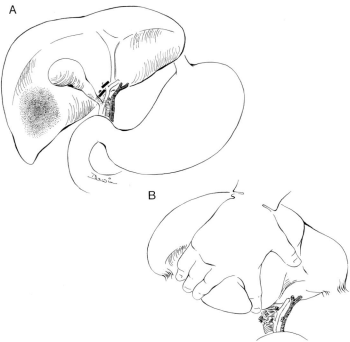

Fig. 8-15. **A:** Dissection of porta hepatis with ligature of bile duct and vascular structures to right hepatic lobe. **B:** Mobilization of right hepatic lobe and ligature of hepatic veins.

sule is incised in the line of proposed liver section and the liver tissue is divided by compression between two fingers. All vessels and bile ducts of any size are easily identified by palpation during this process and they are individually ligated and divided. This method is equally applicable to extended right hepatic lobectomy, right or left hemihepatectomy, or the more limited resection of the lateral segment of the left lobe. This technique has essentially prevented major blood loss during major hepatectomy except for that resulting from surgical misadventures in the porta hepatis or in the region of the hepatic veins.

NONSURGICAL TREATMENT OF PRIMARY LIVER CANCER

The patient with primary liver cancer who is found to be unsuitable for surgical resection is incurable by currently available systemic anticancer agents, and life expectancy is quite short (mean survival in our series was 3.8 months after diagnosis).[34] Both radiotherapy and systemic

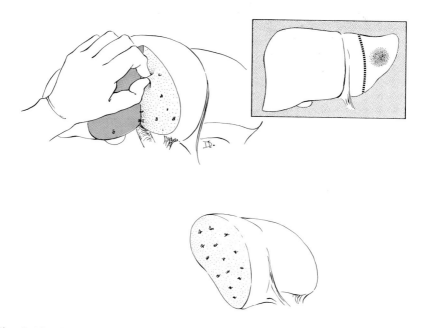

Fig. 8-16. Transection of hepatic parenchyma with clamps and ligatures on major vessels and ducts detected by "finger fracture." **Insert:** left lobe resection.

chemotherapy have been employed for palliative purposes, but neither has demonstrated major benefits thus far.[64]

The technique of continuous intra-arterial infusion chemotherapy has been applied to the liver, and some authors were moderately enthusiastic about responses obtained with this approach for nonresectable primary liver cancer.[5,146,148] Our past experience with regional chemotherapy for primary liver cancer was limited to only 4 patients, but responses to both 5-fluorouracil and methotrexate arterial infusions were discouraging.[75] In 2 patients objective response of the tumor was definite after antimetabolite infusion therapy, but this benefit persisted for only 3–4 months. The other 2 patients had no detectable response. Although some have been more encouraging in their reports of response to regional chemotherapy, improvements in the chemotherapeutic agents are required if this approach is to be worthwhile.

MANAGEMENT OF METASTATIC LIVER CANCER

The diagnosis of liver metastasis from cancers of the gastrointestinal tract or other sites is similar to that described for primary liver cancer with the exception that serum alpha-fetoprotein levels are rarely elevated

and certainly not to high levels. Elevated serum levels of carcinoembryonic antigen may often be a clue to the presence of liver metastasis before clinical findings or other biochemical tests suggest this possibility.
Although the choice of palliative therapy is usually an appropriate regime
employing systemic chemotherapy, various surgical approaches have
been employed in selected cases with benefit.

Resection. It is surprising that some patients undergoing major liver
resection for metastatic cancer have experienced long-term survival, but
this has been clearly documented.[35,42] Favorable factors are solitary
(rather than multiple) metastases, no other evidence of local or systemic
spread of cancer, and a primary tumor that is already controlled or is
readily excised. The major factor of importance is the growth potential
of the particular tumor giving rise to the metastasis.

Patients with colorectal cancer appear to be the most frequent candidates for palliative resection of liver metastases, possibly because they
have a somewhat better prognosis than patients with metastases from
neoplasms arising from other gastrointestinal sites. A 20-percent 5-year
survival rate has been reported after resection of selected metastatic lesions from patients with primary colon or rectal cancer. It is difficult to
prove conclusively that this survival experience is actually owing to liver
resection, in view of the obvious selection of cases suitable for surgery,
but the rarity of long-term survivals without resection suggests some benefit from the surgical approach. It is interesting that patients with
"simultaneous" liver metastasis have an opportunity for benefit from
liver resection similar to those demonstrating metachronous metastasis
with a significant interval. If exploration for colon resection reveals a localized liver metastasis without other metastastic disease, the "timing" of
the liver resection must be considered. If the patient has any clinical features leading to increased operative risk (i.e., cardiac or pulmonary
problems), it is probably best to avoid synchronous resection of the liver
lesion unless this can be accomplished by a relatively limited wedge resection. If associated medical problems do not exist, it seems appropriate to proceed with resection of the liver metastasis, if this requires only a
local resection, or a left lobectomy (left lateral segmentectomy). If the
resection requires hemihepatectomy or extended right hepatic lobectomy
because of the size of the lesion, this is best deferred. After the patient
has fully recovered from the bowel resection, hepatic resection can be
performed. If the interval is prolonged for any reason, systemic chemotherapy can be administered.

Hepatic artery ligation. This approach has been described and employed periodically on the basis that most metastatic lesions receive their

blood supply from the hepatic artery and that selective tumor necrosis has been observed after ligation. Ligation of the common hepatic artery distal to the gastroduodenal artery has been tolerated reasonably well in most series if metastases represent a small proportion of the liver volume (<30 percent).[43,141] Although necrosis of metastatic disease in the liver has been documented after the use of this method, the overall results of this specific measure are somewhat inconclusive because of difficulties in objective assessment of the hepatic lesions and the frequent logical use of this approach in combination with chemotherapy. It seems unlikely that this approach will be of major benefit either to patients with liver metastases or to patients with primary liver cancer.

Regional (hepatic artery) infusion of chemotherapeutic agents. The initial enthusiasm for trials of continuous arterial infusion therapy was based on the anatomy of distribution of blood flow to cancer in the liver. Regional therapy for the portal system has also been employed by catheterization of the umbilical vein.

In our own early experience[26] with intra-arterial infusion chemotherapy for liver metastases, we reported objective responses in 9 of the first 16 patients so treated (1962). Continued trials of this approach led us to conclude that intra-arterial infusion chemotherapy may produce more striking initial results than systemic chemotherapy, but the responses observed are only transient unless maintenance therapy is continued. Our final conclusion after treating 35 patients was that the additional disadvantages and complications of intra-arterial chemotherapy did not justify continued use of this method of administration of anticancer agents.[75] Other groups[5,146,148] have had much greater enthusiasm for this approach to the treatment of liver metastases. Part of the reason for these differences in opinion regarding benefit from regional arterial infusion chemotherapy is the great difficulty in objectively assessing initial response, and the minimal evidence for long-term benefit. It has also been proposed that the hepatic artery be ligated and catheterized distal to the site of ligation for infusion of chemotherapeutic agents,[43] but this is an even less appealing treatment method in our view because of the poor perfusion that must occur in this system.

Systemic chemotherapy. Liver metastasis is a late clinical manifestation of most cancers and is usually associated with an unrelenting course and short survival time. The largest group of patients with gastrointestinal cancer requiring therapeutic management of liver metastasis is the colorectal group, and roughly 10 percent of these patients have an objective response to systemic chemotherapy with 5-FU. Median survival of untreated patients with liver metastasis from colorectal cancer is generally in the range of 5–6 months, but this survival period is extremely variable. It is difficult to observe prolongation of survival as a result of response to 5-fluorouracil. In view of the increased benefit observed with various combinations of agents in the palliative treatment of colorectal and gastric cancer, it is logical to assume there will be increased benefit from this approach to this metastatic site (see Chap. 2).

MANAGEMENT OF BENIGN LIVER NEOPLASMS

Benign tumors of significant size in the liver are relatively rare, with hemangiomas being the most common. Hepatic adenomas are benign, solitary, encapsulated tumors with little or no potential for malignant transformation.[2,92] The major danger of these benign neoplasms is hemorrhage from fracture (hemangioma) or hemorrhagic infarction (adenoma). Malignant vascular tumors and other sarcomas may also arise in the liver.[91]

Liver resection, as described for cancer, is applicable to benign lesions on occasion. Hemangiomas may also be effectively treated by irradiation therapy, and this is the appropriate method if the patient has bilateral hemangioma and an uncomfortably large liver. Hepatic adenomas are best resected if this can be done without hazard. Information on the natural history of this benign lesion is limited, but the excellent prognosis does not warrant exposing the patient to a significant risk from operation.

NEOPLASMS OF THE SMALL BOWEL

A wide range of both benign and malignant tumors has been described in the small bowel,[28,100,112,129,132,138,163] but this portion of the intestine does appear to be relatively immune to neoplasia when compared to the stomach and the large bowel. The frequency of benign tumors is variable, although uniformly low, and malignant neoplasms of the small bowel generally represent only 1–5 percent of all cancers of the gastrointestinal tract.

Clinical Diagnosis

Small bowel neoplasms often are not diagnosed before surgery for symptoms of obstruction (frequently intussusception) or gastrointestinal blood loss, and these lesions are also often incidental findings at the time of surgery for other conditions. The frequent lack of a preoperative diagnosis is not surprising in view of the rarity of the lesions, the nonspecific nature of the symptoms and findings, and the frequent inability of the radiologist to assist in the diagnosis unless the lesion is in the duodenum or distal ileum.

Table 8-4
Small Bowel Neoplasms
(Medical College of Virginia, 1971)[28]

Type	Duodenum	Jejunum	Ileum and Ileocecal Valve	Total
Benign neoplasms				
Adenomas				
Islet cell	5	0	0	5
Brunner's gland	2	0	0	2
Adenoma	1	3	6	10
Leiomyomas	3	3	2	8
Hemangiomas	0	1	1	2
Lymphangiomas	0	1	0	1
Fibromas	0	0	1	1
Lipomas	1	0	4	5
Total	12	8	14	34
Malignant neoplasms				
Adenocarcinoma	2	3	5	10
Leiomyosarcoma	0	2	3	5
Lymphosarcoma	2	0	4	6
Total	4	5	12	21
Carcinoid	5		18	23
Total malignant	9	5	30	44
Grand total	21	13	44	78

A large variety of benign tumors of the small bowel are reported in the world literature. The distribution of benign neoplasms in terms of histology and anatomy in our series[28] is shown in Table 8-4. The most common benign lesions in a larger series reported by the Mayo Clinic were leiomyomas, lipomas, and adenomatous polyps. Of the malignant small bowel tumors (other than carcinoid), adenocarcinoma is always considered the most frequent lesion, followed in incidence by leiomyosarcoma and lymphosarcoma. This distribution was similar in our own series of 21 patients with malignant lesions, but the usual predominance of the adenocarcinoma in the duodenum was not observed. It is of interest that there is a high incidence of second primary cancers both in patients with adenocarcinoma of the small bowel and in patients with carcinoid.

CARCINOID TUMORS

The carcinoid tumor is an unusual gastrointestinal neoplasm that has malignant potential and a wide range of prognostic features.[72,94] Frequency distribution of this lesion throughout the gastrointestinal tract is shown in Figure 8-17. After the appendix, the distal ileum is the most common site of origin. If the tumor is symptomatic, rather than an incidental finding, it is more likely to have metastasized. Moertel et al.[103] state that 93 percent of symptomatic carcinoids in their series has metastasized, whereas only 9 percent of asymptomatic carcinoids had done so. The incidence of metastases is also clearly related to the size of the primary carcinoid, ranging from less than 2 percent for lesions smaller than 1 cm to 80 percent for lesions over 2 cms. McDonald[95] considered depth of invasion of the bowel wall to be another important factor. Lymphatic spread almost never occurred in his series in the absence of muscularis invasion and usually not without serosal involvement. The presence or absence of metastases is of great prognostic significance as shown by the fact that all 13 patients in our series without lymphatic or distant spread at the time of diagnosis and resection have remained well from the stand-

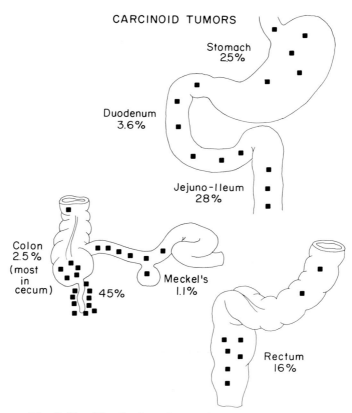

Fig. 8-17.   Distribution of gastrointestinal carcinoids.

point of their carcinoid tumor. Of 10 patients with metastases who underwent segmental resection of the small bowel, 2 are alive less than 5 years afterward, 1 is alive with significant hepatomegaly 14 years afterward, and all the others are dead.[28]

Treatment

Once the diagnosis is established, all small bowel neoplasms are treated by surgical resection. This is often accomplished at the time of operative intervention for examination and biopsy of an abnormality seen on radiographic study, operation for complications such as bleeding or obstruction, or abdominal operation performed for an unrelated disease.

BENIGN LESIONS

A benign small bowel tumor is usually resected easily if the lesion is on a pedicle since local resection is appropriate. Occasionally, adequate excision of a benign lesion of the duodenum without a pedicle requires a major resection of the duodenal wall, and this is more difficult to deal with than a lesion in the jejunum or ileum. Although it has been suggested that large duodenal defects not involving the ampulla of Vater can be closed with the serosal surface of a loop of jejunum or a full-thickness pedicle patch graft of jejunum, these operations are somewhat complex. A simple method of reconstruction that we have employed after extensive duodenal resection is shown in Figure 8-18. Reconstruction of the duodenal defect requires a generous incision across the pylorus into the wall of the stomach to provide tissue for the reconstruction, and the duodenal defect is actually closed with gastric wall—a technique similar to that of Finney pyloroplasty.[79]

MALIGNANT LESIONS

Most malignant neoplasms of the duodenum require pancreatoduodenectomy as outlined earlier in the section on pancreatobiliary cancer. Primary cancers in the jejunum and ileum are more easily resected and should include a wedge of mesentery with accompanying lymphatics, but the extent of feasible lymphatic resection is considerably more limited than with lesions in the large bowel. Malignant tumors of the distal ileum are usually best treated by standard right hemicolectomy since a more reasonable resection of the regional lymphatics can be accomplished for this site by this means. In our series of 21 noncarcinoid malignant tumors of the small bowel, the results were quite disappointing, but there were a few long-term survivors after surgical resection. Generally, patients with localized lymphosarcoma are given radiotherapy postoperatively, but the therapeutic value of this postoperative adjunct is difficult to establish.

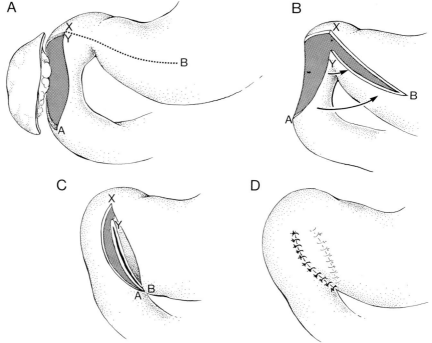

Fig. 8-18. A method of reconstruction after partial duodenal resection.

CARCINOIDS

Although carcinoid tumors have the capacity for metastasis, the differences in behavior of carcinoids in various anatomic sites and the chronic nature of these tumors even when metastasis has occurred necessitate considering carcinoids separately from the other malignant tumors of gastrointestinal tract. Carcinoids of the appendix virtually never develop metastatic disease, and simple appendectomy is adequate treatment. Carcinoids of the stomach, as mentioned previously, may progress to a large size and they are capable of lymph node metastasis. For this reason these lesions have generally been treated in a fashion similar to that employed for adenocarcinoma of the stomach.

Carcinoids of the small bowel also can metastasize; therefore, bowel resection with resection of the adjacent mesentery should be accomplished in a fashion similar to that employed for malignant tumors of the small bowel. In the duodenum, where radical surgery might entail pancreatoduodenectomy, a more conservative procedure seems indicated, if feasible. In the large bowel, particularly the rectum, carcinoid tumors present a particular problem in treatment because of their anatomic location. The choice between a relatively minor local excision of the lesion and a radical abdominoperineal resection of the rectum with permanent colostomy is a major decision. Local resection is adequate for lesions smaller than 2 cm in greatest diameter and without invasion of the muscularis (Orloff).[113] Lesions larger than 2 cm and/or lesions invading the muscularis apparently require a radical resection as employed for adeno carcinoma. The likelihood of lymphatic spread, and the likelihood of survival with these findings, is similar to that observed in patients with carcinoma of the rectum.

The overall survival statistics for carcinoid with metastasis are considerably better than with adenocarcinoma of corresponding sites in the gastrointestinal tract, as exemplified by a 20-percent 5-year survival rate when multiple liver metastases are present.

NONSURGICAL TREATMENT OF SMALL BOWEL NEOPLASMS

The same general approach to systemic chemotherapy used for large bowel cancer is indicated when recurrent or metastastic adenocarcinoma is present. Lymphosarcoma of the small bowel may be treated with systemic chemotherapeutic regimes employed for these same lesions in other sites if there is any evidence of spread away from the primary site at the time of, or subsequent to, surgical resection. Postoperative anticancer chemotherapy for localized lymphosarcoma of the small bowel is an arbitrary decision without helpful data to support it at this time.

Carcinoid tumors that metastasize to the liver may produce a functional syndrome (carcinoid syndrome) because of pharmacologically active tumor products. The details of this fascinating syndrome and its management are described in Chapter 14.

NEOPLASMS OF THE APPENDIX

With the exception of the well-known carcinoid tumor, appendiceal neoplasms are quite rare. Carcinoids constitute 90 percent of all neoplasms of the appendix, and 45 percent of all carcinoids occur in the appendix.[123]

Some unusual neoplasms of the appendix do deserve special mention. Primary adenocarcinoma of the appendix shares all of the characteristics of adenocarcinoma of the large bowel, and it is recommended that this unusual lesion be treated in a fashion similar to that to be described for carcinoma of the cecum.[60] The other neoplasm that deserves particular mention and discussion is mucocele of the appendix. These lesions range in size from 2–12 cm, and approximately 10 percent of mucoceles rupture to form a gelatinous ascites called pseudomyxoma peritonei.

Management of Pseumyxoma Peritonei

The operative findings in patients with ruptured mucoceles of the appendix are usually quite striking. The mucinous deposits coat the abdominal viscera but do not invade them. Histologically, there are a few contiguous well-differentiated neoplastic cells in this exudate in many cases, and this is the basis for considering this an unusual form of low-grade carcinomatosis. In most cases surgical removal of this material is the most effective means of management, but repeated operations are usually required because of the surgeon's inability to remove all of the material. Appendectomy is also indicated if this is the site of origin of the process. A similar process is also associated with some pseudomucinous cystadenocarcinomas of the ovary, and if this is the case, bilateral oophorectomy is indicated.

There has been interest in the past in the use of various substances in the peritoneal cavity to help control this unusual process. Most chemotherapeutic agents, as well as enzymatic agents of various kinds, have been ineffectual. Radiation therapy has also had very limited value for the treatment of this condition.

In view of the concept that this process may be an unusual form of abdominal carcinomatosis, systemic chemotherapy with 5-fluuorouracil or other agents has been recommended. Although there is a logical rationale to this approach, we have observed limited benefits and surgical evacuation of the material is still the preferred treatment when feasible.

CANCER OF THE COLON AND RECTUM

Colorectal cancer is the most common cancer in men and women in the United States today and is challenged in incidence only by lung cancer in men and breast cancer in women. Since the stage of disease clearly affects prognosis, our ability to detect both precancerous lesions and early-stage cancers is of vital importance. The overwhelming majority of cancers of the colon and rectum are adenocarcinomas.

Diagnosis

The routine digital rectal examination has become a part of the general physical examination as a result of widespread educational emphasis. Sigmoidoscopy as part of the routine annual physical examination of the asymptomatic patient is also readily accepted by many physicians, whereas it is rejected by others as having too few significant findings to warrant the time and effort required. However, cancers are occasionally detected in a presymptomatic phase by means of such examinations. It is unlikely that most asymptomatic patients undergoing periodic general physical examinations will have sigmoidoscopy performed as a routine part of the examination, but it is critical that this examination and appropriate radiographic study be performed on all patients with subtle gastrointestinal symptoms, change in bowel habits, rectal blood, and other apparently minor rectal complaints. A positive test of a specimen of stool for occult blood at the time of routine physical examination should also be a firm indication for performing sigmoidoscopy and barium enema x-ray examination.

The development of colonoscopy with flexible endoscopes has greatly expanded our diagnostic capabilities in the colon.[114,166] This technique can be used as an adjunct to standard methods when radiographic examination is required, when colonic x-rays and physical examination are negative despite symptoms or occult bleeding, or when one needs to establish histologic diagnosis of a radiographic lesion above the level of the standard sigmoidoscope. There are some limitations to the procedure, but it is safe and effective in expert hands. The major impediment to its use at the present time is the limited number of physicians who have had adequate training and possess sufficient skill to exploit the method routinely for diagnosis and polyp removal.

Another diagnostic method first employed for cancer of the colon and rectum, and later for other cancers, is the determination of serum titers of carcinoembryonic antigen (CEA).[45,57,65,85,87,167] Virtually all trials with this serodiagnostic method have demonstrated that it is not specific for colorectal cancer as originally hoped and not particularly sensitive. Both of these factors preclude its use as an effective method for either screening or diagnosis of colorectal cancer. Experience has shown, however, that it is a useful tumor marker for following the course of established and treated cancer.[117,127,140] We use it routinely as part of our follow-up procedure for these and other cancers.

DIFFERENTIAL DIAGNOSIS

In addition to the common adenomatous polyp, the differential diagnosis of colorectal cancer also includes diverticulitis, ulcerative colitis, stercoraceous ulcers, lymphogranuloma venereum, and other inflammatory lesions of the bowel. Benign neoplasms that do occur and are rarely a problem in differential diagnosis are lipomas, hamartomas, neurofibromas, and angiomas. Another less common lesion that simulates rectal cancer is the process colitis cystica profunda. Grossly, this lesion appears quite similar to rectal cancer, but it is much softer on palpation. One or two biopsies will usually clarify the diagnosis.[49,139]

In women, both endometriosis and carcinoma of the ovary may produce extrinsic masses that distort the rectal mucosa to such a degree that primary rectal cancer is seriously considered. In men, carcinoma of the prostate is usually quite easy to recognize, but an occasional patient with prostatic cancer develops findings difficult to differentiate from those of rectal cancer. Locally, advanced prostate cancer is extrinsic and encircles and narrows the rectum, but confusion results when actual ulceration of the rectal mucosa occurs. Biopsy of an ulcerated mass on the anterior wall of the rectum will allow easy differentiation of these two primary sites of origin (they are both adenocarcinomas) if acid phosphatase stains on fresh biopsy material are obtained.

Other malignant neoplasms that simulate carcinoma of the colon and rectum are rectal carcinoid, primary lymphoma, malignant melanoma, and sarcoma of muscle origin (either leiomyosarcoma or rhabdomyosarcoma). If the lesion is within range of the anoscope or sigmoidoscope, biopsy is important as it will clarify the diagnosis and may lead to some variation in treatment. If the lesion is more proximal, the diagnosis may not be established until after surgical resection unless colonscopy is performed. In most instances, the surgical treatment of these less-common lesions is similar to that employed for adenocarcinoma, but biopsy before treatment is indicated, particularly if resection of the rectum is one of the considerations (see discussion of rectal carcinoid on page 240).

Treatment of Colorectal Cancer

Although some rectal cancers have been treated successfully by radiotherapy, cryosurgery, or electrocautery, surgical resection has been generally accepted as the standard treatment for most patients with colon and rectal carcinoma. In our view, all patients with colon or rectal cancer, except those with definite evidence of peritoneal metastases or proven distant lymphatic metastases, should be subjected to exploratory celiotomy in order to select the potentially "curable" patients. Even if clinical findings denoting incurability are present, the symptomatology of colon or rectal cancer may well lead to surgical intervention.

At the time of abdominal exploration for colon or rectal cancer, prior spread of the cancer to the peritoneal surfaces is detected by virtue of peritoneal "implants" and/or ascitic fluid. Careful examination of the liver and lymph node basins beyond the possibility of realistic lymph node dissections should also be accomplished as proven spread leads to the abandonment of a radical operative procedure with curative intent. A possible exception is the patient with a solitary hepatic metastasis. This problem can be so conveniently managed by liver resection that we often perform standard "curative" surgical resection of the bowel lesion under these circumstances (see page 234).

If there are no findings of metastasis and no evidence of lymphatic spread beyond the limits of an en bloc resection, standard colon resection with regional lymph nodes should be performed.[145,162] The design of all of our operative procedures for colon and rectal cancer is actually based on the blood supply and anatomy of the lymphatic drainage of the large bowel. Consideration of the hematogenous spread at the time of operation is also important, and this entails avoidance of squeezing or compressing the neoplasm during operative manipulations. This is the genesis of the concept of the so-called no touch technique.[151]

SPECIFIC CURATIVE RESECTIONS FOR CARCINOMA OF THE COLON AND RECTUM

One-stage right hemicolectomy with ileotransverse colostomy (Fig. 8-19A) is considered to be the procedure of choice for lesions of the cecum and ascending portion of the colon. If the primary lesion is the hepatic flexure of the colon, a similar resection should be carried out as well as resecting a generous portion of the transverse colon with the middle colic artery and associated nodes. In each of these instances, a generous segment of mesentery with the regional lymph nodes is included in the resection for the extended segment of bowel that is removed. The same concept is applied to splenic flexure lesions and descending colon and sigmoid lesions above the rectosigmoid area (Fig. 8-19B). Surgical procedures for resection of carcinoma of the rectosigmoid colon and rectum involve other considerations in terms of surgical management as the requirement of an abdominal colostomy stoma in some patients may be a significant factor in the choice of operative procedure.

For lesions of the rectum and rectosigmoid colon, the operator often has the choice of a low "anterior resection" with transabdominal anastomosis between the proximal colon and the rectum, a similar operation through a combined abdominal transcoccygeal approach that allows the anastomosis to be carried out in closer proximity to the anus (Fig. 8-20), the so-called pull through procedure with preservation of the anal sphincter, and the combined abdominoperineal resection of the rectum (see Fig. 8-19C).[163]

Our strategy for making the choice is as follows:

Most lesions arising 12 cm or more from the anal verge in men can be satisfactorily resected and low anterior anastomosis accomplished after mobilization of the rectum from the sacral hollow. The same procedure can be accomplished with the line of resection at a slightly lower level in women.

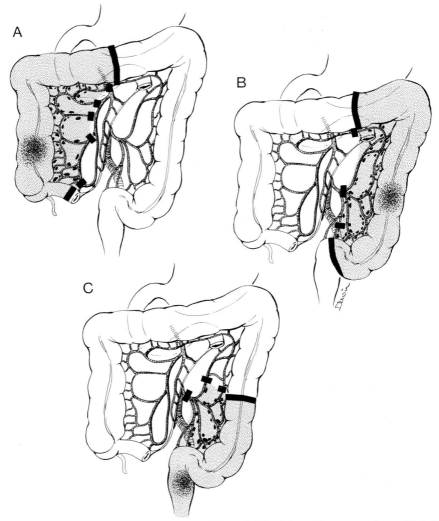

Fig. 8-19. Diagrammatic representation of (**A**) right colon resection, (**B**) left colon resection and (**C**) abdominoperineal resection for carcinoma.

For carcinoma of the rectum extending to a point less than 7 or 8 cm from the anal verge, we prefer abdominoperineal resection rather than any form of sphincter-saving procedure since an unacceptable compromise is required to accomplish an adequate distal margin for lesions at this level without sacrifice of the anus (Fig. 8-19C).

In an effort to obtain a more adequate margin around the local lesion, as well as include the lymphatics within the broad and infundibulopelvic ligaments, we extend our procedure for carcinoma of the rectum and rectosigmoid in women to include total hysterectomy, bilateral salpingo-oophorectomy, and resection of the posterior vaginal wall with more distal lesions.

For carcinoma of the "midrectum" (roughly 7–12 cm from the anal verge), we prefer a combined transcoccygeal approach for resection and anastomosis if the lesion is not large. This allows an adequate distal margin of 5 cm, and the anastomosis can be accomplished several centimeters above the anus by means of the simultaneous incisions and the lateral position for the patient described by Localio and Stahl[86] (Fig. 8-20). Large rectal cancers at this same level are not as adequately resected by this method as by abdominoperineal resection, and we prefer the latter procedure for bulky lesions. Other surgeons prefer the pull through operation instead of the transcoccygeal anastomosis for rectal lesions at this same level. Neither of these two procedures results in as effective bowel function as that achieved with a slightly higher transabdominal colorectal anastomosis, but the result may be superior to a permanent colostomy.

NONSURGICAL TREATMENT OF LOCALIZED RECTAL CANCER

The fact that surgical resection of low-lying rectal cancers requires a permanent colostomy is a major factor in the continued interest in other methods of management of cancers of this site. Radiation therapy by external beam or local radium application has effectively controlled some rectal cancers.[118] Moreover, an increasing number of surgeons employ electrofulguration for highly selected lesions;[8] this technique may be as successful as surgical excision in selected cases. It has been stressed that the small, movable, exophytic type of low-lying rectal cancer (as opposed to the flat, plaquelike lesions with associated local induration) is the ideal lesion for this approach, but others are not particularly enthusiastic.[154] The details of case selection and the conduct of the treatment method are important for success and these have been well described by Madden and Kandaloft[90] and by Crile and Turnbull.[33] We have had limited experience with this technique, but it may well be useful and justifiable for small, localized exophytic lesions that would otherwise require abdominoperineal resection.

ADJUVANT CHEMOTHERAPY FOR SURGICALLY TREATED COLORECTAL CANCER

The possibility of combining therapeutic agents with curative surgical attempts for cancer has received much attention in the management of co-

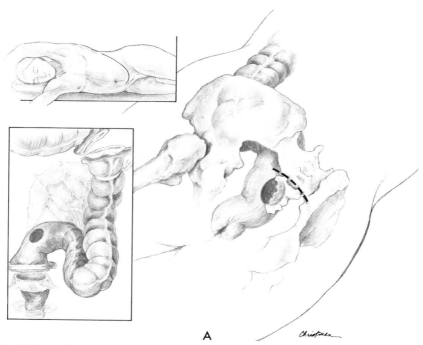

Fig. 8-20. Abdominotranssacral resection of carcinoma of the midrectum (after Localio and Stahl[86]). **A:** Approach. **B:** Anastomosis.

lorectal cancer, and this has been the prototype for this approach to all cancers of the gastrointestinal tract. The rationale is to destroy residual distant or local foci of malignant cells, the "minimal residual disease." Although the principle has been shown to be valid both in animal model systems and in some cancers in man (particularly Wilms' tumor, embryonal rhabdomyosarcoma, and osteogenic sarcoma), a major problem in its application to colorectal cancer has been the relative weakness of available chemotherapeutic agents for this disease.

Extensive clinical trials have been performed using adjuvant chemotherapy with thio-TEPA and with 5-fluorouracil. The latter agent has received the most attention. The trials have employed short-term postoperative intravenous chemotherapy,[39,62,63] intraoperative intraluminal chemotherapy,[52,80,131] long-term postoperative systemic chemotherapy (both oral and intravenous),[48,80] and combinations of these strategies. Beneficial results from this adjuvant approach have not been demonstrated conclusively in any of these clinical trials, although one trial with 5-fluorouracil appeared to demonstrate early (but limited) benefit.[48] On this basis it is not recommended that adjuvant chemotherapy with 5-fluorouracil be employed as standard treatment to follow curative surgical

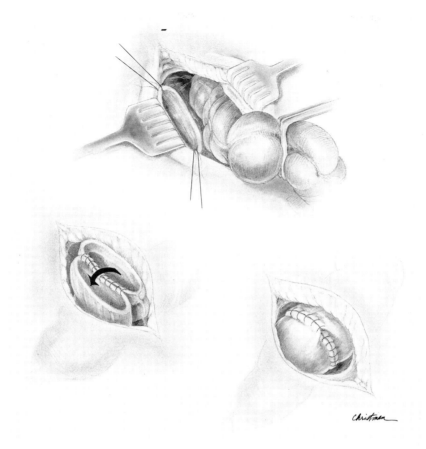

B

Fig. 8-20.   (continued).

resection, but the time is not far off when we will all probably be using adjuvant chemotherapy after surgical resection. This development will require further prospective clinical trials of combination chemotherapy regimes proven to have benefit for advanced disease.

RADIATION THERAPY AS AN ADJUNCT
TO SURGICAL TREATMENT
OF COLORECTAL CANCER

The possibility of using preoperative or postoperative radiation therapy to supplement the benefits of surgical resection for colorectal cancer is suggested by the high "local failure rate," particularly after surgery for rectal cancer. Most clinical data relating to this question concern preoperative radiation therapy, although the concept might well be as valid for postoperative radiation and the latter approach might allow selective use for "high risk" groups.[55] Well-planned clinical trials of low-dose preoperative radiation therapy for rectal cancer have been performed, but, unfortunately, the data are conflicting at this dose level.[38,61,126,143] The reader is referred to this extensive literature on this subject, but it seems appropriate to say that low-dose radiation therapy is not an established adjunct to surgical resection of rectal cancer at this time. The prospect of employing radiation therapy at a high dose level as an adjunct has received some support from the observations of Allen and Fletcher[3] and Kligerman et al.,[71] but convincing data from prospective clinical trials must be obtained before this difficult approach can be recommended for general use.

PRIMARY PALLIATIVE OPERATIONS
FOR COLORECTAL CANCER

If it is determined that the surgical procedure can not be curative, a somewhat more limited removal of the primary lesion itself is usually accomplished as this obviates the major symptoms and allows postoperative systemic chemotherapy to be employed for the residual disease with greater ease. This same principle is as applicable to rectal cancer as it is to lesions in the colon, and we do not hesitate to perform abdominoperineal resection as a palliative procedure.[18]

TREATMENT OF "RECURRENT" OR
METASTATIC CARCINOMA OF
THE COLON AND RECTUM

The patient developing recurrent carcinoma after primary surgical treatment for colorectal cancer frequently manifests intestinal obstruction requiring palliative surgical intervention. This may entail a proximal colostomy for recurrent cancer in the pelvis, a bypass of more proximal obstruction by enteroenterostomy, or a limited bowel resection. These approaches may be required for the acute problem in order to allow the use of other methods of palliative treatment. In some instances this approach to palliation may be totally unsuccessful because of the extent of disease found at the time of exploration, but we feel that surgical intervention for obstruction in these patients is worthwhile (see Chap. 15 for more detailed discussion). Urinary tract obstruction may also require operative relief, but most patients with bilateral ureteral obstruction are not considered candidates for aggressive surgical efforts for palliation because of our inability to correct many of the problems remaining after operation in patients with this type of extensive pelvic recurrence. Surgical resection for selected patients with local, apparently solitary, metastases in the liver or lung is also worthwhile, but most patients with distant metastases are best treated by systemic chemotherapy. Perineal recurrence after resection of the rectum is also treated effectively by surgical excision in highly selected patients, but a surgical approach to this problem usually produces a disappointing result since the apparently localized recurrence is virtually always a manifestation of more extensive recurrent disease in the pelvis.

Radiation therapy. Adenocarcinoma is responsive to radiation therapy and this is an effective method for palliation of localized areas of symptomatic recurrence of colorectal cancer. This is particularly applicable to pelvic or perineal recurrence after surgical resection of the rectum (with or without concomitant systemic chemotherapy) since wound recurrence from local implantation is a distressingly frequent complication of operations for rectal cancer. Other sites of localized symptomic recurrence may well be effectively managed by radiation therapy, but localized metastasis is not the primary problem in most patients with recurrent colorectal cancer.

Systemic chemotherapy. Progress in the development of effective chemotherapeutic agents for the treatment of colorectal cancer (as well as for the treatment of other gastrointestinal cancers) has been distressingly slow, and the standard agent for many years has been 5-fluorouracil. This agent has been shown to produce objective response in 15–20 percent of patients with recurrent and metastastic colorectal cancer, but this is always partial, usually transient, and rarely productive of striking palliation. Variations in dosage schedules and route of administration have been studied extensively, but none of these variations has greatly altered the overall results. Oral administration had some practical advantage over intravenous administration and was even thought to be more effective for liver metastases, but variability in enteric absorption has led to general acceptance of the intravenous route as preferable.[22,56] Intra-arterial administration, when feasible, is still preferred by some physicians, but there is no solid evidence that this is not just another form of continuous infusion without specific benefit from the arterial route. Whatever the route or scheduling of this agent, the best results follow maximally tolerated dosage (from the standpoint of toxicity) and the overall benefits are limited.

Because of general dissatisfaction with 5-fluorouracil, combination chemotherapy regimes have been extensively studied in patients with metastatic colorectal cancer, and prospective clinical trials have demonstrated improvement in palliative results with this combination approach.

Table 8-5
Colorectal Carcinoma: End Results
of Treatment

Dukes' Classification	5-Yr Survival (%)
Dukes' A	85
Dukes' B	55
Dukes' C	40

The combination of methyl-CCNU, 5-fluorouracil, and vincristine has produced an objective response rate of 43 percent in colorectal patients with advanced disease (better than twice the response rate observed in 5-FU control group), and it is hoped that other even more effective combination chemotherapy regimes will be developed. This combination approach should certainly replace single-agent chemotherapy for metastatic colorectal cancer.

PROGNOSIS

The end results of treatment of colorectal cancer in terms of Dukes' classification is shown in Table 8-5.

SPECIAL MANAGEMENT PROBLEMS

Management of Colorectal Polyps

More has been written on the assessment of the colorectal polyp as a potential precursor of cancer than on any other aspect of gastrointestinal neoplasia. A spectrum of ideas has been expressed in the literature regarding the relative cancer risk from the various kinds of colorectal polyps.[51,106] However, data presented by various authors generally agree on the following points:

1. Not all "polyps" are neoplasms (some may be lymphoid polyps, inflammatory polyps, retention polyps, or Peutz-Jeghers polyps, none of which are true neoplasms). A "polyp" is a descriptive term, and the common adenomatous polyp is the key lesion in the long-standing adenoma-cancer controversy.
2. Some individual adenomatous polyps in the colon and rectum must be precursor lesions for cancer, but most individual adenomas are not precancerous.
3. The size of the individual adenomatous lesion is the major factor affecting clinical neoplastic concern. Lesions larger than 1.5 cm, or possibly larger than 1 cm, concern most clinicians and pathologists on

the basis of available data, as the so-called polyp may actually be a small primary cancer.

4. The anatomic location of the "polyp" in question and the presence or absence of a pedicle are the major factors affecting convenience of polyp removal for pathologic diagnosis, but the location is becoming less important as colonoscopy has become more widely available.

5. Villous adenomas (or papillary adenomas) have higher neoplastic potential than more common adenomatous polyps.[125]

6. Multiple adenomatous lesions in the colon are more concerning than solitary lesions, particularly if the number of lesions is great enough to classify the patient within a familial syndrome (i.e., polyposis coli[102] or Gardner's syndrome[159]).

The major problem that is not totally resolved is the assessment of the magnitude of neoplastic risk of an individual clinical "polyp." It seems fair to say that neoplastic risk ranges from small to extremely low. Although the development of the flexible colonoscope has greatly simplified the management decisions for colon polyps, planning management must consider that this technique may not be applicable or available to most patients. Considering all these points, our clinical approach to various "polyps" can be outlined as follows:

1. All polypoid lesions with a stalk, and within the reach of the sigmoidoscope, are excised in toto by cautery snare and submitted to the pathologist for histologic study. Higher lesions of this type are ideal for colonoscopic removal if this technique is available.
   Subsequent actions:
   A. If benign, treatment is complete.
   B. If noninvasive (in situ) cancer is present, treatment is complete.
   C. If invasive cancer is identified microscopically in the polyp, but the stalk is cancer "free," treatment is also complete.
   D. If invasive cancer is identified microscopically in the stalk, the patient is subjected to a secondary operation appropriate for resection of cancer at that location.

2. All *sessile lesions* within reach of the anus or sigmoidscope are biopsied or excised, and colonoscopy, when feasible, extends our capabilities here as well.
   Subsequent actions:
   A. If *benign and small,* the entire lesion can be removed through the sigmoidoscope or colonoscope with fulguration of the base.
   B. If the biopsy is benign from a larger lesion or if noninvasive carcinoma is demonstrated on the biopsy, local excision of the sessile lesion with full thickness of the wall of the bowel is accomplished with an adequate margin at the mucosal level. [This may

be possible transanally or by a transcoccygeal approach for low-lying lesions (up to 12 cm) or transabdominally for higher lesions.]

C. If infiltrating cancer is demonstrated on biopsy, a secondary operation appropriate for resection of cancer is carried out.

3. For lesions identified radiographically above the level of sigmoido-scopy and not approachable by colonoscopy for technical or other reasons, we perform abdominal surgery with colotomy if the lesion is symptomatic (usually bleeding), if multiple lesions are present, or if the asymptomatic "polyp" is 1.5 cm or larger (and no contraindica-tions to surgery are present). Subsequent actions at time of opera-tion:

A. Excise the lesion (and stalk if present) through a colotomy inci-sion and obtain frozen section on stalk.

B. If the frozen section of the stalk is negative, treatment is com-plete whether or not in situ changes are present on the surface of the polyp itself.

C. If no stalk is present, excision of the lesion should include full thickness of the wall of the bowel and frozen section diagnosis to detect infiltrating cancer.

D. If the stalk is involved with cancer or if the sessile lesion on biopsy proves to be an infiltrating carcinoma, appropriate opera-tion for cancer should then be carried out.

4. If colonoscopy is not available or feasible and a polypoid lesion is demonstrated radiologically above the level of the standard sigmoid-oscope, periodic observation by radiologic exam without operation or biopsy is appropriate if:

A. the lesion is asymptomatic and less than 1.5 cm in diameter; or

B. the lesion is either smaller or larger than 1.5 cm in diameter but is on a clear-cut stalk and there is an increase in operative risk in this particular patient because of unrelated medical problems or advanced age. (If the lesion later increases in size as revealed by x-ray examination, or if symptoms develop or increase, opera-tive intervention may be decided on.)

Details of Surgical Techniques for Polyp Management

Transanal removal of polyps. Polyps are usually removed transan-ally under spinal or caudal anesthesia after gentle dilation of the anus. The polyp can usually be brought outside the rectum, exicsed with an ade-quate margin, and the mucosal defect sutured in either a vertical or hori-zontal direction.

Transcoccygeal proctotomy. This is the approach employed for local resection of lesions of the midrectum that cannot be conveniently brought down to the anal region after anal dilation (usually 7–12 cm above the anal verge). With this approach, the coccyx is excised, the levator muscles are incised (similar to the technique shown in Fig. 8-20), and the posterior wall of the rectum is incised transversely. The level of the incision depends somewhat on the location of the lesion, but this general approach does give improved access to the midrectum for lesions requiring limited resection. It is preferable to attempt exposure of the lesion through the anus for possible transanal excision before embarking on this slightly more complex transcoccygeal route.

Cautery snare excision. Probably the most frequently employed technique for excision of polyps is cautery snare excision. A standard sigmoidoscope is used, but a machine for electrocoagulation and a specially shielded cautery snare apparatus are required. The wire loop is tightened over the stalk at the base of the lesion while current is applied and the stalk of the polyp is coagulated. Suction is required for eliminating smoke that develops and reducing the possibility of explosion. A similar technique is employed when polyps are excised through the colonoscope. Most lesions removed by cautery snare excision can be removed on an outpatient basis, but the patient should be observed for a period after the procedure to be certain that hemostasis has been obtained. Hemorrhage may take place several days later at the site of the cauterization, but this is quite rare. Patients should be within the geographic area of the surgeon during the first week after this procedure in view of the remote possibility of late hemorrhage when the small area of sloughing tissue begins to separate. Perforation of the bowel is always a possible complication of polyp removal with this approach when lesions are situated above the peritoneal reflection. Although uncommon, perforation of bowel may be a logical indication for treating polyps at this level in a hospital setting.

Obstructing Carcinoma of the Colon

Carcinoma presenting with obstruction has been managed in several ways, depending on the location of the lesion. Resection considered adequate for elective resection is particularly hazardous for the ill patient with both obstruction and an unprepared bowel.[161] For this reason we always limit the surgical procedure to loop colostomy to relieve the obstruction, except in the rare situation of obstruction produced by cancer of the cecum or ascending colon. In the latter instance, right hemicolectomy with anastamosis generally appears to be more advantageous than proximal ileostomy, unless perforation has already occurred.

The location in the colon of the colostomy performed for obstruction is another decision. We prefer a "two-stage" procedure to the classic three-stage operation under these circumstances. For this reason, we usually place the colostomy at a site in the colon that will be conveniently resected along with the involved colon at the time of the later definitive resection. The proximal site of transection will then serve as the proximal limb for anastomosis, or the limb for permanent end colostomy in the case of cancer of the distal rectum. For obstruction in the transverse colon, the colostomy is constructed in the ascending colon; for splenic flexure obstruction, it is in the right transverse colon; for descending and sigmoid colon obstruction it is constructed in the left transverse colon; and for rectal cancer a proximal sigmoid colostomy is performed. In each case, a more proximal colostomy is usually performed by those surgeons who prefer a three-stage operation consisting of initial colostomy, definitive resection, and later colostomy closure.

Perforated Carcinoma of the Colon

One of the most distressing problems in management of colon cancer is the patient who has perforation at the site of the lesion. This includes lesions that rupture freely into the peritoneal cavity, those that leak locally forming an abscess, and those that form a fistula with another hollow viscus. The immediate morbidity and mortality of the complication are considerable, particularly with free perforation, but they are not as grave as one might think. The surgeon is often forced to perform a compromise procedure of some type to save the patient, but long-term control is possible in some of these patients.

The principle to be followed for free peritoneal perforations is that of excision of the bowel containing the cancer and the perforation. If the right colon is perforated, an ileotransverse colon anastomosis may be performed, despite peritoneal contamination, but an ileostomy and transverse colon mucous fistula might be employed if the amount and time of peritoneal contamination have been excessive. For perforated cancers in the transverse or left colon, we recommend resection of the appropriate length of bowel and mesentery for the site of the lesion, but we believe an end colostomy at the proximal margin of resection is the safest approach. The distal lumen should be brought out through a separate stab wound, unless it is low in the pelvis, when it is closed and covered with a flap of peritoneum. Anastomosis is delayed until the patient recovers from the peritonitis resulting from this complication. Prognosis after free perforation is poor, but long-term control is occasionally achieved.

Perforating cancers of the colon that remain localized and form an

abscess and/or fistula are less catastrophic than the free peritoneal perforations. The morbidity associated with this type of perforation is considerable, but the somewhat better long-term survival rates clearly justify a
"curative" approach. Patients with localized perforations have a prognosis similar to that of patients with standard colon cancers, if they survive the immediate complications.

Pelvic Exenteration for Carcinoma of the Rectum

Some lesions of the rectum and rectosigmoid invade other pelvic viscera by direct extension without developing distant extrapelvic metastasis. In women, the uterus and adnexa usually serve as a "buffer' zone"
between the bowel and bladder, thereby protecting the bladder, and this
allows adequate local resection of the cancer in most instances by inclusion of the uterus, tubes, ovaries, and a portion of the vagina. In men,
anterior extension of the rectal or rectosigmoid cancer is more likely to involve the bladder, and consideration of pelvic exenteration is therefore
more frequent than in women.

Cancer of the rectosigmoid and rectum that involves other pelvic viscera has a greater likelihood of developing distant areas of spread in the
abdominal cavity, but radical resection of the pelvic viscera is still indicated in highly selected cases. With appropriate case selection, long-
term control (more than 5 years) is feasible in approximately 30 percent of
cases.[21,23,24]

CASE SELECTION

Preoperative rectal or rectovaginal examination often suggests the
possibility of involvement of other organs by a rectal cancer, and this
should prompt the surgeon to discuss the possibility of exenteration with
the patient before operation. The preoperative intravenous pyelogram is
another clue to this possibility if complete or partial ureteral obstruction is
demonstrated.

The ability of the patient to deal with the problem of both a colostomy and an ileal conduit is dependent on both age and general condition,
and no chronologic age limit can be set for making this decision. If exenteration is a possible consideration, medical and social factors should be
seriously evaluated before operation as the final decision regarding
acceptability of this approach must be made using both the anatomic findings at operation and this important preoperative assessment.

The anatomic findings of importance in making the decision
regarding pelvic exenteration are the absence of peritoneal or other distant spread, the freedom of invasion by cancer of the lateral pelvic walls,

and the presence of neoplastic invasion of the prostate, the periureteral tissue, and/or the bladder. Although pelvic exenteration may be required for anatomic reasons for men more often than women, the procedure is applicable to selected patients of both sexes.

The procedure of pelvic exenteration for patients with primary carcinoma of the rectum differs somewhat from that employed for advanced uterine or bladder cancer. There is usually no specific need for inclusion of the iliac lymph nodes in the dissection, since these are not the regional lymph nodes for this primary site, but the plane of dissection along the vessels is a convenient one for adequate tissue margins. Another difference when pelvic exenteration is employed for rectal cancer is the more proximal dissection of the sigmoid mesentery required to include the lymph node basin for this site. Total pelvic exenteration is not carried out until it is clear from the dissection that this extensive procedure is actually required to obtain an adequate margin around the neoplasm.

When the resection is completed, an ileal conduit is constructed for ureteral implantation and the stoma constructed in the right lower quadrant. A standard end colostomy is constructed in the left lower quadrant. The details of the technique of this procedure are beyond the scope of this volume since both the operation and the aftercare require experience with this approach to reduce morbidity and mortality to acceptable levels. Patients who appear to be possible candidates for this approach on preoperative assessment should probably be explored in an institution where these procedures are performed on more than an occasional basis.

CARCINOMA OF THE ANUS

Squamous carcinoma of the anus is a relatively infrequent cancer and comprises no more than 2 percent of all malignant lesions of the large bowel.[107,144] Squamous cancers may arise from the perianal skin, the region of the pectinate line, or the lining just proximal to this, the "transitional zone." This last zone has epithelium that is a compromise between the glandular rectal mucosa above and the squamous epithelium below, and cancers arising from this area are often termed "cloacogenic" carcinomas. The key anatomic landmark is the pectinate line since lesions distal to this tend to have a more favorable prognosis. Lesions in the anal area include leukoplakia and in situ carcinoma (Bowen's disease), and both of these are uncommon clinical problems with few distinguishing features on gross examination. Another malignant tumor of the anal region is malignant melanoma, a rare lesion that is sometimes confused clinically with a thrombosed hemorrhoid.

Diagnosis

The lesion in question is usually obvious and diagnosis is established by biopsy. The lymphatic drainage for the anal canal and perianal region is the inguinal lymph node basin, and clinical staging requires careful evaluation of this site.

Treatment

SURGICAL EXCISION

The most frequent anal neoplasm, squamous carcinoma, may be treated in a variety of ways depending on the size and location of the lesion. If the size of a perianal lesion allows local resection, this is clearly adequate treatment for these very low lesions.

The more uncommon noninfiltrative processes (leukoplakia and in situ carcinoma) are also adequately treated by local resection, as is the rare basal cell carcinoma found in this location. Squamous carcinoma at the level of the dentate line or higher requires abdominoperineal resection, as employed for rectal cancer, and malignant melanoma of this site is treated similarly.

The therapeutic decision regarding the surgical management of potentially involved regional lymph nodes is related to the anatomic level of the lesion. Proximal lesions in the anal canal (pectinate line and above) metastasize to the lymphatics of the bowel mesentery, in a fashion similar to that of rectal carcinoma, more frequently than to the groin. This is the primary reason for advising abdominoperineal resection for squamous carcinoma in this location. Involvement of tissues distal to the pectinate line may lead to lymphatic spread to the inguinal nodes, and careful clinical evaluation of the groin nodes is certainly indicated before and after surgical treatment of anal carcinoma. It is generally agreed that the incidence of inguinal node metastasis does not justify prophylactic (elective) removal of these nodes for this disease, but unilateral or bilateral groin dissection is carried out as a secondary procedure if and when clinical involvement of inguinal nodes becomes apparent. Although this finding is not favorable from the prognostic standpoint, some patients with proven extension to the inguinal nodes have had the disease controlled by lymph node dissection.

NONSURGICAL TREATMENT

Radiation therapy has been employed successfully as primary treatment for squamous carcinoma of the anus. The lesion is physically accessible for this treatment method, but radiation change in the perianal skin is often undesirable, and those lesions most suitable for radiation are treated more easily by local surgical excision. Radiation may be an effective method for palliation of patients who are unsuitable for operation for some reason or who develop "recurrence" after surgical excision. No regimes of systemic chemotherapy have been shown to be of particular value in the management of resectable, recurrent, or metastatic anal cancer.

SUMMARY

The general approach to gastrointestinal cancer as summarized in this chapter is the result in general of uncontrolled comparisons of clinical ideas that have developed over past years. Some operative procedures employed that represent an extension of past practice have proved to be worthwhile, and others have produced more morbidity than benefit to the patient population. It is fairly clear that future surgical practice is unlikely to become more aggressive than described here because of this realistic evaluation of past experience by a large number of surgeons operating on patients with gastrointestinal cancer. Future progress, in terms of end results, will undoubtedly come from the combined efforts of members of the other disciplines on the medical team who are concerned with these cancers.

REFERENCES

1. Adson MA, Sheedy PF: Resection of primary hepatic malignant lesions. Arch Surg 108:599–604, 1974.
2. Albritton DR, Tompkins RK, Longmire WP Jr: Hepatic cell adenoma. Ann Surg 180:14–19, 1975
3. Allen CV, Fletcher WS: Observations on preoperative irradiation for rectosigmoid carcinoma. Am J Roentgenol Radium Ther Nucl Med 108:36–40, 1970
4. Almersjo O, Bengmark S, Hafstrom Lo, Rosengren K: Accuracy of diagnostic tools in malignant hepatic lesions: A comparative study using serum tests, angiography, scintiscanning, and laparotomy. Am J Surg 127:663–668, 1974
5. Ansfield FJ, Ramirez G, Skibba JL, Bryan CT, Davis HL, Wirtanem GW: Intrahepatic arterial infusion with 5-fluorouracil. Cancer 28:1147–1151, 1971
6. Aston SJ, Longmire WP Jr: Pancreaticoduodenal resection. Arch Surg 106:813–817, 1973
7. Balasegaram M: Management of primary liver cell carcinoma. Am J Surg 130:33–37, 1975
8. Beahrs OH: Status of fulguration and cryosurgery in the management of

colonic and rectal cancer and polyps. Cancer 34:965–968, 1974

9. Becker WF, Welsh RA, Pratt HS: Cystadenoma and cystadenocarcinoma of the pancreas. Ann Surg 161:845–863, 1965

10. Beltz WR, Condon RE: Primary carcinoma of the gallbladder. Ann Surg 180:180–184, 1974

11. Berci G, Morgenstern L, Shore JM, Shapiro S: A direct approach to the differential diagnosis of jaundice. Am J Surg 126:372–378, 1973

12. Berg JW: Histological aspects of the relation between gastric adenomatous polyps and gastric cancer. Cancer 11:1149–1155, 1958

13. Berry GR, Mathews WH: Gastric lymphosarcoma and pseudolymphoma: Reapprasial of twelve cases of gastric lymphosarcoma. Can Med Assoc J 96:1312–1316, 1967

14. Berry REL, Rottschafer W: The lymphatic spread of cancer of the stomach observed in operative specimens removed by radical surgery including total pancreatectomy. Surg Gynecol Obstet 104:269–279, 1957

15. Bismuth H, Corlette MB: Intrahepatic cholangioenteric anastomosis in carcinoma of the hilus of the liver. Surg Gynecol Obstet 140:170–178, 1975

16. Bloomer JR, Waldmann TA, McIntire KR, Klastskin G: Fetoprotein in non-neoplastic hepatic disorders. JAMA 233:38–41, 1975

17. Blumgart LH: Duodenoscopy and endoscopic retrograde choledochography; Present position and relation to periampullary and pancreatic cancer. J Surg Oncol 7:107–119, 1975

18. Bordos DC, Baker RR, Cameron JL: An evaluation of palliative abdominoperineal resection for carcinoma of the rectum. Surg Gynecol Obstet 139:731–733, 1974

19. Boyce HW Jr: Nonsurgical measures to relieve distress of late esophageal carcinoma. Geriatrics 28:97–102, 1973

20. Brasfield RD, Bowden L, McPeak CJ: Major hepatic resection for malignant neoplasms of the liver. Ann Surg 176:171–177, 1972

21. Bricker EM: Pelvic exenteration. Adv Surg 4:13–70, 1970

22. Bruckner HW, Creasey WA: The administration of 5-fluorouracil by mouth. Cancer 33:14–18, 1974

23. Brunschwig A: Pelvic exenteration for carcinoma of the lower colon. Surgery 40:691–695, 1956

24. Butcher HR Jr, Spjut HJ: An evaluation of pelvic exenteration for advanced carcinoma of the lower colon. Cancer 12:659–681, 1959

25. Camprodon R, Salva JA, Jornet J, Guerrero JA: Successful resection of carcinoma of the common hepatic duct at its superior bifurcation. Am J Surg 128:433–435, 1974

26. Clarkson BD, Lawrence W Jr, Young C, Dierick W, Kuehn P, Kim MC, Berrett A, Clapp P: Effects of continuous hepatic artery infusion of antimetabolites on primary and metastatic cancer of the liver. Cancer 15:472–488, 1962

27. Cohen Y, Tan NC: Liver resection for primary carcinoma. Isr J Med Sci 1:201–213, 1965

28. Cohen A, McNeill D, Terz JJ, Lawrence W Jr: Neoplasms of the small intestine. Am J Digest Dis 16:815–824, 1971

29. Comis RL, Carter SK: A review of chemotherapy in gastric cancer. Cancer 34:1576–1586, 1974

30. Connors J, Wise L: Management of gastric lymphomas. Am J Surg 127:102–108, 1974

31. Crane JM, Gobbel WG Jr, Scott HW Jr: Surgical experience with malignant tumors of the ampulla of Vater and duodenum. Surg Gynecol Obstet 137:937–940, 1973

32. Crile G Jr: The advantages of bypass operations over radical pancreato-duodenectomy in the treatment of pancreatic carcinoma. Surg Gynecol Obstet 130:1049–1053, 1970

33. Crile G Jr, Turnbull RB Jr: The role of electrocoagulation in the treatment of carcinoma of the rectum. Surg Gynecol Obstet 135:391–396, 1972

34. Curutchet HP, Terz JJ, Kay S, Lawrence, W Jr: Primary liver cancer. Surgery 70:467–479, 1970

35. Dillard BM: Experience with twenty-six hepatic lobectomies and extensive hepatic resections. Surg Gynecol Obstet 129:249–257, 1969

36. Douglas HO Jr, Holyoke ED: Pancreatic cancer. JAMA 229:793–797, 1974

37. Dreiling DA: Secretion analysis; secretion testing in pancreatic cancer. J Surg Oncol 7:101–105, 1975

38. Dwight RW, Higgins GA, Roswit B, LeVeen HH, Keehn RJ: Preoperative radiation and surgery for cancer of the sigmoid colon and rectum. Am J Surg 123:93–101, 1972

39. Dwight RW, Humphrey EW, Higgins GA, Keehn RJ: FUDR as an adjuvant to surgery in cancer of the large bowel. J Surg Oncol 5:243–249, 1973

40. Ferrucci JT, Benedict KT, Page DL, Fleischli DJ, Eaton SB: Radiographic features of the normal hypotonic duodenogram. Radiology 96:401–408, 1970

41. Fortner JG: Regional resection of cancer of the pancreas: A new surgical approach. Surgery 73:307–320, 1973

42. Fortner JG, Beattie EJ Jr, Shiu MH, Howland WS, Watson RC, Gastron JP, Benua RS: Surgery in liver tumors. Curr Probl Surg 1972

43. Fortner JG, Mulcare RJ, Solis AP, Watson RC, Golbey RB: The treatment of primary and secondary liver cancer by hepatic artery ligation and infusion chemotherapy. Ann Surg 178:162–172, 1973

44. Gilbertsen VA: Results of treatment of stomach cancer. Cancer 23:1305–1308, 1969

45. Gold P: Antigenic reversion in human cancer. Annu Rev Med 22:85–94, 1971

46. Goldstein HM, Neiman HL, Bookstein JJ: Angiographic evaluation of pancreatic disease; A further appraisal. Radiology 112:275–282, 1974

47. Goodner JT: Surgical and radiation treatment of cancer of the thoracic esophagus. Am J Roentgenol Radium Ther Nucl Med 105:523–528, 1969

48. Grage T, Cornell G, Strawitz J, Jonas K, Frelick R, Metter G: Adjuvant therapy with 5-FU after surgical resection of colo-rectal cancer. Sci Proc Am Assoc Cancer Res 16:1149, 1975

49. Green GK, Ramos P, Bannayan GA, McFee AS: Colitis cystica profunda. Am J Surg 127:749–752, 1974

50. Gregorie HB Jr: Esophagocoloplasty. Ann Surg 175:740–751, 1972

51. Grinnell RS, Lane H: Benign and malignant adenomatous polyps and papillary adenomas of the colon and rectum. An analysis of 1856 tumors in 1335 patients. Surg Gynecol Obstet 106:519–538, 1958

52. Grossi CE, Nealon RF Jr, Rousselot LM: Adjuvant chemotherapy in resectable cancer of the colon and rectum. Surg Clin North Am 524:925–933, 1972

53. Groves LK, Rodriguez-Antunex A: Treatment of carcinoma of the esophagus and gastric cardia with concentrated preoperative irradiation followed by early operation. Ann Thorac Surg 15:333–338, 1973

54. Guernsey JM, Knudsen DF: Abdominal exploration in the evaluation of patients with carcinoma of the thoracic esophagus. J Thorac Cardiovasc Surg 59:62–66, 1970

55. Gunderson LL, Sosin H: Areas of failure found at reoperation (second or symptomatic look) following "curative surgery" for adenocarcinoma of the rectum. Cancer 34:1278–1292, 1974

56. Hahn RC, Moertel CG, Schutt AJ, Bruckner HW: A double-blind comparison of intensive course 5-fluorouracil by oral vs. intravenous route in the treatment of colorectal carcinoma. Cancer 35:1031–1035, 1975

57. Hansen HJ, Snyder JJ, Miller E, Vandevoorde JP, Miller ON, Hines LR, Burns JJ: Carcinoembryonic antigen (CEA) assay. A laboratory adjunct in the diagnosis and management of cancer. J Hum Pathol 5:139–147, 1974

58. Haslam JB, Cavanaugh PJ, Stroup SL: Radiation therapy in the treatment of irresectable adenocarcinoma of the pancreas. Cancer 32:1341–1345, 1973

59. Hicks RE, Brooks JR: Total pancreatectomy for ductal carcinoma. Surg Gynecol Obstet 133:16–20, 1971

60. Higa E, Rosai J, Pizzimbono A, Wise L: Mucosal hyperplasia, mucinous cystadenoma and mucinous cystadenocarcinoma of the appendix. Cancer 32:1525–1541, 1973

61. Higgins GA, Conn JH, Jordan PH, Humphrey EW, Roswit B, Keehn RJ: Preoperative radiotherapy for colorectal cancer. Ann Surg 181:624–631, 1975

62. Higgins GA, Dwight RW, Smith JV, Keehn RJ: Fluorouracil as an adjuvant to surgery in carcinoma of the colon. Arch Surg 102:339–343, 1971

63. Holden WD, Dixon WJ, Kuzma JW: The use of triethylene-thiophosphoramide as an adjuvant of the surgical treatment of colorectal carcinoma. Ann Surg 165:481–503, 1967

64. Holton CP, Burrington JD, Hatch EI: A multiple chemotherapeutic approach to the management of hepatoblastoma. Cancer 35:1083–1087, 1975

65. Holyoke D, Reynoso G, Chu TM: Carcinoembryonic antigen (CEA) in patients with carcinoma of the digestive tract. Ann Surg 176:559–563, 1972

66. Honjo I, Mizumoto R: Primary carcinoma of the liver: Am J Surg 128:31–36, 1974

67. Howard JM: Pancreatico-duodenectomy: Forty-one consecutive Whipple resections without an operative mortality. Ann Surg 168:629–636, 1968

68. Ihde DC, Sherlock P, Winawer SJ, Fortner JG: Clinical manifestations of hepatoma; a review of six years experience at a cancer hospital. Am J Med 56:83–91, 1974

69. Jaffe BM, Donegan WL, Watson F, Spratt JS Jr: Factors influencing survival in patients with untreated hepatic metastases. Surg Gynecol Obstet 127:1–11, 1968

70. Kavlie H, Dillard DH, White TT: Duodenectomy with reimplantation of the papilla into the jejunum as a treatment for benign duodenal lesions. Surgery 73:230–233, 1973

71. Kligerman MM, Urdaneta N, Knowlton A, et al: Preoperative radiation of rectosigmoid carcinoma including the regional lymph nodes. Am J Roentgenol Radium Ther Nucl Med 114:498–503, 1972

72. Kuiper DH, Gracie WA Jr, Pollard HM: Twenty years of gastrointestinal carcinoids. Cancer 25:1424–1430, 1970

73. Lahiri SR, Boileau G, Hall TC: Treatment of metastatic colorectal carcinoma with 5-fluorouracil by mouth. Cancer 28:902–906, 1971

74. Lawrence W Jr: Radical gastrectomy, in Nora PF (ed): Operative Surgery. Philadelphia, Lea & Febiger, 1972, p. 904

✓75. Lawrence W Jr: Regional cancer chemotherapy: An evaluation. Clin Cancer vol. I, pp 341–393, 1965

76. Lawrence W Jr: Reservoir construction after total gastrectomy. Ann Surg 155:191–198, 1962

77. Lawrence W Jr, McNeer G: The effectiveness of surgery for palliation of incurable gastric cancer. Cancer 11:28–32, 1958

78. Lawrence W Jr, McNeer GP: An analysis of the role of radical surgery for gastric cancer. Surg Gynecol Obstet 111:691–696, 1960

79. Lawrence W Jr, McNeill DD, Cohen A, Terz JJ: Benign duodenal tumors (unusual surgical problems). Ann Surg 172:1015–1022, 1970

80. Lawrence WL Jr, Terz JJ, Horsley J, Donaldson M, Brown PW, Lovett W, Ruffner BW, Regelson W: Chemotherapy as an adjuvant to surgery for colorectal cancer. Ann Surg 181:616–623, 1975

81. Leopold GR: Echographic study of the pancreas. JAMA 232:287–289, 1975

82. Lin TY, Chen CC: Metabolic function and regeneration of cirrhotic and non-cirrhotic livers after hepatic lobectomy in man. Ann Surg 162:959–972, 1965

83. Lin TY, Chu SH, Chen MF, Chen CH: Serum alphafetoglobulin and primary cancer of the liver in Taiwan. Cancer 30:435–443, 1972

84. Linder GT, Crook JN, Cohn I Jr: Primary liver carcinoma. Cancer 33:1624–1629, 1974

85. Livingstone AS, Hampson LG, Shuster J, Gold P, Hinchey EJ: Carcinoembryonic antigen in the diagnosis and management of colorectal carcinoma: Current status. Arch Surg 109:259–264, 1974

86. Localio SA, Stahl WM: Simultaneous abdominotranssacral resection and anastomosis for midrectal cancer. Am J Surg 117:282–288, 1969

87. LoGerfo P, LoGerfo F, Herter F, et al: Tumor-associated antigen in patients with carcinoma of the colon. Am J Surg 123:127–131, 1972

88. Longmire WP, Kuzma JW, Dixon WJ: The use of triethylenethiophosphoramide as an adjuvant to the surgical treatment of gastric carcinoma. Ann Surg 167:293–312, 1968

89. Mabogunje O, Rosen PP, Fortner JG: Liver cell carcinoma during the prime of life. Surg Gynecol Obstet 140:75–80, 1975

90. Madden JL, Kandalaft S: Clinical evaluation of electrocoagulation in the treatment of cancer of the rectum. Am J Surg 122:347–352, 1971

91. Makk L, Creech JL, Whelan JG Jr, Johnson MN: Liver damage and angiosarcoma in vinyl chloride workers. JAMA 230:64–68, 1974

92. Malt RA, Hershberg RA, Miller WL: Experience with benign tumors of the liver. Surg Gynecol Obstet 130:285–291, 1970

93. Malt RA, Van Vroonhoven TJ, Kakumoto Y: Manifestations and prognosis of carcinoma of the liver. Surg Gynecol Obstet 135:361–364, 1972

94. Martin RG: Management of carcinoid tumors. Cancer 26:547–551, 1970

95. McDonald RA: A study of 365 carcinoids of the gastrointestinal tract. Am J Med 21:867–878, 1956

96. McNeer G, Berg JW: The clinical behavior and management of primary malignant lymphoma of the stomach. Surgery 46:829–840, 1959

97. McNeer G, Bowden L, Booher RJ, McPeak CJ: Elective total gastrectomy for cancer of the stomach. Ann Surg 180:252–256, 1974

98. McNeer G, Lawrence W Jr, Ashley MP, Pack GT: End results in the treatment of gastric cancer. Surgery 43:879–896, 1958

99. McNeer G, Pack GT: Neoplasms of the Stomach. Philadelphia, JB Lippincott Co, 1967

100. McPeak CJ: Malignant tumors of the small intestine. Am J Surg 114:402–411, 1967

101. Millburn L, Faber LP, Hendrickson FR: Curative treatment of epidermoid carcinoma of the esophagus. Am J Roentgenol 103:291–299, 1968

102. Moertel CG, Hill JR, Adson MA: Management of multiple polyposis of the large bowel. Cancer 28:160–164, 1971

103. Moertel CG, Sauer G, Dockertz MB, et al: Life history of the carcinoid tumor of the small intestine. Cancer 14:901–912, 1961

104. Moertel CG, Childs DS Jr, Reitemeier RJ, et al: Combined 5-FU and supervoltage radiation therapy of locally unresectable gastrointestinal cancer. Lancet 2:865–867, 1969

105. Moossa AR, Anagnost M, Hall AW, Moraldi A, Skinner DB: The continuing challenge of gallbladder cancer. Am J Surg 130:57–62, 1975

106. Morson BC: Evolution of cancer of the colon and rectum. Cancer 34:845, 1974

107. Morson BC: The pathology and results of treatment of squamous cell carcinoma of the anal canal and anal margin. Proc R Soc Med 53:416–420, 1960

108. Motsay GJ, Gamble WG: Clinical experience with hepatic adenomas. Surg Gynecol Obstet 134:415–418, 1972

109. Nakayama K, Orihata H, Yamagach K: Surgical treatment combined with

preoperative concentrated irradiation for esophageal cancer. Cancer 20:778–788, 1967

110. Nevin JE, Moran TJ, King R, Kay S: Carcinoma of the gallbladder —staging, treatment and prognosis. Cancer 37:141–148, 1976

111. Norton L, Eiseman B: Replacement of portal vein during pancreatectomy for carcinoma. Surgery 77:280–284, 1975

112. Olsen JD, Dockerty MB, Gray HK: Benign tumors of the small bowel. Ann Surg 134:195–204, 1951

113. Orloff MJ: Carcinoid tumors of the rectum. Cancer 28:175–180, 1971

114. Overholt BF: Progress in gastroenterology: Colonoscopy. Gastroenterology 68:1308–1320, 1975

115. Pack GT, Baker HW: Total right hepatic lobectomy. Ann Surg 138:253–258, 1953

116. Palmer ED: Peroral prosthesis for the management of incurable esophageal carcinoma. Am J Gastroenterol 59:487–498, 1973

117. Papachristou D, Terz JJ, Lawrence W Jr: Clinical evaluation of the assay for carcinoembryonic antigen. Va Med Mon 101:108–113, 1974

118. Papillon J: Endocavitary irradiation in the curative treatment of rectal cancer. Dis Colon Rectum 17:172–180, 1974

119. Parker EF, Gregorie HB Jr: Combined radiation and surgical treatment of carcinoma of the esophagus. Ann Surg 161:710–722, 1965

120. Paulino F, Roselli A: Carcinoma of the stomach (with special reference to total gastrectomy). Curr Probl Surg 1973

121. Payne WS, Olsen AM: The Esophagus. Philadelphia, Lea & Febiger, 1974

122. Pearson JG: The value of radiotherapy. JAMA 227:181–183, 1974

123. Ponka JL: Carcinoid tumors of the appendix. Am J Surg 126:77–83, 1973

124. Purves LR, Bersohn I, Gaddes WE: Serum alpha-fetoglobulin and primary cancer of the liver in man. Cancer 25:1261–1270, 1970

125. Quan SHQ, Castro EB: Papillary adenomas (villous tumors): A review of 215 cases. Dis Colon Rectum 14:267–280, 1971

126. Quan SHQ, Deddish MR, Stearns MW Jr: The effect of preoperative roentgen therapy upon the 5 and 10 year results of the surgical treatment of cancer of the rectum. Surg Gynecol Obstet 111:507–508, 1960

127. Ravry M, Moertel CG, Schutt AJ, Go VLW: Usefulness of serial serum carcinoembryonic antigen (CEA) determinations during anticancer therapy of long-term followup of gastrointestinal carcinoma. Cancer 34:1230–1234, 1974

128. ReMine WH, Priestly JT, Judd ES, King JN: Total pancreatectomy. Ann Surg 172:595–603, 1970

129. River L, Silverstein J, Tope JW: Collective review: Benign neoplasms of the small intestine, a critical comprehensive review with reports of 20 new cases. Int Abstr Surg 102:1–38, 1956

130. Rohrmann CA, Silvis SE, Vennes JA: Evaluation of the endoscopic pancreatogram. Radiology 113:297–304, 1974

131. Rousselot LM, Cole DR, Grossi CE, et al: Adjuvant chemotherapy with 5-fluorouracil in surgery for colorectal cancer: Eight-year progress report. Dis Colon Rectum 15:169–174, 1972

132. Sachatello RC, Griffen WO Jr: Hereditary polypoid diseases of the gastrointestinal tract. (A working classification.) Am J Surg 129:198–203, 1975

133. Sakita T, Oguro Y, Takasu S, Fukutomi H, et al.: Observations on the healing of ulcerations in early gastric cancer. Gastroenterology 60:835–839, 1958

134. Scanlon EF: The esophagus, in Nora PF (ed): Operative Surgery. Philadelphia, Lea & Febiger, 1972, pp 289–315

135. Scott HW, Law DH IV, Gobbel WG Jr, et al: Clinical and metabolic studies after total gastrectomy with Hunt-Lawrence jejunal food pouch. Am J Surg 115:148–156, 1968

136. Sherlock P, Ehrlich AN, Winawer SJ: Diagnosis of gastrointestinal cancer: Current status and recent progress. Gastroenterology 63:672–700, 1972

137. Sherlock P, Lipkin M, Winawer SJ: Predisposing factors in carcinoma of the colon. Adv Int Med 20:121–150, 1975

138. Silberman H, Crichlow RW, Caplan HS: Neoplasms of the small bowel. Ann Surg 180:157–161, 1974

139. Silver H, Stolar J: Distinguishing features of well differentiated mucinous adenocarcinoma of the rectum and colitis cystica profunda. Am J Clin Pathol 51:493–500, 1969

140. Sorokin JJ, Sugarbaker PH, Zamcheck N, Pisick M, Kupchik HZ, Moore FD: Serial CEA assays: Use in detection of cancer recurrence. JAMA 228:49–53, 1974

141. Sparks FC, Mosher MB, Hallauer WC, Silverstein MJ, Rangel D, Passaro E, Morton D: Hepatic artery ligation and postoperative chemotherapy for hepatic metastases; clinical and pathophysiological results. Cancer 35:1074–1082, 1975

142. Stearns MW Jr: The choice among anterior resection, the pull through, and abdomino-perineal resection of the rectum. Cancer 34:969–971, 1974

143. Stearns MW Jr, Deddish MR, Quan SHQ, Leaming RH: Preoperative roentgen therapy for cancer of rectum and rectosigmoid. Surg Gynecol Obstet 138:584–586, 1974

144. Stearns MW Jr, Quan SHA: Epidermoid carcinoma of the anorectum. Surg Gynecol Obstet 131:953–957, 1970

145. Stearns MW Jr, Schottenfeld D: Techniques for the surgical management of colon cancer. Cancer 28:165–169, 1971

146. Stehlin JS Jr, Hafstrom L, Greeff PJ: Experience with infusion and resection in cancer of the liver. Surg Gynecol Obstet 138:855–863, 1974

147. Strauss AA, Appel M, Saphir O, Rabinovitz AJ: Immunologic resistance to carcinoma produced by electrocoagulation. Surg Gynecol Obstet 121:989–996, 1965

148. Sullivan RD, Zurek WZ: Chemotherapy for liver cancer by protracted ambulatory infusion. JAMA 194:481–486, 1965

149. Tomasulo J: Gastric polyps (histologic types and their relationship to gastric carcinoma). Cancer 27:1346–1355, 1971

150. Turek-Maischeider M, Kazem I: Palliative irradiation for liver metastases. JAMA 232:625–628, 1975

151. Turnbull RB, Kyle K, Watson FR, Spratt J: Cancer of the colon; the influence of the no-touch isolation technic on the survival rates. Ann Surg 166:420–425, 1967

152. VanHeerden JA, Judd ES, Dockerty MD: Carcinoma of the extrahepatic bile ducts. Am J Surg 113:49–56, 1967

153. Vogel CL, Primack A, McIntire KR, Carbone PP, Anthony PP: Serum alpha-fetoprotein in 184 Ugandan patients with hepatocellular carcinoma. Cancer 35:959–964, 1974

154. Wanebo HJ, Quan SHQ: Failures of electrocoagulation of primary carcinoma of the rectum. Surg Gynecol Obstet 138:174–176, 1974

155. Wang CE, Li KT: Surgical treatment of primary carcinoma of liver. Chin Med J 82:65–78, 1963

156. Warren KW, Choe DS, Plaza J, Relihan M: Results of radical resection for periampullary cancer. Ann Surg 181:534–540, 1975

157. Warren KW, Hardy KJ: Cystadenocarcinoma of the pancreas. Surg Gynecol Obstet 127:734–736, 1968

158. Warren KW, Hardy KJ, O'Rourke MGE: Primary neoplasia of the gallbladder. Surg Gynecol Obstet 126:1036–1040, 1968

159. Watne AL, Core SK, Carrier JM: Gardner's syndrome. Surg Gynecol Obstet 141:53–56, 1975

160. Weichert RF, Roth LM, Krementz ET, Hewitt RL, Drapanas T: Carcinoid-islet cell tumors of the duodenum. Am J Surg 121:195–205, 1971

161. Welch JP, Donaldson GA: Management of severe obstruction of the large bowel due to malignant disease. Am J Surg 127:492–499, 1974

162. Welch JP, Donaldson GA: Recent experience in the management of cancer of the colon and rectum. Am J Surg 127:258–266, 1974

163. Wilson JM, Melvin DB, Gray GF, Thorbjarnarson B: Primary malignancies of the small bowel. Ann Surg 180:175–179, 1974

164. Wilson SM, Block GE: Periampullary carcinoma. Arch Surg 108:539–544, 1974

165. Winawer SJ, Sherlock P, Belladonna J, Melamed M, Beattie EJ Jr: Endoscopic brush cytology in esophageal cancer. JAMA 232:1358, 1975

166. Wolff WI, Shinya H: A new approach to colonic polyps. Ann Surg 178:367–378, 1973

167. Zamchek N, Moore T, Dhar P, et al: Immunologic diagnosis and prognosis of human digestive tract cancer. Carcinoembryonic antigens. N Engl J Med 286:83–86, 1972

9

Management of Lymphomas

The term "malignant lymphoma" refers to a large variety of malignant lymphoproliferative disorders arising from lymph nodes and from lymphoid components of various organs. In this chapter we will consider the two major types of lymphoma, Hodgkin's disease and the non-Hodgkin's lymphomas, a series of neoplasms formerly known as reticulum cell sarcoma, lymphosarcoma, giant follicular lymphoma, lymphoblastoma, and undifferentiated lymphoma. Accurate diagnosis and proper classification of lymphomas may be difficult in the initial stages of these diseases when localized adenopathy is the only clinical finding. Since inflammatory and hyperplastic lymph node changes, as well as lymph node metastasis from an undiscovered primary carcinoma, are more common causes of lymphadenopathy, these must be ruled out before making a diagnosis of lymphoma.[15,89]

DIAGNOSIS

The symptoms and physical findings of Hodgkin's disease and non-Hodgkin's lymphoma are similar, but the key feature of the diagnosis is the biopsy. The diagnosis is usually made by excisional biopsy of a peripheral lymph node, although excision of the scalene fat pad, laparotomy, or thoracotomy may be required. An enlarged, palpable lymph node is the usual initiator of these diagnostic procedures since other symptoms are vague or absent.

When the lymph nodes are enlarged in more than one anatomic area, the site of biopsy should be chosen with care. It is better to remove a lower cervical or axillary lymph node than nodes from other sites. The inguinal lymph nodes should be avoided if possible as they often demonstrate atypical changes secondary to inflammatory processes that commonly drain to these nodes. If multiple nodes are present, the largest node should be removed in toto so that the pathologist can thoroughly evaluate the lymph node architecture using paraffin sections. Aspiration biopsy is to be avoided as the distortion of the tissue makes a specific diagnosis difficult. Imprints of the freshly sectioned lymph nodes can be helpful in diagnosis, however.

Under some circumstances the diagnosis requires more detailed procedures such as mediastinoscopy; exploratory laparotomy for an abdominal mass, splenic enlargement, or to determine the cause of an unexplained fever; or even thoracotomy if the disease presents as an isolated mediastinal mass.

HODGKIN'S DISEASE

The incidence of Hodgkin's disease is low in comparison to more common cancers, but its usual occurrence in young adults and its responsiveness to therapy intensify our interest in early diagnosis.[65] This is one cancer for which there has been marked recent improvement in treatment results.

Diagnosis

The most common clinical presentation of Hodgkin's disease is the recently discovered, asymptomatic, painless node in the neck, axilla, or inguinal area, in an otherwise healthy individual. It is not uncommon for the abnormal lymph node to be discovered in young individuals during routine physical examinations or chest x-rays (such as military induction examinations) since the unrecognized adenopathy or mediastinal widening are frequently asymptomatic. In a few patients, systemic symptoms such as fever, night sweats, or pruritus are the initial complaints with or without palpable lymphadenopathy. Pain at the site of adenopathy associated with alcohol ingestion has been frequently described as a finding with Hodgkin's disease, but this clinical presentation is actually quite rare (less than 5 percent of patients). Other clinical manifestations may be the result of large intrathoracic or intra-abdominal lymph nodes producing superior vena cava syndrome, edema of the extremities, or both. Systemic manifestations of Hodgkin's include weight loss, anorexia, weakness, and malaise. Less common clinical findings are bone pain secondary to bone involvement, cord compression owing to extradural involvement, and gastrointestinal bleeding and/or obstruction secondary to visceral involvement by Hodgkin's disease.

The key to the diagnosis of Hodgkin's disease is the biopsy of an involved lymph node or, less frequently, material from extranodal tissues. The specific histologic diagnosis is made by identifying Reed-Sternberg cells, which are large reticulum cells with abnormally basophilic nuclei and a tendency to lobulate and form butterfly or spectacle shapes. These cells appear scattered, forming small clusters surrounded by a mass of reactive stromal cells of various types such as lymphocytes (small and large), eosinophils, plasma cells, and fibroblasts. Although the presence of the Reed-Sternberg cell is the key to the diagnosis of Hodgkin's disease, similar cells have been described also in lymph node biopsies from patients with infectious mononucleosis.[63] It is quite important, therefore, to consider also the overall nodal architecture in the diagnosis.

Within the broad category of Hodgkin's disease, many variations in the histopathology appear to bear a definite relationship to the clinical course. Several histologic classifications have been developed over the last 40 years,[42] but the "Rye classification" (developed at a national conference in Rye, N.Y. in 1966)[60–62,76] has shown good correlation with clinical course and prognosis and it is the currently accepted one. The relationship of the various histologic categories to prior schemes is shown in Table 9-1. Defining the disease in these terms has been helpful both in predicting the clinical extent of the disease in the individual patient and in planning subsequent therapy.

Table 9-1
Interrelationships of the Major Histopathologic
Classifications of Hodgkin's Disease

Jackson and Parker[42]	Rye[62]	Relative Frequency (%)
Paragranuloma	Lymphocytic predominance	10–15
Granuloma	Nodular sclerosis	20–50
	Mixed cellularity	20–40
Sarcoma	Lymphocytic depletion	5–15

Diagnostic Evaluation and Staging

A careful history should be elicited and physical examination performed to detect *systemic* manifestations of Hodgkin's disease (fever, pruritis, night sweats) as well as to evaluate accurately the extent of the disease anatomically. These findings combined with other evaluations will determine the clinical stage as outlined in Table 9-2.

The workup recommended for pretreatment staging of patients with Hodgkin's disease (Ann Arbor Conference, 1971)[16,80] included chest x-rays, tomograms of the mediastinum when indicated, and x-rays of the spine and pelvis. An intravenous pyelogram was also recommended. A bone marrow biopsy is indicated in the presence of an elevated alkaline phosphatase, unexplained anemia, or other blood count depressions, radiological evidence of bone involvement, or systemic symptoms.

ASSESSMENT OF THE INTRA-ABDOMINAL
VISCERA AND LYMPH NODES

A crucial part of the initial pretreatment evaluation is assessment of intra-abdominal viscera and lymph nodes. Intravenous pyelograms and inferior vena-cavograms are relatively inefficient for an early diagnosis of retroperitoneal lymph node involvement. Lee et al.[54] demonstrated in 1964 that these studies carry only a 65-percent and 30-percent reliability,

Table 9-2
Staging of Hodgkin's Disease

Stage I	Disease limited to one anatomic region.
Stage II	Disease limited to two or more anatomic regions on the same side of the diaphragm.
Stage III	Disease on both sides of the diaphragm but not extending beyond lymph nodes, spleen, or Waldeyer's ring.
Stage IV	Involvement of bone marrow, lung parenchyma, pleurae, liver, bone, skin, kidneys, gastrointestinal tract, or any other tissue or organ with or without lymph node involvement.
Anatomic areas	Above the diaphragm: Waldeyer's ring, neck, mediastinal or hilar, supraclavicular, axillary, brachial, and epitrochlear. Below the diaphragm: spleen, para-aortic, mesenteric, celiac, iliac, femoral, popliteal.
Addendum	Denote the suffix letters A or B for the absence or presence of fever, night sweats, and/or unexplained loss of 10 percent or more of the body weight in the 6 months preceeding admission. Identify also with letter suffix all areas of biopsy proven extranodal involvement: M, marrow; L, lung; H, liver; O, bone; D, skin, and subcutaneous tissue; S, spleen (e.g., stage III_{AS} indicates nodal and spleen involvement and absence of systemic symptoms).

respectively. Lymphangiograms, on the other hand, have gained wide acceptance as a reliable indicator of the nodal status in the clinical evaluation of this area[91] (Fig. 9-1). However, the usefulness of this procedure is limited to the visualization of the iliac and aorta caval nodes up to L2 when the injections are made in the feet. Other lymph node groups that can be involved with lymphomas—such as hypogastric, celiac, splenic, portohepatic, and mesenteric nodes—are not visualized by the standard lymphangiogram. Moreover, when the radiological findings were correlated with nodal biopsies obtained during staging laparotomy, there was a 12-percent incidence of false negatives and a 27-percent incidence of false positives in radiological interpretation.[46] Proponents of lymphangiography feel that these studies are certainly useful in the evaluation and staging of Hodgkin's disease because of: (a) a relatively high index of accuracy, (b) the assistance provided to the radiotherapist in outlining radiation ports on the abdomen, (c) the possibility of use as a reference for radiation response after initial therapy is completed, and (d) their potential usefulness to the surgeon in locating abnormal lymph nodes during a subsequent staging laparotomy.

The use of gallium[67] instead of lymphangiography for detecting nodal involvement in Hodgkin's disease has gained wide acceptance since 1969.[28] This method has proven to be of significant value in assessing the status of both mediastinal and intra-abdominal lymph nodes (Fig. 9-2). The results compare favorably with those of lymphangiographic studies. Gallium scans were accurate in 75 percent of the cases when subsequent biopsies of the abnormal lymph nodes were obtained during stag-

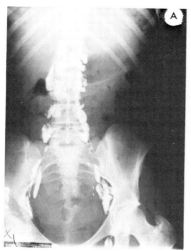 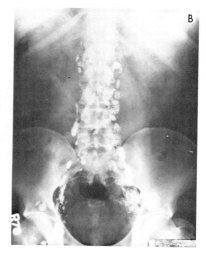

Fig. 9-1. **A**; Normal lymphangiogram. **B:** Lymphangiogram in a patient with Hodgkin's disease demonstrating classic node abnormalities.

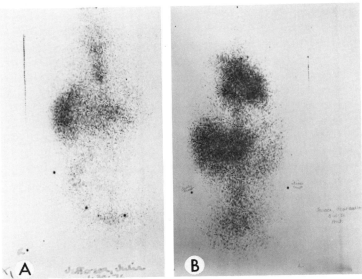

Fig. 9-2. **A:** Normal gallium scan. **B:** Gallium scan demonstrating uptake in lymph nodes involved by Hodgkin's disease (mediastinum).

ing laparotomy.[45,98] Currently, the lymph node scan with gallium[67] is considered a simple, useful, and noninvasive method for assessment of the initial extent of the disease as well as for the subsequent assessment of the patient after therapy.[32]

Once the initial clinical and laboratory studies have been completed on the individual patient, the clinical extent of the disease is categorized according to a clinical staging scheme[16,80] (Table 9-2). The staging process is further refined by a laparotomy in selected patients.

LAPAROTOMY FOR STAGING OF HODGKIN'S DISEASE

Laparotomy was introduced in 1969 for increasing the accuracy of clinical staging of Hodgkin's disease and to shed additional light on the natural history of this neoplasm[46] (Fig. 9-3). The usual steps followed during this surgical intervention are (a) exploration of the abdomen; (b) wedge biopsy and deep needle biopsy from each lobe of the liver; (c) splenectomy with the placement of silver clips at the site of the ligature of the splenic vessels; (d) excisional biopsy of the celiac, aortocaval, iliac, and mesenteric lymph nodes; (e) placement of silver clips at the site of all the lymph nodes biopsied, as well as at the periphery of larger masses to facilitate the outline of subsequent radiation fields; (f) transposition of the ovaries to the midline in women in the childbearing age; and (g) bone marrow biopsy.

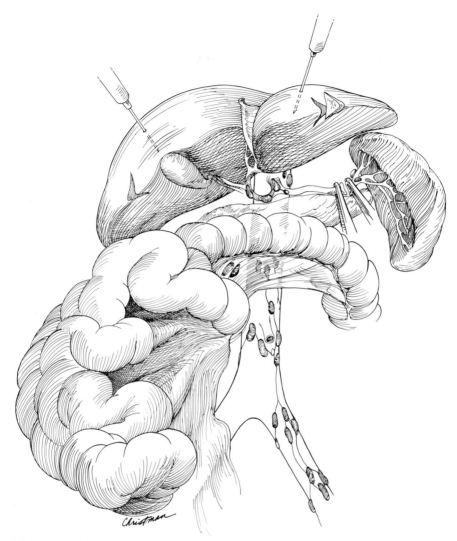

Fig. 9-3.   Diagram of the procedure of staging laparotomy for Hodgkin's disease and non-Hodgkin's lymphoma.   Sites of lymph node and liver biopsies are indicated.

This staging procedure has resulted in important clinicopathological correlations with significant prognostic and therapeutic implications.[24,31,46] Approximately 36 percent of the spleens considered to be normal preoperatively contain Hodgkin's disease.[4]   Liver involvement has been found in only 5 percent of the patients undergoing exploratory laparotomy, and this is always associated with spleen involvement.   The laboratory and isotopic studies of the liver are accurate in predicting this involvement in only 30 percent of the patients. Also, lymph nodes in 12 percent of the patients with normal lymphangiograms and 72 percent of those with abnormal lymphangiograms are found to contain Hodgkin's. The portal, mesenteric, celiac, and splenic hilum nodes are involved in only 7–10 percent of the cases, and on rare occasions these are the only site of intra-abdominal disease.

From these clinicopathological findings, a pattern of behavior can be predicted based on the site of the initial presentation of the disease, the histologic type of the tumor, and the age and sex of the patient. It is also evident from these prior studies that the initial clinical estimation of the extent of the disease is accurate in only 60 percent of the patients. The remaining cases are obviously under- or overstaged. Valuable information has been obtained by this operative extension of the staging process, but there is still no uniform conclusion regarding the desired frequency of application of this operative procedure in pretreatment assessment.

Complications of staging laparotomy. Like any other "invasive" procedure, staging laparotomy is associated with complications directly related to the operation per se. Only one operative mortality (pulmonary embolism) has been reported in over 1000 cases subjected to staging laparotomy, and the overall morbidity has been around 6–8 percent. Pulmonary emboli, intestinal obstruction, and wound infection have been the most common complications. Infectious processes that might be attributed directly to the splenectomy (as observed in children) have not been documented in the reported series of staging laparotomy in adults.[25]

Critique of staging laparotomy. In spite of the significant amount of valuable information obtained with staging laparotomy, this operative procedure has not been unconditionally implemented as part of the management of Hodgkin's disease. The following *objections* to the routine use of abdominal exploration for staging have been raised: (a) the intra-abdominal findings in stage I and II may not greatly alter the therapeutic plan, (b) the surgeon may not be accurate in terms of the biopsy of all involved nodes, (c) intra-abdominal nodal disease outside the retroperitoneum and not seen on lymphangiography is rare, (d) the spleen can be irradiated rather than removed without damage to the surrounding structures, and with the same therapeutic advantage, and (e) the mortality and morbidity of the surgical intervention are still a major threat to the patient, particularly if we consider that the surgical procedure per se will not alter the final outcome of the disease.[43] The following *advantages* have been suggested for this procedure: (a) in the absence of retroperitoneal disease, the pelvis will not need to be irradiated, thereby sparing the ovaries in young women[77,93] (in spite of the oophoropexy and proper shielding, the ovaries receive around 10 percent of the dose delivered to the pelvis, and only 50 percent of the patients maintain normal menses); (b) with the proper assessment of the intra-abdominal disease, the possibility of both under- or overtreatment can be avoided; (c) splenectomy minimizes the possibility of radiation nephritis and pneumonitis; and (d) patients who have undergone splenectomy can tolerate radiation therapy better than those with the spleen in situ. Similar conclusions regarding splenectomy have been reported for patients undergoing chemotherapy,[36,59,75,83] but this conclusion is not shared by others.[29]

It is not yet clear if these described benefits from a staging laparotomy influence the results of treatment of Hodgkin's disease so significantly that it should be carried out routinely on all patients. However, the information that has been gained from the clinical and histologic correlations after a staging laparotomy should suggest criteria for the selection of patients who will benefit from the procedure. We feel the staging laparotomy should be carried out under the following circumstances: (a) in patients suspected clinically of extranodal, infradiaphragmatic disease (histologic verification will change the therapeutic approach significantly); (b) if the therapist believes that only the involved and the adjacent nodal areas should be treated, (laparotomy will determine the status of the infradiaphragmatic areas in view of the 30 percent inaccuracy of the clinical investigation); (c) in young women in whom preservation of ovarian function may supersede the possible benefits of prophylactic irradiation of the pelvis; and (d) in patients with a high probability of intra-abdominal involvement as indicated by a histologic pattern of mixed cellularity or lymphocyte depletion, vascular invasion, or left lower neck disease.

For the present we plan to continue the laparotomy staging approach for patients with Hodgkin's disease unless there is preoperative, objective evidence of stage IV disease or medical disability that would increase the operative risk. This is probably not a procedure for general clinical use, More experience is certainly needed to place this approach in proper perspective from the standpoint of Hodgkin's disease management.

Treatment (Table 9-3)

RADIATION

Radical radiation therapy plays the major role in current therapeutic programs for Hodgkin's disease that appears localized to nodal areas. The principles of primary control of the involved area include the use of: (a) megavoltage (linear accelerator, cobalt 60), (b) doses of 3500–4500 rads at a rate of 1000 rads per week, (c) irradiation fields that include the lymph nodes at the involved site and adjacent nodal groups not clinically

Table 9-3
Therapeutic Outline for Hodgkin's Disease According to Stage
and Histology

Stage	Histology	Therapy
I_A, II_A	Nodular sclerosis, lymphocytic predominance	Mantle field and/or inverted Y (according to location)
I_B, II_B	Nodular sclerosis, lymphatic predominance	Total lymphoid irradiation
I_A, I_B, II_A, II_B	Mixed cellularity, lymphocytic predominance	Total nodal irradiation and 6 cycles of combination chemotherapy (MOPP)
III_A	Nodular sclerosis, lymphocytic predominance	Total nodal irradiation
III_{SA}, III_{SB} III_B, III_S	All histologies	Total nodal irradiation and 6 cycles of chemotherapy (MOPP)
All stages IV	All histologies	3 cycles of combination chemotherapy (MOPP), alternated with selective irradiation to areas with bulky disease; continue MOPP until remission is achieved, then use maintenance chemotherapy (MOPP every 2–3 months)

involved, and (d) proper shielding of vital structures that might be harmed by the radiation beam.[47–49,73,74] Total nodal radiation includes both the "mantle" field—cervical, axillary, supraclavicular, infraclavicular (all bilaterally), and mediastinal nodes down to the diaphragm—and the "inverted Y,"—celiac, aortocaval, iliac, and inguinal areas as well as the splenic hilum. The plan of total nodal irradiation[44] (as opposed to involved field or extended field) has gained wide acceptance as the primary method of therapy for clinical stages I, II, and III, and it has resulted in prolonged disease-free intervals. Many physicians are reluctant to use total nodal irradiation for stage I disease, particularly with the more favorable histologic types, and extended field irradiation (usually the "mantle" field) is used in these instances with some justification.

The large size of the radiation field for either extended field or total nodal irradiation carries some morbidity and requires the expertise of the radiotherapist to keep this at a minimum. Dryness of the throat and dysphagia are frequently seen after the initial treatments, and alopecia, hypothyroidism (10 percent), and radiation pneumonitis have all been observed as an aftermath of the "mantle" field. All of these symptoms usually disappear after a few months. Radiation pericarditis has been observed in 6 percent of cases and is manifested by cardiomegaly, a friction rub, or the presence of pericardial fluid.[88] Very seldom will it progress to cardiac tamponade or chronic pericarditis. Some patients complain of numbness, a tingling sensation without motor dysfunction in the arms and legs, exacerbated by flexing of the neck, but this symptom subsides after several months. Nausea and vomiting are frequently associated with the "inverted Y" field, and they may require temporary interruption of treatment. More severe complications, such as transverse myelitis, are rarely seen. These problems are the reason for diminished enthusiasm for total nodal irradiation on the part of some therapists, but we believe that the therapeutic advantages outweigh this morbidity in most instances.

CHEMOTHERAPY

For many years chemotherapy has been used in the treatment of disseminated Hodgkin's disease (stages IIIb–IV). Single agents[17] are offered in sequential fashion, according to the response or failure of each treatment. The most commonly employed drugs used to be mechlorethamine hydrochloride (nitrogen mustard), cyclophosphamide (Cytoxan®), and chlorambucil (Leukeran®). Also, temporary responses have been obtained with vinblastine (Velban®), procarbazine (mutalane®), and corticosteroids. The overall remission rate in the past was between 10 and 20 percent, and the 2-year survival was less than 50 percent. Recently, it has been shown that the therapeutic index of these drugs can be improved significantly by a more rational manipulation of the dose and duration of the treatment and concomitant use of several drugs in combination.[11,27] A combination program was developed at the National Cancer Institute consisting of six 2-week cycles of therapy with nitrogen mustard, vincristine, procarbazine, and prednisone (MOPP).[27] There is a 2-week rest period between cycles, and the entire course usually requires 6 months. With this regime, complete regression of disease has been seen in 70–80 percent of previously untreated patients, with a mean duration of response of 36 months. Seventy percent of the patients with stages III and IV who achieve remission on combination therapy are alive at 6 years. Forty percent of the complete responders have remained continuously free of disease with no further treatment after 6 years.

In view of the significant success obtained with aggressive radiation therapy, as well as improved response to chemotherapy in the last few years, there has been an increased interest in approaching those cases in stages I and II that fall into a higher risk category with a combination of both modalities rather than radiation alone. A series of clinical trials has been started and the early reports have been encouraging.[36,69,71,82]

Clinical Course

The course of Hodgkin's disease in an individual patient is related to histopathologic classification, clinical stage, and treatment received. Survival after diagnosis can range from prolonged remission or "cure" to rapid disease progression despite the therapy given. When it does progress before or in spite of therapy, the spread occurs in lymphatic tissues adjacent or distal to the primary site, or may include the bone marrow, visceral sites (pulmonary, pleural, peritoneal, or hepatic), bones, or the nervous system.[94]

HEMATOLOGIC ABNORMALITIES

Hematologic abnormalities are usually seen in the patient with advanced disease and/or relapse. Anemia is the most common manifestation and is usually associated with bone marrow involvement or hypersplenism, with or without splenomegaly.[30] A positive bone marrow biopsy and positive Coombs' test establish the diagnosis. Erythrocyte sedimentation rate is usually elevated in patients with active disease, and it has been seen to precede the relapse or remain elevated if the disease is not brought under control by treatment. Eosinophilia is not uncommon and is usually seen in patients with severe and long-standing pruritus, but it has no diagnostic significance. Absolute lymphopenia is not frequently seen, but this hematologic observation is associated with a poor prognosis and severe life-threatening infectious problems. Thrombocytopenia also occurs and may be associated with significant bleeding disorders. When pancytopenia unrelated to therapy occurs, it is usually secondary to hypersplenism and often represents a clinical indication for splenectomy. (See section on treatment of non-Hodgkin's lymphoma on page 289.)

VISCERAL INVOLVEMENT

The liver may become diffusely involved with infiltrates of Hodgkin's disease resulting in serum enzyme changes compatible with biliary obstruction. The importance of liver biopsy as a part of the staging process is emphasized by the grave prognostic significance of liver involvement.

Pulmonary lesions in the course of Hodgkin's disease are frequent and must be differentiated from parenchymal changes secondary to radiation or pneumonitis from a variety of infectious processes that frequently affect patients during therapy. Pleural and peritoneal involvement is usually manifested by effusions or gastrointestinal complications, the latter often producing obstruction or bleeding.

BONE AND CNS INVOLVEMENT

Bone metastases, either blastic or lytic, may develop. These are associated with severe pain but seldom result in fracture. Central nervous system (CNS) involvement is usually manifested by external spinal cord compression by epidural disease. This represents a true emergency and should be suspected in any patient with Hodgkin's disease who develops peripheral neuropathy. The blockage should be documented with a myelogram and the spinal canal must be decompressed, usually by operative means.

IMMUNOLOGIC ABNORMALITIES

Patients with Hodgkin's disease often fail to develop delayed-type hypersensitivity reactions to tuberculin, even in the presence of active tuberculosis.[3,85,102] On tests with a battery of different antigens, these patients also have an incidence of cutaneous anergy higher than that in a normal population. They also have a tendency toward defective development of delayed hypersensitivity to new antigens, failure to elaborate migratory inhibition factor in vitro, decreased response of lymphocytes to transformation after exposure to various mitogens or antigens, and prolonged survival of allogenic skin grafts. These immunologic deficiencies are accentuated in the patient with advanced Hodgkin's disease, and they are also prominent in the patient undergoing radiation therapy and chemotherapy. However, the patient with localized controlled disease usually has an immune response comparable to that of normal individuals.

The immunologic variations described also have some effect on susceptibility to infections.[18] Besides the common bacterial infections, fungal infections that ususally involve the lung and the meninges are of particular importance. The most common agents are *Cryptococcus, Pneumocystis carinii,*[38] and *Toxoplasma*. Among the viral infections, herpes zoster and cytomegalic inclusion infections are frequently associated with this disease.[67,87]

Prognosis

The outlook for patients with Hodgkin's disease has changed significantly in the last decade with the introduction of radical radiotherapy and combination chemotherapy. A proper and detailed study of the extent of the disease at the time of diagnosis has allowed a more realistic and accurate projection of the probability of response to the treatment and the estimation of survival. It has not been definitely established that all foci of Hodgkin's disease are eliminated with appropriate therapy, but it is evident that long-term remissions extending well beyond 5 and 10 years can be accomplished.[74,90]

It has been shown that the therapeutic approach to Hodgkin's disease will influence prognosis. A series of factors that relate to the disease per se are reliable indicators of the natural history of the disease. These variables are the actual extent of the nodal disease, the presence or absence of extranodal involvement, the histologic type, the presence or absence of systemic symptoms, and sex. The best prognosis is seen in younger women with nodular sclerosis or lymphocytic predominant type of disease. With proper therapy, these patients will easily reach a median survival of 10–15 years. On the other hand, in older men with mixed cellularity or lymphoid depletion, extranodal involvement (lung, liver, bone marrow, Waldeyer's ring), and systemic symptoms present at the onset of the disease (fever, night sweats), the median disease-free interval may be no longer than 1 year.[49,74]

Patients judged to have stages Ia and IIa disease after careful diagnostic evaluation, including staging laparotomy and splenectomy, and treated with modern radiotherapy techniques can be expected to have approximately 90 percent chance of disease-free survival for 5 years. However, only about one-third of patients with Hodgkin's disease have such localized disease without systemic symptoms when initially evaluated. More than half of the patients seen have stages Ib, IIb, or IIIa or b, with or without limited extranodal disease (subgroup "e" of the Ann Arbor system).[47] With almost 90 percent of these patients enjoying disease-free survival for periods up to nearly 4 years after the initiation of sequential radiotherapy and combination chemotherapy, the great majority of patients with Hodgkin's disease may be able to look forward to clinical "cure" of their disease. These optimistic results, however, will probably be achieved only at medical centers where experienced pathologists, surgeons, radiologists, radiotherapists, and chemotherapists are working closely together in the evaluation and management of these patients.

NON-HODGKIN'S LYMPHOMA

Non-Hodgkin's lymphoma includes all the malignant lymphoproliferative diseases arising in the lymph glands or extranodal sites with the exception of Hodgkin's disease and Burkitt's lymphoma. Some clinical features separate this group of lesions from the more favorable Hodgkin's disease, but it is often impossible to differentiate these lymphomas before histologic study. The categories of non-Hodgkin's lymphoma have also been reclassified in recent years, and the classification in current use is that of Gall and Rappaport[36] as modified by Berard[8] (Table 9-4). Interpretation of the histologic type is not always clear-cut, and even distinguishing between benign and malignant adenopathy is still difficult in almost 25 percent of the cases. In many instances the interpretation of the lymph node disease must be related to findings in the bone marrow, the

Table 9-4

Classification of non-Hodgkin's Lymphoma

Traditional Terminology	Current Classification
Lymphosarcoma	Lymphoma, lymphocytic type, well differentiated
	Lymphoma, lymphocytic type, poorly differentiated
	Lymphoma, mixed lymphocytic histiocytic type
Reticulum cell	Lymphoma, histiocytic type
sarcoma	Lymphoma, undifferentiated

All forms may be nodular or diffuse.

liver, and the blood, as well as to findings from serum and urine immuno-electrophoresis. Diagnostic problems may arise also as the result of bizarre reactive changes in the lymphoid tissues of the skin or gastric mucosa, and as a result of anatomic variations in the disease morphology.

These lymphomas may also be difficult to differentiate from leukemia. The diagnosis of leukemia implies abnormal cells in the bone marrow and the peripheral blood, whereas in lymphoma morphologic and histologic changes take place primarily in the lymphoid tissue. However, when the marrow as well as the peripheral blood in patients with lymphoma is infiltrated with abnormal cells, it is usually concluded that a leukemic transformation has taken place. At this stage, the diagnosis of lymphoma is changed to that of leukemia, according to the predominant cell type. The well-differentiated lymphocytic lymphoma is changed to chronic lymphocytic leukemia, and the poorly differentiated lymphoma becomes lymphosarcoma cell leukemia. Undifferentiated lymphoma usually leads to an acute leukemia, lymphocytic or stem cell type.

Diagnosis

Non-Hodgkin's lymphoma may present clinically as solitary lymph node enlargement or as a primary mass in a visceral organ. Usually, however, it is characterized as a generalized disease of lymph nodes with eventual involvement of multiple viscera. In only 20 percent of the cases does the disease present as a localized process limited to a single node group or organ. Contrary to Hodgkin's disease, these lymphomas are basically considered multicentric in origin, and they frequently spread to noncontiguous lymphoid areas. This observation has important therapeutic implications.

Painless adenopathy is a common initial manifestation of the disease. In some cases the initial symptoms are those of extranodal involvement (skin nodule, mass in oropharynx or gastrointestinal tract) or systemic symptoms (fever, weight loss, anorexia, malaise). As the disease progresses, the patient may develop pleural effusion, ascites, peripheral edema, multiple skin nodules, renal failure, or jaundice. All of these findings are manifestations of diffuse involvement of multiple organs by the lymphoma. Both pain and neurological symptoms, either radicular or cord compression, are also frequent. Anemia is seen in approximately half of the patients, usually as a result of bone marrow involvement, hypersplenism, autoimmune disease, hemolytic anemia, or gastrointestinal bleeding. There are variations, as with Hodgkin's disease, but the rapid dissemination and the generally poor prognosis of these lesions is striking.

Clinical Evaluation and Staging

As in Hodgkin's disease, it is extremely important to have an accurate assessment of the extent of disease at the time of diagnosis. A careful history, physical examination, and the performance of appropriate laboratory and radiologic studies as outlined in the workup of patients with Hodgkin's disease provide the necessary information for proper staging. For those patients presenting primarily with peripheral node or extranodal involvement, the staging as used in Hodgkin's is followed (Table 9-2).

When positive, the inferior vena-cavogram, lymphangiogram, and gallium 67 scan[55] are accurate in the demonstration of the retroperitoneal lymph nodes in most cases (93 percent, 83 percent, and 80 percent, respectively); however, the incidence of false-negative interpretation is high (47 percent, 67 percent, and 58 percent, respectively).[95] Bone marrow biopsy is of particular importance in non-Hodgkin's lymphoma because of a higher incidence of involvement (10–20 percent) as compared with Hodgkin's disease (1 percent)[79,81,82] at initial diagnosis. Staging laparotomy has also resulted in useful additional information in a number of instances because of the high incidence of extranodal involvement at the onset of the disease.

Sixty percent of untreated patients undergoing exploratory laparotomy were found to have disease below the diaphragm in one or more sites.[38,50,70] In 10 percent of the cases, two different histologic types were coexisting, including Hodgkin's disease. The nodular type of lymphoma had the highest incidence of intra-abdominal involvement (72 percent), whereas the diffuse form had only a 28-percent incidence of subdiaphragmatic involvement at initial evaluation. Unsuspected intra-abdominal involvement was found in mesenteric nodes (56 percent), splenic hilar nodes (54 percent), aortocaval nodes (40 percent), the spleen (34 percent), the liver (16 percent), and the gastrointestinal tract (6 percent). On the basis of these findings, the clinical stage had to be modified in 56 percent of the patients undergoing abdominal staging laparotomy, with 46 percent requiring a reclassification to a higher stage.

IMMUNOLOGIC EVALUATION

Hyperglobulinemia is seen in patients with histiocytic and lymphocytic lymphoma and more frequently in those with chronic lymphocytic leukemia. Peripheral lymphopenia when present is associated with a decrease in production of antibodies. Inhibition of in vitro blastogenesis of lymphocytes to mitogenic stimuli is also present. Despite this, skin reactions to various antigens are usually within normal limits.[66]

Monoclonal peaks of IgM type are associated with diffuse histiocytic or lymphocytic lymphoma in a higher proportion of patients than in the normal population. On the other hand, IgA and IgG are within normal range. These IgM peaks are usually seen in older patients and may return to a normal pattern as the patient responds to therapy.[68] Although these laboratory findings are of interest, the immunologic evaluation of patients with known lymphoma does not need to be this detailed.

Treatment (Table 9-5)

As in Hodgkin's disease, the stage of the disease, the histologic subclassification, and the age and sex of the patient have important prognostic features that will influence the therapeutic approach to these neoplasms. Radiation therapy plays a major role in the initial treatment of Hodgkin's lymphoma and, in many cases, is the only form of treatment required to accomplish permanent control of that disease. In contrast, radiation therapy cannot be relied on as the only treatment in non-

Table 9-5
Therapeutic Outline for
Non-Hodgkin's Lymphoma[95]

Stage	Therapy
I, I_E, II, II_E	Irradiation
III, III_S, III_E	Irradiation, combination chemotherapy
IV	Combination chemotherapy and selective irradiation of bulky tumor

Hodgkin's lymphoma. The latter disease has shown both a multicentric pattern and a higher incidence of extranodal involvement at the time of the initial diagnosis. For these reasons, both radiotherapy and chemotherapy are employed in most patients and surgery is employed for selected cases with primary extranodal lesions.

RADIATION THERAPY

Irradiation is definitely indicated in clinical stage I and II disease, but there is no uniform agreement regarding optimal field size. The concept of using extended fields, as in Hodgkin's disease, is less accepted because of the frequency of generalized dissemination of this disease at initial diagnosis. The dose range of 3000–4500 rads is employed to ensure local control. Several authors have proposed extended fields, or even total nodal irradiation, but the results with this latter approach are disappointing.[34] There is reason to treat all suspected areas of disease with radiation therapy, but the most rewarding approach for patients with extensive disease is cancer chemotherapy.

Radiotherapy in histiocytic lymphoma (reticulum cell sarcoma) is rather disappointing because this disease is uniformly widespread, and the overall 5-year survival rate is around 10 percent.[64] Some patients present with apparently localized lesions in the head and neck area, the soft tissues, or bone, and radical radiation therapy in the range of 5000–6000 rads usually controls the local lesion. In the case of primary gastrointestinal involvement, surgical removal of the involved organs, followed by radiation therapy, yields the best results.

CHEMOTHERAPY

There is a significant correlation among response to chemotherapy, duration of remission, and survival of patients with non-Hodgkin's lymphoma. Continued treatment during remission (maintained remissions) is a well-established concept in the management of these lesions. Of the single agents, cyclophosphamide and nitrogen mustard are the most effective for non-Hodgkin's lymphoma. Other drugs with a lower response rate are vinblastine, procarbazine, and prednisone. The response rate with each of these single drugs is lower than that observed with Hodgkin's disease. Asparaginase and bleomycin have been used more recently but with questionable results. These particular agents are often valuable in the treatment of patients with bone marrow suppression from other treatments, but each has its own toxicity. Asparaginase is known to produce allergic reactions, liver abnormalities, pancreatitis, and renal failure. Bleomycin has a potentially lethal dose-limited toxicity owing to pulmonary fibrosis. Also, it produces alopecia, oral ulcerations, dermatographia, and skin induration.

COMBINATION CHEMOTHERAPY

In spite of initial responses noted, remission of non-Hodgkin's lymphoma resulting from treatment with single agents is infrequent (20 percent) and short lasting. In a comparative study between cyclophosphamide as a single agent and a combination of cyclophosphamide, vincristine, and prednisone, the remission rate rose to 50 percent for lymphocytic lymphoma, and in histiocytic lymphoma the remission rate rose from 13 percent with single agents to 39 percent with multiple agents. Other studies using similar combinations have demonstrated equally improved remission rates.[52,58] The alteration of the nomenclature of the non-Hodgkin's lymphomas to a more dynamic and more prognostic classification has allowed the formulation of therapeutic regimes based on the clinical behavior and expected course of these neoplasms.

Patients with nodular histology have a better response rate to both chemotherapy and radiotherapy, and their clinical course is characterized by a continuous pattern of remission and relapse extending over a period of several years (median survival 3.5–8.5 years). This experience suggests that nodular lymphoma should be treated with radiation therapy followed by a single- or multiple-drug therapy, and this program should be carried out during the remission periods for a long time because of the frequency of late "recurrence." This regimen must be considered in the light of other factors such as the patient's age and normal life expectancy. Most patients over 65 will not tolerate aggressive chemotherapy very well and a single agent should be used for maintenance in this group, whereas younger patients should receive multiple-drug combinations for maintenance. On the other hand, the diffuse histologic types are extremely aggressive and will probably relapse rapidly after initial therapy (median survival of 12–20 months). Late recurrences are rare. In view of this poor prognosis, it seems logical to employ aggressive chemotherapy with multiple-drug combinations as the initial treatment. The addition of cell cycle–specific drugs such as methotrexate and arabinosylcytosine to standard drug therapy has increased the remission rate to 80 percent.[84]

Better understanding of immunologic and morphologic characteristics of lymphoma and the pursuit of prospective trials of aggressive radiotherapy and chemotherapy offer the best chance of improving our current results in the management of these lymphomas.[95]

Clinical Course

During the course of non-Hodgkin's lymphoma, clinical symptoms develop because of therapy or systemic involvement by the neoplasm. Many such conditions are life threatening and require prompt recognition and management.

CENTRAL NERVOUS SYSTEM

Cranial nerve palsies (III, IV, VIII, and XI) are seen in patients with lymphoma arising in the nasopharynx with local extension to the base of the skull. Appropriate physical examination of this area and skull radiographs establish the anatomic diagnosis. In some patients cranial nerve palsy is associated with a leukemic meningitis and symptoms of increased intracranial pressure. The spinal tap will reveal pleocytosis without changes in sugar or protein content of the cerebrospinal fluid. On other occasions, the diagnosis of meningeal involvement has been confirmed by the presence of neoplastic cells in the fluid. Involvement of the spinal canal produces cord compression, and this is usually preceded by symptoms of peripheral neuropathy (laminectomy for decompression and radiation therapy should be carried out immediately).

RENAL FAILURE

Renal failure usually arises as a result of: infiltration of the kidney parenchyma with lymphoma, obstruction of the ureter by large retroperitoneal or pelvic adenopathy, or hyperuricemia with formation of uric acid calculi. Intravenous pyelograms, urinalysis, and serum determination of uric acid will establish the cause. Radiation therapy to the kidney in a dose no greater than 2400 rads improves neoplastic nephritis. Radiation to the retroperitoneum and pelvis relieves ureteral obstruction. Uric acid nephropathy should be treated with increased hydration, alkalinization of the urine, and the use of allopurinal.

CARDIOPULMONARY INVOLVEMENT

Pericardial effusion with tamponade secondary to neoplastic involvement is not infrequent. Direct myocardial invasion, although rare, may also occur.[78] Radiation therapy, appropriate chemotherapy, and pericardiocentesis improve these symptoms. Superior vena caval obstruction is a more frequent manifestation of advanced mediastinal lymphoma. Radiation therapy and chemotherapy produce significant regression of the mediastinal tumor mass with striking relief of symptoms. Pleural effusion is seen in most patients with advanced lymphoma, and thoracocentesis, followed by the instillation of an alkylating agent, is often indicated.[57] When the hematologic effects of these drugs must be avoided, the instillation of quinacrine (Atabrine®), and/or the insertion of a chest tube connected to water seal drainage will usually control the effusion.

INFECTION

Sepsis is the most serious complication observed during this disease and is the leading cause of death. The leukopenia and immunosuppression resulting from chemotherapy and the general reduction in host resistance resulting from the terminal stage of disease encourage bacterial infection. *Pseudomonas aeruginosa, Klebsiella,* and *Escherichia coli* are the most common offenders and will usually respond to the appropriate antibiotics. Fungal infections (candidiasis, aspergillosis) are severe and usually involve the gastrointestinal mucosa and respiratory tract. *Candida* organisms may be recovered from the urine, blood, and sputum, but the presence of aspergilli may be more difficult to demonstrate. Cryptococcal infection is frequently associated with both Hodgkin's disease and non-Hodgkin's lymphoma and involves the meninges and lung parenchyma. It must always be ruled out as a source of fever, central nervous system signs, or lung pathology. Viral infections such as herpes zoster and cytomegalic virus disease are also seen in lymphoma patients, and a series of infectious complication may result from the protozoa *pneumocystis carinii.*[38] The presence of these diseases must be suspected in all lymphoma patients who develop diffuse pneumonia after immunosuppressive chemotherapy. Selective bronchial washings or needle aspirate from the lung will help demonstrate the offending organism.

HYPERCALCEMIA

Hypercalcemia secondary to bone involvement by lymphoma is common. The problem has also been seen in the absence of bone involvement or metastasis, thereby suggesting a hormonal effect of the tumor (parathormone-like hormone). Hydration, steroids, mithramycin, and oral phosphates are effective measures for management.

PANCYTOPENIA

Pancytopenia is a common complication in advanced lymphoma (and leukemia) as a result of increased blood cell destruction by the spleen, bone marrow suppression secondary to radiation and/or chemotherapy, or abnormalities in iron metabolism. Regardless of etiology, this complication interferes with the proper clinical management of the disease. The therapeutic dosage of agents must be lower than optimal in order to prevent further hematologic suppression. The spleen seems to play a major role in these hematologic findings,[12] as shown by the laboratory evidence of red cell and platelet destruction, returning to normal after splenectomy. The role of the spleen in the production of these hematologic problems is further substantiated by the increase in the hematologic tolerance to radiotherapy and chemotherapy in lymphoma patients who have had previous splenectomy. These findings have encouraged us to perform splenectomies in a series of patients with advanced lymphomas and myeloproliferative disease if there is laboratory evidence of hypersplenism, with or without splenomegaly.[20,41] This operative procedure is well tolerated and results in mortality of less than 8 percent and morbidity of around 20 percent. Satisfactory hematologic response to splenectomy is seen in 65 percent of the patients so treated (mean duration 24 months). The hematologic response does not correlate well with the presence of spleno-megaly, involvement of the spleen by the primary disease, or the labora-tory evidence of cell destruction in the spleen.

OTHER LYMPHOPROLIFERATIVE NEOPLASMS

Extranodal Lymphomas

Primary involvement of extranodal anatomic areas, in absence of systemic disease, is a well-established clinical feature of lymphomas. This clinical presentation is extremely rare in patients with Hodgkin's dis-ease, and most extranodal involvement is a manifestation of advanced disease. However, non-Hodgkin's lymphomas may present as localized extranodal disease suitable for local treatment with an overall 30-percent probability of permanent disease control. Both histologic types of non-Hodgkin's lymphoma (lymphocytic and histiocytic) occur in equal pro-portions in this localized extranodal form. Because of the high incidence of extranodal involvement of a secondary nature in the course of lym-phoma,[81] each patient with extranodal disease should be subjected to a thorough workup before a lesion is categorized as an extranodal primary.

The most frequent site for extranodal lymphoma is the gastrointes-tinal tract (see Chap. 8). The diagnosis may be suspected or established by endoscopic biopsy preoperatively, but in most circumstances the di-agnosis is an operative finding. Waldeyer's ring is the second most common anatomic site for primary extranodal lymphoma,[6,7,92] but this process has been described in the parotid gland, the maxillary antrum, and the thyroid gland.[19] Primary extranodal lymphoma lesions have also been described in the lung[72] and the breast,[23,53] but these sites are rare. Splenomegaly,[2,23,56] with or without hypersplenism, may be the only find-ing of lymphoma, and the diagnosis of primary splenic lymphoma is made only after splenectomy and careful evaluation. Primary reticulum cell sarcoma occurs in bone,[86,99] and this lesion represents approximately 5 percent of all malignant bone tumors (see Chap. 10); surgical resection is frequently employed as primary therapy for many of these extranodal sites, but postoperative radiation therapy is normally used in these in-stances.

Burkitt's Tumor

Burkitt's tumor is a malignant lymphoma composed of uniformly undifferentiated lymphoblasts with typical histological and cytological features.[9] The significant features of this tumor are (a) its dramatic and frequently durable response to chemotherapy,[13] (b) its tumor-host immunologic relationships in tumor regression, and (c) the evidence of a viral etiology (Ebstein-Barr virus).[14]

Burkitt's tumor has its highest incidence in East Africa, Papua, and New Guinea where it occurs most often in children 2–14 years of age, but it has been described in adults. Although rare in the United States, over 100 well-documented cases have been reported. It usually presents clinically as a rapidly growing tumor that involves the maxillofacial complex (60 percent), and the remainder appear in the intra-abdominal organs or the central nervous system. Involvement of the peripheral lymph nodes is rare, either initially or later in the course of the disease. The differential diagnosis from other lymphoproliferative neoplasms, particularly the histiocytic and poorly differentiated lymphomas or acute lymphoblastic or myeloblastic leukemia, can be difficult.

TREATMENT

The treatment of choice for Burkitt's tumor is chemotherapy, and cyclophosphamide, methotrexate, and arabinosyl cytosine are effective agents. Radiotherapy in a dose range of 3000–4000 rads induces significant regression of local disease, but chemotherapy plays a major role in management because of the systemic nature of the disease. The overall 2-year survival rate for stages I and II (localized to the maxillofacial area) is 90 percent, and the survival figures for stages III and IV are 62 percent and 52 percent at 1 year.[103]

Mycosis Fungoides

Mycosis fungoides is a chronic, fatal disease that originates in the reticuloendothelial system of the skin and eventually may involve both lymph nodes and viscera.[37] The histologic diagnosis is made from a skin biopsy that shows malignant cells in the reticuloendothelial system of the skin. These are usually lymphocytes, plasma cells, and atypical mononuclear cells (mycosis cells), but many are multinucleate. The epidermis is frequently involved with microabscesses. The clinical course of the disease can be divided into five stages. In the first stage, severe and persistent pruritus is the initial and predominant symptom. The skin changes may resemble eczema or psoriasis and the histologic changes in the skin often are not diagnostic. The second stage is characterized by the formation of well-defined, indurated skin plaques that are irregular in shape. The overall condition of the patient remains good in this stage and the disease may remain in this stage for many years without affecting the well-being of the patient. As the disease progresses, the skin lesions may become ulcerated and infected (stage III). With subsequent nodal (stage IV) and visceral involvement (stage V), the disease enters its final stages and is then associated with a short life expectancy.[97]

TREATMENT

Treatment in the initial stages is primarily symptomatic and is directed to the relief of pruritus. Soothing baths, antihistamines, and topical steroid creams are useful for this purpose. As the skin lesions become more advanced, local improvement can be obtained with the use of radiation therapy[33] to multiple areas or the topical use of nitrogen mustard.[40] The systemic use of nitrogen mustard at low and repeated doses produces significant regression (78 percent) in stages III and IV.[96] Other agents or drug combinations are considered rather ineffective in the treatment of this disease. Mycosis fungoides progresses relentlessly through the years with a minimal expectation of "cure."

Plasma Cell Myeloma

Plasma cell myeloma includes a series of diseases known as multiple myeloma, Waldenstrom's macroglobulinemia, and the heavy chain diseases.[26] This neoplasm arises from the malignant transformation of a cell that resembles the plasma cell morphologically and produces an immunoglobulin (M-protein; M for myeloma, malignant, or monoclonal) that appears as a homogenous peak on serum and/or urine electrophoresis. The M-protein is found in the serum and/or urine of 99 percent of patients with plasma cell myeloma and usually precedes the clinical manifestations of the disease.[10b] This M-protein causes formation of erythrocyte rouleaux, induces elevated sedimentation rate, and interferes with platelet function. The platelet count is normal, but there is an abnormal prolonged bleeding time, a positive tourniquet test, defective clot retraction, and defective prothrombin consumption. Abnormalities in factors V and VIII and in the synthesis of fibrin are also seen.

DIAGNOSIS

The finding of M-protein in the serum should lead to thorough search for this plasma cell neoplasm. A patient with this finding should have bone marrow aspiration, urinary protein measurements (grams per 24 hours, heat test for Bence-Jones, and immunoelectrophoresis on the concentrated urine), and a bone survey. The presence of more than 5 percent plasma cells in the differential count of the marrow aspirate in association with lytic bone lesions and M-protein will establish the diagnosis of plasma cell myeloma. The marrow aspirate should be repeated at different sites if the initial aspirate does not reveal plasmacytosis. The excretion of light chains in the urine at a rate of more than 60 mg/24 hours is strongly suggestive of the diagnosis of plasma cell myeloma if the concentration of M-protein in the serum is greater than 2 gm/100 ml. During this investigation, it should be kept in mind that other neoplasms—such as the other lymphomas, leukemia, or carcinoma—can produce an M-protein. Lytic bone lesions are quite frequent with plasma cell tumors producing G, A, D, E, and light-chain M-proteins, but they are less frequent with tumors producing the IgM and heavy-chain diseases.[10b] These bone lesions are diffuse with minimal bone reaction and are associated with osteoporosis. Hypercalcemia, as a result of bone resorption, is associated with hypercalciuria and negative calcium balance and is also characteristic of the disease.

A single lesion in the bone (rib or sternum) or in the nasal or oral cavity, bronchus, or bowel (solitary plasmacytoma) is the initial manifestation in some patients.[101] Most of these patients have serological evidence of plasma cell myeloma sooner or later and should be treated accordingly. Bone marrow involvement by nucleated plasma cells develops in 95 percent of the patients with this neoplasm.

TREATMENT

Chemotherapy[10] with drugs such as melphalan,[5] cyclophosphamide, and chlorambucil has been useful in the management of this neoplasm.[51] The remission rate is 35 percent and the median survival rate is approximately 20 months from the initiation of therapy. Supportive therapy plays a major role in the overall management of these patients. Transfusion, plasmapheresis, analgesics, hydration, and mobilization and control of hypercalcemia and hyperuricemia are the key features of patient management.

CLINICAL COURSE

The patient may be asymptomatic for years, but as plasma cell myeloma progresses, the patient experiences weakness, weight loss, or severe bone pain. Eventually, infection, anemia, and renal failure become the leading clinical problems and the cause of death.

Immunoglobulin levels are below normal, usually in direct proportion to the volume of the plasma cell tumor rather than the level of M-protein in the serum. Proteinuria, mainly of a light-chain type (Bence-Jones), is seen initially in most patients, but later other forms appear. With the progressive rise of serum M-protein, increase in plasma volume leads to a fall in the hemoglobin concentration, pseudo-hyponatremia, and congestive heart failure. Also, the excess of IgM, IgG, and IgA produces protein aggregates that increase the serum viscosity. As a result, the patient may develop a bleeding diathesis, retinopathy, neurological syndromes, vertigo, nystagmus, paresis, coma, and increased vascular resistance.

The infiltration of the bone marrow with plasma cells eventually leads to bone marrow failure (pancytopenia) and its well-known sequelae.

Increased susceptibility to infections as a result of deficiency in immuno-globulins or bone marrow involvement is also a prominent feature of this disease.

Hypercalcemia and negative calcium balance are accentuated when the patient becomes immobilized because of pain, resulting in increased hypercalciuria, dehydration, and renal failure. Other leading causes of fatal renal failure are hyperuricemia, precipitation of Bence-Jones protein in tubules, amyloidosis, and pyelonephritis.

REFERENCES

1. Adler S, Stutzman L, Sokal JE, Mittleman A: Splenectomy for he-matologic depression in lymphocytic lymphoma and leukemia. Cancer 35:521–528, 1975
2. Ahmann DL, Kiely JM, Harrison EG Jr, et al: Malignant lymphoma of the spleen: A review of 49 cases in which the diagnosis was made at splenec-tomy. Cancer 19:461–469, 1966
3. Aisenberg AC: Studies on delayed hypersensitivity in Hodgkin's disease. J Clin Invest 41:1964–70, 1962
4. Aisenberg AC, Goldman JM, Raker JW, Wang CC: Spleen involvement at the onset of Hodgkin's disease. Ann Intern Med 74:544–547, 1971
5. Alexanian R, Bergsagel DE, Migliore PJ, Vaughan WK, Howe CD: Mel-phalan therapy for plasma cell myeloma. Blood 31:1–10, 1968
6. Banfi A, Bonadonna G, Carnevali C, et al: Lymphoreticular sarcomas with primary involvement of Waldeyer's ring: Clinical evaluation of 225 cases. Cancer 26:341–351, 1970
7. Banfi A, Bonadonna G, Ricci SB, et al: Malignant lymphomas of Wal-deyer's ring: Natural history and survival after radiotherapy. Br Med J 3:140–143, 1972
8. Berard CW: Histopathology of lymphoreticular disorders—conditions with malignant proliferative response lymphoma, in Williams WJ (ed): He-matology. New York, McGraw Hill, 1972, pp 901–912
9. Berard CW, O'Conor GT, Thomas LB, et al: Histopathological definition of Burkitt's tumor. Bull WHO 40:601–607, 1969
10a. Bergsagel DE: Plasma cell myeloma: An interpretative review. Cancer 30:1588–1594, 1972
10b. Bergsagel DE: Plasma cell neoplasms, in Holland JF and Frei E (eds): Cancer Medicine. Philadelphia, Lea & Febiger, 1973
11. Bonadonna G, Zucali R, Monafardini S, DeLena M, Uslenghi C: Combi-nation chemotherapy of Hodgkin's disease with adriamycin, bleomycin, vinblastine, and imidazole carboxamide versus MOPP. Cancer 36:252–259, 1975
12. Bowdler AJ, Prankerd TAJ: Splenic mechanisms in the pathogenesis of anemia. Postgrad Med J 41:748–752, 1965

13. Burchenal JH: Geographic chemotherapy—Burkitt's tumor as a stalking horse for leukemia. Cancer Res 26:2393–2405, 1966

14. Burkitt DP: Etiology of Burkitt's lymphoma: An alternative hypothesis to a vectoree virus. J Natl Cancer Inst 42:19–28, 1969

15. Butler JJ: Non-neoplastic lesions of lymph nodes of man to be differentiated from lymphomas. Natl Cancer Inst Monog 32:233–249, 1968

16. Carbone PP, Kaplan HS, Musshoff K, Smithers DW, Tubiana M: Report of the Committee of Hodgkin's Disease Staging Classification. Cancer Res 31:1860–1861, 1971

17. Carter SK, Livingston RB: Single-agent therapy for Hodgkin's disease. Arch Intern Med 131:377–387, 1973

18. Casazza AR, Duvall CP, Carbone PP: Summary of infectious complications occurring in patients with Hodgkin's disease. Cancer Res 26:1290–1296, 1966

19. Catlin D: Surgery for head and neck lymphomas. Surgery 60:1160–1166, 1966

20. Clendenning WE, Brecher G, Van Scott EJ: Mycosis fungoides. Arch Dermatol 89:785–792, 1964

21. Cooper IA, Ironside PN, Madigan JP, Morris PJ, Ewing MR: The role of splenectomy in the management of advanced Hodgkin's disease. Cancer 34:408–417, 1974

22. Cyr DP, Geokas MC, Worsley GH: Mycosis fungoides. Arch Dermatol 94:558–573, 1966

23. Das Gupta T, Coombes B, Brasfield RD: Primary malignant neoplasms of the spleen. Surg Gynecol Obstet 120:947–960, 1965

24. DeCosse JJ, Berg JW, Fracchia AA, Farrow JH: Primary lymphosarcoma of the breast. A review of 14 cases. Cancer 15:1264–1268, 1962

25. Desser RK, Moran EM, Ultmann JE: Staging of Hodgkin's disease and lymphoma. Med Clin North Am 57:479–498, 1973

26. Desser RK, Ultmann JE: Risk of severe infection in patients with Hodgkin's disease or lymphoma after diagnostic laparotomy and splenectomy. Ann Intern Med 77:143–145, 1972

27. Deutsch HF, Fudenberg HH: Immunoglobulin structure and function. Adv Intern Med 15:377–396, 1969

28. DeVita VT: Hodgkin's disease. Lancet 2:46–47, 1971

29. DeVita VT Jr, Canellos GP, Moxley JH III: A decade of combination chemotherapy of advanced Hodgkin's disease. Cancer 30:1495–1504, 1972

30. Edwards CL, Hayes RL: Tumor scanning with 67 Ga citrate. J Nucl Med 10:103–105, 1969

31. Eisner E, Ley AB, Mayer K: Coombs-positive hemolytic anemia in Hodgkin's disease. Ann Intern Med 66:258–273, 1967

32. Ferguson DJ, Allen LW, Griem ML, et al: Surgical experience with staging laparotomy in 125 patients with lymphoma. Arch Intern Med 131:356–361, 1973

33. Fratkin MJ, Hirsch JI, Sharpe AR Jr: Ga 67 staging of Hodgkin's disease. Va Med Mon 103:257–267, 1976

34. Fromer JL, Johnston DO, Salzman FA, Trump JG, Wright KA: Manage-

ment of lymphoma cutis with low megavolt electron beam therapy: Nine year followup in 200 cases. South Med J 54:769–776, 1961

35. Fuks Z, Kaplan HS: Recurrence rates following radiation therapy of nodular and diffuse malignant lymphomas. Radiology 108:675–684, 1973

36. Gall EA, Rappaport H: Seminar on diseases of lymph nodes and spleen, in McDonald Jr (ed): Proceedings of 23rd Seminar of the American Society of Clinical Pathology. 1958, pp 1–107

37. Gamble JF, Fuller LM, Ibrahim E, et al: Combined chemotherapy and radiotherapy management of stage 3 Hodgkin's disease. Arch Intern Med 131:435–438, 1973

38. Goodell B, Jacobs JB, Powell RD, DeVita VT: Pneumocystis carinii: The spectrum of diffuse interstitial pneumonia in patients with neoplastic disease. Ann Intern Med 72:337–340, 1970

39. Hanks GE, Terry LN Jr, Bryan JA, Newsome JF: Contribution of diagnostic laparotomy to staging non-Hodgkin's lymphoma. Cancer 29:41–43, 1972

40. Haynes HA, Van Scott EJ: Therapy of mycosis fungoides. Prog Dermatol 3:1, 1968

41. Hyatt DF, Skarin AT, Moloney WC, Wilson RE: Splenectomy for lymphosarcoma. Surg Gynecol Obstet 131:928–932, 1970

42. Jackson H Jr, Parker F Jr: Hodgkin's Disease and Allied Disorders. New York, Oxford University Press, 1947, p 177

43. Johnson RE: Is staging laparotomy routinely indicated in Hodgkin's disease? Ann Intern Med 74:459–462, 1971

44. Johnson RE, Glover MK, Marshall SK: Results of radiation therapy and implications for the clinical staging of Hodgkin's disease. Cancer Res 31:1834–1837, 1971

45. Johnston G, Benua RS, Teates CD, Edwards CL, Kniseley RM: 67-Ga citrate imaging in untreated Hodgkin's disease: Preliminary report of cooperative group. J Nucl Med 15:399–403, 1974

46. Kadin ME, Glatstein E, Dorfman RF: Clinicopathologic studies of 117 untreated patients subjected to laparotomy for the staging of Hodgkin's disease. Cancer 27:1277–1294, 1971

47. Kaplan HS: Radiotherapy of advanced Hodgkin's disease with curative intent. JAMA 223:50–53, 1973

48. Kaplan HS: The radical radiotherapy of regionally localized Hodgkin's disease. Radiology 78:553–561, 1962

49. Kaplan HS, Rosenberg SA: Hodgkin's disease: Current recommendations for management. CA 25:306–319, 1975

50. Kim H, Dorfman RF: Morphological studies of 84 untreated patients subjected to laparotomy for the staging of non-Hodgkin's lymphomas. Cancer 35:657–674, 1974

51. Korst DR, Clifford GO, Fowler WM, Louis J, Will J, Wilson HE: Multiple myeloma. II. Analysis of cyclophosphamide therapy in 165 patients. JAMA 189:758–762, 1964

52. Kurnick JE, Robinson WA: Combination chemotherapy of advanced lymphomas. Arch Intern Med 129:908–913, 1972

53. Lawler MR Jr, Richie RE: Reticulum cell sarcoma of the breast. Cancer 20:1438–1446, 1967

54. Lee BJ, Nelson JH, Schwarz G: Evaluation of lymphangiography, Inferior venacavography, and intravenous pyelography in the clinical staging and management of Hodgkin's disease and lymphosarcoma. N Engl J Med 271:327–337, 1964

55. Levi JA, O'Connell MJ, Murphy WL, Sutherland JC, Wiernik PH: Role of 67 gallium citrate scanning in the management of non-Hodgkin's lymphoma. Cancer 36:1690–1701, 1975

56. Long JC, Aisenberg AC: Malignant lymphoma diagnosed at splenectomy and idiopathic splenomegaly. Cancer 33:1054–1061, 1974

57. Lowe DK, Fletcher WS, Horowitz IJ, Hyman MD: Management of chylothorax secondary to lymphoma. Surg Gynecol Obstet 135:35–38, 1972

58. Lowenbraun S, DeVita VT, Serpick AA: Combination chemotherapy with nitrogen mustard, vincristine, procarbazine, and prednisone in lymphosarcoma and reticulum cell sarcoma. Cancer 25:1018–1025, 1970

59. Lowenbraun S, Ramsey HE, Serpick AA: Splenectomy in Hodgkin's disease for splenomegaly, cytopenias and intolerance to myelosuppressive chemotherapy. Am J Med 50:49–55, 1971

60. Lukes RJ: Updated Hodgkin's disease: Prognosis and relationship of histologic features to clinical stage. JAMA 222:1294–1296, 1972

61. Lukes RJ, Butler JJ: The pathology and nomenclature of Hodgkin's disease. Cancer Res 26:1063–1083, 1966

62. Lukes RJ, Craver LF, Hall TC, et al: Report of Nomenclature Committee. Cancer Res 26:1311, 1966

63. Lukes RJ, Tindle BH, Parker JW: Reed–Sternberg-like cells in infectious mononucleosus. Lancet 2:1003–1004, 1969

64. MacMahon B: Epidemiology of Hodgkin's disease. Cancer Res 26:1189–1201, 1966

65. Miller DG: Patterns of immunological deficiency in lymphomas and leukemias. Ann Intern Med 57:703–716, 1962

66. Miller SP, Shanbrom E: Infectious syndromes of leukemias and lymphomas. Am J Med Sci 246:420–428, 1963

67. Moore DF, Migliore PJ, Shullenberger CC, Alexanian R: Monoclonal macroglobulinemia in malignant lymphoma. Ann Intern Med 72:43–47, 1970

68. Moore MR, Bull JM, Jones SE, et al: Sequential radiotherapy and chemotherapy in the treatment of Hodgkin's disease. Ann Intern Med 77:1–9, 1972

69. Muggia FM, Ultmann JE: Exploratory laparotomy in reticulum cell sarcoma. Cancer 30:454–458, 1972

70. Newall J, Freidman M: Reticulum cell sarcoma. Part III: Prognosis. Radiology 97:99–102, 1970

71. O'Connell MJ, Wiernik PK, Brace KC, Byhardt RW, Greene WH: A combined modality approach to the treatment of Hodgkin's disease. Cancer 35:1055–1065, 1975

72. Papaioannou AN, Watson WL: Primary lymphoma of the lung: An

appraisal of its natural history and a comparison with other localized lymphomas. J Thorac Cardiovasc Surg 49:373–387, 1965

73. Peters MV: A study of survivals in Hodgkin's disease treated radiologically. Am J Roentgenol 63:299–311, 1950

74. Peters MV, Middlemiss KC: A study of Hodgkin's disease treated by irradiation. Am J Roentgenol 79:114–121, 1958

75. Prosnitz LR, Fischer JJ, Vera R, et al: Hodgkin's disease treated with radiation therapy: Follow-up data and the value of laparotomy. Am J Roentgenol Radium Ther Nucl Med 114:583–590, 1972

76. Rappaport H, Berard CW, Butler JJ, Dorfman RF, Lukes RJ, Thomas LB: Report of the Committee on Histopathological Criteria Contributing to Staging of Hodgkin's Disease. Cancer Res 31:1864–1865, 1971

77. Ray GR, Trueblood HW, Enright LP, Kaplan HS, Nelsen TS: Oophoropexy: A means of preserving ovarian function following pelvic megavoltage radiotherapy for Hodgkin's disease. Radiology 96:175–180, 1970

78. Roberts WC, Glancy DL, DeVita VT: Heart in malignant lymphoma (Hodgkin's disease, lymphosarcoma, reticulum cell sarcoma, and mycosis fungoides). Am J Cardiol 22:85–107, 1968

79. Rosenberg SA: Hodgkin's disease of the bone marrow. Cancer Res 31:1733–1736, 1971

80. Rosenberg SA, Boiron M, DeVita VT Jr, Johnson RE, Lee BJ, et al: Report of the Committee on Hodgkin's Disease Staging Procedures. Cancer Res 31:1862–1863, 1971

81. Rosenberg SA, Diamond HD, Jaslowitz B, Craver LF: Lymphosarcoma: A review of 1269 cases. Medicine 40:31–84, 1961

82. Rosenberg SA, Moore MR, Bull JM, et al: Combination chemotherapy and radiotherapy for Hodgkin's disease. Cancer 30:1505–1510, 1972

83. Salzman JR, Kaplan HS: Effect of prior splenectomy on hematologic tolerance during total lymphoid radiotherapy of patients with Hodgkin's disease. Cancer 27:471–478, 1971

84. Schein PS, Chabner BA, Canellos GP, Young RC, DeVita VT Jr: Non-Hodgkin's lymphoma: Patterns of relapse from complete remission after combination chemotherapy. Cancer 35:354–357, 1975

85. Schier WW, Roth A, Ostroff G, Schrift MH: Hodgkin's disease and immunity. Am J Med 20:94–99, 1956

86. Shoji H, Miller TR: Primary reticulum cell sarcoma of bone: Significance of clinical features upon the prognosis. Cancer 28:1234–1244, 1971

87. Sokal JE, Firat D: Varicella-zoster infection in Hodgkin's disease. Am J Med 39:452–463, 1965

88. Stewart JR, Fajardo LF: Dose response in human and experimental radiation-induced heart disease: Application of the nominal standard dose concept. Radiology 99:403–408, 1971

89. Strum SB, Park JK, Rappaport H: Observation of cells resembling Sternberg–Reed cells in conditions other than Hodgkin's disease. Cancer 26:176–190, 1970

90. Strum SB, Rappaport H: The persistence of Hodgkin's disease in long-term survivors. Am J Med 51:222–240, 1971

91. Takahashi M, Abrams HL: The accuracy of lymphangiographic diagnosis in malignant lymphoma. Radiology 89:448–460, 1967

92. Terz JJ, Farr HW: Primary lymphosarcoma of the tonsil. Surgery 65:772–776, 1969

93. Trueblood HW, Enright LP, Ray GR, Kaplan HS, et al: Preservation of ovarian function in pelvic radiation for Hodgkin's disease. Arch Surg 100:236–237, 1970

94. Ultmann JE, Moran EM: Clinical course and complications in Hodgkin's disease. Arch Intern Med 131:311–353, 1973

95. Ultmann JE, Stein RS: Non-Hodgkin's lymphoma: An approach to staging and therapy. CA 25:320–333, 1975

96. Van Scott EJ, Grekin DA, Kalmanson JD, Vonderheid EC, Barry WE: Frequent low doses of intravenous mechlorethamine for late-stage mycosis fungoides lymphoma. Cancer 36:1489–1618, 1975

97. Variakojis D, Rosas-Uribe A, Rappaport H: Mycosis fungoides: Pathologic findings in staging laparotomies. Cancer 33:1589–1600, 1974

98. Viamonte M Jr: Current status of lymphography. Cancer Res 31:1731–1732, 1971

99. Wang CC: Treatment of primary reticulum cell sarcoma of bone by irradiation. N Engl J Med 278:1331–1332, 1968

100. Williams HM, Diamond HD, Cravier LF, Parsons H: Neurological Complications of Lymphomas and Leukemias. Springfield, Ill., Charles C Thomas, 1959, pp 1–134

101. Wing EJ, Perchick J, Hubbard J: Solitary obstructing plasmacytoma of the colon. JAMA 233:1298–1299, 1975

102. Young RC, Corder MP, Berard CW, DeVita VT: Immune alterations in Hodgkin's disease. Arch Intern Med 131:446–454, 1973

103. Zigler JL: Burkitt's tumor, in Holland JF, Fried E (eds): Cancer Medicine. Philadelphia, Lea & Febiger, 1973

10

Management of Skin Cancer, Melanomas, and Sarcomas

SKIN CANCER

The skin is the most common site for cancer in our population, the detection and diagnosis of skin cancer are relatively easy, and the treatment of most skin cancers requires only simple outpatient procedures. Our focus will be on exceptions to these statements since most skin cancers will not qualify as "management problems."

The most frequent cancers of the skin in our population are basal cell cancer, squamous cell cancer, and malignant melanoma. Accurate statistics of the true incidence for basal cell and squamous cell lesions are not available since these lesions are characteristically not recorded in our tumor registry statistics and many are treated and then ignored as relatively inconsequential problems. However, the overwhelming proportion of these lesions are basal cell cancers; squamous cancers are next in incidence but are much less frequent than basal cell cancers, and malignant malanomas are relatively rare. Because of major differences in presentation, clinical behavior, and management, malignant melanoma will be considered separately from the more common forms of skin cancer.

Various forms of radiation, particularly the ultraviolet rays of the sun, play a major etiologic role in the development of basal and squamous cancers, and this is supported, to some degree, by the frequency of location of these lesions on surfaces exposed to sunlight and the incidence of these cancers in relation to geographic differences in this exposure. The preponderance of basal and squamous cell cancers in the radiation port of patients receiving radiation therapy is also well established—a hazard that has virtually eliminated the use of this treatment method for benign conditions. The relationship between skin cancer and the ingestion of or exposure to various chemical compounds, particularly arsenic and petroleum products, is also well known. All of these etiologic factors can be effectively controlled with a reasonable hope for reduction in the incidence of skin cancer, but genetic factors that play a role in the predisposition to skin cancer are certainly beyond our control.

Diagnosis

The clinical diagnosis of individual skin lesions is based on the gross pathology of the lesion, with the histology usually playing a later role in the treatment choice. Basal cell cancers are most often either "nodular" or "superficial" in gross presentation. The nodular lesions are moderately firm and elevated with an umbilicated, usually ulcerated, center and a characteristically waxy or pearly border. The superficial lesions have more of a plaque configuration, usually with a crusted erythematous center, and they are often multiple. There are also less-common variations such as the pigmented basal, the cystic variety, or the very subtle barely elevated morphea type.[72] Squamous cell carcinoma usually appears as a scaly ulcerated lesion, a well-defined ulcer, a nodular mass, or a large fungating mass, but most are small lesions and they may be difficult for the physician to differentiate from basal cell cancer. The anatomical location of the lesion is also a useful lead since basal cell cancers are commonly on the nose, eyelids, cheeks, and occasionally on the trunk. Cutaneous squamous lesions are more frequent on the face also, but are less restricted in location than basal cell cancers. They occur frequently on the hands as well as at other sites where basal cell cancer is rarely seen.

During clinical examination the skilled dermatologist observes subtle changes in skin lesions and usually can predict the histology with a great degree of accuracy. However, all physicians must be able to select those skin lesions that are of enough concern to warrant biopsy. The precise classification as basal or squamous cell cancer is certainly not essential before biopsy because that will determine the subsequent management.

Biopsy is effectively accomplished with a small punch biopsy instrument or excision of a small wedge of the lesion if it is large, but total excision is the most practical approach to most small lesions. A small margin of normal skin is advisable with excisional biopsy since this completes the therapy for basal cell cancer in most instances. If a biopsy does demonstrate squamous carcinoma, a chest x-ray is indicated, particularly with large lesions.   It is also important to perform a careful clinical assessment of the regional lymph nodes.[61]   Basal cell cancer, on the other hand, virtually never metastasizes to lymph nodes or distant sites.

Treatment

BASAL CELL CANCERS

The treatment choice depends on the size and extent of the lesion. For small basal cell cancers the alternatives are electrodesiccation with curettage, simple surgical excision with closure, or radiation therapy, and all three are acceptable, efficient methods.   Topical chemotherapy with 5-fluorouracil (or immunotherapy) is favored by some, but this approach is probably more applicable to extensive actinic keratoses or specific diffuse problems (such as xeroderma pigmentosa) and is not recommended for the treatment of solitary skin cancers.   For larger lesions Moh's[83] chemosurgical technique has been recommended as it is effective and produces less sacrifice of normal tissue than surgical excision owing to the stepwise destruction of the neoplasm with careful histologic control. This approach requires prolonged therapy with multiple and extensive pathologic reviews of the treated tissue.   For this reason, chemosurgery has not been widely accepted. Radiation therapy or surgical excision of larger lesions is a more practical approach.

When surgical excision is employed for larger basal cell cancers, skin graft coverage is usually preferred to skin flap rotation after surgical excision since any subsequent recurrence will be less hidden and more amenable to subsequent treatment if a graft is used.   However, specific locations may require local skin flap rotation for optimal results.   It is necessary to obtain a tumor-free margin when surgery is employed for extensive basal cell cancers as demonstrated by the occasional patient with a massive recurrent cancer of the face.   This rare problem is a result of both patient neglect and inadequate initial treatment of a lesion with unusual growth potential.   Fortunately, this type of problem can be prevented and is now rarely seen.

SQUAMOUS CARCINOMAS

Squamous carcinomas are often treated in a fashion similar to the treatment of basal cell cancers.   This histologic diagnosis, however, makes surgical excision or radiation therapy preferable to electrodesiccation and curettage in our view.   When surgical excision is employed, the margin of normal tissue around the lesion should be more generous than that considered acceptable for basal cell cancer because of the possibility of local lymphatic spread, but the frequency of lymph node involvement is too low to warrant elective lymph node dissection.[61] The regional lymph nodes should be evaluated clinically, both initially and on follow-up examination, as regional lymph node dissection is occasionally required.

Specific Management Problems[21]

BOWEN'S DISEASE

Bowen's disease is a superficial intraepidermal carcinoma usually found on the trunk. Characteristically, this lesion undergoes lateral spread within the cutis. There appears to be some association between Bowen's disease and visceral cancers, which suggests a possible carcinogen responsible for both. This process tends to be radioresistant, and limited local surgical resection of the process is considered the treatment of choice.

RADIATION-INDUCED SKIN CANCER

When basal or squamous cancer develops in a field of prior radiation therapy, it is usually associated with other skin changes in the port that are both precancerous and cosmetically disturbing. In many of these patients it is advisable to remove the entire area of skin involved and replace it with a healthy skin flap if these changes are extensive. Fortunately, these problems are less frequent now than they once were owing to the use of higher energy radiation therapy for the treatment of cancer and because x-ray is no longer used for the treatment of benign skin problems.

MARJOLIN'S ULCER

The development of a squamous carcinoma in a chronic ulcer from an incompletely healed full-thickness burn is now a rarity because of the more aggressive approach initially employed for this type of wound. These cancers become particularly virulent in terms of both local and distant spread if the initial treatment of this burn scar cancer is unsuccessful. One gains the impression that the cancer has been released from the confinement of the adjacent scar by incomplete excision and is more capable of growth and spread in the adjacent normal tissues. For this reason, it is important to employ wide surgical resection as the initial treatment, thereby producing a major wound defect. Imaginative reconstruction methods for achieving wound closure are required and must be individualized on the basis of the anatomic location of the problem. In our experience, long-term success after resection is limited despite the frequent statement that these are "low grade cancers." A similar form of cancer occasionally occurs in long-standing chronically draining sinus tracts of osteomyelitis[101] or other chronic infections, and the prognosis of this problem is also poor. Amputation or appropriate aggressive surgical resection is indicated when these lesions are encountered. Prevention of this entire group of cancers is undoubtedly the most successful approach to management.

RARE CANCERS OF THE SKIN ADNEXA

Sweat gland carcinoma is a rare cancer that may metastasize to regional lymph nodes or distant sites. Although it may originate from any site on the skin, it is most commonly seen in the axilla or the anogenital region. Sebaceous gland cancer and carcinomatous degeneration of a sebaceous cyst are also rare clinical problems, and most of these lesions occur on the scalp. All of these rare forms of cancer of the skin adnexa are best treated by surgical excision using the principles described earlier for squamous carcinoma.

XERODERMA PIGMENTOSA

Xeroderma pigmentosa is a rare inherited condition with a high incidence of premalignant keratoses, basal and squamous skin cancers. These lesions on the exposed skin are apparently owing to a genetic biochemical defect in the skin's DNA repair mechanisms that normally respond to heal ultraviolet damage. The lesions that do develop are so extensive that multiple excisions become impractical and total replacement of the affected skin is impossible. A useful approach that has been described is topical treatment with chemotherapeutic agents (5-fluorouracil) or topical immunotherapy.

MULTIPLE BASAL CELL NEVI SYNDROME

This rare syndrome includes multiple nevoid basal cell carcinomas usually appearing in childhood around puberty in both exposed and unexposed cutaneous areas. They are numerous and are flesh colored to brownish nodules, predominately on the face and trunk. This syndrome, which also includes skeletal anomalies, jaw cysts, CNS abnormalities, and a hyporesponsiveness to parathormone, is inherited as an autosomal dominant trait.

MALIGNANT MELANOMA

Malignant melanoma of the skin is a much more concerning skin cancer than the others discussed, despite its relative rarity (1–2 percent of all human cancers), since the frequency of treatment failure and death from melanoma is in the range expected for some visceral cancers. There is even an exaggerated pessimism among many physicians regarding the prognosis of this cancer, probably because the clinical presentation of extensive and visible metastases in a youthful patient is so striking. It is probably fair to say, however, that we accomplish more with surgical therapy for malignant melanoma than we do with some of the more common malignant neoplasms affecting man.

Although malignant melanomas may arise from a number of unusual and unexpected sites, the majority originate in the skin and more than half arise from preexisting benign nevi. Trauma to nevi has often been considered a possible cause of melanoma, but there is no real evidence to support this. Sunlight is also suspected as an etiologic agent.[67] Approximately 70–80 percent of malignant melanomas of the skin occur in light-complexioned, sandy-haired, freckled individuals. This complexion, therefore, might selectively increase our clinical suspicion of melanoma in such patients, but this particular diagnostic factor is far from absolute as shown by the less frequent but definite occurrence of melanoma in blacks. When melanoma does occur in blacks, however, it tends to affect less-pigmented sites such as the palms, soles, subungual areas, or mucous membranes.

All of the skin is vulnerable to the development of malignant melanoma and this lesion shows no strong predilection for specific sites. It is of interest that the distribution of melanoma generally parallels that of nevi.[91] In addition to melanomas in subungual locations (3 percent), where nevi are quite rare, and the genitalia (3 percent), a few malignant melanomas also arise from mucous membranes of the respiratory and gastrointestinal tracts. Although it is sometimes difficult to prove that melanoma is primary in one of these sites, there is little question regarding the validity of many reports of malignant melanoma in the nasal cavity, oral cavity, pharynx, larynx, esophagus, and tracheobronchial tree.[33] Other areas of the gastrointestinal tract (namely, the anorectal canal, rectum, and gallbladder) have also been primary sites for melanoma. Ovaries, cervix, vagina, genitourinary tract, and the leptomeninges have all demonstrated melanomatous lesions thought to be primary in these sites, but it is difficult to obtain proof that many of these lesions are not metastatic. However, the presence of melanocytes in most of these normal tissues establishes the basis for these anatomic areas as possible sites of origin.

Diagnosis

The key word in terms of diagnosis of melanoma of the skin is "change," and any pigmented lesion thought to enlarge, alter in pigmentation, or develop any other subjective or visible change should be evaluated by biopsy and histologic examination. Since the average white adult has 15 benign pigmented nevi, there is a large pool of precursor lesions.[91] Some melanomas present as ulcerating skin lesions, lesions without pigmentation, or lesions with pyogenic features, so the index of suspicion must remain high (Fig. 10-1). The variations in clinical presentation are well illustrated by Mihm et al.[82] Other skin lesions often confused with malignant melanoma include pigmented basal cell cancer, hemangioma, sclerosing angioma, pigmented keratosis, Kaposi's disease, pyogenic granuloma, juvenile melanoma, and blue nevus (Jadassohn), in addition to the more common freckles and benign pigmented nevi. Thus, biopsy is essential for the lesion clinically thought to be a melanoma, as well as for the benign-appearing lesion with subtle clues of potential malignant change. For example, the appropriate therapy for the two lesions shown in Figure 10-2 is markedly different, despite their superficial similarity. Biopsy of the lesion in Figure 10-2A prevented overtreatment of a lesion that proved to be a pigmented basal cell carcinoma, whereas the lesion in Figure 10-2B was a malignant melanoma. Another benign lesion producing great concern on occasion is juvenile melanoma, a spindle cell variant of compound nevus. The usual age group (prepubertal) is a clue, but one must realize that true melanoma can also occur at this age.[70]

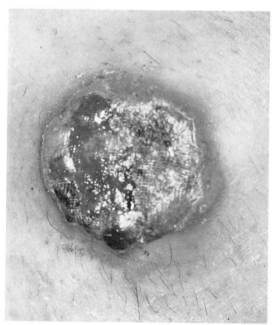

Fig. 10-1.   Ulcerated nonpigmented malignant melanoma.

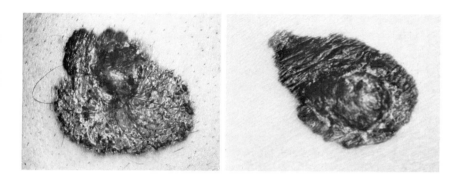

Fig. 10-2. Diagnostic difficulty on clinical examination of pigmented skin lesions. **A:** Pigmented basal cell carcinoma. **B:** Malignant melanoma.

Another special diagnostic problem is that of the patient who has metastatic melanoma in regional nodes without an identifiable skin lesion.[30,106] Spontaneous regression of the primary skin lesion is sometimes difficult to document, but 3–7 percent of patients in most large series present with these findings. In a few patients a tiny, insignificant skin lesion proves to be the primary lesion, but in a number of patients the primary lesion must regress (or disappear) without local therapy.

It is generally considered wise to excise completely a "suspicious" skin lesion for biopsy if the possibility of melanoma exists. However, the actual size of the lesion in a few patients might make this neither feasible nor practical, and despite frequently expressed opinions to the contrary, there is no strong evidence that a preliminary partial biopsy is prejudicial to the patient's prognosis.[42] The major problem with limited biopsy is the distinct possibility that the judgment regarding the depth of the melanoma will be uncertain. This is very concerning since depth of invasion is a major factor in prognosis.[10,16,17,76,81] Biopsy of a portion of pigmented lesion may fail to reveal the area of malignant change that is present, but appropriate and careful selection of the biopsy site will usually avoid this error. If the diagnosis of melanoma is established, appropriate definitive treatment can then be planned if the depth of invasion is more than "superficial" by one of various classifications. However, a melanoma involving only the papillary dermis on partial biopsy may require additional histologic sections after adequte excision of the entire primary lesion before making all of the necessary therapeutic decisions. A wide excision of a "suspicious" lesion for biopsy diagnosis should definitely be avoided. The gross margin obtained is usually less than desired if the lesion is a malignant melanoma and it is unnecessarily radical if the lesion is something else. As with most cancers, the appropriate treatment is best administered after a precise diagnosis is established.

Staging

The choice of treatment approach depends on both the depth of skin invasion on histologic evaluation and the clinical and laboratory evaluation of the possibility of metastatic disease. The most definitive aspect of staging is the histologic assessment of the biopsy material as the depth of invasion is clearly related to both the likelihood of lymphatic metastasis and the prognosis.[10,16,17,81] For years, there were no uniform histologic criteria for this evaluation, and we were limited to the terms "superficial" and "invasive." In recent years, there has been relatively general acceptance of Clark's classification (Fig. 10-3)[16] as it has proven to be useful for communication between pathologists and surgeons, for planning treatment, and for estimating prognosis (Table 10-2). Data reported by Breslow[10] using an optical micrometer for measuring depth of invasion are of similar value in assessing prognosis.

Regional lymph node metastases eventually occur in approximately half of the patients with melanoma of the skin,[78] and clinical evidence of this involvement and evidence of distant metastasis are the bases for the

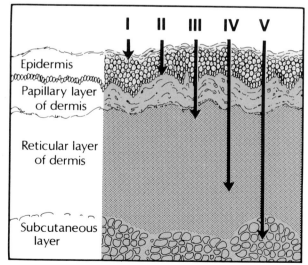

Fig. 10-3.   Diagram of histologic staging (Clark) of malignant melanoma.

Table 10-1
Clinical Stages of Malignant Melanoma

Stage	Description
I	Localized without regional lymph node or distant metastasis (primary untreated or recurrent)
II	Metastasis confined to regional lymph nodes (primary untreated, controlled, locally recurrent or "unknown")
III	Disseminated melanoma (multiple lymphatic sites, multiple cutaneous and/or subcutaneous sites, or organs)

clinical staging categories shown in Table 10-1. Distant metastases may occur to almost any organ, as shown by the following list of sites frequently involved (in decreasing order of frequency): skin, lungs, liver, bone, gastrointestinal tract, brain, kidney, heart, adrenal, and spleen. Careful physical examination, chest radiographs, liver function tests, and other standard examinations are indicated to assist in this staging process. Lymphangiography has not been useful for this purpose in our experience as the radiologic findings are frequently misleading.

Choice of Treatment

Surgery is generally considered optimal treatment for malignant melanoma of the skin, and radiation therapy has often been considered ineffective. Radiation does affect melanoma, however, as shown by the results of Hillriegel.[54] His report of a series of primary melanomas treated by radiation has some defects, particularly the lack of histologic confirmation in some patients; but he clearly demonstrates the ability of radiation therapy to control this disease in a large number of patients. Although there is general consensus that surgical resection has an advantage over radiation for malignant melanoma, the radiation responsiveness that has

Table 10-2
Melanoma: End Results Based
on Depth of Invasion

Level of Invasion (Clark)	5-Yr Survival (%)
I	100
II	72
III	46
IV	31
V	12

been demonstrated suggests that this therapeutic tool may have a significant role in the management of patients unsuitable for operation. There is no evidence that other means of aggressive local ablation (laser, cryosurgery, or electrocoagulation) have beneficial systemic effects, immunologic or otherwise, so "adequte" surgical excision is clearly the treatment of choice.

Surgical Guidelines

THE PRIMARY LESION

For a specific lesion proven to be malignant melanoma, a minimal gross margin might conceivably be "adequate," whereas a much wider and deeper excision would be required for another (apparently similar) lesion in order to avoid local treatment failure. The disability and the cosmetic defect owing to the scar of wide excision with split-thickness graft are limited "costs" for the patient to pay to ensure adequate treatment in comparison to the gravity of the late recurrence obtained in some patients treated by a more limited margin (Fig. 10-4). We believe the limited effectiveness of secondary attempts to control recurrent disease justifies the possibility of "overtreatment" of some local lesions.

Another argument for a wider margin of excision for malignant melanoma than we find acceptable for other malignant skin neoplasms stems from the findings of Wong.[118] His microscopic study of the clinically unaffected epidermal surface surrounding some malignant melanomas demonstrated, using the dopa reaction, an increase in melanocytes, some quite bizarre in both shape and size. These observations may well represent premalignant manifestations of melanoma. Local lymphatic extension of the primary lesion into the immediately surrounding tissue is also a factor encouraging a "wide" margin since this mode of spread is usually not clinically detectable and may not be apparent on histologic study of the biopsy specimen.

If one accepts wide excision as a reasonable concept for the local therapy for malignant melanoma, how wide is actually wide enough? This is an arbitrary decision that cannot be made on histologic grounds before excision for practical reasons, but a 4–5-cm margin in all lateral directions from the periphery of the lesion is generally accepted as a good "rule of thumb" for malignant melanoma in most anatomic locations. Compromise regarding this arbitrary margin is both reasonable and necessary in some anatomic locations (such as a lesion on the digit or on the face), but the margin recommended is an appropriate strategy for most primary melanomas since the size of the skin graft is of minimal practical importance.

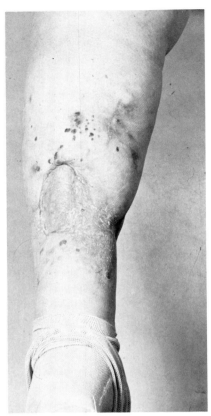

Fig. 10-4.   Recurrent nodules of malignant melanoma after
inadequate primary resection despite use of skin graft.

How deep should the excision be to be considered adequate? This
question is of particular relevance to melanomas extending to Clark's
levels IV and V (Fig. 10-3). It has been noted frequently that the spread
of malignant melanoma is usually limited to the integument and subcutaneous tissue and invades the underlying fascia only in rare instances.
Removing the fascial layer underlying the lesion itself may assist in containing the depth of invasion, particularly with large, deeply ulcerating
melanomas; but excision of the underlying fascia can hardly be considered necessary. The report by Olsen[89] actually appeared to demonstrate
more difficulty with subsequent lymphatic spread when the deep fascia
underlying the lesion was excised. Although Olsen's interpretation of the
data might be open to question, these data do demonstrate that the underlying fascia can be safely preserved in many instances unless the melanoma infiltrates very deeply.

The relationship of the precise histologic classification of depth of invasion to the extent of the local excision required is difficult to establish at this time. It is conceivable that a limited width of excision might be justifiable for superficial level I or II lesions on the basis of a low likelihood of lymphatic extension. On the trunk and extremities the arbitrary skin margin described for more invasive lesions seems indicated for these superficial lesions for both the theoretical and practical reasons outlined previously. However, in a few locations, particularly the digits, underlying soft tissue or bone is so close to the melanoma that amputation is the appropriate excisional procedure.

REGIONAL LYMPH NODES

Malignant melanoma has demonstrated distal spread by both hematogenous and lymphatic routes. Although this is well recognized, most questions regarding surgical management of melanoma center around the regional lymphatics since control of hematogenous spread is currently beyond our therapeutic ability.

Clinically involved nodes. If clinically involved nodes are present in the lymph node basin draining the primary site of the melanoma at the time of initial diagnosis, most surgeons favor a surgical approach to these lymph nodes. It is noteworthy, however, that long-term survival after regional lymph node dissection in this clinical setting is extremely low (approximately 10 percent) if the clinical diagnosis is histologically confirmed (Table 10-3).[78] This could be interpreted as an indication that the synchronous finding of regional lymph node involvement is a clue that distant metastatic disease is present, that local lymph node dissection is inadequate when lymphatic involvement is so grossly apparent, or both. At any rate, clinically apparent regional lymph node involvement at the time of diagnosis of melanoma is surely an indication for careful "staging" procedures designed to detect distant spread of melanoma. A meticulous search for distant disease, possibly including bone marrow

Table 10-3
Prognosis of Cutaneous Malignant Melanoma
in Terms of Regional Lymph Node Status

Clinical Examination	Microscopic Examination	5-Yr Survival (%)
Not palpable	No metastasis	71
Not palpable	Metastasis	53 ⎫ 19
Clinically "positive"	Metastasis	10 ⎭

From McNeer and DasGupta.[78]

biopsy and laparotomy, is indicated before applying aggressive local therapy to the primary site and the regional lymph node basin.

If regional lymph nodes are clinically involved, and if distant spread of disease has not been detected by a careful search of the type described, surgical dissection of the regional lymph nodes is indicated in most instances. However, the very low survival rates achieved by conventional regional lymph node dissection in this clinical situation lead us to consider lymph node excision by a major amputation if the primary lesion is on the distal portion of an extremity rather than on the trunk or proximal extremity, and if age and other aspects of patient status and disease status allow this. This approach naturally requires histologic confirmation of the involvement of the enlarged node or nodes. Data obtained from a major amputation experience in a highly selected series at Memorial Sloan-Kettering Cancer Center (McPeak et al.[80]) demonstrate reasonable survival rates (approximately 33 percent) under these special circumstances, and they are the basis for this approach in a small, highly selected group of patients (Table 10-4). Other clinical data regarding the potential benefit from amputation are less encouraging than this,[25] and a strong argument cannot be made for amputation. The argument for considering amputation in this clinical setting will be weakened further when an effective adjuvant therapy program is developed for melanoma.

Nonpalpable regional nodes. If the regional lymph nodes are not palpable, should "elective" regional lymph node dissection be performed? This is the question most frequently raised in regard to the surgical management of melanoma, and it is quite difficult to answer to everyone's satisfaction. Major factors affecting the surgeon's decision for elective lymph node dissection include: (a) whether the yield of histologically positive lymph nodes is worthwhile in terms of the morbidity and potential mortality associated with the procedures, and (b) whether or not the prognostic advantage of an elective dissection is sufficiently great to choose this over a later therapeutic dissection after palpable lymph nodes appear.

If the primary lesion is clearly "superficial" (i.e., levels I and II in Clark's classification), the incidence of lymphatic spread is certainly too low to warrant the morbidity of regional lymph node dissection. Earlier reports demonstrate less than a 5-percent incidence of lymphatic spread with malignant melanomas having dermal invasion limited to the upper one-third of the corium (or less than 1-mm invasion),[94] and more complete clinicopathologic data from several reports give a similar range for lymphatic metastases in patients with Clark level I and II lesions.[55,115,116] This yield of involved nodes does not justify the morbidity associated with standard regional node dissections.

If the primary malignant melanoma is more deeply invasive, as demonstrated by involvement of the reticular dermis or deeper (levels III–V), the incidence of histologic regional lymph node spread is higher than noted in patients with more superficial lesions.[55,115,116]   Retrospective data from a large, older series reported by Das Gupta and McNeer[34] demonstrate a 25-percent incidence of histologic melanoma in regional lymph nodes of patients thought to have no clinical node involvement.   These were patients with "invasive" melanoma that would probably now fit the category of invasion to level III or deeper (Fig. 10-3).   Further review of these data demonstrated a 5-year survival rate of 53 percent for these patients in this group with clinically negative, histologically positive lymph nodes treated by standard elective regional lymph node dissection.   Retrospective data from results of later therapeutic, rather than elective, lymph node dissection were less favorable (i.e., 20-percent 5-year survival from time of initial diagnosis).   Admitting the vagaries of retrospective examination of nonrandomized patient populations, one can still estimate the potential advantage of regional lymph node dissection from this information.   In simpler terms, 4 out of 16 patients with nonpalpable regional nodes will have a potential advantage from elective lymph node dissection.   The specific patient with these clinical and histologic findings will have a 5-year survival potential of approximately twice that which would have been achieved by a later therapeutic dissection.   Using these approximations, we can predict that 1 of 16 patients in the original elective node dissection group will have benefited in that this 1 patient would not have survived if lymph node dissection had been deferred until nodes were clinically palpable.   However, 12 of the 16 patients will have had regional lymph node dissections with their associated morbidity and without real therapeutic benefit since they would have had histologically negative nodes in the surgical specimen.   Elective regional lymph node dissection does have a small therapeutic advantage, then, in terms of the potential of a modest increase in survival rates, but this is not as

Table 10-4
Major Amputations for Recurrent
and Metastatic Melanoma

Extremity	No. of Cases	Survival 5 Yr with No Evidence of Disease
Lower	46	16
Upper	8	2
	54	18 (33%)

From McPeak et al.[80]

striking an advantage as has been implied by some vigorous proponents of elective node dissection.[49,51,87,107] More recent data using levels of invasion by Clark's levels tend to diminish the likelihood of therapeutic advantage from elective dissection for level III and increase this advantage over the above estimates for levels IV and V.[115]

Are the morbidity and mortality of elective regional lymph node dissection justifiable for deeper melanomas (levels III–V) on the basis of this small potential increase in survival rates for this selected group of patients? The morbidity of axillary lymph node dissection is so low that elective axillary dissection appears to be worthwhile if these treatment results outlined are true estimates of the situation. We also believe that this small therapeutic advantage justifies wide superficial groin dissection in most young or middle-aged, otherwise healthy, patients as well. However, the added morbidity of groin dissection makes this dissection a marginal choice in older or disabled patients, particularly for Clark level III.

We do not include the extraperitoneal iliac portion of the node dissection above Cloquet's node since this extension of the procedure is prognostic but rarely, if ever, therapeutic. Special factors in the individual case—such as the age of the patient, concurrent medical problems, and difficult anatomic problems (e.g., the midline lesion)—may well temper this advice and lead to a decision to observe rather than dissect the regional node area. The majority of surgeons probably favor elective lymph node dissection as described above, but it is difficult to fault the surgeon who argues that the morbidity of an adequate elective groin dissection always outweighs the therapeutic advantages.[20,96] As histologic staging of malignant melanoma becomes generally employed, elective node dissection will probably be reserved for levels IV and V by most surgeons.

Other procedural questions. Other procedural questions regarding elective node dissection for malignant melanoma are discussed below.

Timing: If elective node dissection is planned, the question may arise regarding the timing of this dissection. It was once suggested that a delay of 4–6 weeks between excision of the primary lesion and the node dissection should be allowed so that all cancer cells in transit would reach the lymph node basin. There is no real evidence demonstrating an advantage to delayed lymph node dissection versus immediate dissection at the time of treatment of the primary lesion. Retrospective analysis of data from Memorial Sloan-Kettering Cancer Center failed to show a difference in survival rates between these two groups (Table 10-5).[103] It is certainly practical to carry out both procedures at the same operation, and this is what we prefer when lymph node dissection is included in the operative plan.

Table 10-5
Strategy of Lymph Node Dissection for Malignant Melanoma*

Stage	Simultaneous		Delayed	
	No. of Patients	5-Year Survival	No. of Patients	5-Yr Survival
Stage I				
Incontinuity	63	48(76%)	165	128(78%)
Discontinuity	15	11(73%)	53	40(75%)
Stage II				
Incontinuity	53	22(42%)	167	70(42%)
Discontinuity	20	7(35%)	195	80(41%)

* Effects of incontinuity dissection and of delaying dissection 6 weeks after excision of primary.
From data of Shah and Goldsmith.[103]

Choice of lymph node basin for dissection: This decision is relatively easy when the melanoma originates on either the upper or lower extremity. The study by Fortner et al.[44] demonstrated that certain anatomic guidelines are useful in determining which lymph node basin is the likely site for lymphatic metastasis from melanomas on the trunk (Fig. 10-5). In a few anatomic circumstances, it may be appropriate to consider two lymph node basins for dissection, particularly if one basin has clinical involvement; but available data are inadequate to either support or deny the advisability of this. Bilateral groin dissections or combined axillary and groin dissections are extensive operative procedures, and they have potential wound-healing problems that generally overshadow the theoretical benefits of elective node dissection. The same situation

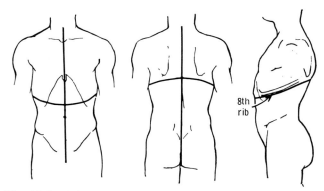

8th rib

Fig. 10-5. Diagram of suitable guidelines for choice of regional node basin for elective node dissection with malignant melanoma of the trunk (from Fortner et al.[44]).

applies to bilateral axillary dissection, but we have carried out combined lymph node dissections in a few select cases.

A few anatomic sites present special problems in terms of lymphatic spread. The lymphatics of the lateral scalp, preauricular, and auricular regions actually drain through the parotid gland en route to the cervical lymph nodes. This is the reason for including parotid resection with the radical neck dissection performed for melanomas of these sites. Another special anatomic problem is the area just below the clavicle as well as the deltoid region. Retrospective clinicopathologic studies by DasGupta and McNeer[34] have shown a significant incidence of neck node metastasis from these sites that are often considered to be primarily in the drainage basin of the axillary nodes. We have employed combined neck and axillary dissection for highly selected cases with melanomas in these locations.

Tissues intervening between regional lymph node and distant primary site: Although it might seem to be a sound theoretical concept to include the tissues containing the intervening lymphatic channels at the time of excision of a malignant melanoma and the regional lymph nodes, there are no data to substantiate this. Shah and Goldsmith[103] could show no benefit in a retrospective comparison of discontinuous and incontinuity procedures (whether the node dissection was simultaneous or delayed) in patients with clinical stage I or II melanoma of the skin (Table 10-5). Nevertheless, individual patients treated by discontinuous lymph node dissection, with the subsequent development of satellite nodules in the tissue between the two surgical incisions, are often presented as examples of the need for incontinuity procedures. However, to include all the lymphatic channels in the specimen of intervening tissue would usually require a much wider resection than is usually considered feasible unless the surgeon is prepared to perform near total integumentectomy as has been described by Hueston.[57] We have had experience with this approach in only 1 patient, but we believe it may have merit in selected patients with clinically involved regional lymph nodes. Being realistic, we should probably reserve the incontinuity approach for melanomas that are quite close to the regional lymph nodes, particularly if the regional nodes are clinically negative.

Variations in lymph node dissection. Combined dissection of the neck and axilla en bloc is occasionally indicated for malignant melanoma and we use the technique described by Bowden[7] (Fig. 10-6). Great pains are taken to preserve the spinal accessory nerve since the resection of the medial clavicle that this procedure requires exaggerates the disability associated with loss of this nerve.

Axillary lymph node dissection can be accomplished with preserva-

A

B

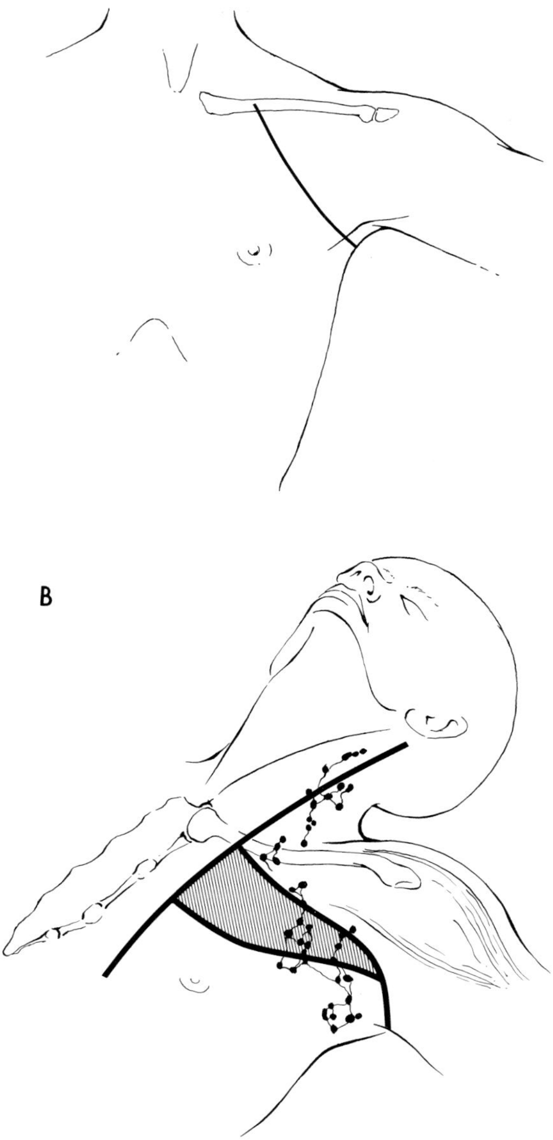

Fig. 10-6. Incisions for axillary dissection (**A**) and for combined neck and axillary lymph node dissection (**B**) (as described by Bowden[7]).

tion of one or both of the pectoral muscles as described for "modified" radical mastectomy. Draping the arm to allow free arm movement in the operative field allows a more thorough procedure when the muscles are preserved.

Internal mammary lymph node dissection (as described by Urban for breast cancer) may be indicated in rare instances, such as a case of primary melanoma in the medial breast skin with axillary lymph node involvement. We have had experience with only 2 patients in whom this procedure seemed indicated, and the actual curative potential of this operation is unknown.

Radical or "simple" groin dissection may be employed in patients with primary melanoma on the trunk or on the lower extremity, and the incisions vary with the location of the primary as well as the factor of "in continuity" versus a separate dissection. In the latter case, we employ an incision that will allow rotation of the abdominal wall skin inferiorly at the time of closure (Fig. 10-7). This allows resection of sufficient skin over the groin itself to limit or eliminate the skin slough so common with standard incisions. The abdominal wall musculature is exposed for the muscle incision to accomplish the deep portion of the groin dissection by elevation of the skin flap at the plane of the external oblique aponeurosis.

By the term "radical groin dissection," we mean excision of the common iliac, external iliac, internal iliac, and obturator lymph nodes in addition to the block of superficial groin tissue containing the femoral and inguinal nodes. Details of the technique of this procedure have been well described by DasGupta.[29] We question the therapeutic value of the deep portion of the dissection and limit the procedure to a wide block dissection of the superficial groin nodes in most cases.

AMPUTATION FOR MALIGNANT MELANOMA

Subungual lesions are in close proximity to bone, and primary digital amputation is the only way to achieve an adequate local resection. This may be true also for other sites on the digits, but melanoma is rarely close enough to bone at other sites on the extremity to raise the consideration of amputation for this reason.

Another group of patients in whom amputation should be considered are those with recurrent melanoma on the extremity after prior local excision with regional lymph node dissection. Lymphatic dissection often seems to localize the "recurrence" temporarily, and it may delay more proximal spread of the disease. Major amputation is justified for this clinical problem in carefully selected patients if a clearly adequate surgical margin can be accomplished by this approach. A patient with gross nodules anywhere near the proposed amputation site is clearly unsuitable for this approach. A meticulous search for distant metastasis, including bone marrow biopsy and laparotomy, is also essential before embarking on amputation in such patients. Other factors such as age, extent of disease, general condition of the patient, time interval since resection of the primary lesion, and presence or absence of distant metastases all play important roles in this decision. With extreme care in case selection, approximately one-third of these patients subjected to major amputation will survive 5 years without recurrence or metastasis.[80] This statistical result for highly selected cases is clearly better than that achieved by palliative treatment with either regional or systemic chemotherapy, and these are the only other options available for this clinical problem with the possible exception of the integumentectomy approach mentioned previously.[57] Except for ideal circumstances, however, regional perfusion or systemic chemotherapy should probably be chosen for this specific clinical problem.

Adjuvant Therapy

REGIONAL PERFUSION FOR EXTREMITY MELANOMA

In 1959, Creech and his associates[26] first described regional chemotherapy using extracorporeal perfusion for the management of recurrent malignant melanoma localized to the extremities. In view of previously disappointing results with systemic chemotherapy, this method of palliative treatment became quite popular for the management of recurrent melanoma clinically limited to the extremity.[65,68] The encouraging early palliative results produced then led to the application of this technique as an adjuvant to the primary surgical therapy for curable extremity melanoma. Extensive experience with this approach by Stehlin and Clark[109] and by Rochlin and Smart[98] failed to yield data demonstrating that results from this approach were superior to those from surgical treatment alone, but more recent data with hyperthermic perfusion suggest possible value.[75,110] There has been no prospective clinical trial which definitely answers this question, and this approach cannot be recommended for routine adjuvant use at this time.

OTHER ADJUVANT THERAPY

Systemic chemotherapy as an adjuvant to surgical therapy is an appealing concept for the improvement of treatment results in melanoma, just as it is for many other "solid tumors" in man. The same holds true for nonspecific or specific immunotherapy for "curable" melanoma. The only convincing evidence of benefit, thus far, from such adjuncts to "curative" therapy is limited to results of treating other cancers—partic-

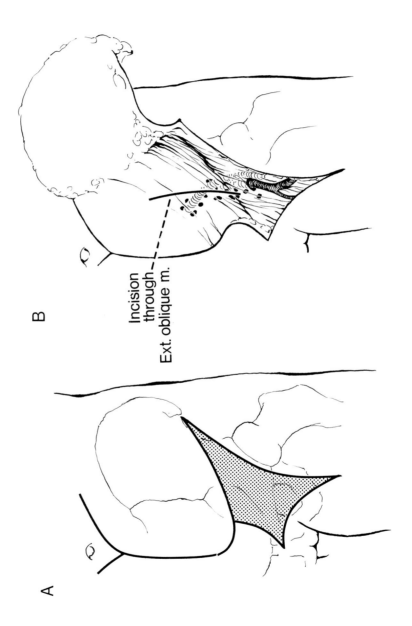

A

B

Incision through Ext. oblique m.

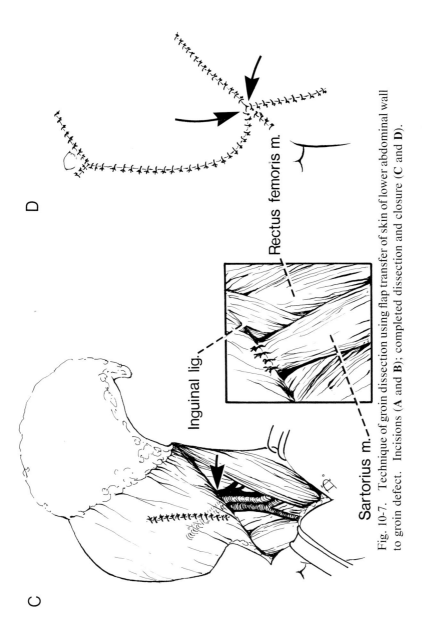

C

D

Inguinal lig.

Rectus femoris m.

Sartorius m.

Fig. 10-7. Technique of groin dissection using flap transfer of skin of lower abdominal wall to groin defect. Incisions (**A** and **B**); completed dissection and closure (**C** and **D**).

ularly tumors in the pediatric age group—that also demonstrate a high response of recurrent and metastatic disease to systemic chemotherapy. Benefit must be demonstrated on prospective, well-planned, randomized clinical trials before this approach can be recommended for general use in the treatment of melanoma. On the other hand, these or other adjunctive approaches are currently the major hope for improvement in the results following the standard surgical approach that has been discussed. Surgeons should follow ongoing clinical trials of adjuvant therapy with great interest and adopt these new methods only when they are proven to be beneficial.

Palliative Treatment of Metastatic Melanoma

SURGERY

In contrast to various other forms of cancer in man for which individual patterns of metastatic spread have been identified, malignant melanoma appears to have the capability of producing metastases in most of the tissues and organs of the body. Usually metastases are multiple and a vigorous surgical approach to these lesions is most inappropriate. On the other hand, some patients with melanoma demonstrate distant metastasis of such a limited nature that there is potential benefit from surgical resection. One example is the occasional patient with an apparently solitary lung metastasis several years after resection of the primary melanoma.[14] This situation is analogous to that occasionally seen after resection of colon cancer or soft part sarcoma. Under these uncommon circumstances, limited pulmonary resection is indicated for such patients in the hope that it will prolong survival. An occasional patient is significantly benefited by surgical resection of a metastatic lesion producing symptoms of localized bone pain, bowel obstruction, or gastrointestinal bleeding; but great care must be exercised in terms of the selection of such patients for palliative operation. Malignant melanoma is less likely to produce clinically localized signs of metastatic disease than most of the other cancers we treat. Nevertheless, palliative surgical therapy is indicated for some patients when careful evaluation reveals limited metastatic disease.

RADIOTHERAPY

Although radiation therapy is not considered the preferable treatment of "curable" melanoma, the experience of Hillriegel[54] and Hilaris et al.[53] has definitely demonstrated radiation response of this lesion. This modality has not been employed frequently for recurrent and metastatic melanoma because of the usual widespread nature of the lesions. However, radiation therapy for localized symptomatic disease, particularly that involving brain and bone, is often of definite benefit and is a palliative tool that should not be overlooked.

SYSTEMIC CHEMOTHERAPY

The effective use of systemic chemotherapy is a relatively recent development since the response rates following the use of most standard agents were disappointing. The agents and combinations of effective agents that have evolved in recent years are shown in Table 10-6. It appears that dimethyltriazino-imidazole carboxamide (DTIC) is equal to any of these currently established regimes and yields a beneficial response in approximately 1 of 4 patients, the responses having some correlation with the pattern of metastatic disease. Visceral metastases are much less likely to respond than soft tissue disease, with the possible exception of lung metastases. Distant metastases from melanoma should be treated initially with DTIC or one of the combinations listed,[23,24,38,39,73,84] until new agents and combinations are shown to be more effective in prospective, cooperative clinical trials. The chemotherapeutic approach for established metastases, particularly visceral lesions, should have priority over a systemic immunotherapy approach because of the frequent inability of this latter experimental method to affect gross disease significantly.

Table 10-6
Chemotherapeutic Agents for Malignant Melanoma

Agent	Response Rates Reported (%)
Single agents	
Cyclophosphamide	21
Vinblastine	20
Vincristine	20
Actinomycin D	14
Procarbazine	28
BCNU	18
DTIC (imidazole carboxamide)	23–29
Combinations	
BCNU and vincristine	23
BCNU and DTIC	19
BCNU, vincristine, and DTIC	28
BCNU, hydroxyurea, and DTIC	27
Cyclophosphamide, vincristine, methotrexate, and 5-fluorouracil	26

From Luce[73] and others.[23,24,84]

IMMUNOTHERAPY

The role of cellular immunity in the control of cancer growth has been recognized with experimental tumor systems since the first demonstration of the existence of tumor-specific transplantation antigens. In recent years, evidence has accumulated for the presence of tumor-specific antigens in a number of human tumors. Both immunofluorescent and complement fixation techniques have demonstrated antigen and antimelanoma antibody in the sera of some patients with malignant melanoma.[86] This is not surprising since there are other examples of host immunity in human malignant melanoma, including the unexpectedly high rate of spontaneous regression of this tumor,[106] the observation that blood transfusions from patients with spontaneous regression sometimes induce regression of melanoma in recipients of these transfusions,[113] and reports that cross-transfusion of leukocytes between sensitized patients with malignant melanoma is occasionally successful.[85]

Immunotherapy for malignant melanoma is obviously an experimental method now, but there is rationale for using host defenses as an adjunct to therapy for melanoma. Clinical trials of immunotherapy using cross-immunization and cross-transfusion of leukocytes produced transient clinical benefit in some patients with advanced melanoma,[58,64,85] but data on immunological factors in human melanoma were probably the major product of these studies. Nonspecific immunotherapy with BCG has been beneficial for recurrent disease in the soft tissues, particularly when administered by local injection of recurrent nodules,[50,86,102] but the poor response to this approach to visceral disease and other forms of metastatic disease of significant volume reduces its value as a palliative method. The most helpful future role for immunotherapy will undoubtedly be an adjuvant one, but more evidence of benefit is required before this approach is adopted for general use.

SARCOMAS

Sarcomas of soft tissues and bone are a rare group of cancers that seldom appear on the usual tables of cancer incidence. Nevertheless, the physician must be aware of the major clinical features and management principles of this group of neoplasms since initial management does play a major role in the outcome.[18,28,90]

The etiology of a few sarcomas is related to inherited factors[27] or prior radiation therapy,[70] but we know little regarding the etiology of the majority of these lesions. Patients often cite trauma as a causative factor, but it is universally agreed that this does not play a role. The recent observations of viral bodies on histologic study, and the presence of antisarcoma antibodies in family members of sarcoma patients, suggest a potentially significant association with a viral agent.[86] The role of these findings has not yet been established.

This discussion will be concerned primarily with the management of sarcomas in adults, and the reader is referred to Chapter 13 for a consideration of sarcomas in the pediatric age group.

SOFT PART SARCOMAS

The classification of soft part sarcomas is based on a presumed histogenetic origin from various nonepithelial mesenchymal structures. Although some lesions can be clearly defined in terms of their origin from fat, muscle, fibrous tissues, synovial membranes, nerve, or blood vessels, a number of sarcomas will not be adequately differentiated to fit into a clear-cut classification and must, therefore, be labeled "spindle cell" sarcomas or sarcomas of unknown histogenesis. The relative proportion of these various forms of soft part sarcoma tends to vary somewhat in the reported series. These differences depend to some degree on the criteria used by the pathologists concerned, but there are general principles of clinical management that apply irrespective of these diagnostic differences. The diagnosis of a specific form of sarcoma usually affects the prognosis to a larger degree than it affects the therapeutic approach.

Diagnosis

Although several sarcomas—particularly those arising from or involving the skin—have clinical presentations of unique character, the typical diagnostic problem is that of a solitary mass in the soft tissues of the extremities, trunk, retroperitoneal space, or head and neck region.

When the mass is accessible and of significant size, our general approach is to perform an open incisional biopsy under general anesthesia. Although others prefer aspiration biopsy to a formal open biopsy, the latter technique has several advantages. First, this approach prevents overtreatment at the first procedure if the diagnosis proves, unexpectedly, to be either a benign tumor or a metastatic lesion from an unrecognized occult primary cancer. Second, a careful attempt at classification using adequate biopsy material may alter the details of the primary therapy to be directed toward the tumor in question. This does not occur frequently, since surgical resection is our usual treatment, but patients with a primary lymphoma of the soft tissues or Kaposi's sarcoma will be managed much more effectively by primary radiation therapy.

Preoperative angiography of soft tissue masses has been employed for evaluation of sarcomas, but it has no real advantage in terms of establishing the diagnosis.[56] This technique has been particularly useful for establishing the extent of disease, however, and it may be helpful also in treatment decisions. The use of a tourniquet at the time of the biopsy procedure has been suggested to reduce the possibility of tumor cell emboli, but this is an ineffective safeguard. It is probably more important to avoid undue manipulation of the primary neoplasm. It has also been suggested that the biopsy should be accomplished by the same surgeon who will eventually perform surgical resection since he will be able to encompass his biopsy wound with first-hand knowledge of the planes that have been entered.

Primary Treatment

SURGERY

Although soft part sarcomas are radiosensitive, their curability by this treatment method is limited, and surgical resection is accepted as the primary treatment of choice for most lesions. The major treatment decision relates to the extent of surgical resection, a factor primarily dictated by the anatomic considerations of the individual lesion; but most sarcomas are on the extremities where the decision regarding amputation must be made.

Many of these soft part neoplasms have the misleading appearance of being encapsulated.[15] This feature of pseudoencapsulation could lead the inexperienced surgeon to enucleate the entire tumor without achieving an adequate margin of normal tissue. Such an inadequate procedure usually leads to a high incidence of local recurrence (80 percent) and seriously jeopardizes the chances of permanent control of the neoplasm. Proper management of soft part sarcomas requires radical resection of the neoplastic mass with an adequate envelope of normal tissue, so all the possible local ramifications of the tumor are eliminated.[9] This resection may include skin, subcutaneous tissue, adjacent muscle and fibrous tissue, and the biopsy site itself. To adhere to this principle in the extremities, it is usually necessary to remove involved and adjacent muscle groups (quadriceps, hamstrings, etc.). However, tumors close to joints or bones, in the distal portion of an extremity, or overlying the shoulder or pelvic girdle usually must be removed by amputation to achieve adequate margins. There are some exceptions to this, such as the anatomic area over the wing of the scapula[97] or the buttock.[8] However, compromise in the effort to achieve desirable margins to preserve a limb (or its vascular supply) will usually result in failure of local tumor control. It may allow distant metastasis also before this failure is clinically evident.

Some surgeons are reluctant to consider soft part resection in lieu of amputation for most sarcomas on the extremities because of the incorrect concept that a large number of these lesions are multicentric in origin. The primary consideration must be complete confidence regarding adequacy of surgical margins, and soft part resection can achieve this in many instances. Preoperative angiography is useful in planning the operative procedure from this standpoint, but preoperative and operative evaluation usually play the major role. The histogenetic classification may also temper the decision regarding the choice of operative procedure, but this is usually a secondary consideration. The principle of including an adequate envelope of normal tissue applies to the less-common primary sites, other than the extremities, but the option of resection by amputation is obviously not applicable. The principle of achieving wide margins has been modified to some extent for rhabdomyosarcomas in the pediatric age group because of the impressive effect of chemotherapy on this neoplasm,[52] but these same benefits are not apparent with other sarcomas.

The regional lymph nodes may be a site of metastasis of sarcomas with a frequency depending on the histologic variety (5–45 percent).[90] However, elective lymph node dissection is not indicated in management of most soft part sarcomas since the majority of these lesions in adults have an incidence of metastasis much too low to justify the morbidity of the procedure unless the primary lesion is anatomically situated in the groin or axilla. Practically speaking, the regional lymph nodes are included in the dissection or with the amputation only if this can be accomplished without significant additional resection, risk, or disability. It is considered an advantage to have removed the regional lymph nodes only in patients with synovial sarcoma and angiosarcoma on the basis of the frequency of metastasis to these nodes.[90]

TECHNICAL FEATURES OF
OPERATIVE PROCEDURES

Soft part resection. The resection must be tailored to fit the individual lesion within the guidelines described, but diagrammatic examples of these resections are shown in Figure 10-8 (anterior thigh), Figure 10-9 (hamstring area), and Figure 10-10 (buttock). In each instance, the procedure of choice is amputation if an adequate soft tissue margin cannot be obtained.

Amputation. The level of amputation depends entirely on the anatomic details of the specific lesion. Interscapulothoracic amputation or hemipelvectomy are frequently required for proximal lesions on the extremity. Diagrams of these procedures are shown in Figures 10-11 and

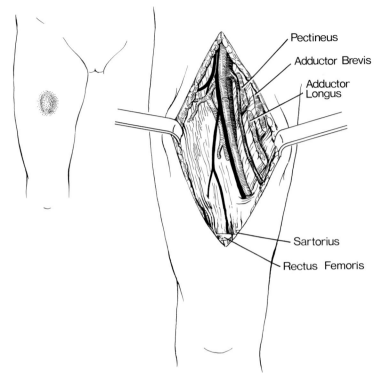

Pectineus

Adductor Brevis

Adductor
Longus

Sartorius

Rectus Femoris

Fig. 10-8.   Diagram of soft part resection for sarcoma arising from soft tissues of anterior thigh (region of quadriceps femoris).

10-12, but it must be stressed that the design of the incision and the limits of the operative procedure must follow the guidelines described for non-amputative soft part resection to avoid the possibility of local failure. These major amputative procedures can be accomplished with minimal risk in experienced hands, but they are not recommended for the surgeon who rarely performs them.   The postoperative facilities for rehabilitation and the proper fitting and training in the use of available prostheses are also essential parts of the treatment program.

RADIATION THERAPY

Although surgery is the preferred means for management of soft part sarcomas, the radiosensitivity of many sarcomas is often unappreciated. Radiation has completely controlled local disease in many patients with soft part sarcoma, and it has also been an effective means of palliative therapy.[35,93,117] Evaluation of the role of radiation in the management of patients with sarcoma unfortunately depends on retrospective data using different types of equipment and varying treatment plans.   Nevertheless,

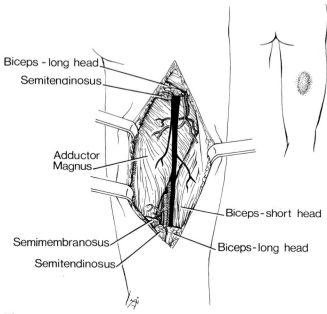

Fig. 10-9.   Diagram of soft part resection for sarcoma arising from soft tissues of posterior thigh (region of hamstring muscles).

histologic sterilization of the local sarcoma was achieved in 24 of 72 patients with various types of sarcoma who were treated preoperatively by radiation at the Memorial Sloan-Kettering Cancer Center.[77]   In the same series, 42 of 58 patients in whom the clinical response could be assessed showed objective signs of response (72 percent).   Some histologic types were particularly responsive (i.e., liposarcoma) and some were relatively resistant, but some responses were observed with all types of sarcomas. These data do support the logic of employing radiation therapy as a palliative tool, and possibly as a preoperative adjunct in selected cases, particularly lesions that are "marginal" from the standpoint of resectability.

CHEMOTHERAPY AND IMMUNOTHERAPY AS ADJUNCTS TO SURGICAL RESECTION

The low level of response of recurrent and metastatic sarcoma in adults to systemic chemotherapy[66] makes this an ill-advised approach at this time.   On the other hand, encouraging progress in both palliative and combined treatment modalities for embryonal rhabdomyosarcoma in children[52] makes this an appealing concept for the future.   Benefit should be demonstrated in prospective clinical trials before adjuvant therapy is recommended for general use.

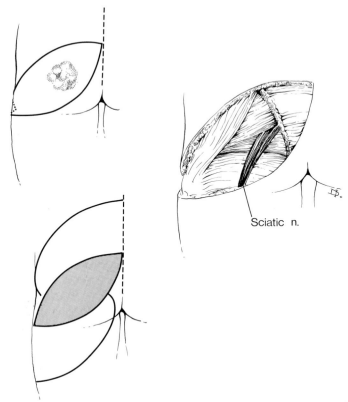

Sciatic n.

Fig. 10-10.   Diagram of soft part resection for lesion arising on the buttock.

Immunotherapy as an adjunct to surgical therapy may well prove useful in spite of the inability of this approach to affect the sarcoma significantly in patients with established disease. This is one of the few human cancers in which tumor antigens and antitumor antibodies have been demonstrated,[86] but the therapeutic application of this information must await further intensive investigation.

Characteristics of Individual Forms of Soft Part Sarcoma (Table 10-7)

LIPOSARCOMA[40,90,92]

Liposarcoma is the most common of the soft tissue sarcomas in adults and it bears no relationship to the benign lipoma. This lesion usually arises along the fascial planes and perivascular spaces in the lower extremities (thigh), the retroperitoneum (around the kidney and mesentery), and the shoulder girdle. Three histologic varieties are recognized: the well-differentiated, the myxoid, and the pleomorphic types. In most circumstances these tumors present as a relatively "pure" form, but it is not unusual to find more than one histologic pattern in the same tumor, or a change in histologic pattern with recurrence or metastasis. The well-differentiated and myxoid types have the best prognosis; the pleomorphic form carries a poorer prognosis. Retroperitoneal liposarcomas are associated with a low survival rate compared with that of liposarcomas in the extremities. This is partly because surgical eradication is seldom as complete as in other sites since the principles of surgical treatment previously described cannot be applied owing to the involvement of, or the close proximity to, vital structures. The 5-year survival of patients with retroperitoneal liposarcoma is 24 percent, and the 10-year survival is in the range of 10 percent. In contrast, the resection of liposarcomas of the extremities produces better results at both 5 and 10 years after treatment in our institution (80 percent and 64 percent, respectively). Liposarcomas are considered quite radiosensitive. Radiotherapy is probably a useful adjuvant in the management of these tumors, particularly if the margins of surgical resection must be compromised in any way.

RHABDOMYOSARCOMAS

Rhabdomyosarcomas that originate from striated muscle are commonly found in the extremities of adults (84 percent), but they may arise in other sites. Together with the liposarcoma and fibrosarcoma, they constitute the most common types of soft tissue sarcomas in adults (80 percent). There are three varieties of rhabdomyosarcoma that differ in histologic pattern, anatomical distribution, age at appearance, and natural history.

Alveolar type.[43] This tumor has a pseudoalveolar pattern, and the presence of solid or medullary areas makes alveolar rhabdomyosarcoma difficult to differentiate from lymphosarcoma, melanoma, poorly differentiated adenocarcinoma, and the other forms of sarcoma. It usually is seen in individuals between the ages of 10 and 20 years, particularly in the arm or forearm, but it may arise in the perirectal or perineal areas. The overall prognosis of this histologic type of rhabdomyosarcoma is bleak, and few patients live 5 years or more.

Pleomorphic type.[63] This variety usually occurs on the extremities of adults who are between 50 and 70 years of age. The survival rate is lower than with most other types of soft part sarcoma at our institution, the 5- and 10-year survival rates being 29 percent and 25 percent, respectively.

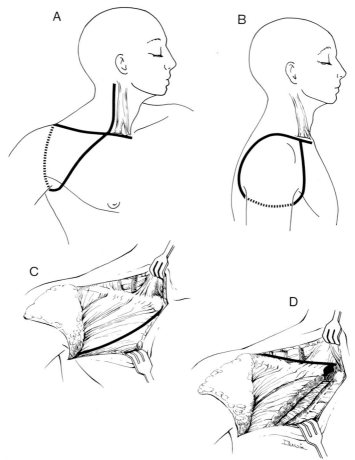

Fig. 10-11.   Technique of interscapulothoracic amputation.   Incision to include neck dissection (**A**), standard incision (**B**), anterior dissection (**C, D** and **E**), and posterior dissection (**F, G,** and **H**).

Embryonal type.[69]   This is the most frequent of the soft tissue sarcomas in children and is discussed in detail in Chapter 13.   This same histologic type of sarcoma is also found in adults, in whom it carries an extremely poor prognosis despite resection, and frequently metastasizes early in the course of the disease.   In contrast, the prognosis of this lesion in children has improved significantly with the aggressive combination of surgery, radiation therapy, and chemotherapy—the last method playing a major role.

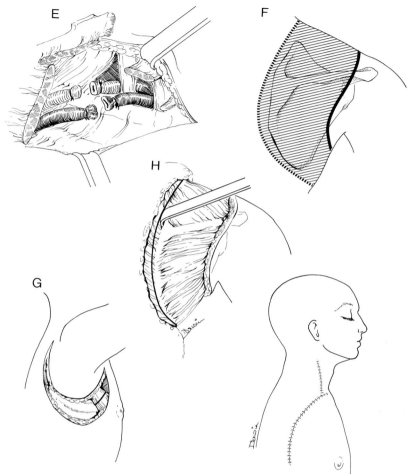

Fig. 10-11.   (continued)

SYNOVIAL SARCOMA[90]

Synovial sarcoma develops in the distal part of the extremities in most cases, but does not usually appear to be associated with a joint lining.   The cellular component shows all stages of differentiation, thereby leading to some difficulty in differential diagnosis.   Because of the proximity to joints, amputation is the treatment of choice in most instances.   Approximately 20 percent of synoviomas metastasize to the regional lymph nodes, and we know of no patient with node metastasis who has enjoyed long-term survival.   The 5 and 10-year survival rates for all synovial sarcomas are 25 percent and 12 percent, respectively.

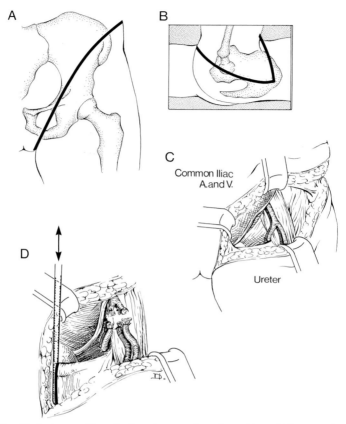

Fig. 10-12. Technique of hemipelvectomy. Incisions (**A** and **B**); anterior dissection (**C**); division of symphisis pubis (**D**); division of sacro-iliac joint (**E** and **F**); division of gluteal muscles (**G**); and closure (**H**).

MALIGNANT SCHWANNOMA[31]

Malignant schwannoma arises from the neurolemma or peripheral nerve tissues and usually appears as a mass on either the trunk or the extremities. The neoplasm seldom involves a major nerve trunk or shows any evidence of regional neurological deficit. The 5- and 10-year survival rates after surgical resection are 65 percent and 58 percent, respectively, and the best results are obtained when the lesion arises on the extremities. Patients with neurofibromatosis (von Recklinghausen's disease) have an increased incidence of malignant schwannoma and, in this particular group of patients, the 5-year survival rate is reduced.

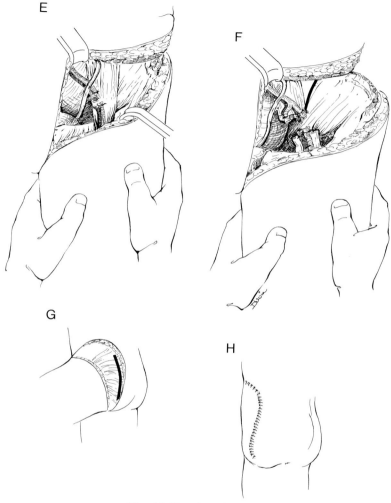

Fig. 10-12. (continued)

FIBROSARCOMA[43]

   Fibrosarcoma may appear at any age, and it usually develops on the trunk, extremities, or head and neck region. Fibrosarcomas are locally aggressive and their ability to metastasize depends on their degree of differentiation. They are often slow growing, but they do infiltrate the surrounding tissues. Conservative surgery is associated with a high incidence of local recurrence (ranging from 30–60 percent), so radical resection is mandatory. The 5- and 10-year survival rates for this neoplasm at our institution are 82 percent and 73 percent, respectively.

Table 10-7
Soft Part Sarcomas: Classification and General Characteristics

Tissue	Benign Neoplasms	Malignant Neoplasms (Sarcomas)			
		Type	Most Frequent Sites	Usual Age Group	Treatment
Fat	Lipoma (solitary or multiple)	Liposarcoma a. Well differentiated b. myxoid c. Pleomorphic (poorly differentiated)	Lower extremity (thigh), retroperitoneum, and shoulder girdle	Middle and older age group	Surgery; radiation therapy often useful
Striated muscle	Rhabdomyoma (rare)	Rhabdomyosarcoma a. Alveolar b. Pleomorphic c. Embryonal	a. Extremities, perineum b. Extremities c. Head and neck region, extremities, trunk, and GU tract	a. Adolescents b. middle age and elderly c. Usually children	a. Surgery, radiation therapy, and chemotherapy b. Surgery c. Surgery, radiation therapy, and chemotherapy
Synovial mesothelium	Giant cell tumor (tendon sheath)	Synovial sarcoma (synovioma	Knees, hands, and feet	Young adults	Surgery (amputation often required)
Nerve	Neurofibroma, neurilemoma	Malignant neurilemoma	No anatomic predilection	Young and middle-aged adults	Surgery

338

Fibrous tissue	Fibroma, fibromatosis, dermatofibroma, nodular fasciitis	Fibrosarcoma			
		a. Desmoid (well differentiated)	a. Abdominal wall, extremities	a. Young adults	Surgery
		b. Undifferentiated	b. Extremities, trunk	b. Any age	Surgery
		c. Dermatofibrosarcoma protuberans	c. Skin of abdomen or back	c. Middle-aged adults	Surgery
		d. Malignant histiocytoma	d. Extremities, trunk, and retroperitoneum	d. All ages	Surgery
Smooth muscle	Leiomyoma	Leiomyosarcoma	Gastrointestinal tract, other soft tissues	All ages	Surgery
Blood vessels	Hemangioma, lymphangioma, glomus tumor, hemangiopericytoma (benign)	Angiosarcoma	Lower extremities, breast, other sites	All ages	Surgery
		Lymphangiosarcoma	Edematous extremity (often arm)	Older adults	Radiation therapy or surgery
		Malignant hemangiogericytoma	Extremities	All ages	Surgery
		Kaposi's sarcoma	Lower extremities (edematous)	Older adults	Radiation therapy
Unknown	Glandular cell myoblastoma	Malignant granular cell myoblastoma	Many sites	Adults	Surgery
		Alveolar soft parts sarcoma	Extremities	Young adults	Surgery
		Epithelioid sarcoma	Extremities (distal)	Young adults	Surgery

The "standard" fibrosarcoma must be differentiated from two other very similar lesions, the desmoid tumor[6,32] (abdominal or extra-abdominal) and dermatofibrosarcoma protuberans[79,114] (a sarcoma of dermal origin). These tumors histologically resemble well-differentiated fibrosarcomas, and identification of each is based essentially on the distribution of fibrous and cellular components. They are both locally aggressive and have a high incidence of local recurrence. They may each cause death by direct invasion of vital structures in the head and neck, trunk, or retroperitoneal regions. Dermatofibrosarcoma is suspected clinically from the appearance of the large bosslike skin nodule involving the adjacent subcutaneous tissues. Distant metastases have been reported with these lesions, but they are uncommon in comparison to those seen with standard fibrosarcomas.

ALVEOLAR SOFT PART SARCOMA[71]

The cell of origin of alveolar soft part sarcoma is not well defined. It is very slow growing, tends to occur in women, and has a high incidence of distant metastasis. Recurrence has been observed even 20 years after the original treatment. The 5- and 10-year survival rates after resection are 50 percent and 47 percent, respectively.

EPITHELIOID SARCOMA[41]

Epithelioid sarcoma, which has only recently been recognized as an entity, usually appears in the soft tissue of the hand, forearm, or leg of younger individuals. The gross lesion has been mistaken clinically for a chronic inflammatory process, a necrotizing granuloma, or squamous cell carcinoma. The 5-year survival free of disease in a small series is only 10 percent, but 40 percent of patients are alive with residual sarcoma after a 5-year period.

MALIGNANT FIBROUS HISTIOCYTOMA (FIBROXANTHOSARCOMA)[61a]

These tumors represent the malignant variant of a series of benign tumors composed of histiocytes and fibroblasts. They develop in the soft tissues of the extremities and retroperitoneal region in all age groups. The malignant form was recognized recently as a separate unity when it became evident that some of the so called "benign" fibrous histiocytomas had a tendency to recur locally and metastasize. The aggressive potential of these lesions is indicated by the presence of bizarre pleomorphic cells with a storiform or cartwheel pattern. Due to the high incidence of local recurrence, a wide local excision as described for other sarcomas is the treatment of choice. Due to the recent categorization of this lesion and the small number of cases reported, it is difficult to define the natural history and prognosis after adequate local treatment, but it appears that only a small proportion of patients survive more than five years free of the disease after resection. An "inflammatory" pattern has also been identified which is virtually always fatal.

LEIOMYOSARCOMA[62,112]

Leiomyosarcomas may arise from the smooth muscle wall of the inferior vena cava or from other vessels, but they may also occur in soft tissues. These neoplasms are identical histologically to their more common counterparts in the gastrointestinal tract. Radical surgery results in 50-percent 5-year survival for most sites, whereas the rare retroperitoneal lesions generally have a very poor prognosis.

ANGIOSARCOMA

The arterial vessels give rise to several forms of sarcoma, all relatively rare. Angiosarcoma may present as a vascular, aggressive soft part tumor, and this uncommon form has a significant incidence of regional lymph node involvement (45 percent).[90] Wide resection with or without regional lymph node dissection and amputation frequently fails to control this disease as there is a high incidence of hematogenous metastasis. Nevertheless, the same principles of resection employed for most soft part sarcomas seem appropriate for this lesion, and we believe (without data) that radiation therapy, either preoperative or postoperative, should be part of the treatment plan. Tumors at some sites (e.g., the breast) are associated with virtually no long-term survivors; but we had one long-term survivor with angiosarcoma of the thigh with soft part resection as the only treatment, and another patient is well five years after radical mastectomy for angiosarcoma of the breast.

HEMANGIOPERICYTOMA

Hemangiopericytoma arising from the capillary pericyte is an indolent neoplasm of blood vessel origin, but it is associated with a much lower survival rate at 10 years than at 5. The general principles of therapy outlined for other sarcomas apply to this lesion, although the late nature of recurrences has led some surgeons to be less aggressive with these lesions.

KAPOSI'S SARCOMA[88]

Idiopathic multiple hemorrhagic sarcoma falls into the category of soft part sarcoma of blood vessel origin. The clinical presentation is so unique that the general principles of diagnosis and treatment outlined for other sarcomas do not apply. Kaposi's sarcoma generally has its onset as a single bluish red macule on the skin of an extremity, and this is not noticed frequently until multiple lesions appear. These gradually coalesce into plaques. Although primary lesions in the viscera or lymph nodes may precede the classic skin lesions on the extremities, the usual presentation is a bilateral stocking distribution of skin lesions on the lower extremities. Kaposi's sarcoma is often associated with chronic lymphedema or venous stasis in the lower extremities, and it is of interest that a similar lesion, lymphangiosarcoma, usually has its origin in either the upper or lower extremity that is the site of chronic lymphedema.[119]   A classic example of this lesion is the lymphangiosarcoma originating in a chronically edematous arm after radical mastectomy (Stewart-Treves syndrome).[111]   In contrast to that of the other sarcomas discussed, the treatment of Kaposi's sarcoma is usually "palliative," but survival may be quite prolonged before terminal visceral dissemination. Radiation therapy has been a useful method of management, but eventual reactivation of the skin lesions is the rule. Regional perfusion with alkylating agents has been useful in a few patients with persistent disease. Also, intra-arterial nitrogen mustard has been used effectively as primary treatment in Africa where this disease is prevalent.

Lymphangiosarcoma in the lymphedematous arm can be treated either by amputation (interscapulothoracic amputation) or by radiation therapy, but the results are generally poor. A review of the world experience [119] (a group of 129 patients with follow-up data that were suitable for this calculation) revealed only 11 patients alive 5 years after treatment. Two of the eleven controlled patients had received radiation therapy, and the others were treated by amputation. We are now following 1 elderly patient who remains well four years after radiation therapy for this disease.

Results of Treatment

Results for individual sarcomas are listed in the preceding text, but these data differ from those in other reports in some instances.

The variations in 5- and 10-year results of treatment that are reported for various sarcomas are undoubtedly owing to variations in the case material included in the different categories. For example, a series of fibrosarcomas that includes a large number of low-grade desmoid lesions will have much better treatment results than another series that categorizes many of the low-grade fibrous lesions as fibromatosis. The inclusion of more "spindle cell sarcomas" in the fibrosarcoma group in some series than in others is another example of a factor that alters the statistics regarding prognosis. For overall 5-year survival, the figure for the entire group of soft part sarcomas is in the 50-percent range.

Although individual series report differing survival rates for the various categories of sarcomas, the overall prognosis for most sarcomas has remained essentially unchanged over the years. An exception to this statement is the improvement in results in children (see Chap. 13) as result of improved chemotherapy. These findings plus the immunologic data mentioned give some hope to the possibility of the future development of effective adjuncts to surgical resection for other sarcomas.

Palliative Treatment of Recurrent or Metastatic Soft Part Sarcoma

RADIATION

Radiation can be quite useful for palliative therapy for recurrent or metastatic sarcoma. The histologic features of the lesion cannot absolutely predict the response or absence of response for the individual case.[77,93] However, radiation therapy is more likely than systemic chemotherapy to produce therapeutic benefits if the pattern of the disease is regional.

SURGERY

Surgery may play a palliative role also in patients with recurrent or metastatic sarcoma. Some of the low-grade tumors (desmoid, dermatofibrosarcoma protuberans, and myxoliposarcoma) are often subjected to multiple surgical procedures for local recurrence before eventual control is achieved. Another palliative role for surgery is resection of lung metastases in selected patients. This has been effective in patients with the primary focus of disease under control, an apparently single metastatic focus in one lung, and a long interval (preferably 3–5 years) between the treatment of the primary lesion and the radiographic appearance of the pulmonary metastasis. With careful case selection, approximately 30-percent 5-year survival can be expected after local resection of the metastasis or lobectomy. This figure is probably indicative more of the growth pattern of the disease in the patients selected for resection than of the operative benefits of excision.

Another guide to the selection of patients who may be benefited by surgical excision of pulmonary metastases is the calculation of "doubling time" of the metastasis from serial radiographic measurements. Under some circumstances (specifically patients with calculated doubling times over 40 days) even bilateral thoracotomy may be indicated for limited metastatic disease.[60] Sarcomas for which we have found pulmonary resection of metastasis useful include liposarcoma, fibrosarcoma, malignant schwannoma, "sarcomas of undetermined histogenesis," and osteogenic sarcoma on rare occasion.

CHEMOTHERAPY

In the past soft part sarcomas in the adult responded poorly to most forms of available systemic chemotherapy.[66] This is in marked contrast to the striking result seen with chemotherapy for some childhood sarcomas. Recently, results in adults have been more encouraging than heretofore, but progress by clinical trials is limited by the low overall incidence of soft part sarcoma. Single-drug studies in patients with established disease have shown response rates to adriamycin in the 25–30-percent range, and the combination of this agent with other agents (DTIC or DTIC plus vincristine) has produced response rates of reasonable duration in 40–50 percent of patients.[48] These developments give hope of future benefit from other drug combinations for this group of cancers.

Regional administration of chemotherapeutic agents, particularly alkylating agents, produced some clinical response in most trials.[68] The incomplete nature of the response usually obtained led to little palliative benefit in our experience. In addition, a frequent problem in the palliative management of sarcomas has been the control of disseminated disease. For these reasons we do not employ regional chemotherapy, but the development of more effective agents and combinations may justify reevaluation of this method in patients who require palliation for local disease on an extremity.

BONE SARCOMAS

Sarcomas of bone are even more infrequent in our population than soft part sarcomas, and roughly half of these uncommon lesions are multiple myelomas, a unique process more appropriately considered with the lymphomas. A useful classification of bone cancer is shown in Table 10-8, but there are a number of somewhat different classifications of this heterogeneous group of neoplasms. Many aspects of the diagnosis and management of this rare group of neoplasms are similar to those discussed for soft part sarcomas, but some unique features of bone cancer deserve special emphasis.

Diagnosis

The clinical suspicion of a primary malignant bone tumor is usually prompted by localized pain and a subsequent abnormality seen on radiographic examination.[37] An absolute diagnosis is not obtained by x-ray examination alone, but the benign or malignant nature of the process is often judged more accurately from this examination than by a limited

Table 10-8
Malignant Neoplasms of Bone

Tumors of Osseous Origin		
Cartilaginous	Osseous	Other
Chondrosarcoma, primary or secondary Chondroblastoma, malignant	Osteogenic sarcoma, sclerosing and osteolytic Parosteal osteosarcoma	Fibrosarcoma Giant cell tumor, with malignant metaplasia
Tumors of Nonosseous Origin		
Marrow and Haversian Systems	Metastatic Deposits	By Inclusion or Direct Invasion
Ewing's sarcoma Primary reticulum sarcoma Multiple myeloma	Metastatic lymphomas and sarcomas Metastatic carcinomas	Chordoma Soft part sarcomas

Modified from Geshickter and Copeland.[46]

pathologic examination. The key radiologic criteria for cancer are beyond the scope of this presentation, but they include an evaluation of the "zone of transition" and the presence or absence of marginal sclerosis. Important also are trabeculation, periosteal reaction, a "moth-eaten" appearance, and the general overall radiologic appearance of the lesion. Other factors such as the site of origin, solitary or multiple nature of the lesions, and the age of the patient are important, but the ultimate diagnosis is dependent on a combination of these observations with an examination of biopsy material. In this situation the surgical pathologist must insist on the benefit of the radiographs and the radiologist's observations before he makes a final diagnosis.

The biopsy may be obtained with a special bone-penetrating needle. Adequate material for diagnosis can be obtained by aspiration in the majority of instances if the surgical pathologist is familiar with, and enthusiastic about, this approach. However, open surgical incisional biopsy is preferred in most institutions. The lack of diagnostic benefit from angiography and the lack of evidence of benefit from use of a tourniquet at the time of biopsy are similar to the situation with soft part sarcomas. The wide range of clinical behaviors observed with bone neoplasms makes it mandatory that both the malignant nature and the classification of the lesion are determined before treatment is initiated. Differentiation of a primary from a metastatic process is particularly important for obvious reasons.

Primary Treatment

Surgical resection is the preferred treatment for most of the primary malignant bone neoplasms, and amputation, until recently, has been almost the uniform choice for extremity lesions. Many variations in the potential of individual bone neoplasms may affect treatment decisions, but operative procedures analogous to extended local resection for soft part sarcoma are not as conveniently performed. In view of the variations in approach for specific diagnoses, the primary malignant bone tumors will be discussed individually.

MALIGNANT CARTILAGINOUS NEOPLASMS[18,22,28,46]

Malignant cartilaginous neoplasms include primary chondrosarcoma, a rapidly growing lesion found chiefly in young adults, and secondary chondrosarcoma. The latter usually arises in a middle-aged patient from a preexisting chondroma, an osteochrondroma, or less frequently from Paget's disease or hereditary deforming chondrodysplasia (Fig. 10-13). Primary and secondary chondrosarcoma are indistinguishable on histopathologic examination, but they differ considerably in both the usual site of origin and the prognosis after treatment. Primary chondrosarcoma

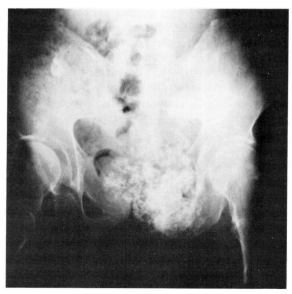

Fig. 10-13. Secondary chondrosarcoma of pubis in patient with multiple osteochondromas (hereditary deforming chondrodysplasia). Patient well 8 years after hemipelvectomy.

arises on the metaphyseal side of the epiphysis of long bones, particularly the lower femur and upper tibia, whereas the secondary tumors are more frequent in the region of the shoulder or pelvic girdle. Evidence of the preexisting benign lesion may also be seen on the x-ray. The preferable treatment for both of these conditions is adequate surgical resection, usually an amputation that includes the entire bone of origin. Major forequarter or hindquarter amputation is frequently required to accomplish adequate resection since local recurrence is a uniform event if there is spillage of tumor cells during surgery for either of these lesions. This is particularly important in the management of secondary chondrosarcoma since distant metastases are rare and local control is the key factor in success or failure.

Overall long-term results after adequate resection of secondary lesions are in the 50-percent range whereas there is marked variation in the reports on prognosis after amputation for primary chondrosarcoma. These results range from a 15-percent 5-years survival upward. Possibly these differences relate to the continued clinical difficulty in differentiating this lesion from osteogenic sarcoma.

Chondroblastomas are primarily benign, vascular, cartilaginous tumors in young adults, but the less-common malignant forms behave like, and are treated as, chondrosarcomas.

MALIGNANT OSSEOUS NEOPLASMS

Malignant osseous neoplasms include the very uncommon, slow growing, more favorable parosteal (or juxtacortical) osteosarcoma in the adolescent or young adult[36] and the standard, more frequent osteosarcoma, or osteogenic sarcoma, which usually occurs in young children. These lesions are differentiated by both radiologic and histologic means. The natural history of each is considerably different, and this has led to somewhat different treatment plans.

The favorable course of parosteal osteosarcoma has led to the recommendation of block resection of the involved bone rather than amputation in selected cases. Five-year survival rates for this rare lesion are probably in excess of 50 percent. A similar lesion, primary fibrosarcoma of bone, has been described,[59] but there is some doubt regarding the identification of this lesion as a separate entity. The treatment approach and results are similar to those for the parosteal variety.

Osteogenic sarcoma, on the other hand, has been a discouraging disease because of the frequency of lung metastases after extremity amputation. Reported results of adequate surgical treatment are in the range of 15–20-percent 5-year survival.[22,28,46] More recently, the addition of aggressive multiple-drug therapy with methotrexate and citrovorum "rescue," vincristine, adriamycin, and other agents in various study protocols has shown marked benefit in conjunction with either amputation or more limited local surgery in children[5,99] (see Chap. 13). It is clear that multimodal therapy is advantageous for this disease, at least in children; but adequate local surgery is still necessary. Amputation may not always be required for these extremity lesions, but it should probably remain the "standard" until more experience is obtained with compromise operative procedures.

MALIGNANT GIANT CELL TUMORS

Malignant giant cell tumors are rare lesions of poor prognosis and represent sarcomatous change in benign giant cell tumors of bone. This change usually follows prior treatment of the benign process, frequently with radiation therapy.[22,48] Radiation is probably contraindicated in the treatment of the benign giant cell tumors for this reason. One major problem is the diagnostic one since osteogenic sarcoma with giant cells may mimic malignant giant cell tumor. Treatment employed for this rare lesion should be similar to that for osteogenic sarcoma.

EWING'S SARCOMA AND RETICULUM CELL SARCOMA OF BONE

Ewing's sarcoma occurs most often in children and adolescents and has classically been treated solely with radiation therapy. The prognosis has been grave, but recent encouraging progress with multimodal therapy is discussed in Chapter 13. A malignant bone tumor with similar histologic appearance is reticulum cell sarcoma of bone, which occurs in the adult age groups.[19] This disease differs markedly from Ewing's sarcoma in prognosis, however. The results of therapy with surgical resection and/or radiation therapy are equally good, generally in the 40-percent 5-year survival range.

CHORDOMA[3,28,108]

Chordoma is a rare malignant neoplasm arising from the notochord, usually in the sacrococcygeal region (50 percent), or the sphenooccipital region (30 percent). It is characterized by slow relentless growth and involves bone only by proximity. Metastases are rare (10 percent) and patient death is caused by local extension of the neoplasm. Palliative benefit is achieved with radiation therapy for lesions in the sphenooccipital region, but surgical resection is preferable for sacrococcygeal lesions if this is feasible. At diagnosis the mass is often so large that surgical resection may require hemipelvectomy or rectal resection in addition to resection of the distal sacrum. Rehabilitation after surgical resection is difficult.

Role of Radiation Therapy

The radiosensitivity of Ewing's sarcoma and reticulum cell sarcoma of bone has been noted, but the cartilaginous and osseous malignant bone tumors are all relatively radioresistant and best treated by surgery as the primary therapy. High-dose preoperative radiation therapy with supervoltage was originally recommended by Cade.[12] Subsequent trials of this approach with several variations[2,11,45,100] have failed to affect overall survival statistics in some instances, but suggested benefit in others. It seems doubtful that radiation therapy will have a major role to play in the therapy for these lesions except for palliation of patients who are not suitable for surgery.

Role of Systemic Chemotherapy and Immunotherapy

The use of high-dose methotrexate with citrovorum "rescue," adriamycin, and various combinations of these with other agents has been shown to have significant benefit.[48,99] Specific combinations and schedules to be recommended are currently being developed. Immunotherapy for bone sarcoma,[74] as for soft part sarcoma, is still in the investigative phase. However, the rationale for adjuvant immunotherapy is a good one, and this may prove to be of benefit in the future.

REFERENCES

1. Allen AC, Spitz S: Malignant melanoma, a clinicopathological analysis of the criteria for diagnosis and prognosis. Cancer 6:1–45, 1953
2. Allen CV, Stevens KR: Preoperative irradiation for osteogenic sarcoma. Cancer 31:1364–1366, 1973
3. Ariel IM, Verdu C: Chordoma: An analysis of twenty cases treated over a twenty-year span. J Surg Oncol 7:27–44, 1975
4. Arlen M, Higinbotham NL, Huvos AG, Marcove RC, Miller T, Shah IC: Radiation-induced sarcoma of bone. Cancer 28:1087–1099, 1971
5. Beattie EJ, Martini N, Rosen G: The management of pulmonary metastases in children with osteogenic sarcoma with surgical resection combined with chemotherapy. Cancer 35:618–621, 1975
6. Booher RJ, Seel DJ, Joel RV: Fibrous tumors of musculoaponeurotic origin. Prog Clin Cancer 2:222–252, 1966
7. Bowden L: A more thorough in-continuity neck and axillary dissection. Ann Surg 143:481–492, 1956
8. Bowden L, Booher RJ: Surgical considerations in the treatment of sarcoma of the buttock. Cancer 6:89–99, 1953
9. Bowden L, Booher RJ: The principles and technique of resection of soft parts for sarcoma. Surgery 44:963–977, 1958

10. Breslow A: Tumor thickness, level of invasion and node dissection in stage I cutaneous melanoma. Ann Surg 182:572–575, 1975

11. Caceres E, Zaharia M: Massive preoperative radiation therapy in the treatment of osteogenic sarcoma. Cancer 30:634–638, 1972

12. Cade S: Osteogenic sarcoma, a study based on 133 patients. J Roy Coll Surg Edinb 1:79–111, 1955

13. Cady B, Legg MA, Redfern AB: Contemporary treatment of malignant melanoma. Am J Surg 129:472–482, 1975

14. Cahan WG: Excision of melanoma metastases to lung: Problems in diagnosis and management. Ann Surg 178:703–709, 1973

15. Clark RL, Martin RG, White EC, Old JW: Clinical aspects of soft tissue tumors. Arch Surg 74:859–870, 1957

16. Clark WH Jr, Ainsworth AM, Bernardino EA, Yang CH, Mihm MC Jr, Reed RJ: The developmental biology of primary human malignant melanomas. Semin Oncol 2:83–103, 1975

17. Clark WH Jr, From L, Bernadino EA, et al: The histogenesis and biologic behavior of primary human malignant melanoma of the skin. Cancer Res 29:705–727, 1969

18. Coley BL: Neoplasms of Bone and Related Conditions (ed 2). New York, Paul B Hoeber, 1960

19. Coley BL, Higinbotham ML, Groesbeck HP: Primary reticulum cell sarcoma of bone, summary of 37 cases. Radiology 55:641–658, 1950

20. Conrad FG: Treatment of malignant melanoma. Arch Surg 104:587–593, 1972

21. Conway H, Hugo NE: The skin, in Nealon TF Jr (ed.): The management of the Patient with Cancer. Philadelphia, WB Saunders Co, 1965, pp 277–332

22. Copeland MM: Primary malignant tumors of bone, evaluation of current diagnosis and treatment. Cancer 20:738–746, 1957

23. Costanza ME, Nathanson L, Lenhard R, Wolter J, et al: Therapy of malignant melanoma with an imidazole carboxamide and bis-chloroethyl nitrosourea. Cancer 30:1457–1461, 1972

24. Costanzi JJ, Vaitkevicius VK, Quagliana JM, Hoogstraten B, Coltman CA Jr, Delaney FC: Combination chemotherapy for disseminated malignant melanoma. Cancer 35:342–346, 1975

25. Cox R: Survival after amputation for recurrent melanoma. Surg Gynecol Obstet 139:720–722, 1974

26. Creech O Jr, Ryan RF, Krementz ET: Treatment of melanoma by isolation perfusion technique. JAMA 169:339, 1959

27. Crow FW, Schull WJ, Neel JV: A Clinical Pathological and Genetic Study of Multiple Neurofibromatosis. Springfield, Ill., Charles C Thomas, 1956

28. Dahlin DC: Bone Tumors. Springfield, Ill., Charles C Thomas, 1967

29. DasGupta T: Radical groin dissection. Surg Gynecol Obstet 129:1275–1280, 1969

30. DasGupta T, Bowden L, Berg J: Malignant melanoma of unknown primary origin. Surg Gynecol Obstet 117:341–345, 1963

31. DasGupta TK, Brasfield RD: Solitary malignant schwannoma. Ann Surg 171:419–428, 1970

32. DasGupta TK, Brasfield RD, O'Hara J: Extra-abdominal desmoids (a clinicopathological study). Ann Surg 170:109–121, 1969

33. DasGupta TK, Brasfield RD, Paglia MA: Primary melanomas in unusual sites (collective review). Surg Gynecol Obstet 128:841–848, 1969

34. DasGupta T, McNeer G: The incidence of metastasis to accessible lymph nodes from melanoma of the trunk and extremities—its therapeutic significance. Cancer 17:897–894, 1964

35. Del Regato JA: Radiotherapy of soft tissue sarcoma. JAMA 185:216–218, 1963

36. Edeiken J, Farrell C, Ackerman LV, Spjut HJ: Parosteal sarcoma. Am J Roentgenol Radium Ther Nucl Med 3:579–583, 1971

37. Edeiken J, Hodes PJ: Roentgen Diagnosis of Diseases of Bone. Baltimore, Williams & Wilkins Co, 1973

38. Einhorn LH, Burgess MA, Vallejos C, Bodey GP Sr, Gutterman J, Mavligit G, Hersh EM, Luce JK, Frei E, Frerieich EJ, Gottlieb JA: Prognostic correlations and response to treatment in advanced metastatic malignant melanoma. Cancer Res 34:1995–2004, 1974

39. Einhorn LH, Luce JK, Gottlieb JA: Result of chemotherapy for disseminated malignant melanoma. Clin Res 22:487, 1974

40. Enterline HT, Culberson JD, Rochlin DB, Brady LW: Liposarcoma (a clinical and pathological study of 53 cases). Cancer 13:932–950, 1960

41. Enzinger FM: Epithelioid sarcoma, a sarcoma simulating a granuloma or a carcinoma. Cancer 26:1029–1041, 1970

42. Epstein E, Bragg K, Linden G: Biopsy and prognosis of malignant melanoma. JAMA 208:1369–1371, 1969

43. Ferrel HW, Frable WJ: Soft part sarcomas revisited. Cancer 30:475–480, 1972

44. Fortner JG, DasGupta T, McNeer G: Primary malignant melanoma on the trunk. Ann Surg 161:161–169, 1965

45. Francis KC, Phillips R, Nickson JJ, Woodward HK, Higinbotham NL, Coley BL: Massive preoperative irradiation in treatment of osteogenic sarcoma in children: A preliminary report. Am J Roentgenol 72:813–818, 1954

46. Geshickter CF, Copeland MM: Bone, in Nealon TF Jr: Management of the Patient with Cancer. Philadelphia, WB Saunders Co, 1965

47. Goldsmith HS, Shah JT, Kim GH: Prognostic significance of lymph node dissection in the treatment of malignant melanoma. Cancer 26:606–609, 1970

48. Gottlieb JA: Proceedings: Combination chemotherapy for metastatic sarcoma. Cancer Chemother Rep 58:265–270, 1974

49. Gumport SL, Harris MN: Results of regional lymph node dissection for melanoma. Ann Surg 179:105–108, 1974

50. Gutterman JU, Mavligit G, McBride CM, Frei EE, Freireich EJ, Hersh EM: Active immunotherapy with BCG for recurrent malignant melanoma. Lancet 1:1208–1212, 1973

51. Harris MN, Gumport SL, Maiwandi H: Axillary lymph node dissection for melanoma. Surg Gynecol Obstet 135:936–940, 1972

52. Heyn RM, Holland R, Newton WA, Tefft M, Breslow N, Hartmann JR: The role of combined chemotherapy in the treatment of rhabdomyosarcoma in children. Cancer 34:2128–2141, 1974

53. Hilaris BS, Raben M, Calabrese AS, Phillips RF, Henschke UK: Value of radiation therapy for distant metastases from malignant melanoma. Cancer 16:765–773, 1963

54. Hillriegel W: Radiation therapy of primary and metastatic melanoma: the pigment cell. Ann NY Acad Sci 100:131–141, 1963

55. Holmes EC, Clark W, Morton DL: Regional lymph node metastases and level of invasion of the primary. Cancer (in press)

56. Hudson TM, Haas G, Enneking WF, Hawkins IF Jr: Angiography in the management of musculoskeletal tumors. Surg Gynecol Obstet 141:11–21, 1975

57. Hueston JT: Integumentectomy for malignant melanoma of the limbs. Aust NZ J Surg 40:114–118, 1970

58. Humphrey LJ, Jewell WR, Murray D, Griffen WO: Immunotherapy for the patient with cancer. Ann Surg 173:47–54, 1971

59. Huvos AG, Higinbotham NL: Primary fibrosarcoma of bone: A clinico-pathologic study of 130 patients. Cancer 35:837–847, 1975

60. Joseph WL: Criteria for resection of sarcoma metastatic to the lung. Cancer Chemother Rep 58:285–290, 1974

61. Katz AD, Urbach F, Lilienfield AM: The frequency and risk of metastases in squamous cell carcinoma of the skin. Cancer 10:1162–1166, 1957

61a. Kempson RL, Kyriakos M: Fibroxanthosarcoma of the soft tissues. Cancer 29:961–976, 1972

62. Kevorkian J, Gento DP: Leiomyosarcoma of large arteries and veins. Surgery 73:390–400, 1973

63. Keyhani A, Booher RJ: Pleomorphic rhabdomyosarcoma. Cancer 22:956–967, 1968

64. Krementz EM, Samuels S, Wallace JH: Clinical experience in immuno-therapy of cancer. Surg Gynecol Obstet 133:209–217, 1971

65. Krementz ET, Ryan RF: Chemotherapy of melanoma of the extremities by perfusion: Fourteen years clinical experience. Ann Surg 175:900–917, 1972

66. Krementz ET, Shaver JO: The treatment of soft tissue sarcoma by che-motherapy. JAMA 184:149–152, 1963

67. Lancaster HO, Nelson J: Sunlight as cause of melanoma: A clinical survey. Med J Aust 1:452–456, 1957

68. Lawrence W Jr: Regional cancer chemotherapy: an evaluation. Prog Clin Cancer 1:341–393, 1965

69. Lawrence W Jr, Jegge G, Foote FW Jr: Embryonal rhabdomysarcoma (a clinical pathologic study). Cancer 17:361–376, 1964

70. Lerman RI, Murray D, O'Hara JM, Booker RJ, Foote FW Jr: Malignant melanoma of childhood. Cancer 25:436–449, 1970

71. Lieberman PH, Foote FW, Stewart FW: Alveolar soft-part sarcoma. JAMA 1047–1051, 1966

72. Litzow TJ, Perry HO, Soderstrom CW: Morpheaform basal cell carcinoma. Am J Surg 116:499–505, 1968
73. Luce JK: Chemotherapy of malignant melanoma. Cancer 30:1604–1615, 1972
74. Marsh B, Flynn L, Enneking W: Immunologic aspects of osteosarcoma and their application to therapy. J Bone Joint Surg 54(A):1367–1387, 1972
75. McBride CM: Management of malignant melanoma. Adv Surg 8:129–150, 1974
76. McGovern VJ, Mihm MC Jr, Bailly C: The classification of malignant melanoma and its histologic reporting. Cancer 32:1446–1457, 1973
77. McNeer JP, Cantin J, Chu F, Nickson JJ: Effectiveness of radiation therapy in the management of sarcoma of the soft somatic tissues. Cancer 22:391–397, 1968
78. McNeer G, DasGupta T: Prognosis in malignant melanoma. Surgery 56:512–518, 1964
79. McPeak CJ, Cruz T, Nicastri AD: Dermatofibrosarcoma protuberans; an analysis of 86 cases—5 with metastasis. Ann Surg 166:803–816, 1967
80. McPeak CJ, McNeer GP, Whitely W, Booher RJ: Amputation for melanoma of the extremity. Surgery 54:426–431, 1963.
81. Mehnert JH, Heard JL: Staging of malignant melanomas by depth of invasion: A proposed index to prognosis. Am J Surg 110:168–176, 1965
82. Mihm MC Jr, Fitzpatrick TB, Brown ML, Raker JW, Malt RA, Kaiser JS: Early detection of primary cutaneous malignant melanoma. N Eng J Med 289:989–996, 1973
83. Mohs FE: Chemosurgery; a microscopically controlled method of cancer excision. Arch Surg 42:279–295, 1941
84. Moon JH, Gaillni S, Cooper MR, et al: Comparison of the combination of 1,3-bis (2-chloroethyl)-1-nitrosourea (BCNU) and vincristine with two dose schedules of 5-(3,3-dimethyl-1-Triazino) imidazole 4-carboxamide (DTIC) in the treatment of disseminated malignant melanoma. Cancer 35:368–371, 1975
85. Moore GE, Gerner RE: Cancer immunity—hypothesis and clinical trial of lymphocytotherapy for malignant disease. Ann Surg 172:733–739, 1970
86. Morton DL, Eilber FR, Joseph WL, Wood WC, Trahan E, Ketchan AS: Immunological factors in human sarcomas and melanomas: A rational basis for immunotherapy. Ann Surg 172:740–749, 1970
87. Mundth ED, Guralnick EA, Raker JW: Malignant melanoma, a clinical study of 427 cases. Am Surg 162:15–28, 1965
88. O'Brien PH, Brasfield RD: Kaposi's sarcoma. Cancer 19:1497–1502, 1966
89. Olsen G: Removal of fascia—cause of more frequent metastases of malignant melanomas of the skin to regional lymph nodes? Cancer 17:1159–1164, 1964
90. Pack GT, Ariel IM: Tumors of the Soft Somatic Tissues: (A Clinical Treatise). New York, Paul B Hoeber, 1958
91. Pack GT, Lenson N, Gerber DM: Regional distribution of moles and melanomas. Arch Surg 65:862–870, 1952
92. Pack GT, Pierson JC: Liposarcoma. Surgery 36:687, 1954

93. Perry H, Chu F: Radiation therapy in the palliative management of soft tissue sarcomas.   Cancer 15:179–183, 1962

94. Peterson RF, Hazard JB, Dykes ER, Anderson R: Superficial Malignant melanomas.   Surg Gynecol Obstet 119:37–41, 1964

95. Phillips PL, Sheline GE: Radiation therapy of malignant bone tumors.   Radiology 92:1537–1545, 1969

96. Polk HC Jr, Linn BS: Selective regional lymphadenectomy for melanoma: A mathematical aid to clinical judgement.   Ann Surg 174:402–413, 1971

97. Ramirez J, Arlen M, Jourdain LM: Total scapulectomy for soft part sarcoma of the shoulder girdle.   Surgery 69:271–275, 1971

98. Rochlin DB, Smart CR: Treatment of malignant melanoma by regional perfusion.   Cancer 18:1544–1550, 1965

99. Rosen G, Suwansirikul S, Kwon C, et al: High-dose methotrexate with citrovorum factor rescue and adriamycin in childhood osteogenic sarcoma.   Cancer 33:1151–1163, 1974

100. Royster RL, King ER, Ebersole J, De Giorgi LS, Levitt SH: High dose preoperative supervoltage irradiation for osteogenic sarcoma.   Am J Roentgenol Radium Ther Nucl Med 114:536–543, 1972

101. Sedlin ED, Fleming JL: Epidermoid carcinoma arising in chronic osteomyelitic foci.   J Bone Joint Surg [Am] 45-A:827–838, 1963

102. Seigler HF, Shingleton WW, Metzgar RS, Buckley CE, Bergoc PM, Miller DS, Fetter BF, Phaup MB: Non-specific and specific immunotherapy in patients with melanoma.   Surgery 72:162–174, 1972

103. Shah JP, Goldsmith H: Incontinuity versus discontinuous lymph node dissection for malignant melanoma.   Cancer 26:610–614, 1970

104. Shingleton WW: Perfusion chemotherapy for recurrent melanoma of extremity.   Ann Surg 169:969–973, 1969

105. Shingleton WW, Seigler HF, Stocks LH, Downs RW Jr: Management of recurrent melanoma of the extremity.   Cancer 35:574–579, 1975

106. Smith JL, Stehlin JS: Spontaneous regression of primary malignant melanomas with regional metastases.   Cancer 18:1399–1415, 1965

107. Southwick HW, Slaughter DP, Hinkamp JF, Johnson FE: The role of regional node dissection in the treatment of malignant melanoma.   Arch Surg 85:63–69, 1962

108. Steckler RM, Margin RC: Sacrococcygeal chordoma.   Am Surg 40:579–581, 1974

109. Stehlin JS, Clark RL: Melanoma of the extremities: Experiences with conventional treatment and perfusion in 339 cases.   Am J Surg 110:366–383, 1965

110. Stehlin JS Jr, Giovanella BC, de Ipolyi PD, Muenz LR, Anderson RF: Results of hyperthermic perfusion for melanoma of the extremities.   Surg Gynecol Obstet 140:339–348, 1975

111. Stewart FW, Treves N: Lymphangiosarcoma in postmastectomy with lymphedema.   Cancer 1:64–81, 1948

112. Stout AP, Hill WT: Leiomyosarcoma of the superficial soft tissues.   Cancer 11:844–854, 1958

113. Sumner WC, Foraker AG: Spontaneous regression of human melanoma. Cancer 13:79–81, 1960

114. Taylor HB, Helwig EB: Dermatofibrosarcoma protuberans (a study of 115 cases) Cancer 15:717–725, 1962

115. Wanebo HJ, Fortner JG, Woodruff J, MacLean B, Binkowski E: Selection of the optimum surgical treatment of stage I melanoma by depth of microinvasion: Use of combined microstage technique. Ann Surg 182: 302–315, 1975

116. Wanebo HJ, Woodruff J, Fortner JG: Malignant melanoma of the extremities: A clinicopathologic study using levels of invasion (microstage). Cancer 35:666–676, 1975

117. Windeyer B, Dische S, Mansfield CM: The place of radiotherapy in the management of fibrosarcoma of the soft tissues. Clin Radiol 17:32–40, 1966

118. Wong CK: A study of melanocytes in the normal skin surrounding malignant melanomata. Dermatologica 141:215–225, 1970

119. Woodward AH, Ivins JC, Soule EH: Lymphangiosarcoma arising in chronic lymphedematous extremities. Cancer 30:562–572, 1972

Warren Koontz, Jr.
and M. J. Vernon Smith

11

Management of Genitourinary Cancer

Neoplasms arising from the prostate, kidney, and bladder are among the more common abnormal growths that affect the human body. Malignant lesions of the ureter, urethra, penis, seminal vesicles, epididymis, and scrotum are quite rare, but cancer of the testicle lies in between in incidence and affects mainly the younger adult male. Cancer of the genitourinary system accounts for 27 percent of all cancers in the male and 4 percent of all cancers in the female.[68]

KIDNEY TUMORS

Tumors of the upper urinary tract are a fascinating and significant problem. An estimated 11,100 new cases are diagnosed each year in the United States, and these tumors constitute some 1–2 percent of all cancers. Like patients with many other cancers, over half the patients with upper urinary tract tumors have metastases at the time of diagnosis.

This discussion is limited to those malignant tumors that occur in adults. All tumors of the kidney should be regarded as malignant until proven otherwise, and only the major tumors of the renal parenchyma and of the collecting system will be presented. These will be discussed separately, as they behave in a different manner, have a different prognosis, and the adjunctive therapy for each varies widely. However, they are similar in that extensive surgical extirpation is the only method of treatment that offers chance of cure.

357

HYPERNEPHROMA

Hypernephroma was first described in 1863 by Grawitz, who observed its yellowish discoloration and striking resemblance to the adrenal cortex. He suggested that it arose from adrenal rests. Over the ensuing years, there have been considerable controversy and disagreement as to its true cell of origin. Today, urologists and pathologists agree that renal tumors arise from the tubular epithelial cells and are correctly termed renal cell carcinoma or renal cell adenocarcinoma. The evidence from light and electron microscopic studies has recently been reviewed, and this further pinpoints the cell of origin as being from proximal convoluted tubular epithelium.[6]

There does not appear to be any specific racial or ethnic incidence; hypernephroma occurs more frequently in men than in women (3:1). There is no evidence for a familial inheritance with this disease except in von Hippel-Lindau's disease; nearly two-thirds of these patients develop adenocarcinoma, which not infrequently is bilateral.

Few epidemiological studies have been undertaken in this disease, although there is some association between tobacco use and an increased danger of renal cancer.[86] The possible underlying agent may be dimethyl-nitrosamine, as this substance among many other chemicals has been shown to produce renal cell carcinoma in animals.

Diagnosis

There are so many ways in which hypernephroma may present in a clinical situation that it rightly deserves its reputation as the internist's tumor.[34] The classic triad of hematuria, pain, and a palpable mass are late findings with a poor prognosis and fortunately are seen in only approximately 10 percent of patients, of whom half already have metastases. About 40 percent of patients have hematuria or other urinary complaints, although just as many if not more have systemic signs and symptoms. A few have problems due to the metastasis (e.g., pathological fractures of a long bone).

Renal tumors may present with *local effects* (hematuria, 60 percent; pain, 50 percent; and flank mass, 20 percent). The presenting finding may be variococele, which is produced by direct pressure of the tumor on the spermatic vein, or because of stasis due to an obstructing tumor thrombus in the main vein. Similarly, distension of the anterior abdominal veins may be noted.

Toxic systemic effects[23] may be pyrexia of an intermittent and variable nature (16 percent), anemia (41 percent) possibly owing to poor erythropoietin production, or abnormal liver function studies (15 percent). Some of these alterations are reversible after nephrectomy.

Erythrocytosis, which occurs in 4 percent, is distinguished from polycythemia vera because there is no elevation of the leukocyte or platelet counts. Hypertension occurs, although a mechanism has not yet been clearly demonstrated, except in patients who have arteriovenous fistulas. Hypercalcemia in the absence of bone metastases is occasionally present and is due to the production of a parathyroidlike hormone by the tumor. Gonadotropin production has also been demonstrated.

Once a renal mass is found or suspected, a number of avenues can be followed in order to evaluate the patient accurately before surgery. The remarkable level of sophistication achieved by these studies has led many physicians to order every study for every patient; recently, these modalities have been reviewed and a rational approach to the diagnostic tests developed so that maximum benefit with minimal testing is achieved.[59]

Intravenous and retrograde pyelograms are seldom specific but will demonstrate evidence of a space-occupying mass with pelviocalyceal displacement and alteration of renal contour. Nephrotomography is a relatively safe method of differentiating renal cysts from tumors with an accuracy of 85 percent. This accuracy will be improved by the use of sonography, particularly when this procedure is used for localization and aspiration of apparent cysts.

Renal arteriography and venacavography also have their place in identifying and staging renal tumors (Fig. 11-1). The degree to which these procedures are used clearly depends on individualized consideration for each patient. The value of these studies to the surgeon in preoperative planning and as a guide during the actual dissection is considerable. When any of the above-mentioned studies are suboptimal, the renal mass should be explored for final diagnosis. However, in the ideal situation where all studies suggest a cyst, percutaneous aspiration and study of the fluid, along with radiographic study of the cyst space should be all that is required.

Further diagnostic evaluation involves a search for possible metastases.

The surgeon must realize that metastases in the chest may be occult, so laminography is important. Bone surveys and isotope scanning are certainly helpful. Any patient who is scheduled for possible nephrectomy should have individual and total renal function assessed preoperatively by means of creatinine clearance and isotopic renography.

Staging

There is still no clear agreement as to whether the grade or the cell type has an influence on survival. Most investigators agree that it probably does, but no single acceptable method of grading the various morphological forms that are seen has yet been agreed on.

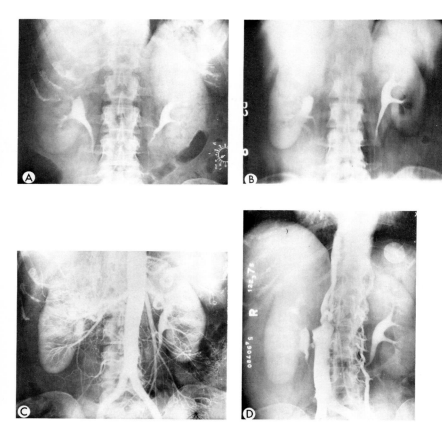

Fig. 11-1. These roentgenographic studies were obtained on a 53 year old patient. **A** shows an upper pole mass in the right kidney which is causing displacement of the upper pole calyces. **B** is a representative cut from a nephrotomogram
which again shows an upper pole mass which may be solid. This finding was confirmed by sonography, which gave the typical appearance of a solid mass; so an
arteriogram was obtained. **C** was taken from the aortic run and clearly demonstrates the presence of a hypernephroma confined to the upper pole on the right.
It is important to note that this study also shows no tumor on the left side. This
can occur in up to 5 percent of patients. **D** is an venacavagram showing complete
obstruction of the vena cava with extensive collateral venous drainage. This
alerted the surgeon to the extensive venous extension of this tumor and we were
able to remove the tumor thrombus from the auricle and cava along with the
surgical specimen. The patient has survived one year so far.

There is no doubt that stage plays a considerable role in the outcome of any form of therapy. The staging classification developed by Robson[65] is probably the most widely accepted:

Stage 1   Tumor confined within the kidney
Stage 2   Perirenal fat involvement but confined within Gerota's fascia
Stage 3   A.   Gross renal vein or inferior vena cava involvement
          B.   Lymphatic involvement
          C.   Vascular and lymphatic involvement
Stage 4   A.   Adjacent organs other than adrenal involved
          B.   Distant metastases

This schema will certainly undergo modification as we learn more about the biology of the tumor. For example, Skinner has shown that renal vein involvement without perinephric involvement or lymphatic spread does not alter the prognosis at 5 and 10 years, whereas lymphatic involvement is an ominous sign.[72]

Treatment

Before discussing the surgical approach to this tumor, it would be more appropriate to discuss the prognosis. The biological potential and the reaction of the host to its presence are extremely variable and at the present time are not entirely predictable. In one series the crude 5-year survival of untreated tumor is 1.7 percent. Occasional patients live for many years with known metastases. Other patients have had a metastasis 31 years after nephrectomy.[64]

There is no convincing evidence that removing the primary tumor affects secondary deposits. However, it must be acknowledged that there has been no case report of regression of secondary deposits when the primary was still present. However, pain, intractable bleeding, or both may require palliative nephrectomy. Occasionally, removal of a solitary metastasis seems justifiable.[70]

SURGICAL APPROACH

There are a variety of approaches to renal adenocarcinoma; the actual incisional approach needs to be individualized on the basis of the surgeon's experience, the location of the tumor, and the body habitus of the patient. The single most significant advance in the technique and its influence on patient survival were pointed out in 1968 by Robson,[65] who maintains that his improved survival rate is due to the combination of early ligation of the renal artery and vein, complete removal of the perinephric envelope (en bloc), and surgical extirpation of the lymphatic field, which extends from bifurcation of the aorta to crus of the diaphragm. Most surgeons have adopted the first two principles and term this procedure radical nephrectomy; however, there is still no general acceptance of the need for excision of the lymphatic tissues. The authors are convinced that this is an essential part of the procedure, and our limited 5-year survival experience has shown dramatic improvement in overall survival. In addition, some 17 percent of specimens have shown lymphatic involvement.

Whichever approach the surgeon elects to use; the foremost principle in the surgery of renal tumors is early location and ligation of the renal vessels. It is important to obtain control of the artery first. If the vein is occluded early in the dissection, then congestion of the kidney and the fragile peripheral veins occurs. Usually it is possible to mobilize and retract the vein that will overlie the artery. At this stage of the operation the preoperative angiogram proves its worth; one can search for the one or more arteries that have been demonstrated. Caution in handling of the vein is also important as unsuspected lumbar vessels or other venous abnormalities may be present, particularly on the left side. If one of these is injured, troublesome bleeding may occur.

The thoracoabdominal approach has the advantage that it gives a wide exposure to the proposed operative field, so the size of the tumor is of little consequence. It is particularly applicable in the patient with an upper pole mass. Also, it allows a planned simultaneous resection of a solitary pulmonary metastasis. The disadvantage is that it cannot be used when there is significant intrathoracic disease or borderline pulmonary function.

There are several modifications of this technique, the most popular of which are those described by Nagamatsu et al.[55] and Turner-Warwick.[81] The techniques that they use to increase the exposure involve creating chest flaps by subperiosteal resection of the rib angle or rib disarticulation. These extra touches are not usually necessary if the approach is through the bed of the 11th rib and the incision is carried well onto the anterior abdominal wall with division of the ipsilateral rectus. Most surgeons begin each one of the foregoing approaches by opening the abdominal cavity first so that thorough exploration can be carried out. Not infrequently, this part of the incision will be perfectly adequate. This has led many surgeons to plan only an abdominal incision for nephrectomy. This may be of a "chevron" type, modified Kocher, or even a long midline. Such a transabdominal incision should be planned so that it can be extended into the chest in order to gain the necessary exposure.

A few surgeons use the approach either through the bed of the 12th rib or via a subcostal pathway, which may be useful in a thin patient with a lower pole tumor. However, it always involves considerable mobilization and manipulation of the kidney before securing the renal pedicle. If there is any development of large venous collaterals (these are friable and bleed easily), then the operative procedure becomes tedious and hazardous. In our opinion, there is little place for this approach to the management of renal cell carcinoma.

As can be seen from the foregoing, surgical excision must be extremely aggressive as it is the only real method available. All other methods are at best palliative. It is extremely difficult to predict the biological behavior of this tumor. Some patients have had primaries that proved inoperable because of the patient's condition, and survival times of up to 15 years have been recorded. On the other hand, there have been patients who have had palliative or apparent curative nephrectomy in whom the secondary did not appear until 25–30 years later.[64]

SURGICAL ADJUNCTS

Recent work has demonstrated that the hazards of surgical manipulation of a vascular tumor can be decreased considerably by preoperative occlusion of the renal artery. One group used an intra-arterial balloon catheter,[45] whereas others are using the Seldinger percutaneous technique to introduce autologous clot or shredded absorbable gelatin sponge to produce infarction.[10] This decreases the necessity for initial ligation of the artery and attention can be directed primarily to the venous supply.

In patients who are unsuitable candidates for surgery, the above technique has also been used in lieu of nephrectomy as a method to control the primary lesion and in hope of stimulating an autoimmune response. Such an approach, although interesting, has not been used sufficiently often to allow study of the immunological response of the patient to autonephrectomy.

Preoperative radiotherapy. Several investigators have advocated the use of preoperative irradiation in the management of renal cancer. Until recently, there has not been a great deal of enthusiasm for such an approach because of the theoretical disadvantage of treating a cancer without a tissue diagnosis. However, the diagnostic accuracy of investigational techniques is now such that it is feasible to submit patients to a course of preoperative radiotherapy. So far, clinical trials have not been in progress long enough to say whether or not long-term survival is improved by preoperative radiation. However, there is little doubt that in certain patients a preoperative course of radiotherapy (3000–4000 rads) to the kidney in 4 weeks and surgical exploration at 6 has markedly decreased the vascularity of the tumor. Isolated reports have also shown that sometimes an apparently inoperable patient can be made operable. At this time, this modality should probably be reserved for cases in which an extremely vascular tumor is present and one is endeavoring to make the surgical procedure somewhat easier.

Postoperative radiotherapy. There is some evidence that postoperative radiotherapy has a beneficial effect on survival statistics. This has usually been used only when there has been extracapsular invasion.[64] Not all surgeons agree that this adjunctive therapy is entirely satisfactory or indeed desirable because liver damage and late liver failure may develop.

Chemotherapy. The use of chemotherapy for the management of metastases from renal cell carcinoma has proven particularly disappointing. However, Bloom[9] in England has had good results using medroxyprogesterone (Provera®) 100 mg t.i.d. He points out that patients show early clinical improvement before there is objective evidence of response. The reader should be reminded that no response has ever been achieved until nephrectomy was undertaken. Also, bony metastases seem to be remarkably resistant to all forms of therapy. A variety of nonhormonal therapies has been used, but none has been particularly effective. A number of cooperative clinical trials are now being carried out in this area.[78]

Immunotherapy. The known biological behavior of hypernephroma and its apparent unpredictable behavior seem to suggest strongly that the host-versus-tumor relationship is real. It is important to remember that the concepts developed by the Hellstroms in regard to blocking and unblocking serum factors were originally derived from a study of renal tumors in hamsters. It would seem, therefore, that as these concepts are refined, immunological manipulation of the host may have an important role to play.[35] Some work in this field has recently been reported, but it has not been established as an effective treatment method.[72]

SPECIAL MANAGEMENT PROBLEMS

Involvement of renal vein and vena cava. Ten percent of patients with hypernephroma show venous involvement at the time of surgery. Therefore, inferior venacavography should be a routine part of the preoperative workup. Initially, many investigators felt that venous invasion was an extremely ominous finding. However, the work of Skinner and his colleagues[71] has brought this time-honored concept into considerable question. Recently, an increasing number of patients with vena caval involvement have been reported to have long-term survival after surgical exploration.

A few patients with total apparent obstruction of the vena cava have been salvaged after heroic surgery because the tumor thrombus that grows out from the renal vein not infrequently invades only the ostium. Throughout the remainder of its course, the thrombus may adhere to the endothelium without invading the vessel wall.

The danger during any surgical resection of renal carcinoma is that the large tumor thrombus may become dislodged and result in death from pulmonary embolus. Control above the level of the distal tip of the thrombus must be established early in the operation if at all possible.

This problem can be approached in two ways. The first is by placing the patient on extracorporal bypass, opening the auricle, and by means of combined dissection from above and below, evacuating the thrombus from both the vena cava and the atrium. The thrombus is then brought out through a large venotomy in the inferior vena cava (IVC), and the retaining renal vein and its ostium are excised. The venous defects are then closed, and radical nephrectomy is carried out as described earlier. Another approach advocated by Fried is to make use of the fact that if one raises the intrathoracic and superior vena caval pressure, it is unnecessary to open either the heart or chest cavity. If the cava itself is involved and a good collateral circulation has developed through the azygos and hemiazygos veins, a few workers have resected the involved portion of the cava. The left renal vein can be ligated because of the good collateral circulation present.

Solitary kidney. Carcinoma arising in a solitary kidney provides a real problem in management. Some surgeons have carried out partial nephrectomy in situ; whereas others have removed the kidney from the body (so-called bench surgery), perfused the kidney, and performed the delicate extirpative surgery required before replantation.[29,77] Others have carried out total extirpation and performed renal transplantation at a later date.[30,77]

RENAL PELVIC TUMORS

Painless hematuria usually prompts the evaluation that leads to the diagnosis of renal pelvic tumors, which constitute approximately 12 percent of upper urinary tract malignancies. About one-third of the patients exhibit flank pain, and a mass is present in one-fifth. These symptoms and signs are sometimes masked by the presence of bladder tumors. These two conditions can and do coexist, so that the possibility of an upper tract tumor "seeding" in the bladder should always cross the alert clinician's mind, particularly when a bladder tumor recurs near the same ureteral orifice as the previous tumor.[5,41]

Eighty percent of renal pelvic tumors are transitional cell papilloma in type, and these are more common in men. Squamous cell carcinoma occurs mainly in women, and approximately 50 percent of these lesions are associated with a stone.

There is some evidence that the metabolites of tryptophan play a role as carcinogenic agents[57] (see section on etiology of bladder cancer, page 368). Recent reports from Yugoslavia have also implicated phenacetin abuse as a cause of transitional cell carcinoma.[3]

Diagnosis

The diagnosis of renal pelvic cancer is usually based on the appearance of a filling defect on intravenous pyelogram that is confirmed by retrograde pyelography. The differential diagnosis from a nonopaque stone or blood clot may sometimes be difficult. Urinary cytological examination is helpful as it is usually positive, and the accuracy of this study can be increased by submitting saline washings obtained from the pelvis at the time of retrograde studies. The recent introduction of a brush that can be passed up the ureter to obtain cytology specimens will certainly enhance our diagnostic abilities.

Arteriography sometimes demonstrates an enlarged tortuous pelviureteric artery, tumor blushing, and very rarely, neovascularity. This study needs further refinement before it is used routinely in known pelvic tumors. It is an essential procedure, however, if the differential diagnosis between a pelvic tumor and an intrarenal tumor has not been established.

Treatment

Nephrectomy and ureterectomy, along with a cuff of bladder, has been the traditional approach to patients with transitional cell carcinoma of the kidney. This procedure requires extensive incisions, and the advantages of single and double incisions have been discussed by Culp.[24] The only cures recorded have been achieved by this radical approach.

Patients with squamous cell carcinoma are usually treated by nephrectomy and partial ureterectomy. This approach is possible because local recurrence in the ureteral stump has not been a problem.

The prognosis depends on the cell grading (75 percent of patients with low-grade tumors are alive after 5 years, whereas the poorly differentiated tumor is associated with an extremely poor prognosis[41]). Follow-up care must always involve repeat urinary cytological examination because this tumor is notorious for its bilaterality or recurrence in the bladder. Local recurrence is also possible and should always be searched for.[5]

Palliative resection may be necessary even in the presence of metastases to relieve pain, severe bleeding, or infection secondary to obstruction.

Unfortunately, radiotherapy and chemotherapy have not been shown to be of much help in the management of this tumor.

URETERAL TUMORS

It is important to remember that ureteral tumors are associated with renal pelvic tumors far more often than they occur as a single entity. Ureteral tumors are rare, but when present they usually occur in the lower ureter.[5,17]

Diagnosis

The presenting symptoms are often owing to the secondary effects of obstruction and may include a dull pain in the loin, fever, or urinary tract infection. Occasionally renal colic is caused by a blood clot, but, as always, a major symptom is hematuria. The diagnosis usually becomes clear when an intravenous pyelogram demonstrates an intraureteral filling defect. Nonfunction on a pyelogram used to be considered one of the characteristics of this problem. That is not so today because of the almost routine use of high-dose or infusion pyelograms. When a retrograde pyelogram is attempted the lesion often causes the catheter to loop back on itself.

Urine cytology is often positive, and this yield can be increased by using ureteral washings, retrograde brushing, or both. With hematuria, the patient must always be cystoscoped, and this aids in lateralization of the disease process.

Treatment

Surgical excision is the treatment of choice, a nephroureterectomy with a cuff of bladder being the standard method.[24] However, there has been a recent resurgence of interest in attempting local excision.[26] The advocates of this latter approach have pointed out that the tumor is multifocal and may subsequently occur on the opposite side. Also, survival is clearly dependent on the grade of the tumor. On the basis of the available evidence, radical surgery seems to be the treatment of choice, although highly selected patients will benefit from a more conservative approach. Patients with bilateral tumors are particularly suitable as these tumors are, fortunately, clinically low grade.

Ureteral tumors are highly radioresistant and chemotherapy has been of no benefit in this disease.

BLADDER CANCER

Bladder cancer accounts for 4–5 percent of all new cancers.[68] It was estimated that in 1975 there were over 28,700 new cases of bladder cancer in the United States with over 9400 deaths. The disease is three times more prominent in men than in women and is four times more common in whites than in nonwhite persons in the United States. The age distribution reveals a peak in persons 75–84 years of age, and 80 percent of these tumors occur after age 50.

Etiology

The known and suspected causes of bladder cancer are grouped into four categories: (a) industrial chemicals; (b) metabolites of foodstuffs; (c) tobacco tar; and (d) chronic mechanical irritation or infection.[3]

In 1894 Rehn noted the occurrence of bladder cancer in men working in a dye factory manufacturing fuchsin. The aniline employed in the process was considered to be the etiologic agent. It is now felt that these tumors were caused by 4-aminobiphenyl, a carcinogen present in aniline residues. At least four compounds are known to produce bladder cancer: b-naphthylamine; 4-aminobiphenyl; 4-nitrobiphenyl; and 4-benzidine.

Metabolism of the essential amino acid tryptophan leads to the excretion of substances that have been demonstrated to produce transitional cell tumors in animals.[57] Some patients with bladder cancers have been noted to excrete excessive quantities of these substances, but it has been difficult to prove that these are individually carcinogenic in man, and inhibition of excretion of these substances has not proven to be beneficial in the prophylaxis of bladder cancer.

The incidence of bladder cancer is high among tobacco smokers. Most of the reports indicate that this problem is confined to cigarette smokers, but the evidence is circumstantial. Other conditions affecting the bladder which give proliferative lesions that have a high association with the development of bladder cancer are cystitis follicularis, cystitis glandularis, leukoplakia, and exstrophy. Five to twenty percent of patients with *Schistosoma haematobium* involvement of the bladder develop cancer. Schistosoma in bladder cancer is usually reported from Egypt, where as many as 90 percent of the inhabitants have been reported to harbor the parasite.[21]

Pathological Type

All but 3–4 percent of bladder tumors originate in the transitional cell epithelium. Transitional cell carcinoma of the bladder occurs in approximately 90 percent of the patients, with squamous cell carcinoma accounting for 6–7 percent and adenocarcinoma 1–2 percent.[40]

Transitional cell carcinoma may be very small and papillary in character, but may be multiple, large, and sessile. The surface may be intact or ulcerated, encrusted, and bleeding.

Squamous cell carcinoma is usually sessile, ulcerated, and sometimes necrotic.

Adenocarcinoma of the bladder appears grossly as transitional or squamous cell and must be differentiated microscopically.

All tumors are graded histologically based on the degree of cellular anaplasia.[13] In transitional cell carcinoma, the 5-year survival for patients with a grade I or well-differentiated tumor is much better than that of patients with a grade III or poorly differentiated tumor. There is no significance in the grading of squamous cell and adenocarcinomas as they pertain to prognosis.

In 1946 Jewett and Strong[38] reported on their observations in autopsy materials. They found that as the tumors were confined to the mucosa and submucosa, all patients were potentially curable. On the other hand, if tumor had extended through the bladder wall and into the perivesical fat, cure was possible in only 26 percent of patients.

Diagnosis

Painless gross hematuria is found in 75–85 percent of patients.[48] As the tumor enlarges, other symptoms such as frequency, urgency, burning, or decrease in caliber or force of the urinary stream may become present. Such symptoms may be secondary to infection in the bladder or they may be irritations caused by the tumor. As the tumor progresses, suprapubic pain and mass may become prominent, leading to signs of uremia associated with obstructive upper urinary tracts. A patient with bladder cancer may have only one minor episode of gross hematuria. Cystoscopic examination is imperative in patients with an episode of gross hematuria in order to rule out an early, low-grade, low-stage cancer.

CYSTOSCOPY

At the time of cystoscopy, if a bladder tumor is seen it should be described and drawn accurately; tumor location, character, number, and distance from ureteral orifices or bladder neck should be noted.

We feel that the tumor should be biopsied under anesthesia since only superficial cup biopsies can be performed without anesthesia. Bleeding may occur during biopsy, and fulguration of bleeding points may be necessary. It is important also that a rectal and bimanual examination be done at the time of the anesthetic examination of the bladder. Palpation of a hard indurated mass is usually a sign of an advanced tumor and a poor prognosis.

At the time of the biopsy and resection, it is important that the extent of the tumor in the bladder be evaluated. It is best to submit separate biopsies from the depth of the bladder wall where obvious tumor has been resected, and in areas containing no obvious tumor, mucosal biopsies should be taken to look for changes of carcinoma in situ.

Cytologic examination of the urine is an important adjunct to the diagnosis during follow-up of these patients. The routine urine Papanicolaou smear can give very poor results if the freshly collected urine is allowed to stand in the patient's room, hospital floor, or physician's office for several hours before reaching the cytologic labotatories. Urinary cytology on voided urine from an outpatient or inpatient is a waste of time and money if the collection is not quickly and accurately processed. Cytologic examinations of the urine can be of great benefit in the followup of patients if urine is obtained at the time of cystoscopic examination and placed directly into fixatives or if bladder washings using saline are obtained and processed quickly. Bladder washings using normal saline can be easily obtained by attaching the syringe to the endoscopic instrument or catheter and irrigating in and out of the bladder four to five times with approximately 30–60 cc of fluid. This fluid can then be submitted for cytologic examination. This procedure, however, is not a substitute for a cystoscopic examination.

RADIOLOGICAL STUDIES

An intravenous urogram is an important step in the preoperative evaluation of patients with bladder carcinoma. The urogram indicates the functional status of the kidneys and the possibilities of ureteral obstruction. The cystogram can be helpful in the evaluation of intraluminal filling defects and bladder wall invasion with use of a triple-phase contrast study. In this study 50–100-cc aliquots of contrast material are instilled into the bladder, and repeated exposures are obtained. By studying three exposures on the same film with the bladder containing increasing amounts of contrast material, one can assess fixation of the bladder wall and the possibility of invasion. Pelvic arteriography has been used in conjunction with perivesical and intravesical gas. Characteristic vascular changes showing increase in vessel size and increased tortuosity or displacement can suggest characteristic tumor staining. We have not found lymphangiography to be of value.

Staging (Fig. 11-2)

Marshall[47] examined carefully 104 surgical specimens obtained after total pelvic exenteration or radical cystectomy and compared the preoperative estimate of the extent of the tumor against that actually proven

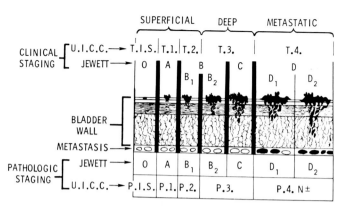

Fig. 11-2. Diagram outlining clinical and pathological staging of bladder cancer according to Jewett compared to staging classification of the International Union Against Cancer (UICC) (Published Atlas Tumor Pathology—Tumors of the Urinary Bladder, AFIP Washington, D.C., 1974).

to be existent. He found that careful assessment of the patient resulted in accurate preoperative staging with regard to whether or not the tumor extended more or less than half way through the bladder wall. The staging criteria as described by Jewett and Strong in 1946[38] (Jewett 1952) and modified by Marshall in 1952[47] are used extensively in the United States. Stage 0 is tumor localized only to the mucosa; stage A is limited to the submucosa; stage B1 indicates that the tumor has invaded the bladder muscles but is less than half way through the bladder wall; stage B2 tumor extends through the bladder muscle but does not invade the perivesical fat. Stage C indicates perivesical fat involvement or involvement of the capsule of another organ. In stage D1 tumor spreads to the pelvic nodes, invades the pelvic wall or rectus muscles, or both. The disease is present extravesically but is below the sacral promentary and medial to the psoas muscle. Stage D2 exists when the tumor has spread beyond these limitations and is outside the pelvis and immediate bladder area.

Bladder cancer usually grows slowly, spreading by direct extension through the bladder wall and into the tissues surrounding the bladder. From here it can spread into adjacent organs or by way of veins or lymphatics through the regional pelvic lymphatics near the pelvic and abdominal blood vessels. Bladder cancer can grow into the prostate, seminal vesicles, ureter, perirectal tissue, rectum, cervix, and vagina. Metastases occur most often in the regional lymph nodes, lungs, liver, and bone.

Gross characteristics are important in that the large papillary tumor having a small peduculated pedicle may be only superficially infiltrated and be a low-stage lesion. However, the larger the base the more opportunity there is for invasion of the bladder wall and therefore dissemination and spread of tumor cells. The biologic potential of a tumor may also differ in different portions of the tumor. In addition, the same apparent histological type of tumor can behave differently in different patients. A seemingly low-grade, low-stage tumor may undergo rapid recurrence and infiltration in one patient, whereas in another patient it may have little biologic potential.

Treatment

The appropriate treatment of a particular patient with bladder carcinoma can be confusing. A careful and thorough examination of the patient will allow for the choice of the treatment plan designed to give the best results and highest rate of cure. The therapy chosen depends on the clinical stage of the tumor and the biological potential of the tumor as determined by its microscopic appearance. A superficial, multifocal, and poorly differentiated tumor may require more radical therapy than a solitary, superficial, and well-differentiated carcinoma. Table 11-1 outlines methods of therapy that we think give the best results when correlated with the clinical stage.

SUPERFICIAL TUMORS

The patient with a single superficial papillary carcinoma is best managed by transurethral resection. This may also apply to a patient with multiple tumors located on the lateral or posterior bladder or on the base of the bladder. Tumors in the dome of the bladder may be difficult to reach transurethrally. These patients may be best managed by suprapubic cystostomy and excision of the neoplasm, if the surgeon feels that adequate removal by the transurethral route cannot be obtained. Careful follow-up examinations with repeat cystoscopy every 3 months for 1 year, every 6 months for 5 years, and every year thereafter are necessary in order that any residual or recurrent tumors may be promptly found and the appropriate therapy instituted.

The patient with rapidly recurring multifocal superficial tumors may benefit from more aggressive surgery; intravesical instillation of thio-TEPA may be of benefit in one-third of these patients, as outlined by Veenema et al.[82] The instillation of thio-TEPA may be therapeutic or prophylactic. The benefit of this therapy is that the entire bladder epithelium becomes bathed with the agent, so the entire bladder is treated. The main toxic effect of the drug is depression of bone marrow, manifested by leukopenia and thrombocytopenia. Radiotherapy appears to have a cumulative effect, and if thio-TEPA is used as an adjunct it must be adminis-

Table 11-1
Therapeutic Choices Available for the Various
Stages of Carcinoma of the Bladder

Superficial tumors
0, A
	Single—TUR B*
	Multifocal—TUR B
	       ? Thio-TEPA
	Papillomatous—TUR B
	       ? Thio-TEPA
	       ? Cystectomy
	       ? Irradiation

Invasive tumors
B1, B2, C
	Localized
	Low grade—Partial cystectomy
	       ? Irradiation
	
	Multifocal
	Large
	Bladder neck
	  to base—? Cystectomy
	       ? Irradiation
	       ? Adjuvant irradiation
	         plus cystectomy

Incurable tumors D1, D2	Irradiation Urinary diversion Chemotherapy

* TUR B, transurethral resections of the bladder lesion.

tered carefully. Before each period of instillation, a complete blood count—including white blood cells and platelets—should be obtained. A white blood cell count below 3000 or a platelet below 50,000 is an indication of toxicity, and therapy should be withheld until the bone marrow has recovered.

The suggested therapeutic program is the instillation of thio-TEPA 60 mg dissolved in 60 cc of sterile distilled water once a week for 4 weeks. After the instillation, the patient is asked to hold the solution in his bladder for 1–2 hours before voiding. Cystoscopy is repeated after the first 1–2 months of therapy. If no effect on the tumor has been noted, no additional therapy is indicated and it is a treatment failure. However, if there has been a partial effect on the tumor, a second course of thio-TEPA is given in 4 weeks. Data so far indicate that more than two courses of therapy are of no additional benefit.

Prophylactic treatment is for the patient who has had all visible tumor removed. Here 30–60 mg of thio-TEPA is instilled in 30–60 cc of distilled water at intervals of 2–4 weeks. Again checks for bone marrow depression are indicated. A course of therapy is for 4–8 instillations. If prophylaxis has been successful as indicated by no recurrent tumor on repeat cystoscopy, then repeat instillation every 6–8 weeks may be of benefit for a prolonged period of time.

INVASIVE BLADDER CANCER

Much controversy continues over the proper mode of therapy for invasive bladder cancer. Palliative therapy for the patient with metastases is less controversial and will be dealt with first. The patient with D1 or D2 bladder carcinoma may receive excellent palliation by urinary diversion consisting of either ureteroileal or ureterocolic diversion. Radiation therapy with tumor dose of 4000–5000 rads may control troublesome symptoms of hematuria, pain, and dysuria. Survival after palliative irradiation is poor, averaging 6–8 months. For the potentially curable patient (B1, B2, and C), the argument centers mainly around surgery, irradiation, or a combination of irradiation and surgery.

SURGICAL TECHNIQUES

The surgical procedures most often used in the management of invasive bladder cancer are segmental resection, simple cystectomy, and radical cystectomy. The advantage of segmental resection is that the patient is left with a portion of his bladder and therefore has urinary control. Simple cystectomy and radical cystectomy require urinary diversion by means of cutaneous ureterostomy, ureteral ileal conduit, ureteral colonic conduit, or ureterosigmoidostomy.

Segmental resection. Segmental resection is indicated if tumor is localized in one area of the bladder with an adequate margin of tissue that can be removed from around the tumor. An adequate cuff of 2–3 cm must be removed with the tumor and then enough bladder remaining to give a functional capacity. A patient with a 50–60-cc capacity bladder after segmental resection would be better off with total cystectomy and urinary diversion.

The operation is performed through a lower abdominal incision, usually from pubis to above the umbilicus. The peritoneum is opened and the abdominal contents inspected for metastatic disease. If liver or lymph node metastases are present, only palliative therapy is indicated. If no evidence of metastases is found, the abdominal contents are packed and the bladder opened in an area well away from the tumor. The tumor is then removed, including the entire thickness of the bladder wall and surrounding perivesical fat. The peritoneum is removed if the tumor is in the dome of the bladder. An important consideration is the spillage of tumor cells into the wound since tumor recurrences have been caused by such spills. Lavage of the bladder preoperatively with distilled water and during the operative procedure may decrease the incidence of viable tumor cells remaining.

The bladder and wound are closed with suprapubic drainage. Bladder healing is usually excellent and not prolonged especially if the mucosa and bladder wall remaining are free of tumor and healthy. This of course must be proven by biopsy before embarking on segmental or partial cystectomy. If the trigone and ureteral orifices are involved in the line of resection, in order to have a good margin around the tumor ureteroneocystostomy or transureteroureterostomy may be performed to reestablish the continuity of the involved upper urinary tracts.

With proper selection, partial or segmental resection of the bladder is an excellent procedure; however, if an adequate resection cannot be carried out and only a small portion of healthy bladder is remaining, we feel that radical cystectomy with urinary diversion is indicated.

Radical cystectomy. Radical cystectomy involves the total removal of the bladder with surrounding perivesical fat and the covering peritoneum.[61] In men the prostate and seminal vesicles are also removed. In women radical cystectomy includes removal of the anterior wall of the vagina, most of the urethra, and, for expediency, the tubes and ovaries. In addition, radical cystectomy means bilateral pelvic lymphadenectomy. This includes removal of the lymph node drainage from the inferior margin of the node of Cloquet in the femoral canal upward to the fossa of Marcelle. The fossa of Marcelle is approximately midway along the common iliac vessels. The obturator fossa is also dissected free of the lymph node–bearing tissue, as are the internal iliac vessels.

After radical cystectomy urinary diversion must be carried out. In most patients construction of an ileal or sigmoid conduit gives the best results. Ureterosigmoidostomy may be an acceptable alternative if no postoperative radiotherapy is thought to be necessary.

Simple cystectomy. A simple cystectomy with removal of only the bladder may be indicated in the patient with rapidly recurring superficial tumor or uncontrolled superficial papillary carcinoma. However, the patient with invasive carcinoma may well have tumor implants in the lymphatic system in the perivesical area, and, therefore, dissection and removal of the lymphatic drainage area immediately adjacent to the bladder are indicated.

RADIATION THERAPY

There is increasing evidence to show that radiation therapy as an adjuvant to surgery may improve the survival for the patient with invasive cancer.[62,82] Preoperative radiation presumably sterilizes microscopic or macroscopic disease in the lymph nodes and periphery of the bladder. This allows surgical removal of the main bladder tumor with no residual tumor remaining. A 3-year survival rate of 40–50 percent without evidence of disease is now being reported with the combined approach. Preoperative doses to the area of the bladder and regional lymph nodes of 4500–5000 rads in 5–5.5 weeks, followed in 4–8 weeks by cystectomy is a suggested treatment.

The survival rate following irradiation for clinical stage B2 and C lesions using 6000 rads is approximately the same as survival in patients following a simple or radical cystectomy alone. The usual cause of failure in both of these groups of patients is residual disease in the bladder or pelvis. If radiation therapy alone is not successful, the appropriate extirpative therapy must then be carried out in the patient who has undergone radiation therapy, and this latter therapy has a much higher risk of morbidity and mortality than the former. Palliative radiation therapy with tumor doses of 3000–6000 rads may be of benefit in terms of controlling bleeding, pain, and dysuria.

CHEMOTHERAPY FOR ADVANCED TUMOR

Long-term survival is rare once the tumor spreads beyond the confines of the bladder. Although improved survival may be possible by combined irradiation and early, more extensive surgery, one means of destroying metastases may be through the use of chemotherapeutic agents. Drugs used in patients with transitional cell carcinoma of the bladder have been 5-fluorouracil, bleomycin, adriamycin, and cyclophosphamide (Cytoxan®) and, more recently, cis-platinum compounds. The response of bladder cancer to chemotherapeutic agents has been far from encouraging.[20]

CANCER OF THE PROSTATE

Cancer of the prostate is the fourth leading cancer in men. Only cancers of the skin, lung, and colon and rectum account for more new cases of male cancer than cancer of the prostate. It is estimated that in 1975 there were more than 56,000 new cases of prostatic cancer in the United States with 18,700 deaths.[69] The mortality rate for non-whites is approximately twice as high as for whites in the United States. The urban incidence is only slightly higher than the rural rate. This would seem to indicate little relationship between prostatic cancer and industrial carcinogens. No relationship has been shown between prostatic cancer and smoking, use of alcohol, disease entities, circumcision, weight, height, blood groups, or hair distribution. Androgenic and estrogenic hormones produce a marked influence on cellular detail and growth of prostatic cancer, but there has been no available evidence to establish a causal relationship between hormonal changes and the development of malignant degeneration.

Approximately 75 percent of all prostatic cancers arise in the posterior lobe or lamella of the prostate.[50] Some 5–20 percent of these tumors are found during the removal of a benign adenomatous enlargement, confirming the origin of some tumors near the urethra. A multicentric origin of the neoplasm has been found also.[8,28]

Prostatic carcinoma is usually classified histologically as proposed by Broders[13] using the percentage of malignant cells to differentiate grades of malignancy. The tumor is graded histologically from well differentiated to anaplastic, depending on the most malignant area identified.[27]

In a series of 195 prostatic carcinomas seen in the Mayo Clinic, the distribution according to grade was as follows: grade 1, 19 percent; grade 2, 50 percent; grade 3, 27.5 percent; and grade 4, 3.5 percent.[60] There is general agreement among a number of investigators (Pool and Thompson,[60] Culp and Meyes,[25] and Schermer et al.[89]) that patients with grade 1 well-differentiated carcinoma survive much longer than those with less well-differentiated tumors. In the Mayo Clinic study only 5.6 percent of patients with grade IV cancer survived 5 years, compared to 60 percent with grade 1 cancer.

Carcinoma of the prostate metastasizes by direct extension, lymphatic invasion, or venous dissemination. Most carcinomas of the prostate when first seen have already exhibited invasion either locally or by metastatic spread. One of the reasons for this is that prostatic cancer is often asymptomatic until it reaches the advanced stage.

Diagnosis

Presenting symptoms in most men are infection or obstruction to urinary flow, which includes hesitancy, straining to initiate the stream, loss of force or caliber of stream, urgency, and dysuria. The best routine diagnostic test for clinical carcinoma of the prostate is the digital rectal examination.[88] Other methods that may be of benefit, but usually only in the late stages, are Papanicolaou smear of the prostatic fluid,[53] detection of elevated serum acid phosphatase levels,[31,32] or the presence of osteoblastic metastases on x-rays of lumbosacral spine. The clinical diagnosis may be confirmed by biopsy: perineal or transrectal needle biopsy or aspiration, open perineal or retropubic biopsy, or transurethral biopsy.

Staging (Fig. 11-3)

Therapy is based on the pathologic stage when the patient is first seen and as he is followed through the course of the disease.[83] Stage A or 1 prostatic cancer by definition is clinically latent. There are no signs or symptoms attributable to its presence. This patient is usually seen for benign prostatic enlargement and undergoes surgery for benign prostatic disease and incidental prostatic cancer found. Stage B or 2 carcinoma is still confined within the prostatic gland. The gland is enlarged and deformed, but the tumor occupies half of the prostate or less and is surrounded by normal prostatic tissue. Stage 3 or C means that the cancer has extended through the capsule of the prostate and there has been local invasion, usually in the area of the bladder neck or seminal vesicles. Stage D or 4 carcinoma of the prostate demonstrates bony or extrapelvic involvement.

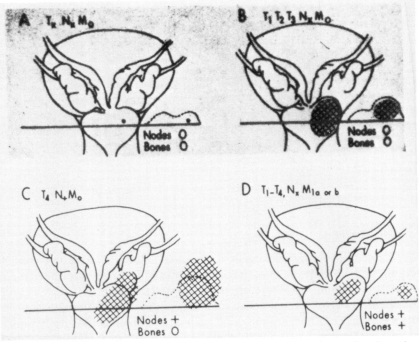

Fig. 11-3. Staging system for prostatic cancer which relates the American system of classification and the classification offered by the Union International Contre Le Cancrum (International Union Against Cancer [UICC]), Reprinted from Rubin P: JAMA 209: 1695, 1969.

Treatment

The treatment of prostatic cancer is generally based on the stage of the disease with consideration given to the histological grading.[37]   Since the prognosis for poorly differentiated tumor is not as good as that for well-differentiated tumor, we feel that a more radical approach may be necessary for therapy for the high-grade tumor.

The therapy for prostatic cancer should be divided into two parts: (a) curative therapy for prostatic cancer, which involves treatment of stage A and stage B cancer, and (b) palliation, which includes stage C and stage D cancer.   Some authors submit that treating a stage C patient with hormones causes the tumor to shrink to operability.[67]   This occurrence is more theoretical than actual since follow-up of these patients after curative surgery reveals no improvement in survival over the patients treated by palliative means.[84]

CURATIVE THERAPY

Curative therapy consists of surgery and irradiation.   A debate rages at this time between urologists and radiotherapists as to which gives the better cure rate.   As of this writing, curative surgery has withstood the test of time.[25]   Radiation therapy for the cure of prostatic cancer is relatively new, and even though its proponents are emphatic about the benefits of irradiation,[2] we do not feel that there have been sufficient cases followed for a sufficient length of time to say definitely that radiation is the treatment of choice.

There are two methods of surgical extirpation of operable prostatic cancer.   The first is by means of the radical perineal prostatectomy introduced by Young in 1905.[18]   The second is the radical retropubic prostatectomy—an approach familiar to most urological surgeons.[22]

Radical perineal prostatectomy has several advantages.   First, the prostate can be approached on its posterior aspect where the majority of prostatic cancer arises.   If further biopsies are needed for diagnosis, these can be easily accomplished by the open perineal route.   In addition, after the prostate has been removed along with the seminal vesicles, the anastomosis of the remaining bladder to the stump of the urethra proximal to the urogenital diaphragm is much more easily accomplished by the perineal than the retropubic route.   There is less blood loss and less postoperative incontinence by the perineal route.   Recovery is quick since there is no abdominal incision.   Impotency occurs in well over 90 percent of the patients by either perineal or retropubic route.

Disadvantages of the perineal procedure over the retropubic are that a lymph node dissection cannot be carried out through this incision, and, therefore, if lymphatic involvement has occurred the surgeon would not know this unless a suprapubic incision and lymph node biopsies had been carried out. However, suprapubic lymphadenectomy for involved nodes has never been shown to increase the 15-year survivalship known to follow the perineal operation in suitable cases. In addition nodes are involved in no more than 7 percent of the cases in the nodule stage.[36] The most difficult technical problems in the perineal operation are encountered during exposure. Here the rectum may be adherent to the prostate and an inadvertent opening made into the rectum. If the rectum and colon have been prepared preoperatively and the opening in the rectum is small, then a three-layer closure of the rectal rent may be accomplished and the radical procedure continued. However, if there is a large rectal opening and the bowel has not been prepared, the procedure should be halted because a rectal fistula into the urinary tract can be quite difficult to treat. In the radical retropubic prostatectomy, one of the most difficult technical problems is bleeding from the subpubic veins. After removal of the prostate, seminal vesicles, and ampulla of the vas, an anastomosis of the bladder to the stump of the urethra is more difficult than by the perineal route. Some surgeons advocate traction sutures through the reconstructed bladder neck down through the urethra and out the perineum to hold the bladder in place. We feel that a direct anastomosis of the reconstructed bladder neck to the stump of the urethra is better and gives better healing, less extravasation, and ultimately better urinary control. We feel that lateral mattress sutures using 2–0 or 3–0 atraumatic chronic catgut for the anastomosis are best. At least four sutures should be placed when doing the anastomosis after radical prostatectomy by either route. Catheter drainage for 10 days to 2 weeks is mandatory, and during the operative procedure the ureteral orifices should be identified and protected. This can best be done by passing a small #5 ureteral catheter up each side in order that the location of the ureteral orifices is known at all times.

The mortality rate for radical prostatectomy by either route is reported between 0 and 5 percent. Impotence is present in greater than 90 percent, and urinary incontinence in 3 percent.

Curative radiotherapy to the prostate has been advocated in recent years, especially by Bagshaw.[2] Radiation dosage of 6000–7000 rads has been advocated as curative. Methods used have been rotating platform or use of coplanar opposed fields with or without a supplemental perineal portal. Radiation sources have been a linear accelerator, betatron Van De Graaff generator, or more commonly a radioactive cobalt source. In addition, seeds containing radioactive gold or iodine may be placed directly into the prostate. The 5- and 10-year survival statistics as reported are small, but survivals appear to approach 60 percent in 5 years. Bagshaw feels that for radiation cure for carcinoma of the prostate, the disease must be restricted to the prostatic area. These modes of therapy for cure are used mostly for stage B lesions.

One widely discussed area in recent years has been how to treat patients who are found to have small areas of carcinoma at the time of resection for benign prostatic hyperplasia. Whitmore[85] has long maintained that these patients survive just as well with no therapy until the carcinoma has become clinically manifest as they do with curative therapy by irradiation or surgery when the tumor is first found. At the Medical College of Virginia we have followed this doctrine except for the young patient with a poorly differentiated occult tumor. Here we feel a more radical approach is necessary to obtain best results. The young man with a poorly differentiated tumor should be offered a radical prostatectomy with the alternative of radiation therapy. A number of these men chose radiation therapy since potency is maintained in 75 percent of the patients postirradiation.

PALLIATIVE THERAPY FOR INOPERABLE CARCINOMA OF THE PROSTATE

Hormonal antiandrogen therapy has been used since 1940 by either the administration of exogenous estrogens or castration.[12,18,66] There is little disagreement today as to the advantage of using this type of therapy in the patient with symptomatic metastatic stage D carcinoma. A favorable symptomatic and/or objective response can be anticipated in not less than 70 percent of the cases. That is, the patient will have improvement in pain, a sense of well being, weight gain, and decrease in urinary symptoms. Objective signs of improvement include lessening of anemia, decrease in serum acid phosphatase, and decrease in size of measurable tumor. There seems to be no advantage in the use of orchiectomy over estrogen therapy since they seem to be equally effective. Relapse may occur, and in general it does within 2–3 years. The relapsed form of the disease is usually hormone resistant. However, there may be indications in certain patients to increase or change the dosage of the estrogenic compound or to use other hormonal modalities such as medical or surgical adrenalectomy or hypophysectomy. A question has been raised by the Veterans Administration Cooperative Urological Research Group that patients on estrogen therapy may have a significantly higher incidence of cardiovascular disease and cardiovascular death. Cardiovascular complications from estrogen therapy seem to be dose related. The most common estrogenic compound used is diethylstilbestrol, and the dosage commonly used is 5 mg by mouth per day. It is apparent that serum testosterone levels can be reduced with 5 mg by mouth per day and be maintained for a varying period of time on the much lower dose of 1 mg per day.[42] There is a possibility that relapse or breakthrough of estrogenic therapy at low levels may occur quicker than if one maintains the 5-mg level. Certainly in the patient with known cardiovascular disease, or-chiectomy is the treatment of choice.

The management of the patient with inoperable stage C carcinoma of the prostate without evidence of metastatic disease continues to be de-bated. The use of hormonal therapy in these patients does not seem to in-crease longevity. Approximately 30 percent of the men presenting to urologists for treatment of carcinoma of the prostate are found in this group. We feel that radiation therapy extends to these patients the best chance for prolonged survival with minimal morbidity.

CHEMOTHERAPY

The patient with diffuse metastases who has suffered exacerbation of disease with bone pain and increasing debility after appropriate surgical, radiation, and hormonal therapy can be a real dilemma. The patient who previously exhibited a good response to hormonal therapy with orchiec-tomy and/or estrogen therapy may benefit from medical or surgical adre-nalectomy or hypophysectomy. The use of testosterone or parathor-mone followed by the injection of radioactive phosphorus (^{32}P) produces regression of bony metastases.[58] Chemotherapeutic agents can be used, and the most common drugs are cyclophosphamide, methotrexate, 5-FU, and nitrogen mustard. A new agent called estracycit [(phenolic bis-[2]-chloroethyl)-carbamate of estradiol-17-phosphate) has the in-triguing possibility of being able to use specific receptor sites for es-trogens within prostatic cancer tissue in order to carry other chemothera-peutic agents within the cancer cell.[54]

TUMORS OF THE TESTIS

All tumors of the testicle should be considered malignant. Most develop in men between the ages of 20 and 35, but they occur also in two other age groups and each type has a distinctive histologic pattern and behavior. Infants less than 1 year old develop embryonal carcinoma and teratoma, which appear to have a slightly different morphology than the same tumors in the adult, and the prognosis is much better. Patients over 50 more commonly develop spermatocytic seminoma and malignant lym-phoma. Only rarely is a testicular tumor benign.

The statistics on this group of patients can sometimes prove con-fusing. In the United States, the incidence is 2.1–2.2 per 100,000 males, but in the 15–34-year age group testicular tumors account for approxi-mately 12 percent of cancer deaths. Testicular tumor is seventh in inci-dence of malignancies among infants. It is alarming that there have been reports recently that mortality from testicular carcinoma has doubled when one compares 1944–1947 to 1958–1962. This disease is rare in American blacks.[51] These numbers, although confusing, indicate that routine testicular palpation should be the rule in all young men. This is particularly true since in recent years one of the major improvements in treatment for patients with cancer has been in the management of those with testicular cancer.

Traditionally, there has always been said to be a higher incidence of tumor in the maldescended testis (14 times greater). The interesting facets of this concept are that the tumor may not necessarily occur in the maldescended testicle, and surgical treatment of this condition does not alter this increased incidence. Significantly, there is, some suggestion that in those with maldescended testicles brought down before 6 years of age, the incidence of testicular tumor is not increased.[51]

Diagnosis

There is a history of painless enlargement of the testis in almost two-thirds of patients. The patient's attention may be drawn to this by a dragging sensation in the scrotum owing to the increased weight of the testicle on that side. On rare occasions a mass may be painful because of intratesticular bleeding. A few patients give a history of trauma or orchitis. If the tumor is elaborating chorionic gonadotropins, gynecomastia may appear. Symptoms from metastases may be lumbar pain, enlarged nodes causing abdominal or supraclavicular masses, cough, and hemoptysis, or generalized weight loss and cachexia.

Physical examination should initially be done with the patient standing as the increased firmness and weight of the affected testis is more readily appreciable in this position. It is important to realize that not infrequently there is a loss of testicular sensation. Occasionally, a nodule is present, but usually the testis maintains its typical ovoid shape. The cord structures usually feel normal and nontender, but a hydrocele is sometimes present (10 percent of cases). The scrotal skin is involved only late in the disease unless there has been prior surgical interference.[46]

The only form of biopsy that should ever be done is a high inguinal or radical orchiectomy. The cord should be isolated through an inguinal incision and cross-clamped with a rubber shod clamp *before* the testis and cord are freed to bring them out of the scrotum into the incision. Usually visual inspection will make the decision, and the cord should be divided as high as possible and tied off with a nonabsorbable suture and marked with a radiopaque clip to facilitate the planning of further therapy. An incisional biopsy should never be performed.[46] The histologic examination of the tissue after resection, and further studies, then form the basis for all future therapeutic decisions.

In addition to routine blood studies and chest roentgenogram, it is desirable to obtain serum and urinary levels of human chorionic gonadotropins. Serum alpha-fetoproteins are probably helpful in prognosis as well as in judging the therapeutic response in individual patients.

Staging

There is still some international disagreement as to nomenclature. However, in the United States, primary testicular tumors are usually classified into two types: germ cell (seminoma, embryonal carcinoma, teratoma, and choriocarcinoma) and stromal tumors (Leydig cell and Sertoli cell). Sixty percent of testicular tumors show a single cell type; the remainder are mixed.[51]

Although there is still no clear agreement on terminology, everyone agrees that staging is important in terms of prognosis and treatment. A useful staging classification is:

Stage A or IA   Tumor confined to the testis
         IB   Tumor confined to the testis plus microscopic foci in lymph nodes
Stage B or II   Spread to retroperitoneal lymph nodes but not above
Stage C or III   Clinical or pathological spread above the diaphragm or to distant body organs

It is important to understand that if there is clinical evidence of retroperitoneal metastases, a left supraclavicular node biopsy should be done. There will be a 15-percent positive yield from this study.

Treatment

Treatment at this time consists of surgery, radiotherapy, and chemotherapy in various combinations for the management of a patient. It is simpler to divide treatment into three phases.

PHASE I

There is universal agreement that high radical inguinal orchiectomy is necessary for treatment and further planning. Presently available information suggests that half of the patients with seminomatous tumors in stage A (IA) are cured by this procedure alone. (However, few surgeons would stop at this phase.)

PHASE II

There is now almost universal agreement that a patient with a stage A or B seminoma is best managed by irradiation of the retroperitoneal nodes (2000–3500 rads).[44] Whether stage A patients should receive further radiation to the mediastinum or chemotherapy is not yet answered. The cure rate in this group is over 95 percent. Stage B patients should probably receive prophylactic therapy to the mediastinum and supraclavicular area. Also, some surgeons advocate retroperitoneal node dissection for this group on the grounds that it will give more accurate staging and reduce tumor bulk. However, it seems to us that there is not enough evidence available to support this approach. Stage C (III) seminomas are managed with combinations of radiotherapy and chemotherapy.[44]

In patients with nonseminomatous germinal tumors, there is considerable disagreement as to the best therapeutic plan. All forms and variations of therapy must be compared with those described in the prospective study begun in 1958 by Staubitz et al.,[76] in which stages A and B were treated by radical bilateral retroperitoneal lymphadenectomy. There appears at this time to be, at best, equivocal evidence that radiotherapy alone or radical lymphadenectomy alone has established superiority over the other.[19] Only prospective randomized trials will establish the formal approach. The same might be said of the use of postoperative radiotherapy and the review by Staubitz et al.[76] should be consulted on this matter. Skinner[69] has recently presented his results in which he recommends using retroperitoneal node dissection combined with chemotherapy, relying mainly on actinomycin D and adding bleomycin and vinblastine (Velban®) if elements of choriocarcinoma are present.

There is little doubt that these various adjuncts have improved survival dramatically. The question at this time is which method offers the best prognosis. There are several ongoing national cooperative studies whose results may answer this. These protocols involve lymphadenectomy with postoperative radiotherapy or radiotherapy given in divided doses before and after surgery.[43] A similar approach using chemotherapy is also under study. The problem with the latter approach is that the actinomycin (the main drug) may interfere with subsequent use of radiotherapy.

As if the above disagreements were not sufficient, surgeons disagree as to whether the retroperitoneal dissection should be bilateral, as advocated by Staubitz et al.,[76] or unilateral, as Whitmore and associates[63] suggest. The reason for this disagreement is that the inevitable removal of the sympathetic ganglia bilaterally results in a total lack of seminal emission. Thus, the patient is infertile while still maintaining libido, erection, and orgasm. Proponents of the unilateral approach maintain that there is excellent removal of lymphatic drainage, and sparing of one sympathetic chain decreases the incidence of this postoperative complication.[11]

PHASE III

Germinal tumors that show evidence of metastasis beyond the retroperitoneum should certainly be managed aggressively with a combination of surgery, radiotherapy, and chemotherapy. The occasional long-term survival in this apparently hopeless situation justifies the effort involved.[72]

CHEMOTHERAPY

New drugs are continually being introduced in the management of germinal tumors. It certainly is true that remissions can be obtained with a variety of drugs, and the recent review by Carter and Wasserman[20] should be consulted for statistics on the more than 20 drugs that have been tried either alone or in combination. The recent reports of the success with *cis*-platinum type of drugs are also very encouraging.

Follow-up

Extremely close follow-up is mandatory. It is good management to obtain chest films at 1- or 2-month intervals for the first 18 months postoperatively. Pulmonary metastases are the commonest site for the appearance of these rapidly growing tumors, and early detection and treatment by the various modalities offer the best hope of cure. It is mandatory that there is close cooperation and exchange of ideas among surgeon, radiotherapist, and medical oncologist in the management of these tumors. This will, of course, provide optimal care, and on many occasions it will even produce cures in patients who would otherwise have been considered hopeless.[56]

CARCINOMA OF THE PENIS

Cancers of the penis are almost always of epithelial origin. Squamous cell carcinoma of the penis accounts for approximately 1 percent of all malignant tumors in the male.[16] The average age of patients with penile carcinoma is 62 years.[33] The disease has been reported in all races but is much more common in Asia and Africa where 10–15 percent of all male cancers are of the penis.

Etiology is unknown, but there is general agreement that circumcision performed in infancy gives almost 100-percent protection against the disease. Although rare, penile carcinoma has occurred in patients circumcised in infancy.[49]

Pathogenesis

A number of precancerous lesions of the penis can be recognized. Leukoplakia rarely involves the penis, but when it does it consists of a white, scaly lesion that causes some thickening of the skin. On microscopic examination there is hyperplasia of the squamous cell layers. Erythroplasia of Queyrat presents as a red, indurated area usually on the glans penis and may progress to ulceration. Microscopic examination reveals overdevelopment of the rete pegs, yet the basement membrane remains intact. There is an increase in vascularity but the epithelial cells are uniform in size even though a number of mitoses are usually present. Bowen's disease or carcinoma in situ may present as a raised, indurated, reddish plaque with an ulcerated center. Light microscopy reveals neoplasia of the epithelial elements with considerable hyperplasia of the squamous cell layers and mitotic activity.

Carcinoma of the penis is nearly always squamous cell and may initially present as a small ulcer, nodule, or verrucous lesion on the glans or inner surface of the prepuce. Advanced lesions may progress to large fungating, ulcerated lesions involving extensive areas of the penis. This tumor may rapidly invade and destroy the glans, prepuce, and portions or all of the shaft of the penis. Pathologically, the tumor may be well to moderately well differentiated and resemble squamous cell carcinoma occurring elsewhere. However, in some foci cells may be disorganized and vary in size, shape, and nuclei, with loss of normal maturation and polarity and demonstrate excessive numbers of abnormal mitoses.[52] Rare tumors are reported such as leiomyosarcoma, melanoma, Kaposi's sarcoma, and vascular tumors.[75]

Metastases occur through lymph channels that drain to the superficial and deep inguinal lymph nodes. The iliac nodes may also become involved. Enlarged lymph nodes are commonly found in these patients; some nodes may be inflammatory but others contain metastatic cancer.

Diagnosis

Beneath the foreskin, patients may notice an enlarging ulcer or mass that is painless unless secondary infection has become pronounced. If the foreskin cannot be retracted, the patient may complain of a purulent discharge coming from beneath the foreskin with a firm lump or mass in the region of the distal penis. Masses in the inguinal region may be noticed. These may be quite painful and tender, especially if they are inflammatory, although metastatic disease may also be present. In stage IV disease the metastatic lymph nodes may be quite large, ulcerated, and can cause death secondary to hemorrhage from the femoral vessels. If the diagnosis is suspected but marked phimosis is present so that biopsy cannot be obtained, a dorsal slit may be made in the foreskin so that the tumor can be exposed and a pathological biopsy made. If doubt exists as to the diagnosis, differential diagnosis is usually between cancer and syphilitic chancre, chancroid, condyloma acuminata,[9] or balanitis xerotica obliterans.

Staging

Penile cancers can be staged in four groups. In stage I the cancer is limited to the glans or foreskin. In stage II the cancer has invaded the shaft or corpora cavernosa, but there is no nodal involvement. Stage III indicates that the cancer has invaded the shaft of the penis, and lymph node metastases are clinically present. Stage IV indicates that inoperable lymph nodes, distant metastases, or both are present.

Treatment

SURGERY

It is important to have a positive tissue biopsy before instituting therapy for this tumor. With a small local stage I lesion, local excision or x-ray therapy may destroy the lesion. It is unusual, however, to find stage I tumor. More extensive lesions require more extensive resection with either partial penectomy or radical total penectomy. If partial amputation is selected, the amputation should be done at a level where there is a 2-cm margin proximal to the tumor. The technique of partial penectomy has been adequately described.[73] Several technical points are important in partial penectomy. First, a red rubber catheter placed around the base of the penis and clamped as a tourniquet eliminates virtually all blood loss. Second, the urethra should be left approximately 1 cm longer than the corpora cavernosa. This allows one to make a spatulated urethral meatus, which lessens the tendency to stenosis. Care should be taken also to leave a good stump of functioning penis. If enough stump remains that the patient can stand and void and direct his stream, this is adequate. However, if the stump of the penis is so short that voiding occurs across and down the scrotum, this will lead to scrotal irritation and an unhappy patient.

When the carcinoma has involved a large portion of the penile shaft, amputation with a cuff of healthy tissue would leave a short stump or no stump at all; therefore, total amputation of the penis is required. A circumferential incision is made around the base of the penis and if necessary extended over the pubis. Since most of these lesions are infected, a small rubber glove or large condom can be tied over the penis after the usual skin preparation, which is then repeated. After the skin incision has been made, all erectile tissue is dissected down to the level of crus of the corpora cavernosa. A transverse incision can be made in the corpora spongiosum to divide the urethra at least 2.5 cm proximal to the malignancy. A catheter can be inserted then through the urethra and into the bladder and sharp dissection used downward to free the proximal corpus spongiosum from the corpora cavernosa. The corpus spongiosum can be used and brought out in the perineum for a perineal urethrostomy.

To complete amputation of the penis, the suspensory ligament is divided dorsally and the dorsal artery and vein are ligated. It is not necessary to separate the crura from the attachments to the ischia pubic ramus, but where the corpora divide one can individually divide across the proximal corpora cavernosa and insure hemostasis with a continuous 2–0 chromic catgut suture to each crural stump. This completes the excision of the penis. The mobilized urethra can then be brought through an opening in the perineal area through an opening 1 cm in diameter made in the skin and subcutaneous tissue. The urethra can be sewn in place with 4–0 chromic catgut to form the new urethral meatus. A small 14 or 16 Foley catheter is left in place for straight drainage for 4–7 days.

LYMPHADENECTOMY

If the primary lesion is small and there is no palpable adenopathy in either groin region, radical resection of the inguinal nodes is not indicated. We do not feel that simultaneous lymphadenectomy adds anything to the operative procedure, and indeed the patient with an inflammatory lesion on his penis may have palpable, inflammatory lymph nodes in the groin. Three to four weeks later these lymph nodes may regress and no longer be palpable. If metastatic inguinal nodes are suspected, a lymphangiogram may be performed for better dilineation. If metastatic inguinal nodes are evident by either clinical examination or lymphangiography, radical inguinal node dissection must be done. This will require bilateral dissection as a staged procedure. One can do the classic radical inguinal dissection of both femoral and iliac vessels on each side through a long incision over the groin. The alternate method is to do bilateral superficial groin dissection and then later an exploratory laparotomy with bilateral iliac node dissections up to the bifurcation of the aorta. We find that this procedure using three incisions and two operative procedures seems to give less problems with skin flaps.

With this approach one can expect an overall 5-year survival from 50–70 percent.   If there are no histologic metastases, a 90-percent 5-year survival can be expected.   However, when histologic examination discloses involvement of regional nodes, 5-year survival ranges from 30–50 percent.[39]

CHEMOTHERAPY

Bleomycin alone or in combination has been used for the advanced case.   This drug can be somewhat toxic and can cause severe pulmonary complications, especially fibrosis.[85]

CANCER OF THE SCROTUM

Malignant tumors arising from the skin of the scrotum are rare. Squamous cell carcinoma of the scrotum was the first neoplasm in the human to be clearly associated with certain hydrocarbons found in soot, oils, and paraffin.[79]   The occupations of chimney sweeps, paraffin workers, and mule spinners have been definitely associated with this disease.   Patients are usually from low socioeconomic groups, and the tumors occur most often in the fifth and sixth decade of life.[14]   Malignant tumors of the scrotum are almost always of the squamous cell carcinoma variety, although one may encounter reticulum cell sarcoma, melanoma, rhabdomyosarcoma, leiomyosarcoma, and liposarcoma.   Cancers of the scrotum metastasize by lymphatic channels to the superficial inguinal and subinguinal nodes as with cancers of the penis but in contradistinction to tumors of the testicle.

Biopsy is necessary before any treatment.   The treatment consists of wide excision, and if lymph node metastases to the groin are proven by radiographic means or aspiration biopsy, then bilateral inguinal lymph node dissection is indicated.   If lymph node metastases are absent, the 5-year survival rate is 50 percent.   If metastatic disease has been found, the 5-year survival rate approaches 25 percent.

TUMORS OF THE SEMINAL VESICLES

Primary cancer of the seminal vesicles is extremely rare.   Most of these cancers are of the papillary adenocarcinoma variety with some being undifferentiated carcinoma.   Metastases have already occurred by the time of diagnosis in the majority of patients.   These tumors cause symptoms suggesting obstruction from an enlarged prostate but bloody ejaculation may be a symptom. Rectal examination reveals a boggy mass above the prostate involving the area of one or both seminal vesicles. Radical extirpative surgery may be indicated, but cures are infrequent.[7,74]

TUMORS OF THE URETHRA

Malignant tumors of the urethra are also extremely uncommon. They do occur more often in women than men. Those arising from the distal portion of the urethra are in general epidermoid or squamous cell carcinoma, and those arising more proximally are characteristically transitional cell carcinoma.

Symptoms are usually secondary to hematuria, bloody urethral discharge, palpable mass, or difficulty in voiding. At times these tumors may be complicated by periurethral abscesses, which lead to the formation of urinary fistulas. Tumors in the distal female urethra can often be cured by local excision, whereas those arising more proximally may require urethrocystectomy and urinary diversion. The same can be said for the male patient who has a distal urethral tumor and is cured by a partial or complete penile amputation, whereas tumors in the more proximal urethra and bulb may require cystoprostatectomy, excision of the urogenital diaphragm, and urinary diversion. Few cures are obtained in the patient with proximal urethral lesions, but the small distal urethral lesion is cured in approximately half of the cases.[30]

ADENOCARCINOMA OF COWPER'S GLAND

Adenocarcinoma of Cowper's gland is a very rare type of tumor: only approximately 12 definite lesions have been reported in the literature.[15] These tumors usually present as a perineal mass separate from the prostate. They metastasize early and are locally invasive.

REFERENCES

1. Arduino LJ, Nuesse WE: Carcinoma of Cowper's gland: Case report. J Urol 102:224–229, 1969
2. Bagshaw MA: Definitive radiotherapy in carcinoma of the prostate. JAMA 210:326–329, 1969
3. Baker R, Masted W: Tumors of the renal pelvis, ureter, and urinary bladder, in: Urology. New York, Harper & Row, 1975
4. Barringer BS, Woodward HR: Prostatic carcinoma with extensive intraprostatic calcification. Trans Am Ass Genitourin Surg 31:363–367, 1938

5. Batata M, Grabstald H: Upper urinary tract urothelial tumors. Urol Clin, North Am 3:1–79, 1976
6. Bennington JL: Cancer of the kidney—etiology, epidemiology and pathology. Cancer 32:1017–1029, 1973
7. Blath RA, Boehm FH: Carcinoma of the female urethra. Surg Gynecol Obstet 136:574–576, 1973
8. Blennerhassett JB, Vickery AL Jr: Carcinoma of the prostate: An anatomical study of tumor location. Cancer 19:980–984, 1966
9. Bloom HJG: Adjuvant therapy for adenocarcinoma of the kidney. Present position and prospects. Br J Urol 45:237–257, 1973
10. Bracken RB, Johnson DE: Sexual function and fecundity after treatment for testicular tumors. Urology 7:35–38, 1976
11. Bracken RB, Johnson DE, Goldstein SW, Ayata AG: Percutaneous transfemoral renal artery occlusion in patients with renal carcinoma. Urology 6:6–10, 1975
12. Brendler H: Therapy with orchiectomy, or estrogens, or both: Current cancer concepts. JAMA 209:28, 1969
13. Broders AC: The grading of carcinoma. Minn Med 8:726–731, 1925
14. Broders AC: Epithelioma of genitourinary organs. Ann Surg 75:574–604, 1922
15. Buck AC, Shaw RE: Primary tumors of the retrovesical region with special reference to mesenchymal tumors of the seminal vesicles. Br J Urol 44:47–50, 1972
16. Buddington WT, Kickman CJ, Smith WE: An assessment of malignant disease of the penis. J Urol 89:442–449, 1963
17. Burger R, Spjut HJ: Primary ureteral carcinoma. Urology 4:40—43, 1974
18. Byan DP: The Veterans Administration Cooperative Urological Research Group Studies of Cancer of the Prostate: Proceedings of the National Conference on Urologic Cancer. Cancer 32:1126–1130, 1973
19. Caldwell WL: Why retroperitoneal lymphadenectomy for testicular tumors. South Med J 62:1232, 1969
20. Carter SK, Wasserman TH: The chemotherapy of urologic cancer. Cancer 36:729–747, 1975
21. Case RAM: Some observations on the alleged casual relationship between infestation with Schistosoma (Bilharzia) haematobium and cancer of the urinary bladder in man. Report to World Health Organization, 1961
22. Ceccarelli FE, Thomas GJ: Techniques of radical retropubic prostatoseminal vesiculectomy and injection of Au 198. J Urol 87:951–963, 1962
23. Chisholm GD, Roy RR: The systemic effects of malignant renal tumors. Br J Urol 43:687–700, 1971
24. Culp OS: Anterior nephroureterectomy: Advantages and limitations of a single incision. J Urol 85:193–198, 1961
25. Culp OS, Meyes JJ: Radical prostatectomy in the treatment of prostatic cancer: Proceedings of the National Conference on Urologic Cancer. Cancer 32:1113, 1973
26. DeWolf WC, Rodgers R, Blackard C: Conservative management of ureteral tumors. Urology 4:44–49, 1974
27. Dixon FJ, Moore RA: Tumors of the male sex organs, in: Atlas of Tumor

Pathology, Sec. VIII Fasc. 316, Armed Forces Institute of Pathology.

28. Franks LM: The spread of prostatic carcinoma to the bones. Pathol Bacteriol 66:91–102, 1953

29. Gittes RF, McCullough DL: Bench surgery for tumor in a solitary kidney. J Urol 113:12–15, 1975

30. Grabstald H: Tumors of the urethra in men and women. Cancer 32:1236–1255, 1973

31. Gutman AB, Gutman EB: Acid phosphatase and functional activity of the prostate (man) and preputial gland (rat). Proc Soc Exp Biol Med 39:529–542, 1938

32. Gutman EB, Sproul EE, Gutman AB: The significance of increased acid phosphatase activity of bone at the site of osteoblastic metastasis secondary to carcinoma of the prostate. Am J Cancer 28:485–494, 1936

33. Hardner GJ, Woodruff MW: Operative management of carcinoma of the penis. J Urol 98:487–492, 1967

34. Holland JM: Cancer of the kidney—natural history and staging. Cancer 32:1030–1042, 1973

35. Javadpour N: Immunologic features of genitourinary cancer. Urology 2:103–108, 1973

36. Jewett HJ: Radical perineal prostatectomy in the treatment of carcinoma of the prostate, current controversies, in Scott R (ed): Urologic Management. Philadelphia, WB Saunders Co, 1972

37. Jewett JH, Bridge RW, Cray GF Jr, Shelley WM: The palpable nodule of prostatic cancer. JAMA 203:115–119, 1968

38. Jewett HJ, Strong GS: Infiltrating carcinoma of the bladder: Relation of depth of penetration of bladder wall to incidence of local extension and metastasis. J Urol 55:366–372, 1946

39. Knudsen OS, Brennhord IO: Radiotherapy in the treatment of the primary tumor in penile cancer. Acta Chir Scand 133:69–78, 1967

40. Koss LG: Tumors of the Urinary Bladder; Atlas of Tumor Pathology. Armed Forces Institute of Pathology, 1974

41. Latham HS, Kay S: Malignant tumors of the renal pelvis. Surg Gynecol Obstet 138:613–622, 1974

42. Mackler MA, Liberti JP, Smith MJV, Koontz WW Jr, Prout GR JR: The effect of orchiectomy and various doses of stilbesterol on plasma testosterone levels in patients with carcinoma of the prostate. Invest Urol 9:423–428, 1972

43. Maier JG, Sulak MH: Radiation therapy in malignant testis tumor: Carcinoma. Cancer 32:1217–1226, 1973

44. Maier JG, Sulak MH: Radiation therapy in malignant testis tumors: seminoma. Cancer 32:1212–1216, 1973

45. Marberger M, Georgi M: Balloon occlusion of the renal artery in tumor nephrectomy. J Urol 114:360–363, 1975

46. Markland C, Kedia K, Fraley EE: Inadequate orchiectomy for patients with testicular tumors. JAMA 224:1025–1026, 1973

47. Marshall VF: The relation of the pre-operative estimate to the pathologic demonstration of the extent of vesical neoplasms. J Urol 68:714–723, 1952

48. Massey BD, Nation EF, Gallups CA, Hendricks ED: Carcinoma of the

bladder: 20 year experience in private practice.   J Urol 93:212–216, 1965

49. Melmed EP, Pyne JR: Carcinoma of the penis in a Jew circumcised in infancy.   Br J Surg 54:729–731, 1967

50. Moore RA: The morphology of the small prostatic carcinoma.   J Urol 33:224–231, 1935

51. Mostofi FK: Testicular tumors: Epidemologic, etiologic, and pathologic features.   Cancer 32:1186–1201, 1973

52. Mostofi FW, Prive ER Jr: Tumors of the genital system.   Atlas of Tumor Pathology (Fascicle 8).   Armed Forces Institute of Medicine, 1973, pp 287–294

53. Mulholland SW: A study of prostatic secretion and its relation to malignancy.   Mayo Clin Proc 6:733–738, 1931

54. Murphy GP: Cancer of the prostate.   Cancer 32:1089–1091, 1973

55. Nagamatsu GR, Lerman PH, Berman MH: The dorsolumbar flap incision in urologic surgery.   J Urol 67:789–795, 1952

56. Nefzger MD, Mostofi FK: Survival after surgery for germinal malignancies of the testis.   Cancer 30:1225–1240, 1972

57. Oyasu R, Hopp ML: The etiology of cancer of the bladder—collective review.   Surg Gynecol Obstet 138:97–115, 1974

58. Pinck BD, Alexander S: Parathormone—potential radiophosphorus therapy in prostatic cancer.   Urology 1:201–206, 1973

59. Pollack HM, Goldberg BB, Morales JD, Bogash M: A systemized approach to the differential diagnosis of renal masses.   Radiology 113:653–657, 1974

60. Pool TL, Thompson GJ: Conservative treatment of carcinoma of the prostate.   JAMA 160:833–837, 1956

61. Prout GR Jr: Radical cystectomy—a photographic seminar of surgical procedures.   Warner-Chilcott, 4:No. 2, 1975

62. Prout GR Jr, Slack NH, Bross IDJ: Pre-operative irradiation and cystectomy for bladder carcinoma: IV.   Results in a selected population, in Proceedings of the Seventh National Cancer Conference, Los Angeles, California, Sept 27–29, 1972.   Philadelphia, JB Lippincott Co, 1973, pp 783–791

63. Ray B, Hajdu SI, Whitmore WF Jr: Distribution of retroperitoneal lymph node metastases in testicular germinal tumors.   Cancer 33:340–348, 1974

64. Riches E: The natural history of renal tumors, in: Tumors of the Kidney and Ureter.   Edinburgh, ES Livingston Ltd, 1964, pp 124–134

65. Robson CJ, Churchill BM, Anderson W: The results of radical nephrectomy for renal cell carcinoma.   Trans Am Assoc Genitourin Surg 60:122–126, 1968

66. Scott BW: Rationale and results of primary endocrine therapy in patients with prostatic cancer: Proceedings of the National Conference on Urologic Cancer.   Cancer 32:1119–1125, 1973

67. Scott WW, Boyd HL: Combined hormone control therapy and radical prostatectomy in the treatment of selected cases of advanced carcinoma of the prostate: A retrospective study based upon 25 years experience.   J Urol 101:86–92, 1969

68. Silverberg E, Holleb AI: Cancer statistics, 1975.   Worldwide epidemiology.   Cancer 25:2–21, 1975

69. Skinner DG: Non-seminomatous testis tumors: Plan of management based

on 96 patients to improve survival in all stages by combined therapeutic modalities. J Urol 115:65–69, 1976

70. Skinner DG, Colvin RB, Vermillon CD, Pfister RC, Leadbetter WF: Diagnosis and management of renal cell carcinoma. Cancer 28:1165–1177, 1971

71. Skinner DG, deKernia JB, Braver PH, Ramming KP, Pilch YH: Advanced
renal cell carcinoma: Treatment with xenogenic immune ribonucleic acid
and appropriate surgical resection. J Urol 115:246–250, 1976

72. Skinner DG, Leadbetter WF: The surgical management of testis tumors. J
Urol 106:84–93, 1971

73. Skinner DG, Leadbetter WF, Kelley SO: The surgical management of
squamous cell carcinoma of the penis. J Urol 107:273–285, 1962

74. Smith BA Jr, Webb EA, Price WE: Carcinoma of the seminal vesicle. J
Urol 97:743–746, 1967

75. Smith DR: General Urology, ed 8. Los Altos, Calif., Lange Medical Publication, 8 1975, pp 286–288

76. Staubitz WJ, Early KS, Magoss IV, Murphy GP: Surgical treatment of non-
seminomatous germinal testes tumors. Cancer 32:1206–1211, 1973

77. Stewart BH, Hewitt CB, Banowsky LHW: Management of extensively
destroyed ureter: Special reference to renal autotransplantation. J Urol
115:257–261, 1976

78. Talley RW: Chemotherapy of adenocarcinoma of the kidney. Cancer
32:1062–1065, 1973

79. Tucci P, Harlambidis G: Carcinoma of the scrotum: Review of literature
and presentation of two cases. J Urol 85:585–590, 1963

80. Turner-Warwick RT: The supracostal approach to renal area. Br J Urol
37:671–672, 1965

81. Van Der Werf MB: Carcinoma of the bladder treated by pre-operative irradiation followed by cystectomy, the second report. Cancer 32:1084–1088,
1973

82. Veenema RJ, Dedn AL Jr, Uson AS, Roberts M, Longo F: Thio-Tepa
bladder instillations: Therapy and prophylaxis for superficial bladder
tumors. J Urol 101:711–715, 1969

83. Veterans Administration Cooperative Urologic Research Group: Carcinoma
of the prostate: Treatment comparisons. J Urol 98:516–522, 1967

84. Whitmore WF: The natural history of prostatic cancer, Proceedings of the
National Conference on Urologic Cancer. Cancer 32:1104–1113, 1973

85. Williams RD, Blackard CE: Chemotherapy for metastatic squamous cell
carcinoma of penis: Combination of vinicristine and bleomycin. Urology
4:69–73, 1974

86. Wynder EL, Mabuck K, Whitmore WF Jr: Epidemiology of adenocarcinoma of the kidney. J Natl Cancer Inst 53:1619–1634, 1974

87. Young HH: Tumors of the prostate, in Karafin L, Kendall AR (eds): Lewis
Textbook of Surgery, vol 1. Hagerstown, Md., W.F. Prior Co, 1951

88. Young HH, Dans DM: Young's Practice of Urology. Philadelphia, WB
Saunders Co, 1926, p. 637

89. Schirmer HKA, Murphy GP, Scott WW: Hormonal Therapy of prostatic
cancer: a correlation between histologic differentiation of prostatic cancer
and the clinical course of the disease. Urol Digest 4:15, 1965

Hugh R. K. Barber, M.D.
and Taehae Kwon, M.D.

12
Management of Gynecologic Cancer

Exclusive of the ovary and the fallopian tube, carcinoma in the female reproductive system can be readily detected early by presently available
diagnostic techniques. The question that is raised (and rightfully so), if
indeed this is the situation, is why are cancers of the vulva, vagina,
cervix, and corpus not diagnosed at any early stage? Why have screening
programs failed to accomplish this? This fault must be shared by the patient as well as the doctor. Despite a considerable outlay of money, effort, and time, the publicity campaigns sponsored by private organiza-
tions as well as the federal government have failed thus far in their goal.
However, only a well-informed public and profession can work coopera-
tively together to search for cancer in its early, more curable stage. Each
doctor's office should serve as a screening clinic for detection of gynecologic cancer.

CANCER OF THE VULVA[34]

Cancer of the vulva accounts for only 1 percent of all cancers and 3 or
4 percent of all gynecological cancers. It is usually encountered late in
life; approximately 85 percent of cases occur after the menopause, particularly in the seventh decade.[19] Cancer of the vulva is rare in women before the age of 45 years and extremely rare in pregnancy. Unfortunately,
the malignant process is sometimes present and ignored by the patient
and/or physician for months or years before treatment.

Little is known of the etiology of cancer of the vulva. Often prior disease states have been present; i.e., leukoplakia, kraurosis vulvae, granulomatous disease, pruritus, pigmented lesions, chronic ulcer, syphilis, and radiation. Potentially malignant states including papillomatosis, erythroplasia, Bowen's disease, and Paget's disease may be present. The majority of cancers of the vulva prove to be squamous cell cancers; only rarely is an adenocarcinoma present, and when it is diagnosed, it usually arises in Bartholin's gland. Fibrosarcomas and myosarcomas have been reported. Mixed tumors, cylindromas, and malignant melanoma are other rare lesions and account for 1–2 percent of vulvar cancers.

Diagnosis

Since the vulva is so easy to inspect and biopsy, there is little excuse for delay in making a diagnosis. Approximately two-thirds of the patients complain of vulvar pruritus, which occurs several years before the onset of cancer and is associated with precancerous lesions (atrophic vulvitis, kraurosis). Cytology may help also in the early detection of a degenerating, precancerous lesion. The use of toluidine blue 1 percent followed by 1 percent acetic acid helps to identify areas at high risk. Studies in which the uptake of radioactive phosphorous was measured in vulvar lesions have been reported, also. Finally, biopsy and histologic examination are all important and should be carried out without delay with any lesion on the vulva that has not responded to medical treatment within 1 month.

The white lesions of the vulva must be viewed with suspicion until a definitive diagnosis is made by biopsy. The diagnosis of leukoplakia is nebulous and nonspecific. One must differentiate between lichen sclerosis et atrophicus, characterized by hyperkeratosis and epithelial atrophy, and hyperplastic vulvitis, a hyperkeratotic lesion with epithelial acanthosis, epithelial hyperactivity, and either dyskaryosis or actual anaplastic cellular changes. The first requires conservative symptomatic therapy and close observation, whereas the latter demands vigilance for malignant changes of the epithelial cells.

One should be especially vigilant for intraepithelial cancer in areas of hypertrophic leukoplakia (5–20-percent malignancy rate), Paget's disease (painful velvet red patches), and granuloma. The lesion is usually elevated, flat, and crusted with sharply defined outlines. The incidence is higher in the forties age group, in contradistinction to the increased median age seen in the group with invasive cancer of the vulva. The diagnosis of intraepithelial carcinoma, or Bowen's disease, is made with greater consistency when one frequently uses vulvar biopsy. The multicentric foci of this disease should not be forgotten.

Staging

The categories of carcinoma of the vulva employing the tumor-node-metastasis classification (International Union Against Cancer) is shown in Table 12-1. This staging system is useful for both planning therapy and estimating prognosis. The frequency of regional lymphatic metastasis is a key factor in planning appropriate therapy since this occurs in 40–50 percent of patients with invasive vulvar cancer.[62] It is found that between 26 and 30 percent have superficial node involvement, 13–15 percent have superficial and deep involvement, whereas another 3 percent have deep node involvement alone.

Treatment

A complete vulvectomy *without* node dissection is considered adequate therapy for noninvasive carcinoma. If thorough study of the specimen reveals invasive cancer, regional lymph node dissection is required at a later date.

Invasive cancer demands wide vulvectomy, bilateral superficial and deep node dissection, and resection of the contiguous organs involved in the process.[42] The survival rate following operation depends primarily on whether or not the regional nodes are positive for cancer. There is approximately 30-percent 5-year survival if the nodes are involved,

Table 12-1
TNM Classification—Cancer of the Vulva
(International Union Against Cancer)

Tumor:
- T-1:   Confined to vulva; <2 cm
- T-2:   Confined to vulva; >2 cm
- T-3:   Any size with spread to urethra and/or vagina and/or anus
- T-4:   Any size with infiltration of bladder mucosa, upper half urethral mucosa, rectal mucosa, or fixation to pelvic bones

Nodes:
- N-0:   No palpable nodes
- N-1:   Discrete, palpable, mobile groin nodes not clinically suggestive of metastasis
- N-2:   Enlarged, firm, mobile groin nodes clinically positive for metastasis

Metastasis:
- M-0:   No clinical evidence of metastases
- M-1a: Palpable clinically positive deep pelvic lymph nodes
- M-1b: Metastases beyond pelvis

whereas 70–80 percent of patients without lymphatic metastasis are free of recurrence or metastasis at 5 years. Other factors that influence the prognosis are the size of the initial lesion (more favorable if less than 3 cm) and its histologic character.

There is some debate as to how important it is to dissect the iliac (or deep) lymph nodes if the lower nodes show positive findings. Since the more extensive dissection greatly increases the morbidity and mortality of the operation, and since the percentage of cures is low even if the positive deep nodes are removed, some men (e.g., Twombly and TeLinde) question whether the additional risks may not cancel out the potential advantage of node dissection. In short, is there any net saving of lives with deep node dissection? The 5-year survival figures generally range from 0–3 percent when the deep lymph nodes are involved, but a large impressive series reported by Way shows a 20-percent 5-year figure when the iliac lymph nodes are involved.

RECURRENT CANCER OF THE VULVA

Several forms of therapy are suggested for the management of locally recurrent cancer of the vulva, but none has yielded impressive survival figures. Treatment includes radiation (either external irradiation or implantation of radioactive substances), cryosurgery, chemotherapy, laser beam, pelvic exenteration, and hemipelvectomy. When secondary surgery can be carried out, it is the form of treatment usually selected.

In those patients in whom considerable time elapses between the initial therapy and recurrence, it can be assumed that either the cancer is of low potency or the patient possesses a high degree of resistance. A well-differentiated cancer is more inclined to remain localized for a longer period of time and have a lower incidence of nodal spread than anaplastic cancer. In evaluating the series at the Memorial-James Ewing Hospitals, it was found that 6 patients (of 30 recurrent cases treated 5 or more years before) presented more than 5 years after initial therapy with recurrent cancer. These patients were treated by pelvic exenteration. Only 1 lived 5 years after secondary treatment, 2 died at 7 months, 1 at 6 months, 1 at 2 months, and 1 other lived only 2 years. None of these patients had lymphatic metastasis at the time of the exenteration. Of the 24 cases developing recurrence less than 5 years after initial therapy, there were three 5-year survivals, but none of the 10 patients in this group with lymphatic metastasis survived this interval.[12]

The operative procedure employed for recurrent vulvar cancer may require resection of a portion of the symphysis or pubic bone to obtain an adequate margin. Of the 37 patients requiring anterior (26) or total (11) pelvic exenteration for recurrent cancer of the vulva, 8 required resection of adjacent bone.

CARCINOMA OF THE VULVA AND PREGNANCY

Primary squamous cell carcinoma in the vulva is a disease of the aged. It is rare in the young and extremely rare in association with pregnancy. Our plan of management for patients who are also pregnant is as follows:

1. First trimester: radical vulvectomy and bilateral superficial and deep node dissection.
2. Second trimester: the same treatment as for the first trimester. However, it may be technically possible to do only the vulvectomy, and, if so, the node dissection should be completed after delivery.
3. Third trimester: if the lesion is small and will not interfere with vaginal delivery, this method of delivery should be permitted. Radical vulvectomy and node dissection should be carried out in the immediate postpartum period (2–4 weeks).

CANCER OF THE VAGINA[55]

Cancer of the vagina is extremely rare, comprising less than 1 percent of all genital malignancies. The ratio of cancer of the cervix to vaginal cancer is roughly 50:1. It is often difficult to tell whether the tumor arises primarily in the vaginal epithelium or extends to it from a primary locus in the cervix. When both are involved together, the cervix is considered the primary locus.

Cancer of the vagina has been found mainly in women over age 50 years. Recently an association between vaginal adenosis and adenocarcinoma has been shown in younger adult women whose mothers were taking diethylstilbestrol during pregnancy. This unusual relationship may alter the normal age distribution described.

Diagnosis

Premalignant lesions of the vagina should be sought especially in women with previous in situ or invasive carcinoma of the cervix. These people should be checked by frequent vaginal smear and Schiller iodine tests. The concept of primary multiple malignant conditions of the genital tract is now assuming general acceptance. Therefore, one should be especially vigilant in women who have had one genital cancer.

Vaginal cancer generally arises in the upper third of the posterior wall of the vagina and involves the rectovaginal septum early. The lesion may be missed when doing a speculum examination unless the speculum is rotated or a plastic speculum is used. The lesion begins as a superficial lesion associated with discharge and/or vaginal bleeding. Leukoplakia of the vaginal mucosa may be regarded as a precancerous lesion. Just as invasive carcinoma of the cervix is preceded by noninvasive (in situ) alterations, so is invasive carcinoma of the vagina. As the disease invades and spreads, the cancer usually destroys the cervix and then invades the parametria. Involvement of the vulva is rare, and spread to the lymph nodes is usually late.

Carcinoma of the vagina is usually of the epidermoid (or squamous)[37] type, but occasionally adenocarcinoma is seen. This may become more frequent as noted previously. When adenocarcinoma is diagnosed, it is important to determine whether the lesion is primary or is actually a metastasis from an unsuspected primary cancer elsewhere. In this regard cancer of the endometrium is prone to metastasize to the vagina and is almost always found on the anterior wall. Less often, secondary vaginal lesions may have their origins from the ovary, paraurethral glands, or gastrointestinal tract (especially the colon), or from hypernephroma or uterine choriocarcinoma. Since many alleged primary vaginal cancers are really metastases from an unsuspected primary cancer elsewhere, it is important to have a careful workup including biopsies and fractional uterine curettage.

Staging and Evaluation

A classification for staging of vaginal cancer is shown in Table 12-2. Excluded from this classification are secondary cancers in the vagina, cervical cancers involving the vagina, and malignant lesions extending into the vagina from the urethra or vulva.

Table 12-2
Staging Classification—Cancer of the Vagina

Stage	Description
Stage 0	Intraepithelial only (in situ)
Stage I	Limited to vaginal wall
Ia	<2 cm in greatest diameter
Ib	>2 cm in greatest diameter but less than entire vaginal wall in longitudinal axis
Ic	Involves entire vaginal wall in longitudinal axis
Stage II	Infiltrates paravaginal tissue but does not reach pelvic wall
Stage III	Extends to and fixed to pelvic wall
Stage IV	Extends beyond true pelvis or involves or extends to mucosa of bladder or rectum
IVa	Extends to or involves mucosa of bladder and rectum
IVb	Extends outside true pelvis to lymph nodes or other sites

In pretreatment evaluation of these patients, it is wise to carry out fractional curettage and cervical biopsies in addition to biopsy of the primary lesion in the vagina. Workup should also include sigmoidoscopy and cystoscopy as well as intravenous pyelography, barium enema examination, and standard assessment for distant metastasis.

Treatment

Since the 5-year survival rate in primary epithelial cancer of the vagina is approximately 45 percent with primary radical surgery with or without supplemental radiation, it behooves the gynecologist to make the diagnosis as early as possible.

GENERAL APPROACH

When carcinoma in situ of the vagina is found, simple excision of the lesion is all that is required. Surgical therapy is generally preferred for invasive vaginal cancer, but many gynecologic oncologists prefer radiation as the primary therapy. Our general approach to these lesions can be summarized as follows:

1. Upper two-thirds of the vagina:
   Stage 0. (carcinoma in situ or intraepithelial). Simple excision or total hysterectomy and total vaginectomy.
   Stage I. Radical hysterectomy, bilateral pelvic node dissection, and total vaginectomy.
   Stage II. Radical hysterectomy, bilateral pelvic node dissection with total vaginectomy. If an extenteration is required to encompass the cancer, primary therapy should be by radiation both external and intracavity. Careful follow-up must be established so that pelvic exenteration can be performed if the patient is not cured by radiation therapy.
   Stage III. Primary radiation therapy. The patient is evaluated in 6 weeks for consideration of radical surgical treatment if deemed necessary.
   Stage IV. Primary radiation, both external and intracavity. It may be necessary to divert the fecal and/or urinary stream before therapy. Primary pelvic exenteration is the treatment chosen if the disease remains central and extends into the bladder.
2. Lower third of the vagina:
   Stage 0. Simple excision or total hysterectomy and total vaginectomy.
   Stage I. Total hysterectomy and total vaginectomy plus radical vulvectomy and bilateral groin node dissection.

Stage II. Radical hysterectomy, bilateral pelvic node dissection, total vaginectomy, plus radical vulvectomy and bilateral node dissection. If pelvic exenteration is required, primary therapy should be by radiation, both external and intracavity. Careful follow-up is indicated to see if pelvic exenteration is indicated for uncontrolled disease.

Stage III. Primary radiation therapy with evaluation in 6 weeks for consideration for radical surgical treatment. In the event that radical surgery in the form of a pelvic exenteration or radical hysterectomy is needed, a radical vulvectomy and bilateral groin node dissection should be added.

Stage IV. Radiation therapy for those patients in whom surgery is not indicated. This therapy may be preceded by diversion of urinary and/or fecal streams. Primary exenteration is chosen for those patients whose disease is central and extends into the bladder causing a fistula and in whom the disease can be encompassed by this procedure. A radical vulvectomy and bilateral groin node dissection should be added.

RADIATION THERAPY

If radiation is chosen as the primary therapy for carcinoma of the vagina, this is usually based on the concept that control of the local disease is tantamount to cure.[27] If the lesion is in the vault, it is treated with a cervical tandem with ovoids applied to the vagina using radium. The total dose given is 8,000–10,000 rads to the tumor. With lesions in locations other than the vault in the upper vagina, a Lucite or Bloedorn vaginal applicator may be used with a total tumor dose of 8,000–10,000 rads. This is usually given in two or three applications at 1–2-week intervals, followed by external radiation of 3000 rads from an external cobalt source. With lateral wall lesions some physicians prefer a radon needle implantation, giving a total dose to the tumor of 3000 rads locally. This is followed by external cobalt beam, giving an additional 3000–4000 rads. This routine is also followed with urethral lesions. In lesions of the lower vagina, it is most important to limit the dose to the bladder and rectum to less than 5000 rads or severe complications may result. Finally, if large lesions of the vagina are found, it is perhaps best to use external cobalt as preliminary therapy before using local radium. Basically, one tries to achieve control of the disease (without harming contiguous organs) while still salvaging a functioning vagina.

So far as the prognosis is concerned, endophytic cancers have the worst outlook, with 15–20-percent 5-year survival regardless of therapy. With an exophytic lesion, there is a 75-percent likelihood of 5-year survival. The best prognosis as far as location is concerned is with tumors in the fornices, and lesions in the upper two-thirds of the vagina generally have better 5-year survival figures than those of the lower third. The size of the cancer is equally important in determining prognosis. Those that are less than 3 cm in diameter have a much better 5-year survival rate than larger lesions.

CLEAR CELL ADENOCARCINOMA
(MÜLLERIAN[45] TYPE) AND ADENOSIS

Herbst et al. reported 7 girls, 15–22 years of age, with adenocarcinoma of the vagina (clear cell or müllerian type) between 1966 and 1969.[45,46] Before this, they report that not a single case was recorded in the files of the Massachusetts General Hospital. Because these cases occurred within a brief period of time and were rather unique, a careful retrospective study of the patients and their families with matched controls was undertaken. The results of the study revealed a highly significant association between the treatment of their mothers with diethylstilbestrol during pregnancy and the later development of adenocarcinomas in their daughters.

In 1938 a synthetic nonsteroidal estrogen, diethylstilbestrol (DES), was introduced into clinical medicine. It was inexpensive, potent orally, and was used for a great number of hormonally associated problems including threatened abortion and the pregnant diabetic. As a result, thousands of women during the 1940s and early 1950s received stilbestrol for a variety of complaints and many for problems related to their pregnancy. With only 275 cases of vaginal and cervical clear carcinomas reported to date, it is obvious that not every female fetus whose mother took stilbestrol is affected. Futhermore, teen-age patients are reported with this type of cancer in whom it has not been documented that their mothers took stilbestrol. The natural estrogens have apparently not been associated with this problem. However, other nonsteroidal estrogens—i.e., dienestrol (nestrol®, synestrol®), hexestrol, and benzetrol—have also been associated with this type of vaginal cancer.

The incidence rate for the development of clear cell carcinoma of the vagina or cervix is approximately 0.1 percent in the female fetus whose mother took stilbestrol. However, about 80–90 percent of these patients develop adenosis of the vagina or have a congenital anomaly of the cervix and/or vagina. From these observations it has been suggested that diethylstilbestrol acts as a teratogen rather than as a carcinogen.

Since young girls often have irregularities of their menses, a diagnosis of anovulatory bleeding is commonly made and hormonal treatment instituted. In view of the present reports, all teen-age girls with irregular bleeding should receive a thorough pelvic examination, including palpation and direct visual inspection of the cervix and vagina plus cytological studies. Daughters of mothers who received stilbestrol should also be examined prophylactically at the menarche even if there are no symptoms and at any age if there is increasing discharge or any staining or bleeding. If it is impossible to insert a small speculum, the patient should be advised to use tampons for a month to 6 weeks and then return for a vaginal examination. If there is a great deal of suspicion that a pathologic condition is present and it is impossible to complete a vaginal examination in the office, it is justifiable to do an examination under anesthesia. Although the cytology studies are often negative because the tumors have a low-grade malignancy and are often covered with either intact mucosa or slough, the studies should still be carried out, and it is suggested that the lesions or fornices be scraped with a spatula.

On examination the anterior fornix often appears shortened and is less elastic than usual. A cervical hood may be present and gives the appearance of a coxcomb. The cervix appears red. There is often a red granular mucosa, small cysts, or a papillary lesion that may be multicentric in appearance. On palpation there is a sandy irregularity. The involved area takes Schiller's or Lugol's stain poorly, if at all. The same findings may exist in patients with adenocarcinoma. Usually the findings are more marked, and often polypoid, nodular, or papillary lesions are present.

In all cases of clear cell adenocarcinoma with a history of diethylstilbestrol ingestion by the mother, adenosis has been found. However, there is no current evidence that indicates that adenosis is a precursor of clear cell adenocarcinoma. In studies carried out with the microspectrophotometer, all clear cell adenocarcinomas had aneuploid DNA distribution; all the areas of adenosis had a diploid to tetraploid distribution pattern, which is usually seen in proliferating epithelium.

Following representative biopsies, the general program for managing adenosis is close observation and repeated examinations. Acijel and the use of intravaginal progesterone have been beneficial in accelerating the metaplastic changes that normally occur as the adolescent gets older. It is felt that current data do not warrant excision of this tissue or other types of destructive surgery. Adenosis is benign and there is currently no evidence to indicate that it will turn directly to cancer. Based on present knowledge, close follow-up is the preferred method of management.

The patient with clear cell adenocarcinoma of the cervix is probably best treated with radical surgery. Early lesions (stage I vaginal or cervical carcinomas) can and do metastasize to regional pelvic lymph nodes. Regional nodal involvement was found in 16 percent of stage I vaginal tumors. For most patients with early-stage tumors, therapy chosen has usually been radical hysterectomy, vaginectomy, pelvic lymph node dissection, and placement of a split-thickness graft from the buttock into the area from which the vagina was excised. The ovaries are preserved unless they are diseased. Pelvic exenteration has been employed to encompass disease too extensive to be cured by a less radical surgical procedure.

The clear cell adenocarcinoma can also be treated and cured by radiation. However, many radiotherapists do not like to deliver large doses of cancerocidal radiation to a young woman because of the potential late-stage complications of radiation and the necessity of the sacrifice of ovarian function. Also, the vaginas that result may often become dry and stenotic and are less satisfactory than those that result after surgery. However, radiation therapy is considered by some to be preferable to pelvic exenteration as therapy for the more advanced lesion.

The important criteria for a good prognosis depend on (a) the degree of mitotic activity (one or more mitoses per high-power fields carries a bad prognosis), (b) the presence of involved regional lymph nodes, and (c) the stage of disease. The recent observation of pulmonary and/or supraclavicular lymph node metastases indicates that prolonged follow-up of treated individuals is essential.

CANCER OF THE CERVIX

Cancer of the cervix develops in approximately 2 percent of all women. In the United States there are approximately 30,000 new cases per year with 10,000 deaths a year,[71] or one death each hour. Although the incidence has remained about the same, the mortality rate from cancer of the cervix has dropped in the last 40 years in the more industrialized countries of the world. The high-risk group includes those starting intercourse in their teens, having multiple sexual partners, or having many children, as well as non-whites and women from low socioeconomic groups. With the knowledge available to us, it should be possible to practically eradicate cancer of the cervix by the turn of the century.

The peak incidence for carcinoma in situ of the cervix is between 30 and 40 years of age, whereas for invasive squamous cancer it is between the ages of 40 and 50 years. However, cervical cancer may occur at any age, and an incidence of 15 percent has been given for those developing cancer of the cervix before age 30. Currently the literature is emphasizing an increasing number of patients diagnosed at age 20 years and under, probably because of the sexual revolution and the sexual emancipation of the teen-age female. There are rare reports of cervical cancer in the newborn.

Diagnosis

It must be emphasized that there are no symptoms characteristic of cancer of the cervix. A high index of suspicion is necessary. Bleeding is probably the most common symptom associated with cancer of the cervix and is usually bright red and "lawless." Bleeding is not predictable as to time, amount, or duration, and is more frequent after intercourse or any vaginal manipulation. Less frequently, there is a serosanguinous or serous discharge, and if associated with an overgrowth of saprophytes, it has a foul odor. Pain, swelling of legs, weight loss, and marked anemia are associated with advanced lesions. In this day and age when the potential to eradicate cancer of the cervix is available to us, the diagnosis of advanced cancer of the cervix is intolerable and unacceptable.

It is of prime importance to pinpoint the area of bleeding. However, the remainder of the physical examination is also important and should include a careful rectal examination. The cervix should be examined carefully with rotation of the speculum in order to see all the fornices as well as the cervix proper. A cervix involved with a malignant process may show nothing if the disease is localized in the canal or if the lesion is smaller than an ulcerated mass. The spectrum of findings may include red areas, erosions, ulcers, nodularity, an exophytic or endophytic lesion, or nodularity with ulceration.

An accurate histologic diagnosis is essential before definitive treatment is instituted. A differential diagnosis should rule out chancres, tuberculosis, granuloma inguinale, lymphogranuloma venereum, condyloma accuminata, and radium eschars. A point to emphasize is that each of these lesions can be present concurrently with cancer, and this argues strongly for biopsy proof of disease.

"PAP SMEAR"

The Papanicolaou smear is merely a screening method and has its greatest application in the asymptomatic woman. Any lesion visible on the cervix should be biopsied since an obvious lesion may result in a negative Pap smear, despite the invasive nature of the lesion. The combination of the Pap smear and biopsy will give a high yield of positive results in those patients in whom "early" cancer is present. Pregnant patients represent a captive group and afford the physician the opportunity of not only doing a vaginal smear but also for training the patient in the need for routine physical examinations and cytologic and biopsy screening.

It is important to have an accurate histologic diagnosis once positive or suspicious cells are reported on Pap smear examination. Our plan for workup is as follows:

1. Repeat smears are submitted to another laboratory.
2. On an outpatient basis, punch biopsies of the Schiller's—or toluidine

blue—treated cervix and vagina are taken. Endocervical curettage with a small curette may be performed.
3. Hospital admission for fractional D&C, further biopsies, or conization of the cervix if it is deemed necessary.
4. Biopsy revealing invasive cancer avoids the need for conization.

EVALUATION OF VAGINAL BLEEDING

It is recommended that all women with vaginal bleeding have an examination under anesthesia and fractional D&C. This first curettage must be done properly in order to stage the disease properly:

1. Curettage of endocervix with small curette. Any tissue is kept separate from endometrial curetting.
2. Determine depth of uterine cavity with a sound.
3. Dilate cervix.
4. Explore uterine cavity with polyp forceps.
5. Curette endometrial cavity. Try to identify site of tumor.
6. Multiple punch biopsies of the cervix.

Clinical Staging and Evaluation[2]

Many classifications have been proposed for staging the extent of disease among patients with cancer of the cervix, showing that no completely satisfactory classification has been established. However, it is important for purposes of reporting experiences, comparing results, and determining prognosis to have a uniform classification that is generally accepted. After World War I a committee of experts was appointed by the League of Nations organization to set guidelines for staging cancer of the cervix. Although the classification has been modified often since that time, the basic part has remained and is referred to as the International Classification (FIGO). The most recent edition is shown in Table 12-3.

QUALIFICATIONS IN STAGING CERVIX CANCER

A case should be classified as stage Ia after microscopic diagnosis of the earliest stromal invasion, but there is a great deal of controversy over what constitutes early stromal invasion. Up to a depth of 5 mm is accepted by most, but the American College of Obstetrics and Gynecology suggests 1-mm penetration as the outside limit. In the remainder of stage I cases, a clinical diagnosis on the basis of inspection and biopsy will be possible.

A patient with extension of the growth to the pelvic wall by a short and indurated but not nodular parametrium should be alloted to stage II. The patient should be placed in stage III only if the parametrium is nodular *out on* the pelvic wall or if the growth itself extends *out on* the pelvic wall.

Table 12-3
Figo Classification—Cancer of the Cervix

Stage	Description
Stage 0	Carcinoma in situ, intraepithelial carcinoma
Stage I	Carcinoma confined to the cervix (disregard extension to the corpus)
Ia	Microinvasive carcinoma (early stromal invasion)
Ib	All other cases of stage I; occult cancer is marked ''occ''
Stage II	Carcinoma extends beyond the cervix but has not extended to the pelvic wall; carcinoma involves the vagina, but not the lower third
IIa	No obvious parametrial involvement
IIb	Obvious parametrial involvement
Stage III	Carcinoma extends to the pelvic wall; on rectal examination there is no cancer-free space between the tumor and the pelvic wall; tumor involves the lower third of the vagina; all cases with hydronephrosis or nonfunctioning kidney
IIIa	No extension to the pelvic wall
IIIb	Extension to the pelvic wall and/or hydronephrosis or nonfunctioning kidney
Stage IV	Carcinoma extends beyond the true pelvis or has clinically involved mucosa of the bladder or rectum; bullous edema is not classified as stage IV
IVa	Spread to adjacent organs
IVb	Spread to distant organs

The presence of bullous edema or a growth bulging into the bladder or the rectum does not permit consignment of a case to stage IV unless bladder invasion is proven by biopsy. Ridges and furrows in the bladder wall should be interpreted as signs of involvement if they remain fixed to the growth at examination, thus bearing out that the carcinoma has invaded the submucosa of the bladder.

The above is strictly a clinical classification for untreated patients, and classification is not changed after therapy is initiated. There is an error rate of 10–15 percent between the clinical staging and extent of disease found at surgery. The surgical-pathological classification is included for cases of cancer of the cervix treated by surgery[58] (Table 12-4).

PATIENT EVALUATION

Before therapy is begun, the patient with carcinoma of the cervix should have intravenous pyelography and barium enema examination in addition to standard evaluations for medical status and possible metastatic disease. The patient should be brought to treatment in the best

Table 12-4
Surgical Pathological Classification—Cancer of the Cervix

Class*	Description
Class 0	Carcinoma in situ, microcarcinoma
Class A	Carcinoma limited to the cervix
Class Ao	After positive biopsy specimen of infiltrating carcinoma, no tumor in the cervix in the surgical specimen
Class B	Carcinoma extends from the cervix to involve the vagina, except the lower third; carcinoma extends into the corpus; carcinoma may involve the upper vagina and corpus; vaginal or uterine extension, or both, may be by direct or metastatic spread
Class C	Carcinoma involves paracervical or paravaginal tissue, or both, by direct extension or by lymphatic vessels, or in nodes within such tissues or direct extension, or both, into the lower third of the vagina
Class D	Lymph vessel and node involvement beyond paracervical and paravaginal regions; this includes all lymphatic vessels or nodes, or both, in the true pelvis, except as described in class C; metastases to the ovary or tube
Class E	Carcinoma penetrates to the serosa, musculature, or mucosa of the bladder, colon, rectum, or some combination of these
Class F	Carcinoma involves the pelvic wall (fascia, muscle, bone, or sacral plexus, or some combination)

From Meigs and Brunschwig.[58]

* Combinations are used: for example, DC, node at the periphery of the pelvis and parametrial or paracervical extension; CN, parametrial or paracervical extension as well as a positive node in the parametrial or paracervical area. D is reserved for positive nodes at the periphery of the pelvis.

physical condition possible. This includes appropriate bowel preparation if operation is planned, antibiotic vaginal suppositories, high caloric diet, and correction of any anemia or electrolyte imbalance.

Treatment

DYSPLASIA

Marked dysplasia is usually adequately treated by conization or multiple biopsies plus endocervical curettage. This is followed postoperatively by Pap smears.

CARCINOMA IN SITU

The proper treatment of patients with carcinoma in situ is based on the clinical and histologic findings. It is important to reemphasize that carcinoma in situ may occur in multiple sites and may be found in the cervix, vagina, vulva, perineum, and urethra. Therefore, careful clinical evaluation (adequate exposure, use of Schiller's test, and histologic evaluation) must be carried out in each patient and treatment individualized. Careful, planned, and systematized follow-up over a long period is necessary. It is obvious that all suspicious smears and even positive smears should be carefully repeated because laboratory errors are made occasionally. Repeat positive smears require additional evaluation.

In young women desirous of having children, a well-planned cone (following outline by Schiller's stain) is removed, anticipating that it will be a therapeutic cone. This form of therapy is acceptable only if the patient is cooperative and will accept careful long-term follow-up. There is universal agreement that therapy should be surgical and not by irradiation. After conization, it is permissible to follow the patient if the smears remain negative. However, with positive smears indicating residual disease, the patient is a candidate for either another cone or hysterectomy. In those patients treated by hysterectomy, it is important to include approximately 2 cm of vagina in the resection, which we believe is best done by the vaginal route. Attempts to obtain additional cuff by the abdominal route have an increased urinary fistula rate unless the ureters are exposed and carefully dissected. The ovaries should be preserved in young patients. In patients over 40 years of age with a positive smear, either multiple biopsies with careful curettage of the endocervix or a cone biopsy is indicated. If invasive cancer is ruled out, a total hysterectomy with vaginal cuff and bilateral oophorectomy is indicated.

INVASIVE CARCINOMA—GENERAL APPROACH

Before 1895 the only therapy offered for cancer of the cervix was application of chemical caustics, cauterization, or amputation of the cervix. This limited therapy produced predictably poor results. In 1895 John G. Clark introduced a more radical operative procedure, and by the early part of the twentieth century, Wertheim reported approximately 500 cases of radical hysterectomy with encouraging results. Abbe, in 1903, introduced radium into clinical practice and showed that cancer of the cervix was a radiocurable lesion with a low mortality and low immediate morbidity. Its popularity was such that sentiment swung to radium as the preferred therapy. Meigs[57] then combined the Wertheim hysterectomy with pelvic lymph node dissection for stages I and II cervical cancer, and this proved to be an effective treatment method with low morbidity and mortality. Brunschwig confirmed these findings in a large unselected group of patients. The controversy as to whether surgery or radiation was the preferable treatment for cervix cancer raged from 1939 until the early 1960s, when it became evident that results were similar and that both approaches had exhausted their potential for further improvement in end results.

CHOICE OF TREATMENT METHOD
FOR STAGES Ib–IV

Radiation has been the treatment of choice for the country as a whole. However, there has been a change in attitude in the last few years reflected in a review of the 14th Annual Report collected by Kottmeir. From 1934–1938, only 4 percent of the patients were operated on in 20 percent of the institutions reporting; whereas in 1953–1957, a total of 33 percent of the patients were operated on in 74 percent of the institutions listed. In the 14th Annual Report, only 11 of the 124 institutions reporting had no operated cases, whereas at 5 institutions, the operation percentage in stage I exceeded 90 percent. These figures demonstrate clearly a change in philosophy from treating the disease to treating the patient and a swing away from standardization to individualizing treatment. Whatever treatment is chosen, it should be based on a knowledge of the natural history of the disease as well as on an understanding of the treatment chosen and its complications. Poor radiation is no better than poor surgery and is fraught with the same high morbidity and mortality.

This new orientation changed the emphasis from, Which is better—surgery or radiation?, to the more enlightened attitude, Which is *better for a given patient*—surgery or radiation? In turning from treating the cancer to treating the patient, the philosophy has swung from "standardization" to "individualized therapy." Our general approach is as follows:

1. Stage Ia
   A. Early stromal invasion. In general, this lesion is to be treated as invasive cancer. When invasion is indefinite or only 1–2 mm in depth, does not cover a wide area, and involves no vascular or lymphatic area, the treatment is the same as that suggested for carcinoma in situ.
   B. Occult cancer (carcinoma hidden in the cervix). In general, the treatment is radical hysterectomy and bilateral pelvic node dissection, *or* primary radiation therapy.
   C. Post-surgical. The management is best individualized and consists of a combination of radical surgery including bilateral pelvic lymphadenectomy and radiation therapy, *or* primary radiation therapy.
2. Stage Ib
   Radical hysterectomy and bilateral pelvic lymphadenectomy.
   Radiation therapy in those patients in whom surgical therapy is not to be performed because of age or general health.
3. Stage IIa
   The same treatment as for Stage Ib.

4.   Stages IIb, IIIa, and IIIb
     Primary radiation therapy.
5.   Stage IV
     A.   Primary radiation therapy. This therapy may require preradia-
          tion diversion of the fecal and/or urinary stream.
     B.   Primary pelvic exenteration may be selected for those patients
          with central disease that extends into the bladder and in whom it
          is possible that the disease can be totally removed.

There are some problems and controversies related to the above management outline. Microinvasion in stage Ia is defined in different ways, leading to some differences in opinion regarding the optimal type of operative procedure for this group of patients. Microinvasion has a predominant histologic picture of carcinoma in situ but has, in addition, a focus of invasion confined to the most superficial stroma. Microinvasion is found in approximately 6–10 percent of those patients presenting with carcinoma in situ. A review of the literature reveals only a handful of such patients in which there was involvement of submucosal lymphatics or lymph nodes. The survival rates in patients with microinvasion treated by total hysterectomy and a cuff of vagina have been excellent. The infinitesimal risk of node metastases is adequately balanced by the small mortality associated with radical hysterectomy. If on serial or step biopsies there is lymphatic involvement, or the invasion is more than 5 mm in depth, the disease should be treated as stage I cancer of the cervix. Our preference for treating microinvasion is a classic Wertheim hysterectomy with a cuff of the paravaginal and paracervical areas and the upper one-quarter of the vagina. The ovaries are managed according to the age of the patient.

An apparently normal-appearing cervix that proves to have invasive carcinoma is not necessarily a "micro-carcinoma." A sizeable lesion may be hidden within the endocervical canal, and this should be termed "occult" carcinoma. Occult cancer may be found in a cone or in the specimen from a large wedge biopsy performed in cases of carcinoma in situ or dysplasia. Obviously, such carcinomas are invasive and should be treated with the appropriate radical operation or planned cancericidal radiation therapy.

RADIATION THERAPY

Most plans of treatment are modified forms of one of the three leading schools: Paris, Stockholm, or Manchester. Todd and Meredity (Manchester) reported that the dosage should be related to two theoretical points—A, defined as 2 cm lateral to the axis of the uterine canal and 2 cm above the vaginal fornix; and B, a point 3 cm lateral to A. The rationale for this approach is that the dosage at point A represents a convenient method of expressing the dosage received by the primary carcinoma in the cervix, and the dosage at point B represents the dosage received in the lymph-bearing area. Although this approach provides a convenient plan to follow, it has not been universally accepted.

In order to achieve successful irradiation of cancer of the cervix, it is necessary to deliver a high dose of radiation to the tumor and the tumor-bearing areas. The cervix and the vagina can tolerate extremely high doses, although the bladder and rectum have a lower radiation tolerance. Careful calculation of the dosage to be administered as well as well-planned and executed technique are essential if radiation damage to normal tissue is to be avoided. A systematic and careful pelvic and rectal examination should be carried out under anesthesia. Fractional curettage and biopsies must precede the insertion of radium. A rigid application—i.e., that of Campbell, Ernst, or Manchester—should be employed in order to minimize the variation in dose. Consistency in dosage promotes even distribution of radium and permits delivery of 12,000 rads to the cervical canal, 6000 rads to point A, and 2000 rads to point B without an inordinately high morbidity. Scintillation probes and ionization chambers should be used to check the dosage delivered to the bladder and the rectum. A flat plate of the abdomen should be done to check the position of the radium. After-loading techniques have been introduced, and they eliminate radiation exposure to the personnel in the operating room. By means of a computer, it is now possible to acquire information on dose distribution around an applicator within the pelvis far beyond the limited information available by using points A and B as the only references.

Recently, there has been a swing from the use of radium followed by pelvic external radiation to radiation of the whole pelvis by megavoltage technique (delivering 4000 rads in stages I and II) and followed by radium insertion (6000–9000 mg hours). The technique is changed for stage III, reducing the milligram hours of radium and supplementing an additional 1000 or 1500) rads to the involved side; stage IV is treated with 7000 rads, reducing the size of the field after 5000 mg hours to the cervix. However, in most clinics, radium is inserted in divided doses (Stockholm or Manchester techniques) and is left in place for 36–50 hours at 2–3-week intervals, attempting to deliver a total dose of 6000 mg hours at point A. Two or three weeks after the final radium application, external therapy is started.

SURGERY

When Meigs reintroduced radical surgery for cancer of the cervix in 1939, an additional useful modality became available. In order to follow a surgical program, it is necessary to employ a wide range of total operations from radical hysterectomy to pelvic exenteration. The latter is a

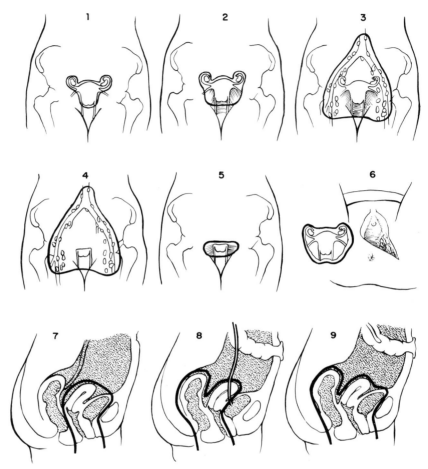

Fig. 12-1.   Surgical procedures used for carcinoma of the cervix: (1) total hysterectomy and bilateral salpingo-oophorectomy; (2) Wertheim hysterectomy; (3) hysterectomy, salpingo-oophorectomy, and pelvic lymph node dissection; (4) excision of cervical stump with pelvic lymph node dissection; (5) radical resection of cervical stump; (6) radical vaginal hysterectomy (Schauta operation); (7) anterior pelvic exenteration; (8) posterior pelvic exenteration; (9) total pelvic exenteration.

synthesis of three major procedures: (a) radical hysterectomy with bilateral pelvic node excision and bilateral salpingo-oophorectomy, (b) total cystectomy, and (c) combined abdominoperineal resection of the rectum. Anterior exenteration is removal of the above structures with preservation of the rectum, and posterior exenteration is removal of the above structures with preservation of the bladder.   The specific indications for radical surgery of some type have been appreciated as a result of the extensive experience of the gynecologic service at Memorial Sloan-Kettering Cancer Center under the late Alexander Brunschwig[29]. From a review of the results of this surgical program, it is now evident that selection of patients for the different forms of treatment is not only justified but indicated (Fig.12-1). The rationale and indications for radical surgery in lieu of radiation therapy for cancer of cervix may include the following:

1. patients in stages I and IIa, and selected patients with stage IV cervix cancer;
2. patients who are young and/or pregnant;
3. patients with an atrophic, conical, inelastic vagina;
4. patients with radioresistant cervical cancer;
5. patients with pelvic infections (salpingitis), or simultaneous ovarian or uterine pathology;
6. patients with recurrent cervical cancer after prior radiation;
7. patients with prior radiation for other reasons; and
8. obese patients.

CAUSES OF DEATH FROM CANCER OF THE CERVIX

In understanding the natural history of cancer of the cervix, it is important to know the cause of death from the disease. Uremia, infection, and hemorrhage are usually given as the leading causes of death from invasive cancer of the cervix. Although these are the most common causes, some women die from distant metastases. In a Memorial Hospital study of patients dying with cervical cancer, 50 percent had no disease beyond the pelvis. Other studies have confirmed this observation, which emphasizes the importance of adequate local treatment of this particular cancer.

Special Management Problems

ADENOCARCINOMA OF THE CERVIX

Adenocarcinomas constitute approximately 5 percent of cancers of the cervix. The average age of affected women is slightly higher than in squamous cancer. On the other hand, cancers of the cervix occurring at an early age (20 years and under) are almost universally adenocarcinoma. The same diagnostic measures are carried out as for squamous cancer. Opinion has been divided about whether adenocarcinoma responds to radiation as well as squamous cancinoma. After a review of the literature, it is concluded that the treatment is probably the same as for squamous cancer. If surgery is chosen as the method of treatment, it must be radical; if irradiation is selected, it must be well planned and carried to a cancericidal dose.

ENDOCERVICAL CANCER

Carcinoma involving the endocervix affects the corpus more often than is commonly realized. These cases should be treated as carcinoma of the cervix rather than corpus carcinoma. The attack should include radical hysterectomy and node dissection, or complete cancericidal doses of radiation both with radium and with external therapy, plus hysterectomy and an extended vagina cuff. Cases of endocervical carcinoma spreading into the corpus are usually diagnosed correctly only after hysterectomy. Myometrial invasion is an obvious source of clinically recurrent cancer if hysterectomy is not performed.

CANCER OF THE CERVIX
COMPLICATING PREGNANCY[8,36]

Approximately 1 pregnancy in 3000 is complicated by cervical cancer. The disease is not different from that found in the nonpregnant state. A comparison of cure rates in comparable stages of disease between pregnant and nonpregnant patients shows no difference. Prognosis depends on the extent of the disease. If surgery is employed as primary treatment, the plan should be:

1. First trimester and early second trimester: radical hysterectomy and pelvic node dissection with fetus in utero.
2. Late second trimester: await viability of the fetus and then do a classic cesarean section followed immediately by radical hysterectomy and pelvic node dissection.
3. Third trimester: classic cesarean section followed immediately by radical hysterectomy and pelvic node dissection.
4. Postpartum: radical hysterectomy and pelvic node dissection.

If radiation therapy is employed, the following plan is suitable:

1. First and second trimesters (nonviable fetus): Heyman stressed the poor results associated with inducing abortion before beginning irradiation. Five-year survival results were reduced by this procedure to 11 percent, compared to 56.7 percent when spontaneous abortion followed radiation therapy.

    Treatment is given as if pregnancy were not present: (a) tandems and colpostats; (b) alternative is to direct 3000 rads by means of external therapy to the uterus. Await spontaneous evacuation, or, if necessary, do a hysterectomy and then complete the therapy with radium application and additional x-ray therapy as needed for a cancericidal dose.

2. Third trimester (viable fetus): classic cesarean section at viability and followed immediately with external therapy. After this is completed, radium insertion is carried out.

3. Postpartum: Radiate as in the nonpregnant patient. Because of the danger of infection, external radiation is usually completed before radium is inserted.

CERVICAL STUMP CANCER[29]

Cervical stump cancer constitutes approximately 4 percent of all cancers of the cervix. If cancer is found within 2 years of the subtotal hysterectomy, it probably was present at the time of hysterectomy. Total hysterectomy obviously prevents the subsequent development of stump cancer.

Stump cancer can be treated by either surgery or irradiation. A review of the literature reveals that the survival rate after either modality of treatment is essentially the same as if the uterus were present with only slight increase in morbidity. However, in pursuing a surgical program, we have found that approximately 15 percent of patients required some type of pelvic exenteration to encompass the disease.

RECURRENT OR PERSISTENT CANCER OF THE CERVIX

Brunschwig[28] demonstrated that an appreciable salvage of patients demonstrating recurrence after radiation therapy is possible by appropriate surgery if extrapelvic metastases have not occurred. However, the problem of recurrent or persistent cancer of the cervix after a prior attempt at cure by irradiation is a serious problem and one that taxes both the ingenuity of the responsible physician and the resources of the hospital. Treatment, either palliative or curative, should be offered only if there is no inordinate increase in morbidity and mortality.

Early diagnosis of recurrent cancer is as important for salvaging the patient with recurrence as it is for the treatment of those with previously untreated cancer of the cervix. Any new symptoms or signs, as well as the development of uterine asymmetry or nodularity or pyelogram changes, should be suspect.[10]

Recurrent cancer is best treated by a surgical approach. Reradiation has little to offer in terms of cure and is accompanied by a high complication rate and augmentation of symptoms. A point to be emphasized in the surgical treatment of recurrence is that not all patients require pelvic exenteration to encompass their disease. Approximately 20 percent can be managed by less than a pelvic exenteration. For those requiring a pelvic exenteration, the 5-year survival rate is 20 percent and it jumps to 40 percent among those treatable by less than a pelvic exenteration.[9]

CANCER OF THE ENDOMETRIUM

Adenocarcinoma of the endometrium is increasing in incidence and is now the second most common gynecologic cancer. Although it was once considered to be about one-tenth as common as carcinoma of the cervix, the figures have become nearly the same in the last few years, particularly in the middle and more affluent classes. There are now more than 11,000 new cases per year (4.3 percent of female cancer incidence). The overall "cure rate" for New York State is 70 percent. Generally speaking, endometrial cancer is characterized by its apparent slow growth and is successfully treated with relatively unsophisticated techniques.

Cancer of the endometrium is usually an adenocarcinoma that is predominantly a disease of the peri- and postmenopausal age groups. However, it does occur in 5 percent of cases in women less than 40 years of age and has been found as early as age 17. Over 75 percent of cases occur after age 50, and 20 percent occur between ages 40 and 50. There is an increasing number of adenosquamous cancers of the endometrium occurring in the same age groups.

Diagnosis

Attention must be focused on early diagnosis. Knowledge available to us provides us the opportunity to identify clinically the patient at high risk for developing endometrial cancer. Garnet has suggested several parameters, i.e., obesity, nulliparity, reduced glucose tolerance, hypertension, hyperestrogenism, continuous uninterrupted estrogen stimulation, bloody menopause over age 50, dysfunctional uterine bleeding, and a long history of anovulation.[38]

Although the above parameters help identify the high-risk patient, screening methods employing cytology have been more elusive. Screening programs by cytology have yielded considerably inferior results as compared to those reported from the cervix. In asymptomatic women, only 3 percent of all endometrial cancers are detected by routine Pap smear technique. In symptomatic women, however, employing the routine vaginal smear plus endometrial aspiration, the success rate in identifying cancer of the endometrium is 90 percent or more. By examining an endometrial aspiration specimen, the cytologist can tell whether the smear is negative or positive for malignancy, but he cannot identify the high-risk group with the accuracy that he can when there are early abnormalities of the cervix. The pathologist can detect the in-between groups such as those with hyperplasia, dysplasia, anaplasia, and in situ carcinoma when tissue is obtained for paraffin block and histologic examination. Unfortunately, this cannot always be obtained without general anesthesia. A curettage (fractional) should be carried out in every postmenopausal patient with vaginal bleeding.

Staging and Evaluation

The clinical staging system for endometrial cancer is shown in Table 12-5. Each patient should be examined under anesthesia and a fractional curettage with sounding of the uterus should be carried out. The pre-treatment evaluation described for cervix cancer is appropriate for these patients, but endoscopy of the bladder and large bowel is not as essential.

Treatment

The concepts of therapy for endometrial cancer are based on an understanding of the natural history of the disease. It arises as a local-ized or diffuse lesion and remains in the uterine cavity for a long time, spreading within the endometrium. As it grows, it invades the myome-trium, spreading toward the endocervix, or goes directly through the myometrium to the serosa and then to the peritoneal cavity. Deep pene-tration of the myometrium is associated with an increased incidence of lymph node involvement.[53] The myometrium in the postmenopausal woman is much thinner than in the premenopausal woman, and relatively superficial penetration may bring the cancer into contact with the lym-

Table 12-5
Staging Classification—Cancer of the Endometrium

Stage	Description
Stage 0	Confined to endometrial epithelium (in situ)
Stage I	Confined to corpus of uterus
Ia	Present in a uterus measuring up to 8 cm from external os to upper limit uterine cavity
Ib	Present in a uterus measuring more than 8 cm from external os to upper limit uterine cavity
Stage II	Involves corpus and cervix but does not extend beyond uterus
Stage III	Extends beyond uterus but confined to true pelvis
Stage IV	Extends outside true pelvis or involves mucosa of bladder or rectum (not bullous edema)

phatics and account for the greater potency of endometrial cancer among this age group.[18,20] The high-risk group for extrauterine spread are those with (a) involvement of the lower uterus or cervix, (b) histologic grade III lesions, and (c) myometrial invasion. Our general approach to therapy is described in the following paragraphs.

Stage 0—carcinoma in situ. The management should be tailored to fit the needs of the patient, her age, and desire for future childbearing. In selected young patients with minimal disease, an alternative to hysterectomy may be repeat curettage in 3–4 months or a course of progestational agents followed by repeat curettage.

Stage Ia, G1. Total hysterectomy and bilateral salpingo-oophorectomy are followed by postoperative vaginal radiation. Some oncologists prefer radical hysterectomy.

In patients in whom the histologic grade is G2 or G3, external pelvic radiation should be given preoperatively, followed by total hysterectomy, bilateral salpingo-oophorectomy, and vaginal radiation postoperatively.

If preoperative external radiation has not been given and the surgical specimen reveals a histologic grade of G2 or G3 (instead of G1) or moderate or extensive myometrial invasion (one-third or more of myometrial penetration), postoperative external radiation should be given.[40]

Stage Ib. In Stage Ib G1, total hysterectomy and bilateral salpingo-oophorectomy are performed, followed by postoperative vaginal irradiation. In Stage Ib G2 or G3, preoperative external irradiation is given followed by total hysterectomy and bilateral salpingo-oophorectomy 6 weeks later. Postoperative vaginal radiation is indicated. An alternative to total hysterectomy is radical hysterectomy. A few gynecologists still insert Heyman capsules in the uterus and colpostats in the vagina and then follow this in 6 weeks with total hysterectomy and bilateral salpingo-oophorectomy.

Stage II. Preoperative external pelvic radiation is followed in 6 weeks by a modified radical hysterectomy and pelvic node dissection. Postoperative vaginal radiation is given. Since there is an increased incidence of pelvic nodes (up to 37 percent) among this group, careful biopsies are taken of the para-aortic nodes.

Stage III. If the lesion involves only the adnexal structures, preoperative x-ray therapy is followed by total hysterectomy and bilateral salpingo-oophorectomy. Postoperatively, vaginal radiation is given. An alternative plan to total hysterectomy is modified radical hysterectomy.

Stage IV. Primary therapy is external and intracavitary radiation treatment. The patient is evaluated to ascertain whether supplementary progestational agents should be used. If the cancer is limited to the pelvis but involves bladder, rectum, or both, the patient is evaluated for pelvic exenteration. External therapy may be employed before pelvic exenteration.

Distant metastases. Primary progestational therapy is indicated. Localized disease without response to progestational therapy is treated with x-ray therapy.

In the presence of widespread disease and no response, chemotherapy should be tried.

RECURRENT ADENOCARCINOMA OF THE ENDOMETRIUM[75]

Primary therapy is started with progestational agents. Localized symptomatic cancer is treated with radiation. Selected patients may be candidates for pelvic exenteration. Of 36 patients receiving pelvic exenteration for recurrent corpus cancer 5 or more years ago, 7 received their initial treatment less than 1 year before treatment for recurrence and none survived more than 15 months. Of 29 patients who were free of disease for at least 1 year after initial treatment and before receiving exenteration for recurrence, 5 lived 5 or more years.

Although there are fewer indications for pelvic exenteration[13] among patients with cancer of the corpus than in those with cervical cancer, pelvic exenteration has a place among the methods of treatment used as definitive therapy for this cancer. If, indeed, the progestins[66] are able to provide a 5-year cure in advanced cancer of the corpus uteri, this will become the treatment of choice. Although certain spectacular results have been recorded, there is no series of any magnitude currently reported. Nonhormonal chemotherapy for endometrial cancer is reviewed by Donovan.[35]

Adenosquamous Cancer[65]

The increasing number of mixed adenosquamous cancers detected in the endometrium is of some importance. This cancer has both malignant-appearing squamous and glandular components. Venous involvement is observed in one-half of the cases, and blood vascular and transtubal routes may be involved in the dissemination of the neoplasm. In mixed adenosquamous cancer of the endometrium, the mean age at detection is 65.5 years. The duration of symptoms tends to be short, and abdominal

or distant spread is observed more frequently than with endometrial adenocarcinoma or adenoacanthoma. Adenosquamous tumors respond
poorly to ionizing radiation. The five-year survival rate is 19.2 percent.
This is significantly lower than the survival rates for the other types of endometrial cancer.

SARCOMA OF THE UTERUS

Klempson and Bari[47] have modified Ober's[61] classification of uterine sarcomas as shown in Table 12-6. Sarcomas are not commonly observed, however, and the main varieties are (a) leiomyosarcomas—true
malignant neoplasms of smooth muscle cells (most common form); (b) endometrial stroma sarcomas, which are composed of rounded and fusiform

Table 12-6
Sarcomas of the Uterus

I. Pure sarcomas
  A. Pure homologous
    1. Leiomyosarcoma[1]
    2. Stromal sarcoma
    3. Endolymphatic stromal myosis*
    4. Angiosarcoma
    5. Fibrosarcoma
  B. Pure heterologous
    1. Rhabdomyosarcoma (including sarcoma botryoides)
    2. Chondrosarcoma
    3. Osteosarcoma
    4. Liposarcoma
II. Mixed sarcomas[3,4]
  A. Mixed homologous
  B. Mixed heterologous
    Mixed heterologous sarcomas with or without homologous elements
III. Malignant mixed müllerian tumors (mixed mesodermal tumors)
  A. Malignant mixed müllerian tumor, homologous type
    Carcinoma plus leiomyosarcoma, stromal sarcoma, or fibrosarcoma, or
    mixtures of these sarcomas
  B. Malignant mixed müllerian tumor, heterologous type
    Carcinoma plus heterologous sarcoma with or without homologous
    sarcoma
IV. Sarcomas, unclassified
V. Malignant lymphomas

* This tumor was benign in this series[47] but has been classified as sarcoma because of
reported recurrences and metastases.

cells arising from mesoblastic elements of the endometrium itself; (c) mixed mesodermal tumors of the corpus, the counterpart in the adult of sarcoma botryoides of infants and children; and (d) very rare forms such as fibrosarcomas and carcinosarcomas (mixture of leiomyosarcoma and endometrial carcinoma).

It would appear that two clinical forms of leiomyosarcoma may be recognized. In the first, the entire tumor mass is sarcomatous and seems to have been so since its inception. In the second, the uterus removed for fibroids shows an area in a fibroid that is softer and redder than the surrounding tissue, immediately causing suspicion of sarcomatous change, which is confirmed by histologic study. The prognosis in the former is very poor because few instances of 5-year survivors are recorded. Among those who have survived, the lesion was probably endometrial stromal sarcoma, the prognosis of which is less grave than that for leiomyosarcoma. The prognosis for leiomyosarcoma that arises in a leiomyoma is not as serious as that for the one that originates from the myometrium.[22]

Diagnosis

There are no characteristic signs or symptoms of sarcoma. Early bleeding does not occur unless polypoid lesions project into the endometrial cavity. On physical examination the uterus is enlarged, suggestive of fibroids. Rapidly enlarging masses in the uterus, especially of soft consistency, suggest sarcoma, but eventual histologic study may not confirm this.

Treatment

Sarcoma in a myoma, diffuse nonencapsulated sarcoma, endometrial sarcoma, and mixed mesodermal sarcoma (carcinosarcoma) are all best treated by total abdominal hysterectomy and bilateral salpingo-oophorectomy.[77] All of these lesions except the sarcoma developing in a myoma should receive postoperative external radiation therapy and/or combination chemotherapy. The treatment of sarcoma botryoides in children is described in more detail in Chapter 13.

CHORIOCARCINOMA

Choriocarcinoma is a highly malignant neoplasm arising from the embryonic chorion, both layers of the trophoblastic epithelium being involved. The uterus is the most common site for the primary growth, but it is not the only site. There is a clear association with pregnancy, since 50 percent of choriocarcinomas are preceded by a mole, 25 percent by abortion, and approximately 22 percent by normal delivery or ectopic pregnancy. However, choriocarcinoma is rare in the United States and occurs about 1 in 40,000 pregnancies. It is much more common in the Orient. Pregnancies in rapid succession and malnutrition with protein deficiency are thought to be involved in the etiology of the neoplasm. In addition, crowded conditions may predispose to a carcinogen—whether viral, physical, or chemical—that may play a role in tumor production.

Choriocarcinoma reproduces the capacity for invasion and spread characteristic of trophoblastic tissue. The course of the disease is highly malignant, and rapid local growth and distant metastases—chiefly to lungs, liver, brain, vagina, and various pelvic organs—are seen. The clinical symptoms may simulate those of several gynecological conditions such as abortion or dysfunctional bleeding. The demonstration of choriocarcinoma cells in the curettings suggests but does not confirm the diagnosis. However, when the growth lies in the myometrium, beyond reach of the curette, biopsy yields a false-negative report. In such cases, and in all cases where the diagnosis is suspected, the urine, blood, or both must be examined for chorionic gonadotropin (HCG).[32]

It has been shown that if the duration of disease is less than 4 months and the titer less than 100,000 IU/liter of urine, the 5-year survival rate with chemotherapy will be between 85 and 90 percent, whereas with a duration of disease greater than 4 months and a titer of more than 100,000 IU/liter of urine, the survival rate drops to 61 percent.[44,52]

The high-risk metastatic disease group meets one or more of the following criteria: metastatic disease in multiple sites—including liver or brain or both, and small intestine; gonadotropin excretion over 100,000 IU/24 hours; and duration of disease over 4 months from the termination of the antecedent pregnancy or the onset of symptoms. All other patients with choriocarcinoma are classified as having low-risk metastatic disease.

Treatment[5,25,26,54,67]

NONMETASTATIC TROPHOBLASTIC DISEASE[63]

Hydatidiform mole in situ. A 5-day course of actinomycin D is given, and the mole is evacuated on the third day of chemotherapy.

Postevacuation mole. Follow with HCG titers every 2 weeks. If they are not reduced to pituitary gonadotropin levels at 8 weeks or if they rise at any time, begin treatment. Treatment consists of chemotherapy alone if the patient desires more children or hysterectomy during a course of chemotherapy if no more children are desired. If chemotherapy is to be used, dilatation and curettage is performed during the first course to rule out transition to choriocarcinoma.

Choriocarcinoma after abortion or term delivery. Treatment consists of either an intermittent 5-day course of actinomycin D, or hysterectomy on the third day of chemotherapy if preservation of childbearing is no longer desired.

METASTATIC TROPHOBLASTIC DISEASE
(REGARDLESS OF HISTOLOGY)

An intermittent 5-day course of methotrexate, actinomycin D, or "triple therapy" is administered if the liver or brain is involved. If cerebral or hepatic metastases have been demonstrated, we suggest the immediate institution of whole-brain or whole-liver irradiation (2000 rads) simultaneously with combination chemotherapy and delivered over 10–14 days. The administration of cortisone at the same time decreases the incidence of edema in the treated organ. The follow-up should include weekly HCG measurements until titers are negative for 3 consecutive weeks, then monthly for 6 months, and then every 6 months. A subsequent pregnancy is acceptable after HCG titers have been normal for 1 year.

CANCER OF THE FALLOPIAN TUBE[70]

Primary cancer of the fallopian tube is the rarest carcinoma of the female genital tract. The incidence is less than 0.1 percent of the cancers of the reproductive system.[30] At the Mayo Clinic there were only 16 cases over a 45-year period. At the Free Hospital for Women in Boston there were only 12 cases among over 90,000 admissions during a 45-year period. The average age was 49 years among the cases reviewed in the American literature up to 1959, and the range was 18–80 years of age.

The commonest form of fallopian tube carcinoma is that arising from the mucosa and forming papillary or medullary anaplastic lesions.[41] Metastases develop in the opposite tube and the vagina; they spread widely in the omentum and liver, and over the abdominal peritoneal surfaces. Primary sarcoma arising from the muscularis is very rare and among the reported cases is uniformly fatal. The fallopian tube is commonly involved secondarily in advanced cases of endometrial and ovarian cancer also.[24]

Diagnosis

There are usually no or only slight symptoms until the disease is advanced. Abnormal vaginal bleeding and/or discharge may be noted. A profuse, intermittent, watery discharge, often blood-tinged, the so-called hemohydrops tubal profluens, is often reported as being common in the presence of carcinoma of the tube. A positive Pap smear in the presence of a negative curettage should alert the clinician to this possibility also. The cancer cells on the smear are sometimes arranged in alveoli. On pelvic examination an adnexal mass is discovered, with the corpus and cervix seemingly normal, but the exact diagnosis is rarely made preoperatively. Staging for cancer of the fallopian tube is similar to that for ovarian cancer.[68]

Treatment

Most patients with cancer of the fallopian tube are diagnosed at the time of laparotomy with histologic confirmation by frozen section. The resection employed is similar to that for ovarian cancer; total hysterectomy, bilateral salpingo-oophorectomy, and omentectomy. Any peritoneal fluid present should be studied for malignant cells, and intraperitoneal administration of radioactive phosphorous (^{32}P) should be considered in the postoperative period. With extended disease, external radiation therapy, chemotherapy, or both are given as individualized.[23]

The prognosis depends on the histologic type and the extent of spread. The most favorable prognosis is for a papillary type confined to the tube, without permeation into the muscularis. In general, 5-year survivors are few indeed, and the majority of patients recorded died within 6 months to 2 years after the cancer was discovered.

OVARIAN CANCER[43]

Deaths from ovarian cancer have slowly increased over the last 40 years, and the rate is now 2.5 times that of 1930.[64] More than 10,000 women die from ovarian cancer each year, and this is now the leading cause of death from gynecological cancer.[39] Early diagnosis is the key to successful treatment, but this is a matter of chance rather than a scientific method. When ovarian cancer is diagnosed in its early stages, it is considered a surgical disease; the standard treatment is total hysterectomy, bilateral salpingo-oophorectomy, and omentectomy. However, there is a definite role for radiation and chemotherapy for most patients and there have been definite benefits from the latter.

Ovarian cancer is considered a family of tumors. The tumors are made up of epithelial cells, germ cells, gonadal stromal (sex cord), and mesenchymal cells. The majority are of surface epithelial and ovarian stromal origin. These are the common epithelial tumors. For purposes of orientation, a brief outline of ovarian tumors is presented:

1. Common primary epithelial tumors of the ovary[69] (benign, borderline, or malignant)
   Serous
   Mucinous
   Endometrioid
   Mesonephric
2. Germ cell tumors
   Dysgerminoma
   Extraembryonal teratomas
   Adult teratomas
   Carcinoids
   Struma ovarii
3. Gonadoblastoma
4. Gonadal stromal (sex cord-mesenchymal) tumors
   Female type
      Granulosa cell tumor
   Male type
      Sertoli-Leydig
5. Tumors not specific for the ovary
   Lymphoma
6. Metastatic tumors
   Krukenberg
   Adenocarcinoma of large intestinal origin
   Miscellaneous

Natural History of Ovarian Cancer

Although cancer of the ovary is considered to arise bilaterally in a high percentage of cases, this is not confirmed in early cases where the cancer has not extended beyond the uterus, tube, or ovary. The cancer eventually spreads to the upper abdomen, and this is a characteristically surface type of spread. The omentum may be invaded before the macroscopic appearance of metastases over the peritoneal surface is noted, but in most instances peritoneal seeding and ascites are present by the time omental masses have appeared. The mesentery of the bowel is involved, and although the lumen may be patent clinically, the patient often reveals a picture of an intestinal obstruction. This unique type of simulated obstruction has been referred to as carcinomatosis ileus. Death usually results from inanition and repeated bouts of intestinal obstruction.

Diagnosis

There are no early symptoms of ovarian cancer.[7] This alone is a major contributing factor to the poor therapeutic results. The usual symptoms of abdominal swelling, pain, and a mass are associated with an advanced state of the disease. The earliest symptom is vague abdominal discomfort and mild digestive disturbances and may be present for months before the diagnosis is made. In the high-risk group between ages 40 and 60 years, the diagnosis of ovarian cancer should be considered in patients with bouts of dyspepsia, indigestion, and abdominal pain in whom no definite diagnosis can be made. Early ovarian cancer is often drowned in a sea of bicarbonate of soda.

The early diagnosis of ovarian cancer is a matter of chance and not a triumph of a scientific approach.[17] Means of early detection are extremely limited. In the majority of cases the finding of a pelvic mass is the only available method of diagnosis, with the exception of functional tumors, which may manifest endocrine activity with minimal ovarian enlargement. In some cases the pelvic findings may be uncertain even late in the disease. Pain in the early stage is associated with a complication such as torsion or rupture. Later, pain occurs when adjacent organs or nerve sheaths are infiltrated by tumor.

Menstrual disorders may be seen with endocrine-producing tumors. In the menopause patient, vaginal bleeding may occur. This has been attributed to the functioning stroma in the malignancy. Ascites with positive cells is a sign of advanced disease.

The pelvic findings are of limited help in making the diagnosis. However, combined with a high index of suspicion, the following pelvic findings may alert the physician to the diagnosis:

1. A mass in the ovarian area.
2. Relative immobility because of fixation and adhesions.
3. Irregularity of the tumor.
4. Shotty consistency with increased firmness.
5. Tumors in the cul-de-sac described as a handful of knuckles.
6. Relative insensitivity of the mass.
7. Increasing size under observation.
8. Bilaterality (70 percent in ovarian carcinoma versus 5 percent in benign cases).
9. In late disease, palpation of the omental cake, nodular hepato-

megaly, and ascites are common findings. (See Table 12-7 for staging classification.)

The diagnostic procedures include the Pap smear, which has been reported to be positive in 40 percent of patients with advanced disease, and cul-de-sac taps, which are associated with 90-percent finding of positive cells. The authors' results are very poor when compared to these figures. The diagnostic value of laparoscopy remains to be determined.[4] It has value in staging cancer of the ovary since it affords an opportunity to view the area between the liver and diaphragm on the posterior abdominal wall.

The major diagnostic tool is exploratory laparotomy on the basis of a high index of suspicion of ovarian cancer. Any adnexal mass that is enlarging or is more than 10 cm in size, or any mass that that cannot be accurately defined as a uterine fibroid should be examined at the operating

Table 12-7
Staging Classification—Ovarian Cancer

Stage	Description
Stage I	Growth limited to the ovaries
Ia	Growth limited to *one* ovary; no ascites
1	No tumor on the external surface; capsule intact
2	Tumor present on the external surface and/or capsule ruptured
Ib	Growth limited to *both* ovaries; no ascites
1	No tumor on the external surface; capsule intact
2	Tumor present on the external surface and/or capsule(s) ruptured
Ic	Tumor either stage Ia or Ib but with ascites* or positive peritoneal washings
Stage II	Growth involving one or both ovaries with pelvic extension
IIa	Extension and/or metastases to the uterus and/or tubes
IIb	Extension to other pelvic tissues
IIc	Tumor either stage IIa or IIb, but with ascites* or positive peritoneal washings
Stage III	Growth involving one or both ovaries with intraperitoneal metastases outside the pelvis and/or positive retroperitoneal nodes; or tumor limited to the true pelvis with histologically proven malignant extension to small bowel or omentum
Stage IV	Growth involving one or both ovaries with distant metastases; if pleural effusion is present, there must be positive cytology to allot a case to stage IV; parenchymal liver metastases
Special category	Unexplored cases thought to be ovarian carcinoma

* Peritoneal effusion which in the opinion of the surgeon is pathologic and/or clearly exceeds normal amounts.

table. In postmenopausal women, even a small palpable ovary is suspect.

POSTMENOPAUSAL PALPABLE OVARY (PMPO) SYNDROME

The PMPO syndrome (Fig. 12-2) is simply the palpation in a postmenopausal patient of what would be interpreted as a normal-sized ovary in the premenopausal woman.[16] We feel that the postmenopausal palpable ovary is an ovarian tumor and is a most significant finding. If our goal is to diminish the mortality rate from ovarian cancer, we must be more liberal in our indications for operation. The important concept is that palpation of what appears to be a normal-sized ovary in a patient 3–5 years postmenopausal is indicative of an ovarian tumor and should be investigated promptly. These patients should *not* be followed and reevaluated but, rather, examined operatively for the presence or absence of an ovarian cancer.

Treatment

Tumors of surface epithelial and ovarian stromal origin make up approximately 90 percent of ovarian cancers.[21] Only about 8 percent occur in women under age 35 years and most are in women between 40 and 60 years of age. In the latter group, conservative surgery is not indicated and treatment consists of total hysterectomy, bilateral salpingo-oophorectomy, omentectomy, appendectomy, and instillation of ^{32}P. Radiation therapy has been reserved for selected stage IV patients in whom disease involves supraclavicular and/or inguinal nodes.[15,31,48] Chemotherapy is currently being given prophylactically when all disease

POSTMENOPAUSAL PALPABLE OVARY SYNDROME
The PMPO Syndrome

Normal ovary
Premenopausal
3.5 x 2 x 1.5 cm

Early menopause
(1 - 2 years)
2 x 1.5 x 0.5 cm

Late menopause
(2 - 5 years)
1.5 x 0.75 x 0.5 cm

Fig. 12-2. Postmenopausal palpable ovary syndrome.

has been removed in stages I and II and to control the disease in stages III and IV. The subsequent management of patients with epithelial ovarian cancers includes chemotherapy for stages III and IV using alkylating agents.[74]

Special Problems in Management

GERM CELL TUMORS

Germ cell tumors, with the exception of the dermoids, are encountered mostly in childhood and adolescence.[76] The decision for radical or conservative treatment of this group of tumors must be based on a knowledge of the natural history of each tumor in the group.

Among the germ cell tumors, the dysgerminoma generates the greatest amount of discussion about treatment, and physicians are confused about whether to treat it conservatively or not. In the patient over 35 years of age, treatment should include total hysterectomy, bilateral salpingo-oophorectomy, omentectomy, appendectomy, and biopsy of nodes in the para-aortic area with postoperative x-ray therapy given to the pelvis and the para-aortic area. In the young patient with evidence of spread or in patients with gonadal dysgenesis or testicular feminization, this is also the treatment of choice. However, in the patient with a unilateral, encapsulated dysgerminoma who is young and wants to have a family, there is controversy over the ideal treatment. Since the bilaterality rate is only 5–10 percent and a good survival rate can be anticipated, there is some justification for a conservative operation. The treatment then is unilateral salpingo-oophorectomy, bisection, and biopsy of the opposite ovary with exploration of the para-aortic area with frozen section examination of any nodes encountered. These patients should then be followed carefully, and an argument can be made for reevaluation at approximately 8 months after initial surgery for the dysgerminoma. A 5-year survival of up to 90 percent can be expected from this treatment.

Therapy for the highly malignant forms of germ cell tumors such as entodermal sinus, embryonic teratoma, choriocarcinoma, and polyvesicular vitelline tumor is usually excision of the uterus, tubes, and ovaries. However, the results are so poor from treatment that there is no advantage over a more conservative unilateral oophorectomy in the absence of spread. Generally, these tumors are not radiosensitive. The role of chemotherapy remains to be evaluated, but preliminary work with multiple antitumor drugs given intermittently over several months has yielded promising results.

The solid adult teratomas, which are comprised of mature adult tissue derived from all three layers, are relatively benign tumors. Since they occur in the over 35-year-old group, excision of the uterus, tubes, and ovaries is the treatment chosen. The adult cystic teratoma usually occurs in the younger patient. Conservative therapy may be selected in those patients desirous of preserving their childbearing ability. Resection of the tumor and splitting the other ovary is adequate therapy. In the older patient, there is no indication for being conservative, and bilateral oophorectomy is carried out.

GONADAL STROMAL TUMORS

Gonadal stromal tumors of the female cell type are often referred to as feminizing tumors, although a certain number do not function.[59] The granulosa cell is the most important malignant tumor of this group, presenting as a bilateral tumor in approximately 5 percent of the cases. The diagnosis is occasionally made after rupture of the cyst with the production of a hemoperitoneum. When childbearing is not a consideration, treatment is total hysterectomy and bilateral salpingo-oophorectomy. When the patient is young and has a unilateral encapsulated ovary, unilateral salpingo-oophorectomy with bisection and biopsy of the opposite ovary is acceptable. This treatment is justified because the tumor is rarely bilateral, has a late recurrence rate beyond 5 years, recurs locally, and is highly responsive to additional therapy in the form of external x-ray therapy.

The gonadal stromal tumors of the male type are represented by the Sertoli-Leydig tumors, formerly called arrhenoblastoma. This term has been abandoned since the tumors are not all masculinizing and, indeed, those with an abundance of Sertoli cells may estrogenize the patient. Although these male gonadal stromal tumors may be slightly more malignant than granulosa cell tumors, their management and response are about the same.

The gynandroblastoma is made up of approximately equal elements of unquestionable granulosa cells and hollow tubules characteristic of the tubular adenoma of Leydig cells. Their natural history and management are similar to that reported for the granulosa and/or Sertoli-Leydig cell cancers of the ovary.

GONADOBLASTOMA

The gonadoblastoma is an exotic tumor that occurs most commonly in patients with an intersex problem such as gonadal dysgenesis or testicular feminizing syndrome. Since the patient's gonads are useless, removal of both ovaries is indicated, followed by adequate hormonal replacement.

METASTATIC OVARIAN CANCER[50,72,78]

Five to ten percent of ovarian carcinomas are metastatic. Most arise from the gastrointestinal tract, breast, and thyroid. In terms of survival, it makes little difference whether the tumor is primary or metastatic to the ovary. Although these tumors are referred to as Krukenberg tumors, few really qualify by having a significant number of signet-ring cells and a cellular stroma derived from the ovarian stroma. If possible, the primary site as well as the seat of the metastases should be excised. It is rare for a patient with a primary gastrointestinal cancer complicated by ovarian metastases to survive for a long time even though the gross disease has been removed. However, at the time of surgery for ovarian cancer, a thorough exploration should be carried out. Incidentally, some Krukenberg[50] tumors are reported as primary in the ovary. These can be completely excised with a reasonable chance of cure in early cases.

OVARIAN CANCER IN PREGNANCY[56,79]

If the surgeon finds an ovarian cancer at the time of abdominal exploration, his first obligation is to stage the disease, collect peritoneal fluid for block diagnosis, and remove the lesion for immediate frozen section for definitive diagnosis and documentation. This is followed by whatever further surgery is indicated, depending on the type of tumor, its histological grading, and the degree of anatomic spread. Biopsies of omentum, peritoneum, or any other intra-abdominal area where one suspects tumor are indicated.

If the tumor is unilateral, well encapsulated, shows no anatomical evidence of spread, and is reported as one of those listed with a comparatively low degree of malignancy, and if the peritoneal fluid shows no malignant cells, it is permissible to do a unilateral oophorectomy and permit the pregnancy to continue. The other ovary, however, should be split and biopsied to ensure its freedom from disease. This procedure is permissible with a histologically low-grade mucinous cystadenocarcinoma, dysgerminoma, granulosa-thecal cell tumor, arrhenoblastoma, gynandroblastoma, and possibly a low-grade papillary tumor when it is doubtful whether it is a cystadenoma or possible cystadenocarcinoma. The fetus is then delivered from below at term. Six weeks post-partum, the patient is reexplored and a total hysterectomy and bilateral salpingo-oophorectomy are done.

If the cancer is beyond stage Ia or if the cancer is any other than those enumerated above, therapy at the initial operation must be immediate total hysterectomy, bilateral salpingo-oophorectomy, and omentectomy. Implantation of polyethylene tubes for postoperative instillation of radioactive chromic phosphate (^{32}P) plus postoperative cobalt irradiation if the disease is localized to the pelvis is our usual routine. Chemotherapy is instituted promptly if the disease is beyond the pelvis. If the entire tumor cannot be removed, the pregnancy should still be terminated and as much tumor as possible removed surgically. Irradiation or chemotherapy is instituted as soon as feasible. The pregnancy is secondary.

In most reported series, approximately one-third of the cases are stage III or IV at operation. One must be prepared for this contingency before the initial operation. The most aggressive cancers in terms of early spread are the solid adenocarcinomas and serous cystadenocarcinomas. Survival in patients with ovarian cancer and pregnancy is no different than in the nonpregnant group. The type of tumor and its anatomical spread determine the 5-year cure rate.

Role of Pelvic Exenteration

Barber and Brunschwig[11] reviewed results in patients who had received pelvic exenteration in order to ascertain whether this operation should be carried out in the presence of locally advanced ovarian cancer. They studied 14 patients who had been operated on 5 or more years previously, and 13 had received total pelvic exenteration. Only 1 of these patients survived 5 years without recurrence. In the last 5 years of the study, 8 patients received pelvic exenteration. Of these, one patient is living and well nearly 5 years, 1 was cancer free for approximately 3 years, and the remaining 6 had cancer present at the time of death. Ovarian cancer lends itself to pelvic exenteration only if it violates the usual method of spread characteristic of its natural history. There is no experience with endometrioid ovarian cancer. Since it is less frequently bilateral and does not spread to the upper abdomen as readily as other epithelial ovarian cancers, an argument may be made for treatment of the locally advanced endometrioid ovarian cancer by pelvic exenteration. However, in general, patients with advanced ovarian cancer are an unfavorable group for pelvic exenteration except in extremely rare instances.

Role of Radiation Therapy in Adult Ovarian Cancer

In stage I, external x-ray therapy has not added to the survival rates. However, the use of radioactive phosphorus ^{32}P in a 15-mCi dose given intraperitoneally has increased the survival rate. Stage IIa is usually treated as is stage I. Although one author (HRKB) reserves radiation therapy only for highly selected stage IV patients in whom disease involves supraclavicular and/or inguinal nodes, the method is chosen by some and therefore the two leading radiation approaches are outlined.

In stage III, the whole pelvis and abdomen are irradiated, care being exercised to avoid radiation to the kidneys. At the M.D. Anderson Hospital in Houston, Luis Delclos uses a moving strip technique in which lines 2.5 cm apart are marked on the front and back of the patient. Each day an area 2.5 cm in width is treated first on the front and then on the back, advancing after this to the next 2.5-cm strip. Approximately 2600–2800 rads is delivered at each treatment. The time span is 30–40 days, during which time 12 treatments are given. This high dose has a greater biologic effect than the whole-abdomen type of static-field technique. The area radiated by the moving strip technique is small, and therefore the side effects from the radiation are minimal.

Kottmeier reports that by adding postoperative x-ray therapy, he has increased his survival rate as follows: when the surgery was considered to be complete, the 5-year survival was 16.9 percent, and by the addition of postoperative x-ray therapy, survival was increased to 61.5 percent. In those cases in whom it was impossible to remove all the disease or in those considered inoperable, there were no survivors; but by the addition of x-ray therapy he salvaged 2.4 percent. Kottmeier administers x-ray therapy through two large anterior and two corresponding posterior fields and keeps the total dose to 2000 rads delivered over 6 weeks. The x-ray therapy is restricted to the pelvis and lower abdomen in cases of completely removed ovarian cancer. In cases considered inoperable, radiation therapy led to marked clinical improvement in 45 percent of the cases, although 35 percent had no noticeable improvement. The latter group died within 6 months of therapy.

Chemotherapy for Ovarian Cancer

Chemotherapy has provided another useful modality to attack the tumor. It may have increased the overall survival rates, and it has made life much more comfortable for a moderate number of unfortunate patients with stage III and IV disease. In general, patients with disease spread, ascites, and masses of tissue that cannot be removed surgically have been chosen for chemotherapy. Radiation to the upper abdomen is accompanied by an increased morbidity, but chemotherapy given in a well-controlled manner avoids this problem. After a response to chemotherapy, and in the absence of palpable disease, repeat surgery may be undertaken to see whether the patient is a candidate for excision of any remaining cancer, radiation therapy, or continuation of chemotherapy.

The alkylating agents have proven to be the best chemotherapeutic agents for the treatment of ovarian cancer. Before initiating treatment, the physician should carefully evaluate the bone marrow, liver, and kidney. Cyclophosphamide (Cytoxan®) has been the agent most commonly used by the authors. After a pretreatment workup, Cytoxan® is given in doses of 200 mg intravenously for 5 days and then 50 mg twice a day by mouth if leukopenia does not require modification of the treatment plan. The M.D. Anderson Hospital group uses L-phenylalanine mustard (Melphalan®) 1 mg/kg body weight, given in divided doses over 5–6 days postoperatively and repeated monthly. The total white count should be above 3000/cu mm and the polymorphonuclear leukocyte count above 1500/cu mm. The platelets should be 100,000 or above. It has been observed that combinations of drugs give results no better than those seen with the alkylating agents alone. However, the embryonal tumors are different, and they do respond better to triple therapy. Chemotherapy and radiation as a combined therapy has not proved to be any more successful than either given alone.

OVARIAN TUMORS IN CHILDREN[4]

Ovarian tumors comprise about 1 percent of all new growths in the field of pediatric gynecology. The problem of diagnosis is surpassed only by the problems and confusion about treatment. In this age group it is difficult to accept the diagnosis of ovarian cancer and even more difficult for the surgeon to carry out surgery that would deprive a child of her reproductive potential. Since the treatment of ovarian cancers in children is such an emotionally charged problem, an outline for the management of the different broad classes of tumors is presented.

Epithelial Tumors

Although epithelial tumors comprise 90 percent of all ovarian tumors, they are rarely encountered in children, particularly before puberty. If an encapsulated, unilateral mucinous or serous cystadenocarcinoma is found in the absence of positive cells in the pelvis, unilateral salpingo-oophorectomy with bisection and biopsy of the opposite ovary is adequate treatment. However, if there is any evidence of spread beyond the ovary, a total hysterectomy, bilateral salpingo-oophorectomy, appendectomy, and omentectomy (if an omentum has been developed) should be carried out.

Germ Cell Tumors

The germ cell tumors are almost always found in children and adolescents. Fortunately, more than one-third of all ovarian tumors in children are benign cystic teratomas that can be handled by simple excision of

the cyst with preservation of the ovary in most instances. The dysgerminoma is also more common in children and adolescents, is radiosensitive, and has a bilateral rate of 5–10 percent. Although treatment is controversial, most gynecologists agree that the treatment of an encapsulated
unilateral dysgerminoma in a young girl is unilateral oophorectomy. This
treatment is based on the assumption that there are no positive cells in the
pelvis, no tumor is in the opposite ovary, and the para-aortic nodes are
negative. However, if there is any evidence of spread, total hysterectomy and bilateral salpingo-oophorectomy is the treatment despite youth
of the patient. Whether postoperative x-ray therapy is indicated is best
individualized for each patient. The embryonal teratoma, choriocarcinoma, entodermal sinus tumor, and polyvesicular vitelline tumor are
highly malignant as in the adult and if unilateral and encapsulated, are
treated as successfully by unilateral oophorectomy as by a more aggressive surgical approach. In the rare malignancies (2 percent) in cystic
teratomas, a unilateral oophorectomy is indicated if there is no evidence
of spread.

Gonadoblastoma

The gonadoblastoma is composed of both germ cells and gonadal
stromal cells. Most affected children are intersexual and have primary
amenorrhea. The malignant potential has not been established but is
probably determined by the type of germ cell present. Since these
tumors are commonly found in the intersexual patient, bilateral oophorectomy is indicated.

Gonadal Stromal Tumors

The gonadal stromal tumors include tumors that have the potential to
produce either an estrogenizing or masculinizing effect. The only important malignant tumor of the female cell type is the granulosa cell cancer.
It is usually unilateral, has a late recurrence rate beyond 5 years, and typically has local spread or recurrence confined to the pelvis. Since the
tumor has a low grade of malignancy and is seldom bilateral, conservative
surgery in the form of unilateral oophorectomy is indicated when the
tumor is unilateral and encapsulated with a normal ovary on the opposite side.

Among the male cell types the Sertoli-Leydig cell tumor (arrhenoblastoma) is the most important. When it functions endocrinologically, it
defeminizes and then masculinizes the patient. It is probably more often
found clinically than the granulosa cell tumor, although the incidence of
the granulosa cell tumor is greater. When the Sertoli-Leydig cell tumor
is malignant, this is usually manifested by spread within the pelvis and

rarely by distant metastases. The indications for conservative surgery are the same as those outlined for granulosa cell tumors.

The gynandroblastoma is composed of cells from both the male and the female cell types in about equal proportions. This tumor comprises about 10 percent of all gonadal stromal tumors. It should be managed the same as the granulosa or Sertoli-Leydig cell tumors.

Metastatic Ovarian Cancer

Metastatic cancer does occur in the ovaries in childhood. There are reports of Krukenberg tumors with a primary cancer in the upper gastrointestinal tract. The surgical treatment is the same as in the adult with removal of as much tumor as possible, including the primary cancer.

Sarcoma of the Ovary

Ovarian sarcoma is relatively rare, but when present it is usually found in children. It is usually primary but may be the result of secondary malignant change in a preexisting fibroma or teratoma. The tumor is highly malignant and it is rare to have a patient survive 5 years. If the tumor is encapsulated and unilateral, there is no advantage of radical over conservative surgery. However, if there is spread or involvement of the other ovary, a total hysterectomy and bilateral salpingo-oophorectomy are indicated.

Other sarcomas that are not specific for the ovary are lymphosarcoma, lymphoma, and Burkitt's lymphoma.[3] If the lesion is unilateral and encapsulated, unilateral oophorectomy is appropriate and adequate. Removal of an ovarian lymphoma in a child should be followed by antitumor chemotherapy as these lesions are highly sensitive to this approach.

CHEMOTHERAPY IN GYNECOLOGIC CANCER[49,51,72]

The chemotherapy regimen for trophoblastic disease and ovarian cancer was discussed earlier in the chapter. However, the actual drug regimens will be given in this section. Gestational trophoblastic disease is the most responsive of all human neoplasms, and this may be directly related to the precise method available to monitor the disease. Epidermoid cancer of the cervix, vagina, and vulva are the least sensitive. Endometrial cancer, pelvic sarcoma, and carcinoma of the fallopian tube often give spectacular results, but the results are not as predictable as those associated with gestational trophoblastic disease or even ovarian cancer.

Adenocarcinoma of the Endometrium[35]

Adenocarcinoma of the endometrium has not responded well to cytotoxic agents, but some spectacular results have followed treatment with progestational agents. The patients with well-differentiated lesions metastasizing to the lung receive the greatest therapeutic response from progestational agents. However, they may also benefit patients with endometrial metastases to other sites. The drug has practically no toxic effects and is well tolerated by most patients. The personal preference of the authors is to give 1250 mg of hydroxyprogesterone (Delalutin,® 250 mg/ml) intramuscularly every day for 10 days and then once a week for an indefinite and extended period of time. Megestrol acetate is also given orally in dosages up to 200 mg per day. Depo-Provera® may be given instead of Delalutin,® and the dosage advised is slightly higher than that usually recommended by others. A dose of 400 mg of Depo-Provera® is given intramuscularly each day for 10 days and then once a week as prescribed for Delalutin.® Medrogestone is also given following the above regimen. It is important to continue the regimen for at least 2 months before concluding that the results are not satisfactory. If one progestational agent fails, another may be tried or a trial with a cytotoxic or anticancer drug is indicated, followed by a return to therapy with the progestational agents at a later date.

Sarcomas

Patients with pelvic sarcomas have a dismal survival rate. After initial surgery, irradiation therapy, or both, recurrences have usually not responded to additional therapy. However, recently a combination of cyclophosphamide 200–400 mg IV, actinomycin D 0.5 mg IV, vincristine 1 mg, and adriamycin 50 mg IV has been given on the first day. Cyclophosphamide and actinomycin D are repeated daily for 4 additional days. The regimen is repeated every 4 weeks if the white blood count remains above 3000/cu mm, polymorphonuclear leukocytes above 1500/cu mm, and the platelet count above 150,000/cu mm. The electrocardiogram should be checked to detect any changes prior to the use of adriamycin, and the total dosage of adriamycin should not exceed 600 mg/sq m. Some of the stromal sarcomas are benefited by the addition of progestational agents as outlined for endometrial carcinoma. Adriamycin has shown promise especially when used as one drug of a combination regime, particularly in embryonal sarcomas. Progestational agents have been given in addition to the patients with leiomyosarcoma with an occasional response.

Epidermoid Carcinoma of the Cervix, Vagina, and Vulva

Epidermoid carcinoma of the lower genital tract is relatively insensitive to the anticancer drugs. Single agents such as the alkylating agents, 5-fluorouracil, vincristine, methotrexate, hydroxyurea, porfiromycin, adriamycin, and bleomycin have been universally unpredictable in their results, and most often they offered very little. Multiple-drug therapy has not produced any better response than that achieved with a single drug except in rare instances. Adriamycin has just recently been introduced as an additional drug for therapy, and it will take time to judge its contribution. The intra-aortic infusion of agents in the management of these tumors will be discussed separately.

Gestational Trophoblastic Disease[44]

Gestational trophoblastic tumors are the most responsive. Nevertheless, expertise is important in the management of these patients, and they are best treated in a center.

Methotrexate and actinomycin D are the two drugs most often used as single-agent therapy. Methotrexate, 15–25 mg, is given intramuscularly for 5 days. Repetitive 5-day courses are administered every 10 days to 2 weeks, depending on the blood count and blood chemistries. The progress of the patient is monitored with weekly gonadotropin assays. If the patient fails to show a decline in gonadotropin secretion through two courses of the chemotherapeutic drug or fails to achieve a normal HCG titer after four or five courses of the drug, the alternate drug is chosen. Methotrexate is contraindicated in the presence of decreased renal or hepatic function.

Actinomycin D, 12 μg/kg, is given intravenously over 5 days. The same repetitive plan is followed as for methotrexate. The same regimen for blood counts and chemistries must be followed.

In the high-risk patient or one categorized as having a poor prognosis, the initial chemotherapy should be of a combination variety. Triple therapy most often chosen is methotrexate 15 mg intramuscularly, actinomycin D 10 μg/kg intravenously, and chlorambucil 10 mg orally, each drug being given daily for 5 days. The interval between courses should be longer than 10 days but shorter than 21 days. The same safety criteria should be followed as for single-agent treatment, but they are not as effective in predicting impending imbalances. Therefore, extreme caution must be exercised. After two or three courses of triple therapy, treatment is altered to single-agent therapy with actinomycin D at a dosage of 13 μg/kg for 5 days.

Ovarian Cancer and Adenocarcinoma of the Fallopian Tube[72]

These two entities have similar clinical pictures and therefore are discussed together. The single alkylating agents have given the best results. Cyclophosphamide and melphalan (Alkeran®) are most often chosen. Cyclophosphamide may be administered intravenously, 200 mg a day for 5 days and then 50 mg orally twice a day. The white count and differential must be followed daily during the intravenous administration of the drug and every 2–3 weeks during oral therapy. An alternative plan is to give cyclophosphamide 8 mg/kg body weight intravenously for 5 days with repetitive treatments at 6-week intervals, providing the white count remains above 3000/cu mm, polymorphonuclear leukocytes above 1500/cu mm, and the platelet count above 150,000.

Melphalan is given for 5 days, 0.2 mg/day orally in divided doses. The treatment is repetitive at 4-week-intervals if the white count and platelets are maintained as outlined for cyclophosphamide.

When the single-agent therapy has failed, a limited success rate has occurred after the use of triple therapy. The regimen most often chosen is actinomycin D 0.5 mg intravenously (push), 5-fluorouracil 8 mg/kg as an intravenous drip, and cyclophosphamide 7 mg/kg intravenously (push). The treatment is given daily for 5 days and each 5-day cycle is repeated at 4-week intervals. The drugs are given sequentially on the same day. The blood and platelet counts and blood chemistries must be carefully monitored.

The role of adriamycin remains to be evaluated. Some early reports are promising, but the data are too limited at this time to make a firm statement.

Intra-aortic Chemotherapy[1]

After a catheter is inserted in the aorta through the femoral or brachial arteries and placed at any level desired, anticancer drugs are infused. Approximately 40 cases have been treated; 32 have been recently studied. Seven are living and three are free of disease. All of the patients presented with far-advanced disease and had previously received multiple and a variety of treatments. The original plan was to deliver the drugs in sequence, hopefully to attack the cell by using a drug most likely to damage the cell in a given phase of the cycle. The treatment has been altered and a standard plan is now employed. Epidermoid carcinomas of the cervix, vagina, and vulva as well as of the corpus receive one regimen, whereas cancer of the ovary and tube are treated by another regimen. The epidermoid cancers and cancer of the endometrium are given cyclophosphamide 200 mg a day for 2 days, actinomycin D 1 mg in 8 hours, bleomycin 15 units a day for 2 days, vincristine 1 mg in 6 hours, and recently adriamycin 50 mg in 24 hours has been added. Cancers of the ovary and the fallopian tube are treated with a similar regimen but bleomycin is not included. In the early part of the project methotrexate 50 mg was given in 24 hours and repeated. Later, the dosage was reduced to 30 mg. From time to time methotrexate is still included as part of the regimen.

Before therapy is begun, the blood count, platelets, chemistries, and bone marrow must be evaluated. The blood count and chemistries are evaluated approximately three times a week during treatment.

Each series of treatments is interrupted for 48 hours or until the blood count and chemistries return to normal, and then the regimen is repeated. The average time for giving the regimen is 6 weeks. One patient received therapy for about 5 months and is now free of disease. The primary cancer was squamous cell of the cervix. The patients presenting with pain were almost universally free of pain within a short time after starting therapy, and some have remained free of pain for extended periods of time. Most of the patients had a sense of well being and were improved. Unfortunately, the response is usually short-lived. This may be the direct result of the natural history of the disease or it may be owing to a lack of understanding at this time of the optimal dosages and methods of administration of the anticancer drugs.

REFERENCES

1. Aaro LA, Dockerty ME: Leiomyosarcoma of the uterus. Am J Obstet Gynecol 77:1187, 1959
2. Averette HE, Ford JH Jr, Dudan RC, Girtanner RE, Hoskins WJ, Lutz MH: Staging of cervical cancer. Clin Obstet Gynecol 18:215, 1975
3. Azoury RS, Woodruff JD: Primary ovarian sarcoma: report of 47 cases from the Emil Novak Ovarian Tumor Registry. Obstet Gynecol 37:920, 1971
4. Bagley CM, Young RC, Schein PS, Chabuer BA, DeVita VT: Ovarian carcinoma metastatic to the diaphragm, frequently undiagnosed at laparotomy: a preliminary report. Am J Obstet Gynecol 116:397, 1973
5. Bagshawe KD: Choriocarcinoma and trophoblastic tumors. In Halnan KE (ed): Recent Advances in Cancer and Radiotherapeutics: Clinical Oncology. Baltimore, Williams and Wilkins, 1972, p 45
6. Barber HRK: Cancer of the vulva and vagina. Lecture outlines. Postgraduate Course on Malignant Disease in the Female Pelvis, 53rd Annual Clinical Congress, Oct. 2–6, 1967, Chicago, American College of Surgeons
7. Barber HRK: Foreword. Clin Obstet Gynecol 12:929, 1969
8. Barber HRK: Gynecologic cancer complicating pregnancy. In Gynecological Oncology. Amsterdam, Excerpta Medica, 1969, p 283

9. Barber HRK: Relative prognostic significance of preoperative and operative findings in pelvic exenteration. Surg Clin North Am 49:431, 1969
10. Barber HRK: Results of surgical treatment of cancer of the cervix at the Memorial-James Ewing Hospitals, New York. Adv Obstet Gynecol 1:622, 1967
11. Barber HRK, Brunschwig A: Pelvic exenteration for advanced and recurrent ovarian cancer. Surgery 58:935, 1965
12. Barber HRK, Brunschwig A: The role of radical surgery in gynecological cancer. Acad Med NJ Bull 16:102, 1970
13. Barber HRK, Brunschwig A: Treatment and results of recurrent cancer of corpus uteri in patients receiving anterior and total pelvic exenteration. Cancer 22:949, 1956
14. Barber HRK, Graber EA: Gynecological tumors in childhood and adolescence. Obstet Gynecol Survey 28:357, 1973
15. Barber HRK, Graber EA: Surgical aspects of ovarian cancer, in: Selected Topics of Cancer—Current Concepts. Miami, Symposia Specialists, 1974, pp 161–183
16. Barber HRK, Graber EA: The PMPO syndrome (postmenopausal palpable ovary syndrome). Obstet Gynecol 38:921, 1971
17. Barber HRK, Graber EA, Kwon T: Ovarian cancer. CA 24:339, 1975
18. Barber HRK, Kwon T: Cancer of the endometrium. *In* Nealon TF Jr (ed): Management of the Patient with Cancer. Philadelphia, WB, Saunders, 1976, ed. 2 (in press)
19. Barber HRK, Kwon T: Carcinoma of the vulva, in Conn HF (ed): Current Therapy. Philadelphia, WB Saunders Co, 1975, p. 769
20. Barber HRK, Reisman B, Sommers SC, Graber EA: Cancer of the endometrium. Tex Med 70:41, 1974
21. Barber HRK, Sommers SC, Snyder R, Kwon T: Histologic and nuclear grading and stromal reactions as indices for prognosis in ovarian cancer. Am J Obstet Gynecol 121:795, 1975
22. Bell HG, Edgehill H: Sarcomas developing in uterine fibroids: review of literature and presentation of 3 cases. Am J Surg 100:416, 1960
23. Boronow RC: Chemotherapy for disseminated tubal cancer. Obstet Gynecol 42:62, 1973
24. Boutselis J, Thompson J: Clinical aspects of primary carcinoma of the fallopian tube. Am J Obstet Gynecol 111:98, 1971
25. Brewer JI, Eckman TR, Dolhart RE, Torok EE, Webster A: Gestational trophoblastic disease. Am J Obstet Gynecol 109:335, 1971
26. Brewer JI, Gerbie AB, Dolhart RE, Skom JH, Nagle RG, Torok EE: Chemotherapy in trophoblastic disease. Am J Obstet Gynecol 90:566, 1964
27. Brown AR, Fletcher GH, Rutledge FN: Irradiation of ''in situ'' and invasive squamous carcinoma of the vagina. Cancer 28:1278, 1971
28. Brunschwig A: Complete excision of pelvic viscera for advanced carcinoma. Cancer 1:177, 1948
29. Brunschwig A, Barber HRK: Surgical treatment of carcinoma of the cervix. Obstet Gynecol 27:21, 1966

30. Cancer Facts and Figures. American Cancer Society, 1975
31. Delclos L, Smith JP: Tumors of the ovary, in Fletcher G (ed): Textbook of Radiotherapy. Philadelphia, Lea & Febiger, 1973
32. Delfs E: Quantitative chorionic gonadotropin: Prognostic value in hydatidiform mole and chorioepithelioma. Obstet Gynecol 9:1, 1957
33. DiSaia PJ, Castro JR, Rutledge FN: Mixed mesodermal sarcoma of the uterus. Am J Roentgenol Radium Ther Nucl Med 117:632, 1973
34. DiSaia PJ, Morrow CP, Townsend DE: Cancer of the vulva. West J Med 118:13, 1973
35. Donovan JF: Nonhormonal chemotherapy of endometrial adenocarcinoma: a review. Cancer 34:1587, 1974
36. Dudan RC, Ford JH Jr, Yon JL, Averette HE: Carcinoma of the cervix and pregnancy. Gynecol Oncol 1:283, 1973
37. Frick HC Jacox, HW, Taylor HC: Primary carcinoma of the vagina. Am J Obstet Gynecol 101:695, 1968
38. Frick HC, Munnell EW, Richart RM, Berger AP, Lawry MF: Carcinoma of the endometrium. Am J Obstet Gynecol 115:663, 1973
39. Gibbs EK: Suggested prophylaxis for ovarian cancer: a 20 year report from cases at Butterworth Hospital. Am J Obstet Gynecol 111:756, 1971
40. Graham J: The value of preoperative or postoperative treatment by radium for carcinoma of the uterine body. Surg Gynecol Obstet 132:855, 1971
41. Green TH, Scully RE: Tumors of the fallopian tube. Clin Obstet Gynecol 5:886, 1962
42. Green TH, Ulfelder H, Meigs JV: Epidermoid carcinoma of the vulva. Am J Obstet Gynecol 75:834, 1958
43. Greenwald EF: Ovarian tumors. Clin Obstet Gynecol 18:61, 1975
44. Hammond CB, Lewis JL Jr: Gestational trophoblastic neoplasms, in: Davis' Gynecology and Obstetrics, vol 1. New York, Harper & Row, 1972, p 1
45. Herbst AL, Green TH, Ulfelder H: Primary carcinoma of vagina. Am J Obstet Gynecol 106:210, 1970
46. Herbst AL, Kurman RJ, Scully RE, et al: Clear cell adenocarcinoma of the genital tract in young females: Registry report. N Engl J Med 287:1259, 1972
47. Kempson RL, Bari W: Uterine sarcomas: Classification, diagnosis and prognosis. Hum Pathol 1:331, 1970
48. Kottmeier HC: Ovarian cancer with special regard to radiotherapy. Am J Roentgenol Radium Ther Nucl Med 3:417, 1971
49. Krakoff JH: Cancer chemotherapeutic agents. CA 23:209, 1973
50. Krukenberg F: Fibrosarcoma ovarii mucocellulare. Arch Gynak 1:287, 1893; Über das fibrosarcoma ovarri mucocellulare (carcinomatodes). Arch Gynak 30:287, 1896
51. Lawrence W Jr: Current status of regional chemotherapy, Part I and Part II. NY State J Med 63:2359, 2518, 1963
52. Lewis J Jr: Chemotherapy for metastatic gestational trophoblastic neoplasms. Clin Obstet Gynecol 10:330, 1967
53. Lewis BV, Stallworthy JA, Cowdell R: Adenocarcinoma of the body of the

uterus. J Obstet Gynecol Br Commonw 77:343, 1970

54. Li MC, Hertz R, Spencer DB: Effects of methotrexate therapy upon choriocarcinoma and chorioadenoma. Proc Soc Exp Biol Med 93:361, 1956

55. Marcus SL: Primary carcinoma of the vagina. Obstet Gynecol 15:673, 1960

56. McGowan L: Cancer in Pregnancy. Springfield, Ill., Charles C Thomas, 1967, p 84

57. Meigs JV: Surgical Treatment of Cancer of the Cervix. New York, Grune & Stratton, 1954, pp 83–84

58. Meigs JV, Brunschwig A: A proposed classification for cases of cancer of the cervix treated by surgery. Am J Obstet Gynecol 64:413, 1952

59. Morris J MacLean, Scully R: Endocrine Pathology of the Ovary. St. Louis, CV Mosby Co, 1958, p 65

60. Morrow CP, DiSaia PJ, Townsend DT: Current management of endometrial carcinoma. Obstet Gynecol 42:399, 1973

61. Ober WB: Uterine sarcomas: Histogenesis and taxonomy. Ann NY Acad Sci 73:568, 1959

62. Parry-Jones E: Lymphatics of vulva. J Obstet Gynecol Br Commonw 67:919, 1960

63. Queenan JT (ed): Symposium: Managing the hydatidiform mole patient. 3:117, 1974

64. Randall CR: Background of statistical data on ovarian cancer, in Barber HRK, Graber EA (eds): Gynecological Oncology. Amsterdam, Excerpta Medica, 1970, p 211

65. Reagen JW: The changing nature of endometrial cancer. Gynecol Oncol 2:144, 1974

66. Reifenstein ED Jr: The treatment of advanced endometrial cancer with hydroxy-progesterone caproate. Gynecol Oncol 2:377, 1974

67. Ross GT, Goldstein DP, Hertz R, Lipsett MB, Odell WD: Sequential use of methotrexate and actinomycin D in treatment of metastatic choriocarcinoma and related trophoblastic diseases in women. Am J Obstet Gynecol 93:223, 1965

68. Schiller H, Silverberg S: Staging and prognosis in primary carcinoma of the fallopian tube. Cancer 28:389–395, 1971

69. Scully R: Recent progress in ovarian cancer. Hum Pathol 1:73, 1970

70. Sedlis A: Carcinoma of the fallopian tube, in Barber HRK, Graber EA (eds): Symposium on Gynecological Oncology, A Comprehensive Review and Evaluation. Amsterdam, Excerpta Medica Foundation, 1969, p 198

71. Silverberg E, Holleb A: Statistics. Cancer Bull 23: No. 1, 1973

72. Smith JP: Chemotherapy in gynecologic cancer. Clin Obstet Gynecol 18:109, 1975

73. Smith JP, Rutledge FN: Metastatic ovarian cancer. Clin Obstet Gynecol 16:286, 1973

74. Smith JP, Rutledge F, Wharton JT: Chemotherapy of ovarian cancer. New approaches to treatment. Cancer 30:1565, 1972

75. Stander RW: Vaginal metastases following treatment of endometrial carcinoma. Am J Obstet Gynecol 71:776, 1956

76. Teilum G: Tumors of germinal origin. Ovarian cancer. *In* International Union against Cancer Monograph Series, vol. II. Berlin, Springer-Verlag, 1968, p 58

77. Thornton WW, Carter JP: Sarcoma of the uterus: A clinical study. Am J Obstet Gynecol 62:294, 1951

78. Webb MJ, Decker DG, Mussey E: Cancer metastatic to the ovary: Factors influencing survival. Obstet Gynecol 45:391, 1975

79. White KC: Ovarian tumors in pregnancy. Am J Obstet Gynecol 116:544, 1973

Harold M. Maurer, M.D.
and Nancy B. McWilliams, M.D.

13

Management of Pediatric Solid Tumors

Although cancer is less common in children than in adults, it kills more children than any other disease in the 1–14-age group. Leukemia, the most common malignancy in childhood, is not considered in this chapter. Only those "solid tumors" outside the central nervous system that occur with some degree of regularity are described.

Substantial progress has been made in the treatment of childhood solid tumors during the last two decades with the notable exception of neuroblastoma. Improved survival is a result of many factors that include careful disease staging, improved histological classifications, new techniques for accurately defining disease extent, effective chemotherapy coordinated with improved radiation therapy and surgery to maximize the benefit of each, and finally, vigorous supportive therapy. The importance of active rehabilitation programs and continuing emotional support of the children and their families throughout the treatment cannot be overemphasized.

Certain principles of therapy have gradually evolved during this period:

1. Combined-modality therapy is superior to therapy with any single modality by itself.
2. Adjuvant chemotherapy, radiation therapy, and immunotherapy are of maximum benefit when the body burden of tumor cells is lowest. Thus, surgical excision of bulk disease, if feasible, is an important component of therapy.
3. "Prophylactic" chemotherapy, better termed chemotherapy of micrometastases, prolongs remission and increases survival.

4. Combination chemotherapy is superior to single-agent chemotherapy.
5. Maintenance chemotherapy given during the period of greatest risk of recurrence prolongs remission and increases survival.
6. Intermittent chemotherapy schedules are superior to continuous chemotherapy schedules.
7. Drug and treatment schedule selections should be based on the knowledge of the proliferative behavior of the malignant cell and the cell cycle specificity of the drug whenever possible.
8. For childhood solid tumors, 2-year disease-free survival is usually equivalent to cure.

Treatment of childhood solid tumors will obviously remain in a dynamic state until "the cure" is found. As new knowledge becomes available, existing treatment programs are modified and new ones are developed. Thus, recommendations made in this chapter, although appropriate at present, are by no means fixed.

In contrast to the management of cancer in adults, surgical and other treatment procedures employed for children must be aimed at preserving normal growth and development in addition to saving lives.

WILMS' TUMOR

Wilms' tumor is the most common intra-abdominal tumor of childhood.[84] In 1899 Max Wilms compiled and reported cases of this tumor and described it as a clinical entity. Although the tumor may present at birth, the median age at diagnosis is approximately 43 months, with the disease being slightly more common in males than in females (1.2:1). Approximately 15 percent of patients are black.

Clinical Features and Diagnostic Studies

In the majority of patients an abdominal mass is the first abnormality noted and is frequently discovered by the parents. Less-common symptoms include abdominal pain, hematuria, anorexia, nausea, vomiting, diarrhea and/or fever. The tumor arises in the left kidney in over half of the cases. Because of the greater length of the left renal vein, a left-sided Wilms' tumor is less difficult to remove than one involving the right kidney. In 10–12 percent of children, tumors occur bilaterally. Two-thirds of bilateral tumors are usually discovered at the time of initial diagnosis, and one-third become apparent 6–15 months after the first tumor is diagnosed.[57] A variety of congenital malformations may be found with increased frequency among children with Wilms' tumor. These include hemihypertrophy, bilateral aniridia, hypospadias, cryptorchidism, horseshoe kidney, and other renal anomalies.[49] Although the genesis of each anomaly and its association with the origin of Wilms' tumor are unknown, children with these high-risk malformations should be observed carefully for the appearance of this tumor.

Pathology

The histologic appearance of Wilms' tumor shows a wide variation in growth pattern. It is usually characterized by growth of undifferentiated embryonic renal tissue in various stages of tubular and primitive glomerular differentiation. In some cases, nonepithelial components also appear in varying proportions. There is a greater degree of nonepithelial differentiation (fibrous, striated, and smooth muscle components) and a decrease in the tubular and glomerular differentiation in the metastases as compared to the primary tumors. Irradiation appears to accelerate and possibly induce nonepithelial differentiation. Tumors with a predominance of epithelial elements, well-formed glomeruloid structures, and tubules appear less prone to metastasize and have been associated with a better prognosis than tumors with a predominance of undifferentiated spindle cells.

More recently, mesoblastic nephroma of infancy has been distinguished histologically from Wilms' tumor.[29] Mesoblastic nephroma may have constituted as many as 50 percent of the renal tumors of infancy previously reported and may account for the improved survival of children less than 1 year of age misdiagnosed as having true Wilms' tumor in the past. Although mesonephroma generally is histologically benign, instances of malignant clinical behavior have been described.[29]

Staging Classification

Clinical and anatomic staging of Wilms' tumor is important since it determines in large measure the type of therapy to be given. Staging is done by the surgeon in the operating room and is confirmed by the pathologist. Although the scheme devised by the National Wilms' Tumor Study (NWTS) provides for "clinical groups" rather than "stages," it remains the staging system of choice at this time.[11] Details of this scheme and the recommended current therapy for each clinical group are shown in Table 13-1. Meticulous examination of the surgical specimen is required since it is well established that the extent of disease at diagnosis is the most important factor in prognosis.

Preoperative evaluation should include the following: chest x-ray

Table 13-1
Wilms' Tumor: Clinical Grouping and Treatment After Surgery

Clinical Group[11]	Estimated Percentage of Cases	Postoperative Treatment*
I. Tumor limited to kidney and completely resected. Surface of renal capsule intact	35	Dact, 15 µg/kg, IV, for 5 days; 5-day course repeated at 6 weeks, and at 3, 6, 9, 12, and 15 months Vcr, 1.5 mg/sq m on day 7 and then weekly for 7 weeks; then 2 doses are given every 3 mo from 3–15 mo postoperatively, administered on the 1st and 5th day of the Dact course
II. Tumor extends beyond the kidney but is completely resected; penetration beyond pseudocapsule; periaortic lymph nodes involved; renal vessels outside kidney substance involved	25	Radiotherapy to tumor bed Chemotherapy as with I
III. Residual nonhematogenous tumor confined to abdomen Any one or more of following occur: 1. Biopsy or rupture 2. Implants on peritoneal surfaces 3. Involved lymph nodes beyond periaortic chains 4. Tumor incompletely resected	20	Radiotherapy to entire abdomen with shielding of the opposite kidney Chemotherapy as with I
IV. Hematogenous metastases (e.g., lung, liver, bone, brain)	20	Radiotherapy to tumor bed and metastases Chemotherapy as with I
V. Bilateral renal involvement	—	Radiotherapy to tumor bed Chemotherapy as with I

* Dact, dactinomycin; Vcr, vincristine.

(and possibly tomography), intravenous pyelogram with simultaneous inferior venacavagram, liver and bone scans, complete blood count, urinalysis, BUN, SGOT, LDH, uric acid, alkaline phosphatase, and bone marrow examination. Blood pressures should be monitored and if hypertension exists medical treatment should be instituted before surgery is undertaken.

Treatment

SURGERY

Surgery is the cornerstone of therapy and should be undertaken without undue delay. Tumor can usually be removed even if it has already extended to adjacent viscera. Every effort should be made to remove as much tumor bulk as possible, even if distant metastases are present, to afford greater success with postoperative radiation therapy and chemotherapy. At the present time, surgery usually precedes all chemotherapy and radiation therapy. The following aspects of the surgical procedure deserve emphasis:

1. A generous transverse transperitoneal incision is the most desirable. The incision lends itself well to thorough inspection of the abdominal contents and identification of the renal artery and vein, which should be dissected carefully and ligated as quickly as possible.

2. The contralateral kidney should be inspected and palpated both anteriorly and posteriorly, and any suspicious nodule must be totally excised if possible, or the site marked with metallic clips for the radiotherapists.

3. The entire mass, including the perirenal fascia and fat, should be removed and the margins of any tumor not amenable to resection marked with metallic clips. The tumor bed should also be marked with clips so that postoperative radiation therapy fields can be well delineated.

4. Thorough and complete lymph node dissection from the level of the diaphragm to the aortic bifurcation is recommended for both staging of disease and removal of any residual tumor.

5. When the disease is bilateral, bilateral partial nephrectomy, when possible, should be performed. If one tumor is large and not amenable to partial nephrectomy, the entire kidney should be removed and the opposite side treated with partial nephrectomy. In either case surgery would be followed by radiation therapy and chemotherapy.

6. In contrast to the treatment of many other types of malignancies, Wilms' tumor metastases should be attacked vigorously. Surgical excision of pulmonary metastases should be considered if metastases are lim-

ited to a solitary nodule or a resectable anatomic segment of the lung after a trial of radiation therapy and chemotherapy. Solitary liver metastasis have been successfully treated in some cases by resection.

RADIOTHERAPY

Recommended cobalt radiotherapy techniques and dosages are those employed in the NWTS. Irradiation of the postoperative tumor bed is recommended for clinical groups II through V to eradicate any residual disease. The tumor confines on the affected side are considered "contaminated," and all this volume is included within the treatment fields. The field is extended across the midline to include all of the vertebral bodies at the levels concerned, but the field does not overlap any portion of the contralateral kidney. Opposing anterior-posterior portals are used. Treatment is given 5 or 6 days a week at a rate of 1000–1200 rads per week. The doses to be employed are as follows:

Age	Total Tumor Dose
Birth to 18 months	1800–2400 rads
19–30 months	2400–3000 rads
31–40 months	3000–3500 rads
41 months or older	3500–4000 rads

For group III patients, abdominal bath treatment is delivered shielding the opposite kidney after 1500 rads and the liver after 3000 rads. Pulmonary metastases are treated by total thoracic irradiation regardless of the number and location of visible metastases. The recommended dose is 1400 rads. Liver metastases may be treated with doses of 3000 rads in 3.5–4 weeks, and metastases to brain, bone, lymph nodes, and other sites are treated using doses comparable to those delivered to the liver. Chemotherapy is of course administered concurrently.

CHEMOTHERAPY

The major advance in the treatment of Wilms' tumor has been the development of effective chemotherapy, although optimal chemotherapy has not yet been defined.[71,86] Current recommendations are shown in Table 13-1. Dactinomycin and vincristine are the most active agents now available and are recommended in combination. Adriamycin, a new agent, has promising antitumor effect and is currently being investigated in combination with the dactinomycin and vincristine. Cyclophosphamide also has antitumor activity but its activity is of low order in Wilms' tumor.

Complications of dactinomycin include myelosuppression, abdominal pain, nausea, vomiting, ulceration of the buccal mucosa, and alopecia. Erythema of the skin in the radiation portals has been induced by this agent. Vincristine causes constipation, alopecia, and a constellation of neuromuscular problems including paresthesias in the fingers and toes, jaw or throat pain, muscle weakness, ptosis, and eventual disappearance of the deep tendon reflexes. Adriamycin causes alopecia, myelosuppression, and at total doses above 600 mg/sq m, cardiac toxicity. Each of these agents is given intravenously and can cause severe skin irritation when extravasation occurs.

Prognosis

The outlook in Wilms' tumor has changed considerably during the last few decades, and now approximately 80 percent of children can be cured provided they receive the benefits of a coordinated treatment program using surgery, radiation therapy, and chemotherapy. Generally speaking, a disease-free survival of 2 years is equivalent to a cure. According to the NWTS, the following 2 year disease-free rates might be expected: group I, 86 percent; groups II and III, 79 percent. The 2-year survival rate overall is above 90 percent for each of these groups and is approximately 60 percent for group IV patients.

NEUROBLASTOMA

Although the concept of cure is now a reality in many childhood tumors, neuroblastoma still represents a major stumbling block on the road to complete control of pediatric malignancies.

Neuroblastoma is the commonest form of solid tumor in children after tumors of the central nervous system. It is a disease of infants and young children, and some 75 percent of cases are diagnosed during the first 3 years of life.[38] There is a preponderance of males to females in a ratio of approximately 1.4:1 among white children.[89] Although no hereditary factor is proven, a number of cases of familial neuroblastoma have been reported.[7,78,88]

Neuroblastoma and its variants, ganglioneuroblastoma and ganglioneuroma, represent a unique spectrum of human neoplasms and comprise a biologic continuum.[32] They arise from cells derived from embryonic sympathetic neuroblasts, which migrate ventrally during fetal life to give rise to the sympathetic ganglia and adrenal medulla.

Neuroblastoma has many curious features. It has been reported in situ in autopsied infants under 3 months of age, and it was found in the adrenals of 1 of every 200 infants in a study by Beckwith and Perrin[2] and in 1 out of 39 adrenals scrutinized by Guin and associates.[21] Spontaneous regression in neuroblastoma is reported, as is benign transformation to ganglioneuroma.[17,82]   The association between these phenomena and the presence of a complex host immune response in neuroblastoma is intriguing.[23]

Pathology

Histologically neuroblastoma consists of sheets of small round cells with scant cytoplasm and central densely staining nuclei.   Rosette-like arrangements of cells are found in the less-undifferentiated tumors with neurofibrils occupying the center of each rosette.

The ganglioneuroblastoma contains varying numbers of mature ganglion cells admixed with immature neuroblasts, whereas the benign ganglioneuroma contains aggregates of mature ganglion cells and neurofibrils scattered throughout collagenous tissue.

Clinical Features and Diagnostic Studies

Approximately 60 percent of neuroblastomas arise in the abdomen or pelvis; hence, overall an abdominal mass is the most common presenting sign.   Other signs and symptoms of the disease are legion and may be related to: metastases, e.g., bone pain, anemia, proptosis; direct extension of the tumor, e.g., spinal cord compression, tracheal-bronchial obstruction, lower urinary tract obstruction; or presumed biochemically mediated effects from excess catecholamine secretion, e.g., chronic diarrhea, polymyoclonia-opsoclonia.

Neuroblastoma must be considered in any child with an unexplained neurological finding, unexplained limp, or prolonged unexplained fever.

Complete hematologic examination including bone marrow aspiration is crucial.   A skeletal survey and/or bone scan, a chest radiograph, and an intravenous pyelogram (IVP) must all be done in a patient suspected of having neuroblastoma.   Injection of contrast material for the IVP through a vein in the foot frequently yields more information about the extent of the tumor and its relationship to the inferior vena cava than the standard antecubital vein injection.   A 24-hour urine sample should be collected before surgery and examined for catecholamines, their metabolites, or both.

Staging Classification

The widely accepted staging system of Evans and associates[16] is based on patterns of origin and clinical behavior.

Stage I: Tumor confined to organ or structure of origin.

Stage II: Tumors extending in continuity beyond the organ or struc-
                ture of origin but not crossing the midline, with or without
                regional lymph node involvement on the homolateral side;
                or tumors in midline structures, e.g., the organs of Zucker-
                kandl with penetration beyond the capsule and involvement
                of lymph nodes on the same side.
Stage III: Tumors extending in continuity beyond the midline, with or
                without bilateral lymph node involvement, or bilateral ex-
                tension of tumors arising in midline structures.
Stage IV: Remote disease involving skeleton, organs, soft tissues, or
                distant lymph nodes.
Stage IV-S: Patients who would otherwise be stage I or II but who have
                remote disease confined to one or more of the following
                sites: liver, skin, or bone marrow (without radiographic evi-
                dence of bone metastases).

Treatment

Total surgical excision is the ideal treatment for neuroblastoma; but
tumor size, invasion of or adherence to vital structures, extension through
neural foramina, and frequent presence of distant metastases at the time
of diagnosis limit the number of patients who will be cured by surgery.
For children with stage I, II, or IV-S disease, however, surgery alone may
be curative. The role of adjunct chemotherapy and radiation therapy
after surgery is not well defined in these groups.

The role of surgery in patients with unresectable widespread tumor
should be limited to biopsy only. In those patients with large bulk tumor
(stage III) we recommend removal of as much tumor as possible without
jeopardizing normal organs and placement of silver clips around the remaining lesions. If response to radiation and chemotherapy is favorable, a second operation may be considered.

Vincristine, cyclophosphamide, daunomycin, and adriamycin have
been shown to have some effect in neuroblastoma.[27,65,66,79] We recommend courses of combination chemotherapy at 4-week intervals starting
with vincristine 1.5 mg/sq m IV weekly ×2, cyclophosphamide 500
mg/sq m IV, and adriamycin 25 mg/sq m/day ×3 IV. At week 4, or after
marrow recovery, vincristine 1.5 mg/sq m is again given weekly ×2,
adriamycin is omitted, and cyclophosphamide is given in a dose of
1000 mg/sq m IV. This schedule is repeated at 4-week intervals and
should be continued for 12 months. When the cumulative adriamycin
dose reaches 540 mg/sq m, it should be discontinued and vincristine and
cyclophosphamide continued for an additional 6–12 months.

In patients with stage III disease or stage IV with bulky tumor, radia-

tion therapy should be started after the first two courses of chemotherapy, i.e., week 5. The dose must be adjusted for age and should not exceed 2400 rads in children less than 18 months or 4000 rads in children
older than 40 months. It should be given in 180–200-rad fractions 5 days
a week.

Prognosis

Prognosis for survival in neuroblastoma has been estimated by site,
histologic criteria, age of the patient, and stage of the disease. Studies on
the relationship between the degree of histologic differentiation of the
tumor and survival indicate improved survival with greater differentiation, and, in general, thoracic lesions are more favorable than abdominal
tumors.[16,42]

Breslow and McCann[4] analyzed the joint influence of age and disease
state on survival in 134 children with neuroblastoma. They concluded
that both were highly significant in determining prognosis, even after an
adjustment was made for the effect of the other variable. The older the
child, the worse the prognosis in each stage except stage I. The 2-year
disease-free survival was 74 percent for children less than 1 year and only
12 percent for those older than 2 years. They found that 85 percent of
the children with stage I disease, 77 percent with stage IV-S, 63 percent
with stage II, 37 percent with stage III, and only 5.8 percent with stage IV
survived free of disease for 2 years.[4]

These grim statistics indicate that new agents are needed for the
treatment of neuroblastoma. Compounds that stimulate immune responsiveness might prove useful if truly effective chemotherapy were available to reduce tumor cell burden substantially.

RHABDOMYOSARCOMA

Rhabdomyosarcoma is the most frequent soft tissue sarcoma found
in children.[48] Surprisingly, based on patient accrual rates in national
studies [National Wilms' Tumor Study and Intergroup Rhabdomyosarcoma (IRS)], rhabdomyosarcoma appears to occur at least as frequently
as Wilms' tumor.[45] Improved understanding of the histologic features of
the tumor probably accounts for the increase in its recognition. Survival
rates have increased dramatically from less than 20 percent one and one-
half decades ago to over 70 percent at the present time coincident with the
change in treatment from surgery or radiation therapy to a multidisciplinary approach using surgery, radiation therapy, and intensive chemotherapy at diagnosis.[34,47]

Clinical Features and Diagnostic Studies

Approximately 70 percent of the cases present before age 10, with the peak incidence being between ages 2 and 5. The disease is more common in males than females. The abnormality most frequently noted is a mass. Signs and symptoms relate primarily either to the location of the primary tumor, which can arise virtually anywhere, or to the metastases. The common sites of origin in order of frequency are the head and neck region (36 percent), extremities (24 percent), genitourinary tract (18 percent), trunk (8 percent), retroperitoneum (7 percent), gastrointestinal-hepatobiliary tract (3 percent), intrathoracic region (2 percent), and perineum-anus (2 percent).

Orbital tumors produce proptosis. Nasopharyngeal tumors cause airway obstruction, sinusitis, epistaxis, local pain, and dysphagia. Middle ear involvement is associated with a polypoid mass in the external auditory canal with pain and unremitting otitis media. Cervical and nasopharyngeal masses may extend directly into the central nervous system causing cranial nerve palsies, meningeal symptoms, and respiratory paralysis owing to infiltration of the brainstem. The tumor can arise in the prostate and bladder causing urinary tract symptoms. Paratesticular lesions usually present as masses. In girls, the classic sarcoma botryoides may arise from the vagina or uterus and present as a hemorrhagic polypoid mass protuding from the introitus or cervix.

Rhabdomyosarcoma extends locally and margins are indistinct. Metastases result from lymphatic and hematogenous spread. Common sites of metastasis include lung, bone, bone marrow, lymph nodes, brain, and heart.

Noteworthy is an increased incidence of carcinoma of the breast in relatives of children with rhabdomyosarcoma.[36] There is also a high frequency of soft tissue sarcoma, brain tumor, and adrenocortical carcinoma among siblings.[36]

Histological Classification

Rhabdomyosarcoma arises from embryonic mesenchyme. Five histologic variants have now been identified in children.[67] The most common form, the embryonal type, is more frequently encountered in the head and neck regions. These lesions are composed primarily of small, round, and spindle-shaped rhabdomyoblasts.

The alveolar type is more often found in the deep tissues of the trunk and extremities. Rhabdomyoblasts are often mixed with larger round cells that exhibit more prominent eosinophilic cytoplasm. The tumor cells tend to grow in cords that often present cleftlike spaces.

The botryoid type is usually seen in the urogenital tract but is occasionally found in other regions, for example, in the head and neck region. A layer of small round cells is apparent at the periphery of the polypoid tumor. A zone of myxoid stroma is followed by a deeper compact zone composed of round and spindle-shaped cells that can usually be readily recognized as rhabdomyoblasts.

The pleomorphic type (adult form) occurs most often in the somatic soft parts of the extremities and trunk. It is composed of larger, more pleomorphic cells, often described as strap-shaped cells with multiple nuclei in tandem, racket-shaped cells with cytoplasmic tails, large round cells with giant size nucleus, and multinucleated giant tumor cells.

Recently, a fifth variant occurring in soft tissues but considered histologically indistinguishable from Ewing's sarcoma of bone has been described and is referred to as "extraosseous Ewing's."[1,68] This type is found in only a small number of cases. The tumor is composed of round or slightly elongated cells that exhibit a scant amount of cytoplasm containing glycogen. The cells are larger than those seen in Ewing's sarcoma and are not clearly identifiable as rhabdomyoblasts.

There is a tendency for some rhabdomyosarcomas to show mixtures of the different tumor types, particularly the embryonal and alveolar types. Pleomorphic foci are also seen occasionally. Cross striations are frequently not found in a given tumor and are not essential for diagnosis.

When the diagnosis is questionable, electron microscopy may reveal thin and thick myosin filaments and primative Z-bands not visible by light microscopy. Antimyosin immunofluorescence can be used to confirm the presence of myosin in the tumor cells.

Staging Classification

A clinical staging classification for rhabdomyosarcoma has recently been established by the Intergroup Rhabdomyosarcoma Study and is described in Table 13-2.[45] The amount of residual disease after surgical resection plus the status of the regional lymph nodes are to a large extent determinants of clinical stage. Staging is extremely important for treatment planning and prognosis.

In addition to a complete history, physical examination, CBC, and urinalysis, preoperative evaluation should include chest film, bone scan and/or skeletal survey, bone marrow aspiration or biopsy, liver scan, brain scan, and CSF examination for those with head and neck tumors; lymphangiography for children with lower extremity and genitourinary lesions; and, as indicated, angiography for deep-seated tumors, full-lung tomography, and gallium scan. Chemistries should include BUN, LDH, SGOT, uric acid, bilirubin, creatinine, and alkaline phosphatase.

Table 13-2
Rhabdomyosarcoma: Clinical Grouping and Treatment After Surgery

Clinical Grouping[45]	Estimated Percentage of Cases	Postoperative Treatment*
I. Localized disease, completely resected; no lymph node involvement a. Confined to muscle or organ of origin b. Contiguous involvement with infiltration outside the muscle or organ of origin, as through fascial planes; microscopic confirmation of complete resection	20	Dact, 15 µg/kg, IV, for 5 days; 5-day courses repeated at 12, 24, 36, and 48 weeks Vcr, 2 mg/sq m, IV weekly for 12 doses Cyclo, 2.5 mg/kg/day, orally starting on day 42 and continuing up through 24 months
II. a. Localized tumor, grossly resected, but with micro-scopic residual disease; no lymph node involvement b. Regional disease, completely resected without micro-scopic residual; regional nodes involved or extension of tumor into an adjacent organ c. Regional disease with involved nodes, grossly resected, but with residual microscopic disease	25	Radiotherapy to tumor bed Chemotherapy as with I
III. Incomplete resection or biopsy with gross residual disease	35	Dact, 15 µg/kg IV for 5 days; 5-day courses repeated at 18, 30, 42, and 54 weeks Vcr, 2 mg/sq m IV weekly for 12 doses Cyclo, 10 mg/kg/day, IV for 5 days; a second 5-day course is given at 13 weeks (oral); from the 21st week through 24th month, 2.5 mg/kg/day, orally; radio-therapy to tumor bed at 6 weeks
IV. Distant metastatic disease present at onset (lung, liver, bone, bone marrow, brain, and distant muscle and node)	20	Chemotherapy as with III plus Adr, 60 mg/sq m IV at 5, 18, 27, 39, and 51 weeks Radiotherapy to tumor bed and to metastases at 6 weeks

* Dact, dactinomycin; Vcr, vincristine; Cyclo, Cyclophosphamide; Adr, Adriamycin.

Treatment

SURGERY

Surgical management of rhabdomyosarcoma currently is undergoing change in parallel with improved survival from combined chemotherapy and radiation therapy programs. Evidence is accumulating that limited surgical excision with preservation of the organ involved may be all that is required for selected sites of origin.[31,60] Radical surgical excision, heretofore employed exclusively, may at times not be necessary for disease control. The operative procedure employed depends on the primary site of involvement and the extent of local and distant disease.

The basic principle of wide excision of the primary tumor with an "envelope" of normal tissue is best adhered to whenever possible, but this approach is generally more applicable to extremity lesions and certain trunk lesions than to those of the head and neck. If the surgeon leaves "microscopic residual," as judged by positive histologic examination of resected margins, a second resection may not be required if chemotherapy and radiation therapy are to follow.

Recent evidence suggests that regional lymph node involvement occurs with sufficient frequency to justify lymph node biopsy or elective node dissection for genitourinary (particularly paratesticular lesions) and extremity primaries.[35] Although the variety of anatomic possibilities is too great to establish a firm guideline for lymph node management, the regional nodes should be considered for biopsy if the surgeon does not plan regional lymph node dissection as part of his definitive procedure. Metal clips should be placed in areas of node removal that might prove to be positive, at the periphery of unremoved tumor, or at sites of possible residual tumor tissue during operations in the abdomen or thorax to aid in directing subsequent radiotherapy. Pedal lymphangiography may be helpful in staging patients with pelvic, inguinal canal, and paratesticular lesions.

Further guidelines for surgery depend on disease site.

Orbit. Simple biopsy followed by radiation therapy and chemotherapy is appropriate for orbital cancers, although some centers still prefer exenteration.[64]

Head and neck. Wide excision is appropriate, but the possibility of achieving wide margins is quite restricted.[14] Biopsy is often the only procedure possible short of radical surgery.

Extremity. Amputation or wide local excision is required to avoid recurrence when surgery alone is used. More conservative surgical procedures are under study in which the emphasis is placed on removal of tumor bulk only, relying on postoperative chemotherapy and radiation therapy for control of local residual disease.

Pelvis. The preservation of one or more of the major pelvic organs, i.e., the bladder or rectum, is an important goal in therapy, and if the tumor is grossly completely removed, it is probable that microscopic residual tumor in the walls of these organs may be controlled by chemotherapy and radiation therapy.[60]

Paratesticular tumors. Inguinal orchiectomy with high ligation of the spermatic cord is coupled with retroperitoneal lymph node dissection. The remaining testicle may be spared exposure to irradiation by relocating it into the tissues of the ipsilateral thigh, subcutaneously. After irradiation is completed, the testicle is returned to its normal position.

Recurrent disease. The patient should definitely be submitted to a "curative" surgical procedure if this is anatomically feasible and if there are no distant metastases. Persistent metastatic disease in the lung following chemotherapy and radiation therapy should be resected if this can be accomplished and if it is warranted by the general status of the patient.

RADIATION THERAPY

A dose of 5000 rads in 5 weeks to 6000 rads in 6 weeks to the primary tumor is recommended.[77] Lower doses of irradiation might be considered in the very young child, especially under 3 years of age, when the primary site is to be irradiated. However, no less than 4000 rads in 4 weeks should be given in this latter instance. It is important to protect such vital structures as lung, kidney, and liver whenever possible, so that normal tissue tolerance is not exceeded.

"Prophylactic" irradiation of adjacent lymph node areas is not recommended.

When the whole abdomen must be included in the volume for irradiation, the dose to the abdominal contents should be limited to 3000 rads in 4 weeks. Local areas of the abdomen that contain the "bulk" of disease should be "boosted" to the prescribed doses listed above for primary tumors at other sites.

When secondary disease is present in a lung, bilateral lung irradiation is recommended (1400–1800 rads) even in the event of total regression of all demonstrable lesions by initial chemotherapy. Localized pulmonary nodules that persist may be treated through coned-down "postage stamp" portals to a *total* dose of 5000 rads.

Solitary bone metastasis may also be treated with local irradiation; doses of 5000–6000 rads in 5–6 weeks should be used.

After complete excision of localized disease, postoperative irradiation to the tumor bed does not appear to enhance local disease control
over that afforded by chemotherapy alone.[46] Thus, postoperative irradiation is not recommended for stage I disease when chemotherapy is given.
This recommendation is based on recent data derived from the IRS.

With the availability of effective chemotherapy programs, attempts
are being made to evaluate lower doses of irradiation (4000 rads) combined with chemotherapy for local disease control. Results using this approach are not yet available.

CHEMOTHERAPY

The evidence is compelling that all rhabdomyosarcoma patients
should receive chemotherapy routinely. Heyn and associates[24] showed
that the 2-year disease-free survival rate increases from 47 percent to 82
percent when 12 months of chemotherapy is given after total surgical removal of the primary tumor supplemented by postoperative radiation
therapy. The efficacy of such "prophylactic" chemotherapy, better
termed chemotherapy of micrometastases, has been demonstrated now
by several groups.

The role of chemotherapy in rhabdomyosarcoma is gradually changing from one of adjuvant therapy to one of primary therapy with the ad-
vent of effective drugs used in intensive combinations and schedules. In
the presence of gross residual or metastatic disease at diagnosis, a 6-week
course of chemotherapy is appropriate to reduce tumor burden before irradiation. The *complete* response rate from this "induction" chemotherapy alone in these children with advanced disease is approximately
25 percent with the overall response rate being about 80 percent. Chemotherapy should be continued for 2 years.

Drugs active against rhabdomyosarcoma are dactinomycin, vincristine, cyclophosphamide, and adriamycin and are best used in 2–4-drug
combinations. Although optimal chemotherapy schedules and doses
have not been defined, current recommendations based on the experience
of the IRS are shown in Table 13-2.

Drug toxicities have already been described in the discussion of
Wilms' tumor.

Prognosis

Younger children (below age 7) have a better prognosis than older
children according to Sutow and associates.[73] Younger children also
have less-advanced disease at diagnosis, possibly accounting for their
better prognosis.

Prognosis also varies with the location of the primary tumor. Lesions of the orbit and genitourinary tract have a comparatively good prognosis as they tend to infiltrate locally, metastasize late, and give rise to signs and symptoms early. Tumors originating in the prostate, middle ear, and extremity have a poorer outlook. Extremity and head and neck lesions tend to metastasize to the central nervous system.

Whether histologic type is of any prognostic value has yet to be determined. The historically "unfavorable" types (alveolar, pleomorphic) tend to occur in older children who as a group tend to have more advanced disease at diagnosis.

Although location provides a helpful prognostic clue, the extent of disease at diagnosis (stage) is the most important factor. At present, the 2-year survival rate is approximately 90 percent for stage I, 90 percent for stage II, 75 percent for stage III, and 45 percent for stage IV disease.

MALIGNANT LYMPHOMAS IN CHILDREN

The malignant lymphomas can be divided into two distinct groups: Hodgkin's disease and the non-Hodgkin's lymphomas. These two groups have in common an origin in lymphoid tissue but are otherwise dissimilar, in particular with regard to presentation, evolution, and response to treatment. Current methods of management are described in this section. A comprehensive review of these diseases is beyond the scope of this section and can be found elsewhere.[30]

Hodgkin's Disease

Similar patterns of disease are observed in adults and children. Thus, many of the decisions regarding management of childhood cases are based on the larger adult experience. Two notable areas where the philosophies of management differ concern the extent of irradiation to be delivered to a growing child and the need for splenectomy. Because of the deleterious effects of total nodal irridation on growth, involved field irradiation supplemented with chemotherapy is now being advocated.[76] Growth problems are minimized without sacrificing disease control. Late severe infection, usually pneumococcal, is the specific complication most feared after splenectomy in children, especially those under age 5 at diagnosis. This procedure is best avoided in the few cases falling into this age group.

STAGING CLASSIFICATION

Treatment decisions and prognosis are stage dependent. The Ann Arbor[69] classification has replaced the Rye[51] classification and is the one currently in use:

Stage I.   Involvement of a single lymph node region (I), on a single extralymphatic organ or site (I_E).

Stage II.   Involvement of two or more lymph node regions on the same side of the diaphragm (II), or localized involvement of extralymphatic organ site and of one or more lymph node regions on the same side of the diaphragm (II_E).

Stage III.   Involvement of lymph node regions on both sides of the diaphragm (III), which may be accompanied by localized involvement of extralymphatic organ or site (III_E), or by involvement of the spleen (III_S), or both (III_{SE}).

Stage IV.   Diffuse or disseminated involvement of one or more extralymphatic organs or tissue with or without associated lymph node enlargement.

Each stage is subdivided into "A" or "B" categories. A indicates that there are no systemic symptoms, and B indicates the presence of one or more of the following symptoms: (a) unexplained weight loss of more than 10 percent of the body weight in the prior 6 months, (b) unexplained fever with temperature above 38° C, (c) night sweats. Pruritus alone is no longer considered to warrant B status.

Staging laparotomy with splenectomy is appropriate in most circumstances for accurate classification.[22,63] Preoperative investigations that provide anatomical details of disease extent and assess organ function should also be included. Staging laparotomy results in a substantial increase in the proportion classified as stage III, mainly in children considered to have clinical stage II or I disease with supraclavicular localization. When laparotomy and lymphangiography are included in a careful evaluation, approximately one-half the children are found to have stage I or II disease and approximately one-third have stage III disease.

HISTOLOGICAL CLASSIFICATION

Hodgkin's disease is divided into four histological subgroups: lymphocytic predominance, nodular sclerosis, mixed cellularity, and lymphocytic depletion.[6,40] Nodular sclerosis appears to be the most common subgroup, although this varies a good deal from one report to another. Each histologic subgroup has certain clinical hallmarks. Lymphocytic predominance type is often found in stage I disease and is rarely associated with mediastinal involvement. Regional cervical disease with mediastinal lymphadenopathy is quite characteristic of the nodular sclerosis pattern, whereas lesions in nonadjacent regions above the diaphragm, with mediastinal sparing in combination with occult abdominal disease may be seen with the mixed cellularity variant. The lymphocyte depletion subgroup occurs infrequently in children.

TREATMENT

Treatment is outlined by stage and pattern of disease in Table 13-3. Irradiation fields are either total nodal—i.e., a combination of the mantle (nodal regions above the diaphragm) and the inverted Y (nodal regions below the diaphragm)—or involved fields only. Results of a large cooperative clinical study in adults show no significant difference in survival between patients treated with these two techniques.[50] Total nodal irradiation offers the least chance of relapse by disease extension to unirradiated lymph nodes. Involved field irradiation supplemented with chemotherapy may offer the same advantage.[76] A comparative trial of these techniques in childhood Hodgkin's disease has not yet been done.

The standard chemotherapy employed is the regimen introduced by DeVita et al.[13] and known as MOPP therapy. This consists of six 2-week cycles of nitrogen mustard (6 mg/sq m IV) and vincristine (1.4 mg/sq m IV) on days 1 and 8 of each cycle. Procarbazine (100 mg/sq m) and prednisone (40 mg/sq m) are taken daily by mouth in cycles 1 and 4. Each cycle is followed by a 2-week rest period. Recent experience indicates that this combination may be improved by substituting CCNU for nitrogen mustard, and by continuing on maintenance therapy (BCNU, vinblastine) after the six cycles.

B-DOPA is a second combination that shows promise and is active in patients who fail on MOPP therapy.[39] Drugs are given in the following schedule: bleomycin, 4 units/sq m, IV days 2 and 5; vincristine, 2 mg/sq m, IV days 1 and 5; adriamycin, 60 mg/sq m, IV day 1 only; prednisone, 40 mg/sq m, orally days 1 through 5; and DTIC, 150 mg/sq m IV

Table 13-3
Management of Hodgkin's Disease in Childhood*

Stage	Sites	Volume Irradiated	Chemotherapy	Sequence
I A	Upper neck (NS, LP)	⎱IF	No	
	Other neck		⎱Yes	RC
	Supraclavicular		⎰2 yr	
	Axilla			
	Femoral			
I B	All	IF	Yes—2 yr	RC
II A	All	IF	Yes—2 yr	RC
II B, III A, III B, IV A, IV B	All	IF	Yes—2 yr	CRC

* IF, involved field irradiation, 3500–4000 rads; NS, nodular sclerosis; LP, lymphocytic predominance; R, radiation therapy; C, chemotherapy.

days 1 through 5. The cycle is repeated every 21 days for six courses.

The role of immunotherapy is unknown at the present time; clinical trials are in progress.

PROGNOSIS

The 5-year survival rate for stages I and II is approximately 90 percent with further moderate attrition between 5 and 10 years. For all stages, the 5-year survival rate is approximately 75 percent. Although the results of combination chemotherapy are impressive for advanced Hodgkin's disease (53–100-percent complete response rate with MOPP therapy), approximately half of the patients still relapse during the first 3–4 years of follow-up. The use of irradiation combined with multiple drug chemotherapy programs holds promise for the best results.

Non-Hodgkin's Lymphomas

Non-Hodgkin's lymphomas occur in childhood most commonly between ages 2 and 12. Males predominate with the sex ratio being 3.5:1. Tumors may arise from nodal, extranodal lymphatic, or nonlymphatic sites. Nonlymphatic primaries account for between 5 and 20 percent of cases. Initial symptoms relate to site of involvement and include dyspnea, abdominal pain, and bone pain.

Histologically, non-Hodgkin's lymphomas have been classified as lymphocytic (approximately two-thirds of all children with about two-thirds of these undifferentiated), histiocytic, and stem cell or mixed. Nodular and diffuse forms of each subtype are present, the latter occurring infrequently in children. The prognostic significance of histologic classification in children under 12 years is still uncertain.

STAGING CLASSIFICATION

Non-Hodgkin's lymphomas in childhood disseminate early and should be managed accordingly at diagnosis. To date, cure has been confined to children with disease limited to the primary site, whether extranodal, nodal, or nonlymphatic. Up to 70 percent of children develop CNS disease with the exception of children with small bowel lesions, in whom CNS involvement is uncommon. Whether staging laparotomy is of value in treatment and prognosis is not clear as yet. At best it can serve to separate two groups, one having localized or regional disease with a modest cure rate and the other having occult disseminated disease with only a few long-term survivors. The role of surgery is primarily for intra-abdominal lymphomas where resection of the primary tumor and regional nodes is possible. Biopsy of other abdominal nodes, liver, and kidney may be performed, and ovaries transposed when the bulk of the disease to be irradiated is in the pelvis. The value of splenectomy for these patients has not been demonstrated.

A simplified staging system has been proposed by Wollner and associates[87] and is as follows:

Stage I.   One single site
Stage II.   Two or more sites on the same side of the diaphragm
Stage III. Disseminated disease without marrow or central nervous system involvement
Stage IV.   Any of the above with bone marrow and/or central nervous system involvement

TREATMENT

The most successful therapeutic regimen reported to date is the LSA_2-L_2 Memorial Hospital multiple drug–radiation therapy protocol.[87] The protocol is designed to provide (a) intensive induction chemotherapy to reduce bulk disease rapidly; (b) simultaneous radiation therapy to the primary or bulk disease tumor (any tumor measuring 5 cm or more) early in the disease; (c) intensive consolidation, and maintenance chemotherapy as for leukemia; and (d) prophylactic treatment of the central nervous system. Details of the protocol are shown in Table 13-4.

For disease confined to the gut and regional mesenteric nodes, segmental excision is appropriate. In such cases, when excision is grossly complete a 10-percent cure rate may be achieved by surgery alone. When whole-abdominal irradiation is given promptly postoperatively, the cure rate is markedly improved to approximately 80 percent. It is not clear whether chemotherapy adds benefit.

PROGNOSIS

An important prognostic factor in therapy is the achievement of a complete response, i.e., disappearance of all measurable tumor within 1–2 months from onset of therapy. When this is not accomplished, regrowth of tumor and/or dissemination is the rule.

Of the 43 children treated with the LSA_2-L_2 protocol, 76 percent are surviving free of disease with a median observation time of 25 + months. Fifty-one percent of the survivors are off therapy without evidence of disease.

BONE TUMORS

Bone tumors are the sixth most common malignant tumor in childhood.[89]

Until a few years ago, the outlook for children with osteogenic sar-

Table 13-4
LSA$_2$-L$_2$ Protocol for Non-Hodgkin's Lymphoma[87]

---

1. Induction
   Day 1. Cyclophosphamide 1200 mg/sq m single IV push
   Days 3–31. Prednisone 60 mg/sq m PO divided into 3 daily doses
   Days 3, 10, 17, 24. Vincristine 1.5–2.25 mg/sq m IV
   Days 5, 27, 30. Spinal tap and intrathecal injection of methotrexate 6.25
     mg/sq m
   Days 12, 13. Daunorubicin 60 mg/sq m IV
Concomitant radiation therapy is given to bulky sites
2. Consolidation
   Day 34 or 36. Cytosine arabinoside 150 mg/sq m daily IV for 15 injections
   Day 34 or 36. Thioguanine 75 mg/sq m daily PO, 8–12 hr after the cytosine
     arabinoside
   Day 70. L-Asparaginase 60,000 U/sq m daily IV for 12 injections
   Day 85. Spinal tap and two intrathecal injections of methotrexate, 6.25
     mg/sq m, 2 days apart
   Day 90. BCNU 60 mg/sq m IV
Rest 3–4 days
3. Maintenance
   Cycle I. Thioguanine 300 mg/sq m PO for 4 days
             Cyclophosphamide 600 mg/sq m on day 5
             Rest 7–10 days
   Cycle II. Hydroxyurea 2400 mg/sq m PO for 4 days
              Daunorubicin 45 mg/sq m on day 5
              Rest 7–10 days
   Cycle III. Methotrexate 10 mg/sq m PO for 4 days
               BCNU 60 mg/sq m IV on day 5
               Rest 7–10 days
   Cycle IV. Cytosine arabinoside 150 mg/sq m IV for 4 days
              Vincristine 1.5 mg/sq m IV on day 5
              Rest 7–10 days
   Cycle V. Two doses of methotrexate 6.25 mg/sq m
             intrathecally, 2–3 days apart
             Rest 7–10 days and restart with cycle I
   Stages I, II, and III are treated for 2 years from onset of treatment and
stage IV for 3 years

---

coma or Ewing's sarcoma was uniformly grim. Five-year survival rates
in osteogenic sarcoma were in the range of 12–18 percent,[33,43,56] whereas
those in Ewing's sarcoma were only 8 percent in one large series.[18] In
both tumors the patients succumbed with respiratory failure from pulmonary metastases, although bony metastases contributed to the overall
morbidity.

Both tumors are most common in the second decade of life, and in both there is a predominance of males to females of 1.6:1 to 2.25:1. The mortality rate for osteogenic sarcoma is similar for whites and non-whites. Ewing's sarcoma, however, is a distinct rarity among blacks.[89] Osteogenic sarcoma and Ewing's sarcoma account for almost 90 percent of malignant bone tumors in the pediatric age group.

Osteogenic Sarcoma

PATHOLOGY

Osteogenic sarcoma is a primary malignant tumor of bone thought to arise from bone-forming mesenchyme. Grossly the tumor is bulky and infiltrating and commonly invades the cortex and soft tissue. Histologically it consists of malignant osteoid and bone and malignant stroma with varying degrees of anaplasia. Lesions have been subclassified into osteoblastic, chondroblastic, and fibroblastic types. Metastases occur hematogenously, usually to the lungs or other bones. Involvement of regional lymph nodes and viscera is rare. Variants include paraosteal osteogenic sarcoma, a slow-growing tumor that usually does not manifest cortical invasion and is associated with a good prognosis and multicentric osteogenic sarcoma, characterized by numerous tumors throughout the skeleton.

The etiology of osteogenic sarcoma is unknown. A viral agent has been suggested from animal studies but has not been proven in man.[59] Mounting circumstantial evidence, however, strongly implicates ionizing radiation as one causative factor.[3]

CLINICAL FEATURES AND
DIAGNOSTIC STUDIES

Osteogenic sarcoma may arise in any bone but is most common in the metaphyseal portion of long bones, especially the distal femur. Other long bones frequently involved with primary tumor are the tibia and humerus at their proximal ends.

Pain alone or pain with swelling is the most frequent presenting complaint. The patient may report that the pain started only after a traumatic episode, attribute the pain to the injury, and delay seeking medical care. Malaise and weight loss usually indicate widespread disease.

Physical examination usually discloses a painful mass over the affected bone with or without venous engorgement, local heat, or limitation of motion at the neighboring joint.

Roentgenographs may reveal bony destruction of both cortex and medulla as well as proliferation of new bone. An extraosseous mass may

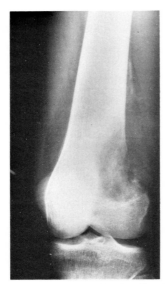

Fig. 13-1. Osteogenic sarcoma in the distal femoral meta-
physis. Moth-eaten pattern of bone destruction with tumor;
new bone formation in the soft tissue mass. A Codman's tri-
angle is also seen.

be visible contiguous to the involved bone (Fig. 13-1). Approximately
two-thirds of the films are considered characteristic of osteogenic sarcoma, whereas the remainder may suggest malignancy but lack characteristic features.[37]

Definitive diagnosis can be made only by biopsy. Preoperative
workup should include a complete history and physical examination, he-
mogram, and measurement of alkaline phosphatase, creatinine, SGOT,
LDH, and bilirubin levels. Other studies should include a complete skeletal survey, bone scan, chest x-ray, and full lung tomograms. Angiography may be helpful in determining the degree of tumor infiltration into
soft tissues.

TREATMENT

Until very recently, radical ablative surgery alone or radiation of the
tumor followed by radical ablative surgery were the so-called treatments
of choice. Studies comparing the two modalities failed to show any
improvement in survival with the addition of radiation. The median time
to development of pulmonary metastases was 10 months with death
usually occurring within the next 6 months.[74]

In 1971 Martini and associates[44] reported results of a study in 22 patients treated with multiple wedge resections or lobectomies for pulmonary metastases from osteogenic sarcoma. The 50-percent survival in this group of patients, 26 months to 3 years after amputation and 15–24 months after resection of pulmonary metastases, indicates that aggressive surgical intervention has a definite role in the management of patients with metastatic disease.

With the exception of sporadic reports of limited responses, most chemotherapeutic agents have in the past failed to change the inexorable progression of the disease.[19]

In 1972 Cortes and associates[9] reported the results of adriamycin therapy in 13 patients with pulmonary metastases of osteogenic sarcoma. One patient achieved complete remission, three had partial remissions, and another had 25-percent tumor regression. Since that time patients with metastatic tumor have been reported to respond favorably to adriamycin,[9] high-dose methotrexate,[26] or combinations of these agents.[62]

For patients without metastases a note of justified optimism now seems allowable[10,25,55,72,81] (Table 13-5). The literature is replete with depressing historical controls, and there seems little doubt that aggressive adjunctive chemotherapy can eradicate tumor microfoci. The results of Acute Leukemia Group B using adriamycin alone, 30 mg/sq m/day for 3 days every 4 weeks for six courses starting 4–14 days after radical amputation, indicate a projected 77 percent of the patients who receive full doses of the drug at intervals no longer than 6 weeks apart will be free of disease at 18 months.

Although successful attempts to preserve limbs are now reported using chemotherapy followed by en bloc resection and prosthetic bone

Table 13-5
Nonmetastatic Osteogenic Sarcoma: Results of Chemotherapy

Reference	Patients Treated (No.)	Chemotherapy*	Patients Disease Free (No.)	Disease-Free Period (Mo)
Cortes[10]	15	VCR, HDMtx	11	2–23
Jaffe et al.[25]	21	ADR	16	1+–32+
Pratt et al.[55]	5	ADM, CTX, HDMtx	5	4–11
Sutow et al.[72]	5	HDMtx, VCR, ADM, CTX	4	7+–12+
Wilbur et al.[81]	18	CTX, VCR, ADR, PAM	10	24+
Total	64		46	

* VCR, vincristine; HDMtx, high-dose methotrexate with citrovorum factor rescue; ADR, adriamycin; CTX, cyclophosphamide; PAM, phenylalanine mustard.

replacement,[61] we advocate incisional biopsy followed by radical amputation, i.e., removal of the entire affected bone. Until cooperative studies indicate the superiority of combinations of drugs over adriamycin alone in nonmetastatic disease, we advocate the use of adriamycin in the dosage and time course given above. Toxicity is tolerable and consists of skin necrosis with extravasation of the drug during administration and nausea and vomiting for approximately 24 hours after the drug is administered. The patient should be told that the drug will make the urine red and that some increased pigmentation of the nails may develop. Alopecia, stomatitis, and/or esophagitis and transient marrow depression are common side effects. The total cumulative dose of adriamycin is 540 mg/sq m, a safe level in terms of myocardial toxicity.[20]

Rehabilitation can begin before surgery. We introduce the child facing an amputation to another young amputee who is skilled at crutch-walking or using a prosthesis. Crutch-walking should be started as soon as possible after surgery and the child fitted for a prosthesis as soon as the stump is well healed.

For children with pulmonary metastases at the time of diagnosis, aggressive surgical therapy, i.e., amputation and resection of lung lesions, should be undertaken when feasible to remove as much bulk tumor as possible. Chemotherapy consisting of adriamycin alone or in combination with high-dose methotrexate with citrovorum factor rescue may then be used.

Ewing's Sarcoma

PATHOLOGY

The exact histogenesis of Ewing's sarcoma is not known, but it is thought to arise from immature reticulum cells or the primitive mesenchyme of the medullary cavity. Grossly the tumor tissue is soft and areas of hemorrhagic necrosis are often found. Microscipically it consists of closely packed uniform cells in cords or nests. Cell membranes are indistinct and cytoplasm scanty. PAS-positive material can be demonstrated in well-preserved tissue. Osteoid and chondroid are not found.

CLINICAL FEATURES AND
DIAGNOSTIC STUDIES

Ewing's sarcoma arises most commonly in bones of the trunk, including the pelvis, ribs, sternum, and scapula, or in the midshaft or metaphyseal portions of the long bones, especially the femur.

Pain or discomfort relating to the involved bone with or without swelling is the usual presenting symptom. Fever, weight loss, and anemia are also occasionally seen. Physical examination may disclose a palpable mass over the affected bone, but this sign was present in only 55 percent of the patients reported by Pomeroy and Johnson.[53]

The radiographic features of the tumor are nonspecific and may simulate eosinophilic granuloma, osteomyelitis, metastatic tumor, or reticulum cell sarcoma of bone. An onion skin appearance secondary to reactive bone production with elevation of the periosteum is seen most often in the diaphyses of long bones. Lesions may be either lytic or sclerotic, but a mixture of the two with or without an associated soft tissue mass was seen in two-thirds of tumors in one series.[53]

Workup before biopsy should include a complete blood count, determination of LDH and alkaline phosphatase, complete skeletal survey and/or bone scan, full lung tomograms, and bone marrow aspiration.

In cases of suspected Ewing's sarcoma, the biopsy should be directed at a soft tissue mass with removal of only small amounts of bone. Overzealous removal of bone compounds morbidity and may result in fractures, especially in lesions of the femur. No generally accepted staging system is available at this time, and patients are usually categorized as to whether metastases are clinically evident or not.

TREATMENT

Although between 76 and 86 percent of patients have no clinical or radiographic evidence of metastases at the time of diagnosis,[3,80] the dismal survival rate even after treatment of the tumor with radiation therapy or ablative surgery has led investigators to the inevitable conclusion that Ewing's sarcoma is a generalized disease at the time of diagnosis.

Radical surgery, as a result, has only a small role and should probably be limited to lesions within a rib where danger of compromise of pulmonary tissue precludes high-dose radiation therapy using conventional techniques.

Treatment should be aggressive and aimed not only at the primary lesion but also at the clinically inapparent metastases. To accomplish this we recommend that radiation be given to the entire involved bone in a dose of 4500 rads for children under 5 or 5000–5500 rads for older children over a 5–6-week period. An additional 1000 rads should then be directed at the initial tumor with a 5-cm margin in each dimension sparing the epiphyseal centers whenever possible.

Combination chemotherapy should be started simultaneously with radiation, and we recommend weekly doses of vincristine 1.5 mg/sq m IV per week for 6 weeks along with cyclophosphamide 500 mg/sq m. At week 6 adriamycin 60 mg/sq m should be given IV with the other agents. A 6-week rest period is then allowed before the reinitiation of 7-week courses of chemotherapy, which are continued at 3-month intervals for a total treatment period of 18 months. These courses consist of dactinomycin 15 μg/kg/day IV for 5 days followed by a 9-day rest period. Vincristine and cyclophosphamide are then given weekly for 5 weeks in the doses above with adriamycin again added in the final week of the course. Preservation of a functional limb should be a prime consideration in treatment. Judicious biopsies and a program of active exercise will help reduce morbidity and preserve muscle function.

For some pelvic lesions, the bladder must be included in the radiation field, and the potential for cyclophosphamide bladder toxicity with hemorrhagic cystitis is thereby enhanced. If radiation ports include the bladder, cyclophosphamide should not be given until the second course of chemotherapy, when radiation is completed. If hemorrhagic cystitis then develops in the face of good fluid intake, chlorambucil may be given daily in a dose of 0.1 mg/kg orally.

When pulmonary metastases are present at diagnosis, 1500–2000 rads to the lungs may be given over a 3-week period. A single bony metastasis should be vigorously treated with radiation as for the primary tumor and chemotherapy continued. Even with multiple metastatic lesions, survival may be prolonged by judicious use of chemotherapy and radiation. Recurrence of tumor at the primary site after radiation therapy and without evidence of distant metastasis is an indication for amputation.

In addition to the presence or absence of obvious metastasis at diagnosis, site of the primary tumor is another useful prognostic indicator with the most favorable lesions being in the distal long bones.[54]

Multimodality therapy for Ewing's sarcoma is promising. Of 19 patients from the M.D. Anderson Hospital treated with 6000–7000 rads to the primary tumor with adjuvant vincristine and cyclophosphamide, 10 remain free of disease from 6–42 months (median 28 months). In those who relapsed, the median time to diagnosis of first metastasis was 14 months, compared to a control of 8 months in patients treated with radiation alone or with single-agent chemotherapy.[70] Fifty percent of patients entered on a large cooperative study and treated with radiation to the primary tumor with or without prophylactic pulmonary radiation and multiagent chemotherapy are surviving longer than 18 months. The results are encouraging, but longer follow-up is required to determine with certainty if the onset of metastases is merely delayed or if these patients are indeed cured.

RETINOBLASTOMA

Retinoblastoma is the most common intraocular tumor of childhood. The average annual incidence is estimated at 11 per million children less than 5 years of age at diagnosis, or a frequency of 1 in 18,000.[12] It is primarily a tumor of infants and young children. In the large epidemiologic study of Jensen and Miller,[28] 81 percent of white children with the disease were diagnosed by age 3. In contrast, only 72 percent of black children were diagnosed by age 3, and the peak mortality was 2.5 times greater than in white children. Retinoblastoma has been associated with D-group deletion syndromes, and a greater than expected incidence of severe mental retardation has been reported.[52,85] In contrast, survivors blinded from retinoblastoma were found to have a significantly higher IQ than children blinded from other causes.[83] Of particular interest is the increased risk of a survivor of bilateral retinoblastoma developing a second primary tumor, either radiation induced or in an area remote from the field of treatment.[33]

Genetics

That retinoblastoma may occur in several members of one family has been appreciated since the turn of the century. The paucity of survivors of the tumor who went on to have their own children initially prevented complete genetic studies. Early, vigorous treatment has, however, resulted in a large number of survivors and has permitted critical genetic analysis.

In a study of 598 patients with retinoblastoma, Briard-Guillemot et al.[5] found that 10.5 percent of cases were familial and that of these, 60 percent had bilateral disease as compared to only 33.1 percent in sporadic cases. In reviewing the literature she found 23 cases (5 percent) of retinoblastoma among 397 children of 177 survivors of unilateral sporadic disease, whereas there were 25 cases (52.1 percent) among the 48 offspring of 27 survivors of bilateral disease. It is now generally accepted that bilateral retinoblastoma is transmitted as an autosomal dominant gene and results from a germinal mutation. Unilateral sporadic cases are regarded as somatic mutations, although the 1.2–11.8-percent recurrence risk in their offspring raises the possibility of a carrier state or incompletely expressed bilateral retinoblastoma.[5]

Pathology and Staging

Although retinoblastoma may present as a single tumor, more characteristically it arises in multiple foci in the retina. Two or more retinal tumors were found in 84 percent of patients reported by Ellsworth.[15] The tumor may be endophytic, growing into the vitreous cavity, or exophytic, growing into the subretinal space.[75]

Microscopically, retinoblastoma consists of small cells with scant cytoplasm and deeply staining nuclei, undifferentiated cells, or large cells that form rosettes. Metastasis to the subarachnoid space occurs by direct extension along the optic nerve. Blood-borne metastases may be found in bones, liver, lymph nodes, and bone marrow.

The staging classification of Reese and Ellsworth is generally accepted and is related to the size and extent of tumor within the fundus. The prognosis within each group relates to the potential of preserving useful vision.[5,58]

Group I.   Very favorable
  1. Solitary tumor, less than 4 disc diameters in size, at or behind the equator
  2. Multiple tumors, none over 4 disc diameters in size, all at or behind the equator

Group II.   Favorable
  1. Solitary lesion, 4–10 disc diameters in dize, at or behind the equator
  2. Multiple tumors, 4–10 disc diameters in size, behind the equator

Group III.   Doubtful
  1. Any lesion anterior to the equator
  2. Solitary tumors larger than 10 disc diameters behind the equator

Group IV.   Unfavorable
  1. Multiple tumors, some larger than 10 disc diameters
  2. Any lesion extending anteriorly to the ora serrata

Group V.   Very unfavorable
  1. Massive tumors involving over half the retina
  2. Vitreous seeding

Clinical Features and Diagnostic Studies

The most common presenting sign in children with retinoblastoma is a white or yellowish appearance of the pupil—the so-called cat's eye reflex—usually discovered by the parents. Pain from secondary glaucoma, redness of the eye, strabismus, and vision loss may also occur. Enlargement of the globe and proptosis usually indicate advanced disease (Fig. 13-2).

Workup should include a careful general medical and family history and a complete physical examination. Both eyes must be scrupulously examined with a binocular indirect ophthalmoscope under general anesthesia. All lesions should be carefully plotted on a diagram and classified according to the system of Reese and Ellsworth. The tumor may appear

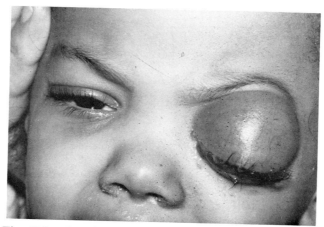

Fig. 13-2.   Massive proptosis in a 3-year-old child with advanced retinoblastoma.

as a round pink mass with fine vasculature on its surface or as a white
avascular mass if vitreous rupture has occurred, or multiple spherical
masses may be seen seeding throughout the eye.

Important laboratory studies include a complete blood count, liver
function tests, urinary VMA and HVA, and chromosome analysis if possible. Roentgenographic studies should include coned-down views of the
orbit and a complete skeletal survey in addition to routine x-rays of the
chest. A marrow aspirate should be obtained from one or more sites and
examined for tumor cells, and careful cytological examination of the spinal fluid should be performed. Every effort must be made to rule out
conditions that may mimic retinoblastoma, e.g., nematode infection, vascular malformations, Coats' disease, or endophthalmitis.

Treatment

Large cooperative studies in retinoblastoma are not available and
certain questions remain unanswered, e.g., the exact role of chemotherapy in group IV and V lesions.

Most newly diagnosed sporadic unilateral retinoblastomas are stage
IV or V. Enucleation is the treatment of choice followed by 6 months of
combination chemotherapy with intravenous cyclophosphamide and vincristine.

For unilateral stage I, II, and III lesions, careful retinal mapping is
done as a baseline, and 3500 rads is delivered to the posterior pole of the
retina in three fractions a week over a 3-week period.

When the patient presents with bilateral tumor, the most severely involved eye is enucleated and the remaining eye radiated with 4000–4500 rads over a 4-week period, treating 3 days a week. After the completion of radiation, any residual anterior tumor can be treated with photocoagulation. The chance of preserving vision in such instances is approximately 60 percent for stage IV tumors and 30 percent with stage V.

For patients with metastatic disease, the primary tumor may be removed or treated with radiation. If enucleation is done, 5000 rads should be given to the orbit and optic foramen in 15 fractions over 5 weeks treating three times a week. Combination chemotherapy, as for neuroblastoma, should be used and if the central nervous system is involved, intrathecal methotrexate 12 mg/sq m weekly for 6 weeks should be added. Cranial or cranial-spinal radiation, 3500 rads in 4 weeks to 5000 rads in 6 weeks, depending on age, may also be given.

Prognosis

Except for metastatic disease or intracranial spread, the prognosis in retinoblastoma is very good with only an 18-percent mortality rate. The control rate of local tumor and preservation of vision even in patients with bilateral or orbital tumor ranged from 34 percent in patients with stage V tumor to 95 percent in those with stage I.[15]

Indefinite follow-up care is essential as late recurrences of retinoblastoma are reported and secondary malignancies may develop.

REFERENCES

1. Angervall L, Enzinger FM: Extraskeletal neoplasm resembling Ewing's sarcoma. Cancer 36:240–256, 1975
2. Beckwith JB, Perrin EV: In situ neuroblastomas. A contribution to the natural history of neural crest tumors. Am J Pathol 43:1089–1100, 1963
3. Bhansali SK, Desai PB: Ewing's sarcoma. Observations on 107 cases. J Bone Joint Surg 45A:541–553, 1963
4. Breslow N, McCann B: Statistical estimation of prognosis for children with neuroblastoma. Cancer Res 31:2098–2103, 1971
5. Briard-Guillemot ML, Bonaiti-Pellie C, Feingold J, Frezal J: Etude genetique du retinoblastome. Humangenetik 24:271–284, 1974
6. Butler JJ: Relationship of histological findings to survival in Hodgkin's disease. Cancer Res 31:1770–1775, 1971
7. Chatten J, Voorhess ML: Familial neuroblastoma—report of a kindred with multiple disorders, including neuroblastoma in four siblings. N Engl J Med 277:1230–1236, 1967

8. Cortes EP, Holland JF, Wang JJ, Sinks LF: Chemotherapy of advanced osteosarcoma. Colston Paper No. 24, in Price CHG, Ross FGM (eds): Bone—Certain Aspects of Neoplasia. London, Butterworth & Co, 1972, pp 265–280

9. Cortes EP, Holland JF, Wang JJ, Sinks LF: Doxorubicin in disseminated osteosarcoma. JAMA 221:1132–1138, 1972

10. Cortes EP, Holland JF, Wang JJ, Sinks LF, Blom LF, Senn H, Bank A, Glidewell O: Amputation and adriamycin in primary osteosarcoma. N Engl J Med 291:998–1000, 1974

11. D'Angio GJ, Evans AE, Breslow N, Beckwith B, et al: The treatment of Wilms' tumor: Results of the National Wilms' Tumor Study. Cancer 38:633–646, 1976

12. Devesa SS: The incidence of retinoblastoma. Am J Ophthalmol 80:263–265, 1975

13. DeVita VT, Serpick AA, Carbone PP: Combination chemotherapy in the treatment of advanced Hodgkin's disease. Ann Intern Med 73:881–895, 1970

14. Donaldson SS, Castro JR, Wilbur JR, Jesse RH: Rhabdomyosarcoma of head and neck in children: Combination treatment by surgery, irradiation, and chemotherapy. Cancer 31:26–35, 1973

15. Ellsworth RM: The practical management of retinoblastoma. Trans Am Ophthalmol Soc 67:462–534, 1969

16. Evans AE, D'Angio GJ, Randolph J: A proposed staging for children with neuroblastoma. Cancer 27:374–378, 1971

17. Everson TC, Cole WH: Spontaneous Regression of Cancer. Philadelphia, WB Saunders Co, 1966, pp 11–87

18. Falk S, Alpert M: Five-year survival of patients with Ewing's sarcoma. Surg Gynecol Obstet 124:319–324, 1967

19. Finklestein JZ, Hittle RE, Hammond GD: Evaluation of a high dose cyclophosphamide regimen on childhood tumors. Cancer 23:1239–1242, 1969

20. Gilladoga AC, Manuel C, Tann CC, Wollner N, Murphy ML: Cardiotoxicity of adriamycin (NSC-123127) in children. Cancer Chemother Rep 6:209–214, 1975

21. Guin GH, Gilbert EF, Jones B: Incidental neuroblastoma in infants. Am J Clin Pathol 51:126–136, 1969

22. Hays DM, Karon M, Isaacs H, Mittle RE: Hodgkin's disease. Technique and results of staging laparotomy in childhood. Arch Surg 106:507–512, 1973

23. Hellstrom KE, Hellstrom IE, Bill AH, Pierce GE, Yang JPS: Studies on cellular immunity to human neuroblastoma cells. Int J Cancer 6:172–188, 1970

24. Heyn RM, Holland R, Newton WA, Tefft M, Breslow N, Hartmann JR: The role of combined chemotherapy in the treatment of rhabdomyosarcoma in children. Cancer 34:2128–2141, 1974

25. Jaffe N, Frei E, Traggis D, Bishio Y: Adjuvant methotrexate and citrovorum factor treatment of osteogenic sarcoma. N Engl J Med 291:994–997, 1974

26. Jaffe N, Paed D: Recent advances in the chemotherapy of metastatic osteogenic sarcoma. Cancer 30:1627–1631, 1972
27. James DH Jr, Hustu O, Wrenn EL Jr, Pinkel D: Combination chemotherapy of childhood neuroblastoma. JAMA 194:123–126, 1965
28. Jensen RD, Miller RW: Retinoblastoma: Epidemiologic characteristics. N Engl J Med 285:307, 310, 1971
29. Joshi VV, Kay S, Milstein R, Koontz WW, McWilliams NB: Congenital mesoblastic nephroma of infancy: Report of a case with unusual clinical behavior. Am J Clin Pathol 60:811–816, 1973
30. Kaplan HS: Hodgkin's Disease. Cambridge, Mass., Harvard University Press, 1972
31. Kilmay JW, Clatworthy HW, Newton WA, Grosfeld JL: Reasonable surgery for rhabdomyosarcoma: A study of 67 cases. Ann Surg 178:346–351, 1973
32. Kissane JM: Pathology of Infancy and Childhood. St. Louis, CV Mosby Co, 1975, p 770
33. Kitchin FD, Ellsworth RM: Pleiotrophic effects of the gene for retinoblastoma. J Med Genet 11:244–246, 1974
34. Lawrence W, Jegge G, Foote FW: Embryonal rhabdomyosarcoma, a clinicopathological study. Cancer 17:361, 1964
35. Lawrence W, Hays D, Moon T: Lymphatic metastasis with childhood rhabdomyosarcoma. Cancer (in press)
36. Li FP, Fraumeni JF: Rhabdomyosarcoma in children: Epidemiologic study and identification of a familial cancer syndrome. J Natl Cancer Inst 43:1365–1373, 1969
37. Lindom A, Soderberg G, Spjut HJ: Osteosarcoma: A review of 96 cases. Acta Radiol (Stockh) 56:1–19, 1961
38. Lingley JF, Sagerman RH, Santulli TV, Wolff JA: Neuroblastoma–management and survival. N Engl J Med 277:1227–1230, 1967
39. Lokich JJ, Jaffe N, Moloney WC, Frei E: MOPP resistant Hodgkin's disease: New multiple agent chemotherapy (B-DOPA). Amer Soc Hematol 17th Annual Meeting, Atlanta, Dec 7–10, 1974
40. Lukes RJ, Craver LF, Hall TC, Rappaport H, Rubin P: Report of the Nomenclature Committee. Cancer Res 26:1311, 1966
41. McKenna RJ, Schwinn CP, Soong KY, Higinbotham NL: Sarcomata of the osteogenic series (osteosarcoma, fibrosarcoma, chondrosarcoma, parosteal osteogenic sarcoma and sarcomata arising in abnormal bone). J Bone Joint Surg 48-A:1–26, 1966
42. Makinen J: Microscopic patterns as a guide to prognosis of neuroblastoma in childhood. Cancer 29:1637–1646, 1972
43. Marcove RC, Mike V, Hajek JV, Levin AG, Hutter RVP: Osteogenic sarcoma in childhood. NY State J Med 71:855–859, 1971
44. Martini N, Huvos A, Mike V, Marcove RC, Beattie E J Jr: Multiple pulmonary resections in the treatment of osteogenic sarcoma. Ann Thorac Surg 12:271–280, 1971
45. Maurer HM: The Intergroup Rhabdomyosarcoma Study (NIH): Objectives and clinical staging classification. J Pediatr Surg 10:977, 1975

46. Maurer HM: Intergroup Rhabdomyosarcoms Study: Progress report. Proc Am Soc Clin Oncol, Toronto, May 4-5, 1976, p 24

47. Maurer HM: Rhabdomyosarcoma in children: Progress and problems, in Sinks LF, Godden JO (eds): Conflicts in Childhood Cancer. New York, Alan R Liss, 1975, p. 345

48. Miller RW: Fifty-two forms of chldhood cancer: United States mortality experience, 1960 to 1966. J Pediatr 75:685–689, 1969

49. Miller RW, Fraumeni JF, Manning MD: Association of Wilms' tumor with aniridia, hemihypertrophy, and other congenital malformations. N Engl J Med 270:922–927, 1964

50. Nickson JJ: Hodgkin's disease clinical trial. Cancer Res 26:1279–1283, 1966

51. Obstacles to the control of Hodgkin's disease (Rye Conference). Cancer Res 26:1047, 1966

52. O'Grady RB, Rothstein TB, Romano PE: D-group deletion syndromes and retinoblastoma. Am J Ophthalnol 77:40–45, 1974

53. Pomeroy TC, Johnson RE: Combined modality therapy of Ewing's sarcoma. Cancer 35:36–47, 1975

54. Pomeroy TC, Johnson RE: Prognostic factors for survival in Ewing's sarcoma. Am J Roentgenol Radium Ther Nucl Med 123:598–606, 1975

55. Pratt CB, Hustu O, Shanks E: Cyclic multiple drug adjuvant chemotherapy for osteosarcoma. Proc Am Assoc Cancer Res 15:19, 1974

56. Price CHG, Zhuber K, Salzer-Kuntschik M et al: Osteosarcoma in children. J Bone Joint Surg 57-B:341–345, 1976

57. Ragab AH, Vietti TJ, Crist W, Perez C, McAllister W: Bilateral Wilms' tumor. A review. Cancer 30:983–988, 1972

58. Reese AB, Hyman GA, Meriam GR Jr, Forrest AW, Klingerman MM: Treatment of retinoblastoma by radiation and triethylene melamine. Arch Ophthalmol 53:505–513, 1955

59. Reilly CA, Pritchard DJ, Biskis BO, Finkel MP: Immunologic evidence suggesting a viral etiology of human osteosarcoma. Cancer 30:603–609, 1972

60. Rivard G, Ortega J, Hittle R, Nitschke R, Karon M: Intensive chemotherapy as primary treatment for rhabdomyosarcoma of the pelvis. Cancer 36:1593–1597, 1975

61. Rosen G, Murphy ML, Huvos AG, Gutierrez M, Marcove RC: Chemotherapy, en bloc resection and prosthetic bone replacement in the treatment of osteogenic sarcoma. Cancer 37:1–11, 1976

62. Rosen G, Suwansirikul S, Kwon C, Tan C, Wu SJ, Beattie EJ Jr, Murphy ML: High-dose methotrexate with citrovorum factor rescue and adriamycin in childhood osteogenic sarcoma. Cancer 33:1151–1163, 1974

63. Rosenberg SA: A critique of the value of laparotomy and splenectomy in the evaluation of patients with Hodgkin's disease. Cancer Res 31:1737–1740, 1971

64. Sagerman RH, Tretter P, Ellsworth RM: The treatment of orbital rhabdomyosarcoma of children with primary radiation therapy. J Roentgenol Radium Ther Nucl Med 114:31–34, 1972

65. Samuels LD, Newton WA Jr, Heyn R: Daunorubicin therapy in advanced neuroblastoma. Cancer 27:831–834, 1971
66. Sawitsky A: Vincristine and cyclophosphamide therapy in generalized neuroblastoma. A collaborative study. Am J Dis Child 119:308–313, 1970
67. Soule EH, Mahour GH, Mills SD, Lynn HB: Soft tissue sarcomas of infants and children. Mayo Clin Proc 43:313–326, 1968
68. Soule EH, Newton WA: Intergroup Rhabdomyosarcoma Study. Identification of a histologic subgroup: Ewing's tumor of soft tissue. Proc Am Soc Clin Oncol (in press)
69. Staging in Hodgkin's disease (Ann Arbor Conference). Cancer Res 31:1712, 1971
70. Suit HD, Sutow WW, Martin RG: Bone tumors, in Bloom, HJG, Lemerle J, Neidhardt MK, Voute PA (eds): Cancer in Children: Clinical Management. Berlin, Springer-Verlag, 1975, p 209
71. Sullivan MP, Sutow WW, Cangir A, Taylor G: Vincristine sulfate in management of Wilms' tumor, replacement of preoperative irradiation by chemotherapy. JAMA 202:381–384, 1967
72. Sutow WW, Sullivan MP, Fernbach DJ, Cangir A, George SL: Adjuvant chemotherapy in primary treatment of osteogenic sarcoma. Cancer 36:1598–1602, 1975
73. Sutow WW, Sullivan MP, Reid HL, Taylor HG, Griffith KM: Prognosis in childhood rhabdomyosarcoma. Cancer 25:1384–1390, 1970
74. Sweetnam R, Knowelden J, Seddon H: Bone sarcoma: Treatment by irradiation, amputation or a combination of the two. Br Med J 2:363–367, 1971
75. Tapley N duV, Tretter P: Retinoblastoma, in Sutow WW, Vietti TJ, Fernbach DJ (eds): Clinical Pediatric Oncology. St. Louis, CV Mosby Co, 1973, p 413
76. Tefft M: Radiotherapeutic management of Hodgkin's disease in children, in Sinks LF, Godden JO (eds): Conflicts in Childhood Cancer. New York, Alan R Liss, 1975, p 93
77. Tefft M, Fernandez C, Moon T: Rhabdomyosarcoma: Response with chemotherapy prior to radiation in patients with gross residual disease. Cancer (in press)
78. Wagger J, Aherne G: Familial neuroblastoma. Arch Dis Child 48:63–66, 1973
79. Wang JJ, Holland JF, Sinks LF: Phase II study of adriamycin (NSC-123127) in childhood solid tumors. Cancer Chemother Rep 6:267–270, 1975
80. Wang CC, Schulz MD: Ewing's sarcoma—a study of 50 cases treated at the Massachusetts General Hospital, 1930–1952 inclusive. N Engl J Med 248:571–576, 1953
81. Wilbur JR, Etcubanas E, Long T, Glatstein E, Leavitt T: Four-drug therapy and irradiation in primary and metastatic osteogenic sarcoma. Proc Am Assoc Cancer Res 15:188, 1974
82. Wilkerson JA, Van de Water JM, Gaepfert H: Role of embryonic induction in benign transformation of neuroblastomas. Cancer 20:1335–1342, 1967

83. Williams M: Superior intelligence of children blinded from retinoblastoma. Arch Dis Child 43:204–210, 1968

84. Wilms M: Die Mischgeschwülsete der Nieve. Leipzig, A. Georgi, 1899

85. Wilson MG, Towner JW, Fujimoto A: Retinoblastoma and D-chromosome deletions. Am J Hum Genet 25:57–61, 1973

86. Wolff JA, Krivit W, Newton WA, D'Angio GJ: Single versus multiple dose dactinomycin therapy of Wilms' tumor. N Engl J Med 279:290–294, 1968

87. Wollner N, Burchenal JH, Lieberman PH, Exelby P, D'Angio GJ, Murphy ML: Non-Hodgkin's lymphoma in children. A comparative study of two modalities of therapy. Cancer 37:123–134, 1976

88. Wong KY, Hanenson IB, Lampkin BC: Familial neuroblastoma. Am J Dis Child 121:415–416, 1971

89. Young JL Jr, Miller RW: Incidence of malignant tumors in U.S. children. J Pediatr 86:254–258, 1975

Heber H. Newsome, Jr., M.D.

14
Neoplasms of the Endocrine Glands

INTRODUCTION

Neoplasms of the endocrine glands are a challenge because of their relative rarity, their occasionally complex diagnostic features, and the specific hormonally related therapeutic problems. Because of their rarity the busy physician may not suspect their presence in a given patient. Once the disease is suspected, the diagnostic process may in some cases be long and tedious. Then treatment may be made more difficult by the hormonally produced changes in the patient and the consequent risks that may accompany treatment.

In the following sections hormonally active neoplasms of the pancreas, parathyroids, adrenals, and thyroid gland are considered. The familial associations of these neoplasms as well as such topics as carcinoids and ectopic production of hormones are also discussed. It is hoped that for each of these entities a brief survey of the pathology, pathophysiology, clinical features, diagnosis, treatment, and prognosis will help raise the awareness of the practicing physician, simplify the diagnostic complexities when possible, and point out some of the pitfalls in patient management.

PANCREATIC TUMORS[51,64,141,150]

Endocrine tumors of the pancreas arise from the islet cells. Although pancreatic islet cell neoplasms can be found in 1–2 percent of carefully performed autopsies, few of these neoplasms become clinically significant. Islet cell carcinomas probably occur in fewer than 1 in 100,000 people. The type of clinical syndrome produced by islet cell tumors depends on the cell of origin. The three cell types of the islets are designated beta, alpha, and delta. Special stains can usually identify these types. For example, only the beta cell stains with aldehyde fuchsin. The alpha-1 (or delta cell) can be distinguished from the alpha-2 cell by failure of the latter cell to stain with silver nitrate. These distinctions are sometimes blurred, and electron microscopy is necessary to identify unequivocally the cell of origin of the islet cell tumors.

Beta cells secrete insulin and the consequent syndrome produced by tumors of this type is characterized by hypoglycemia and its manifestations. Alpha-1 (or delta) cells may secrete gastrin, and these tumors produce the well-known Zollinger-Ellison syndrome of severe peptic ulcer disease. Only a few alpha-2 or glucagon-secreting tumors have been documented in the literature, and these apparently can produce diabetes mellitus, an eczematoid rash, and a raw tongue.[39,97,101] A fourth clinical syndrome, seen with pancreatic islet cell tumors, is that of severe diarrhea. The cell type for this syndrome has not been identified. Lastly, ectopic production of several other hormones has been reported in association with pancreatic neoplasms. The ectopic hormones are mentioned again in a later section of this chapter.

Beta Cell Neoplasms (Insulinomas)[53,73,81,86,90,96,142,148,159,177,178]

Insulinomas are small discrete neoplasms, slightly firmer than normal pancreatic tissue, and can range in color from gray or yellow to orange-brown. Approximately 90 percent are benign and 80 percent are single. Both the single and multiple tumors are homogeneously distributed throughout the pancreas. About 1–3 percent of cases of hyperinsulinism are caused by islet cell hyperplasia. In 10 percent of the cases metastases are evident at the time of exploration. Unfortunately, metastases are the only sure criteria of malignancy. No microscopic features reliably distinguish benign from malignant islet cell neoplasms. Microscopically, both benign and malignant tumors are composed of cords of cells interspersed with capillaries and vascular channels. Although many appear grossly to be encapsulated, areas of interdigitation of the tumor with surrounding pancreatic tissue may be seen. At surgery the tumor can rarely be "shelled-out" along a capsule. Only 1–2 percent of islet cell tumors are found outside the pancreas, usually in or near the duodenum. It should also be noted that 20–25 percent of islet cell carcinomas may be nonfunctioning and present as obstructive jaundice, abdominal pain, or an abdominal mass.

Clinical manifestations of the insulinoma most often result from depriving the brain of glucose. Confusion, drowsiness, irritability, personality changes, seizures, and coma are seen especially during the fasting state. Some of the other symptoms are a reflection of the increased catecholamine release invoked by the hypoglycemia and include sweating, palpitations, pallor, headache, and tremor. Obesity is common because of hypoglycemia, voracious appetite, and overeating. Such a clinical picture should bring to mind the possibility of hypoglycemia and a blood glucose should be done immediately. Whipple's[177] triad—a hypoglycemic attack during fasting, a blood glucose concentration of 50 mg/100 ml or less during the attack, and prompt relief of the symptoms by glucose—is a good diagnostic starting point. Other organic causes of fasting hypoglycemia[24,103] must be considered, and the differential diagnosis should include decreased liver glycogen (cirrhosis, hepatitis, carcinomatosis), enzyme defects (glycogen storage disease, galactosemia), defects in hyperglycemic responses (adrenal insufficiency, hypopituitarism), non-beta cell neoplasms (sarcomas, mesotheliomas, hepatomas, bronchial adenomas), and miscellaneous causes (alcoholism, salicylates, and factitious cases with sulfonylureas or insulin).

The simplest and most reliable method for establishing the diagnosis is to measure simultaneously the blood glucose and serum insulin concentrations. Normally, the serum insulin falls to extremely low concentrations during hypoglycemia. With the autonomous, unregulated production of insulin by the insulinoma, concentrations of serum insulin remain inappropriately elevated in the face of hypoglycemia. Regardless of the blood glucose concentration, there is a relative hyperinsulinemia. The ratio of blood glucose (mg/100 ml) to serum insulin (μU/ml) is usually greater than 3.0 in normal subjects. In patients with insulinomas, a ratio of less than 2.0 is almost always found. The normal insulin:glucose relationship and that of a hypothetical patient with an insulinoma are depicted in Figures 14-1 and 14-2. Caution must be taken to note the lower limits of assay sensitivity and accuracy of some of the commercially available insulin assay kits. In some cases of very low blood glucose due to other causes, the inaccurate measurement of serum insulin at low concentrations may give falsely positive glucose:insulin ratios. In unusual cases of insulinomas that produce only proinsulin, standard insulin assays may not detect the proinsulin and a falsely negative test is obtained. Patients who surreptitiously self-administer insulin or hypoglycemic agents present a special problem in diagnosis. Patients with a medical relationship or background are prime candidates for this. The presence of insulin antibodies and the absence of proinsulin in serum are two indications of hypoglycemia from exogenous insulin injection, but these assays are not widely available. Screening of the urine for derivatives of hypoglycemic drugs can be done at many toxicology centers.

NORMAL SUBJECTS

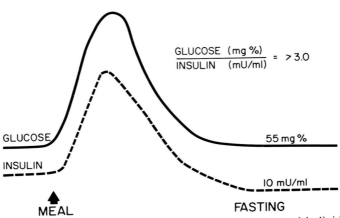

$$\frac{\text{GLUCOSE (mg \%)}}{\text{INSULIN (mU/ml)}} = > 3.0$$

GLUCOSE   55 mg %

INSULIN

                                                        10 mU/ml

▲
MEAL   FASTING

Fig. 14-1.   Response of plasma insulin and glucose in a normal individual after ingestion of carbohydrate (meal).   Note insulin and glucose ratio during fasting.

As mentioned above, hypoglycemia produced after a 12–72-hour fast (the patient should be observed closely during this fast) and inappropriately high serum insulin concentrations are the simplest means to establish the presence of an insulinoma.   However, several other functional tests may be of some help in borderline cases.   Stimulation tests using tolbutamide or glucagon as secretagogues of insulin can result in exaggerated hypoglycemia or hyperinsulinemia in patients with insulinomas.[89,184]

PATIENT WITH INSULINOMA

$$\frac{\text{GLUCOSE (mg \%)}}{\text{INSULIN (mU/ml)}} = < 2.0$$

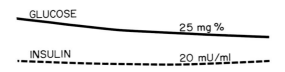

GLUCOSE
                                        25 mg %

INSULIN
                                        20 mU/ml

FASTING

Fig. 14-2.   Glucose-insulin pattern during fasting in a patient with insulinoma.

With these tests false negatives occur in 20–30 percent of patients with insulinomas. The tests are difficult to interpret if the initial blood glucose is low. There may be a falsely positive fall in blood glucose in cirrhosis or other diseases and a falsely positive rise in serum insulin in obese individuals. If the hypoglycemia in a given patient occurs a few hours after meals, an oral glucose tolerance test can be done to confirm this reactive type of hypoglycemia, which may be idiopathic, early diabetes mellitus, or postgastrectomy in nature. Suppression tests[170] have not had wide clinical acceptance, as yet.

Preoperative localization of the tumor is hindered by the small size of the neoplasms and by the occasional avascularity encountered. Nevertheless, overall experience with celiac angiography suggests that approximately 60 percent of tumors are visible by this means.[35,50,63,151] Arteriography has also been useful in some cases to demonstrate hepatic metastases. Pancreatic scans with selenium have not proved to be worthwhile.

Once the diagnosis of insulinoma has been made and arteriography performed, a direct surgical approach to the pancreas is indicated.[39] Since about 80 percent are single and two-thirds of these are in either the body or the tail of the pancreas, distal pancreatectomy is the maximum resection required in about 50–60 percent of cases. In practice, many insulinomas including those in the head of the pancreas can be removed by simple wedge resection. Probably less than 5 percent require pancreaticoduodenectomy. Since 10 percent of insulinomas are multiple, finding of a single one may not terminate the case. It is extremely useful to measure blood glucose at frequent intervals during the case. This can be done with acceptable accuracy by a "Dextrostix" method. The rise in blood glucose after the removal of a lone insulinoma usually occurs within the first hour.[51] Such a rise indicates that an insulinoma is indeed single and no others are left behind. A slight rise in blood sugar may occur as a normal response to surgical trauma. Also, the anesthetist must maintain a constant rate of glucose infusion from the start, and a steady baseline of serum glucose values should be established before pancreatic manipulation is begun. Carcinomas (insulinomas with metastases) should be removed when simple excision is possible. This is consistent with the general principle of always removing as much functioning endocrine tissue as possible commensurate with low morbidity or mortality.

Because insulinomas may be small and hidden within the pancreatic tissue, the neoplasms may not be palpable even after thorough mobilization and careful bimanual palpation of the pancreas. The customary approach is to remove sequentially sections of the pancreas starting with the tail. Examination of the tissue and monitoring of the blood glucose will indicate removal of the insulinomas. It is problematic whether or not to do a "blind" pancreaticoduodenectomy if no tumor is found in the body and tail of the pancreas and/or the blood glucose has not risen. The use of diazoxide in the treatment of insulinomas has opened other therapeutic possibilities. This drug, although introduced primarily as an antihypertensive agent, also suppresses insulin secretion. It affords a useful alternative to a blind resection in the case of the occult neoplasm. One may choose to follow the patient on diazoxide therapy until the neoplasm becomes arteriographically evident. In addition to drug intolerance, diazoxide treatment alone (especially without initial abdominal exploration) must be undertaken with the understanding that an islet cell carcinoma may be growing and metatasizing. It also should be remembered that, in the case of an occult insulinoma, the duodenum and surrounding areas including the omentum, splenic hilum, gallbladder, and small bowel should be searched for an ectopic neoplasm before a decision is made for either a blind resection or diazoxide treatment.

Complications of surgery include cyst formation, fistulas, acute pancreatitis, peritonitis, and abscesses. Any of these events has occurred with even enucleation of the neoplasm. Careful suturing of cut portions of pancreatic tissue and thorough drainage of the area are recommended in even the simplest resections.

Carcinoma with metastases can be treated with either diazoxide or streptozotocin. Experience with either treatment is not large, but symptoms can be controlled effectively with diazoxide for long periods of time. Although diazoxide can control the hyperinsulinemia, the lack of antitumor activity means that tumor growth continues during therapy. Streptozotocin, on the other hand, can control the growth of the tumor. The objective remission rate has been reported at 15 percent for a median survival of 500 days in untreated patients with islet cell carcinomas. Those cases responding to streptozotocin survived a median of 1268 days.

Non-Beta Cell Neoplasms (Gastrinomas)[46,47,56,80,122,167]

Although somewhat similar to insulinomas in both gross and histologic appearance, gastrinomas are functionally quite different. The excessive autonomous production of gastrin by these neoplasms results in hypersecretion of gastric fluid and acid, the secretion of pancreatic fluid to a lesser extent, and inhibition of salt and water reabsorption in the intestine. The resultant syndrome is one of fulminant peptic ulcer disease and, in over half the cases, severe diarrhea. Another important feature of gastrinomas is that 50–60 percent of them are malignant and 30–40 percent are multiple. In 10–20 percent of cases the syndrome may be caused by diffuse hyperplasia of the islets. Because of the malignancy and multiplicity of gastrinomas, it is usually not possible to eradicate the disease by attempting to remove the neoplasm.

Several clinical characteristics of the disease should be noted. The severity, intractability, and rapid postsurgical recurrence of the peptic ulcer disease may raise suspicions of the syndrome. Unusual locations of the ulceration are very suggestive. Ulcerations in the jejunum, as presented in the original 2 patients reported by Zollinger and Ellison,[187] are virtually pathognomonic. However, in approximately 20–30 percent of patients the clinical picture may not be significantly different from that of the standard peptic ulcer disease, and in about 75 percent of cases the ulcers are confined to the usual locations. Other endocrinopathies may exist and hyperparathyroidism has been reported in as high as 20 percent of cases with gastrinomas. Characteristic radiologic features of the syndrome include ulcers distal to the duodenal bulb, multiple ulcers, marginal ulcer appearing soon after partial gastrectomy, prominent gastric and duodenal mucosal folds, and a dilated, hypotonic duodenum.

Several means for diagnosis can be used as outlined in Table 14-1, but the most reliable ones are derived from measurement of serum gastrin by radioimmunoassay.[25,104,185] Exact units and concentrations vary with laboratories, but serum gastrin concentrations of fasting patients with gastrinomas are usually at least four times the normal fasting concentrations. In any given patient gastrin concentrations may fluctuate, and in borderline cases paired samples should be collected on two separate mornings. Other causes of hypergastrinemia with gastric hypersecretion are retained gastric antrum after initial partial gastrectomy, gastric outlet obstruction, chronic renal failure, short-bowel syndrome, and the rare antral gastrin cell hyperplasia. This last disease may prove to be distinguishable preoperatively from gastrinoma in that in gastrin cell hyperplasia a standard test meal stimulates gastrin production, whereas secretin or calcium do not. Gastrin stimulation tests can be very helpful in the borderline cases.[85] Infusion of Ca^{++} 5 mg/kg over 3 hours with hourly gastric acid and serum gastrin measurements results in at least a twofold rise in gastrin with an absolute value usually greater than 500 pg/ml.[8,117,136,169] Secretin stimulation[17] produces a more rapid rise in serum gastrin than does calcium stimulation, but the more widespread availability of calcium as compared to that of secretin is a factor in choice.

Table 14-1
Gastrinoma: Diagnostic
Tests

Gastric acid secretion BAO/MAO >0.6
Serum gastrin
Provocative tests
  Calcium
  Secretin

Criteria for acid secretion in the diagnosis of gastrinoma were emphasized in the era before the availability of gastrin assays. A 12-hour overnight secretion of > 1000 ml volume or > 100 mEq acid was first used. An hourly basal acid output (BAO) of > 15 mEq has also been used. Comparing the BAO to maximum acid output (MAO) after histamine stimulation appears to be the most accurate means of diagnosis using secretory studies.[93] A BAO/MAO of > 0.6 is taken to be diagnostic of gastrinoma. Few false-positive results are obtained, but false-negative tests are common perhaps because of the fluctuations in serum gastrin levels. The acid secretion tests are mainly useful when measurement of serum gastrin is unavailable.

The treatment of choice for gastrinoma continues to be total gastrectomy.[47,181,182] Because of the high rate of malignancy and multicentricity of the tumors, removal of the pancreatic source of gastrin is usually incomplete. Partial gastrectomy almost invariably results in recurrence of ulcer due to persistence of acid-producing cells under the continued stimulus of gastrin.

A food reservoir can be satisfactorily reconstructed after total gastrectomy by the Hunt-Lawrence pouch. A feeding tube jejunostomy can be used and, if leak at the esophagojejunal anastomosis is identified by the barium swallow (usually obtained 7–10 days postoperatively), feeding can be instituted via the tube.

In 1967 a follow-up by Ellison and Wilson of 348 patients with gastrinoma revealed that 27 percent of patients with no resection, 53 percent with partial resection, 73 percent with partial resection and subsequent re-resection, and 87 percent with total resection of the stomach were surviving. An interesting but unquantitated phenomenon is the slow growth, even remission of these tumors seen after total gastrectomy.[57]

WDHA Syndrome

Special mention should be made of the diarrheogenic tumors of the pancreas.[138,186] Although the ulcerogenic tumors may be associated with diarrhea because of intestinal "flooding" by excessive gastric and pancreatic secretions, the Verner-Morrison syndrome[172] or watery diarrhea, hypokalemia, and achlorhydria (WDHA) is a different entity. The WDHA syndrome can be due to non-beta cell pancreatic adenoma, hyperplasia, or carcinoma.[142] The etiology of this syndrome is unclear, but production of gastric inhibitory polypeptide[45] and vasoactive intestinal peptide (VIP)[16,134] has been demonstrated in this syndrome. It is of interest to note that other neoplasms such as bronchogenic carcinomas, medullary carcinoma of the thyroid, pheochromocytomas, and carcinoids may be associated with WDHA.[157] In some of these patients elevated plasma concentrations of VIP have been documented.[134] The treatment of choice is surgical removal of the neoplasm, if possible.

PARATHYROID TUMORS[5,41,61,67,78,87,111,116,123,137]

The immediate consequences of hyperfunctioning tumors of the parathyroid glands are hypercalcemia and hypophosphaturia. These chemical abnormalities result from the hypersecretion of parathyroid hormone by adenomas (80 percent), hyperplasia (20 percent), or the rare carcinoma of the parathyroid glands. These chemical abnormalities over a period of time produce target-organ changes that characterize the clinical entity of primary hyperparathyroidism.

The color of normal glands varies from yellowish-tan to light reddish-brown, and glands are about $2 \times 3 \times 6$ mm in dimension.[30,162] The normal weight of each is about 40–60 mg. Adenomas are similar to normal glands in color but can grow to sizes of 7–10 grams. Hyperplastic glands can range in size from less than 100 mg to several grams. Each of the four glands may be of various sizes in the same patient. The glands in clear cell hyperplasia are sometimes chocolate brown, whereas in chief cell hyperplasia they appear more like adenomas in color. As more experience has been gained with parathyroid surgery, there has been an awareness, on the basis of light and electron microscopy, of a high incidence of both hyperplasia alone and hyperplasia of "normal" glands in the presence of adenomas.[66,162] In several large series,[111,123,137] however, removal of a single adenoma has resulted in cure of the hypercalcemia in over 90 percent of patients, so that the clinical significance of the histologically determined hyperplasia is currently unclear. Parathyroid carcinoma is indistinguishable grossly from adenoma unless invasion of surrounding structures or spread to distant sites has occurred. Microscopically, mitoses within parenchymal cells are the best indicators of malignancy, although a trabecular pattern, thick fibrous bands, and capsular and blood vessel invasion are other features sometimes seen.[82,139]

Diagnosis

In the present era, asymptomatic hypercalcemia is the usual presentation of the patient. Even with the widespread use of serum calcium determinations, however, some patients are first seen because of clinical consequences of hypercalcemia or of parathyroid hormone's actions on bones. These manifestations are listed in Table 14-2. The hypercalcemia of parathyroid carcinoma is persistent and generally of a higher degree than that produced by benign disease. In one series of patients,[139]

Table 14-2
Clinical Signs and Symptoms in Hyperparathyroidism

Genitourinary
  Calculi, nephrocalcinosis, polyuria, polydipsia
Skeletal
  Fractures, osteitis fibrosa cystica, brown tumors
Gastrointestinal
  Anorexia, nausea, vomiting, constipation, peptic ulcers, acute pancreatitis
Neurologic
  Fatigue, muscle weakness, depressed tendon reflexes, disorientation, coma,
  death
Psychiatric
  Apathy, depression, psychotic behavior

the average serum calcium concentration was 15.2 mg/100 ml, and in only 22 percent of patients were the values below 13 mg/100 ml. The hypercalcemia of benign hyperparathyroidism may fluctuate considerably and occasional normal serum calcium values in a patient do not rule out the disease. In fact, some cases of persistently normocalcemic hyperparathyroidism have been reported.[70,149,179] Also, in interpreting serum calcium values, one should be aware that only the ionized (non-protein-bound) fraction of the circulating calcium is physiologically active and, for example, a high serum protein concentration will result in a high total serum calcium value even though the ionized calcium fraction (and the patient) remains normal. In making the diagnosis of hyperparathyroidism, it is also important to consider other causes of hypercalcemia. Some of these are listed in Table 14-3. The hypercalcemia of malignancies, both metastatic and nonmetastatic to bone, is quite interesting and is discussed in more detail below.

In addition to the demonstration of the presence of hypercalcemia and hypophosphatemia and the absence of other causes, the positive diagnosis of hyperparathyroidism can be made by measurement of urinary excretion of cyclic adenosine monophosphate (cAMP).[110,112] Approximately 50 percent of urinary cAMP comes from the renal tubular cell and is under the control of parathyroid hormone (PTH). The urinary cAMP excretion is reported in terms of μM/gm creatinine per 24 hours and, depending on which lab is reporting, is less than about 5.5/day in normal people. As renal clearance rates diminish, the test becomes less reliable, so results are difficult to interpret when the serum creatinine is greater than 2.0–3.0 mg/100 ml.

The measurement of circulating PTH may hold promise in the future as a test for primary hyperparathyroidism. Since concentrations of PTH are extremely low, measurement has been difficult even with radioim-

Table 14-3
Causes of Hypercalcemia

Malignancy with bone metastases
Primary and "tertiary" hyperparathyroidism
Hyperthyroidism
Thiazide therapy
Multiple myeloma
Sarcoidosis
Hypervitaminosis D
Milk–alkali syndrome
Leukemia
Addisonian crisis
Malignancy without bone metastases (ectopic PTH or pseudohyperparathyroidism)

munoassays. To compound the difficulty, the various circulating forms and fragments of PTH make assay specificity a problem.[4] Antisera developed in several research laboratories confer suitable specificity to the PTH radioimmunoassay, but these assays are not, as of this writing, available for widespread clinical use. The assay has been used also for preoperative localization of parathyroid adenomas by measuring PTH in blood obtained from selective catheterization and sampling of veins draining the neck area. The expense of this has been estimated at $500–$700 per patient and seems impractical except in the search for residual hyperfunctioning parathyroid tissue after initial unsuccessful neck explorations. The same statement can be applied to arteriography in terms of indications.[18,147] Other means of preoperative localization such as selenomethionine scan have been unsuccessful except in large glands.[40] Occasionally a barium swallow will detect a large adenoma indenting the esophagus. As a rule, physical examination is unrewarding since the benign adenomas or hyperplastic glands are almost never palpable, but the unusual parathyroid cyst can be felt externally[84,174] and approximately 30 percent of parathyroid carcinomas are palpable preoperatively.[139]

Treatment

The standard surgical exploration of the neck in hyperparathyroidism[23] is done through a "collar" incision about 2–3 cm above the suprasternal notch. Since locating the glands is problematical in many instances, attention must be given to meticulous dissection, hemostasis, and anatomical relationships. Since the upper glands come along embryologically with the thyroid lobes from the fourth branchial pouch, they are more constant in location and are usually found on the posterolateral surface of the thyroid lobes somewhere between the inferior thyroid artery and the upper pole of the thyroid gland. The lower glands, on the other hand, arise and migrate with the thymus. Although the lower parathyroid glands usually do not follow the thymus beyond the lower pole of the thyroid, they may be found anywhere from the upper pole of the thyroid down to the lower mediastinum. Other ectopic locations of parathyroid glands include the underside of the sternohyoid or sternothyroid muscles, within the thyroid gland itself, in the tracheoesophageal groove, behind the esophagus, and within the carotid sheath. If a single adenoma is found, this is removed. An attempt should be made to identify and biopsy all four glands because of the incidence (1–3 percent) of multiple adenomas and because of the possibility of hyperplasia in all four glands. In the case of hyperplasia all but the 50–70 mg of parathyroid tissue in one remaining gland should be removed. Some cases of hyperplasia may be asymmetrical and one or more glands will be minimally enlarged. Since no absolute criteria have been established for identifying hyperplasia by frozen section, resection of these "normal" asymmetrical glands may be necessary to prevent persistent postoperative hypercalcemia.[66] The entity of hyperplastic normal-sized glands is currently an unresolved issue from the standpoint of both histopathologic identification and clinical importance.

When an "adenoma" is adherent to or invading surrounding tissue, a carcinoma is the most likely diagnosis. An en bloc resection of surrounding tissue is favored in an attempt to decrease the incidence of local recurrence. Lymph node metastases are unusual and late, so prophylactic neck dissection is not indicated.

Treatment of Parathyroid Cancer

Recurrent parathyroid carcinoma appears locally in about one-third of cases and can be managed by re-resection in some instances. Metastases typically occur late in the disease and are to lung, liver, and bone in addition to local nodes. An attempt should be made to resect all functioning tissue reasonably accessible to the surgeon since reasonably good palliation[60] or cure[139] can be achieved. Successful removal of single metastases has been reported.[34] For recurrent disease not amenable to resection, temporary control of hypercalcemia has been reported with either oral phosphate, calcitonin, or mithramycin. Because of the rarity of the disease, no large series are available, but the overall 5-year survival is approximately 55 percent.[139] Roughly one-third of patients who have only local recurrence are cured by the second resection; all of these cures occur in patients who have recurrences appear more than 2 years after the initial surgery.

Pseudohyperparathyroidism

Special note should be made of the occurrence of hypercalcemia produced by nonparathyroid tumors in the absence of metastases to bone. In many of these cases ectopic production of a parathyroid hormonelike substance is responsible for the hypercalcemia and hypophosphatemia.[12] The term pseudohyperparathyroidism has been introduced to describe this syndrome which is indistinguishable by the usual means from primary hyperparathyroidism. The specificity of certain PTH radioimmunoassays allows tumor-produced PTH to be distinguished from that arising from parathyroid glands,[11] but these assays are not yet widely available. Hypernephromas and bronchogenic carcinomas account for over 60 percent of the cases, but many other malignancies including head and neck squamous cell carcinomas,[3,166] leukemias,[113] and sarcomas can produce this syndrome associated with elevated PTH-like activity in plasma. In one report very few cases with pseudohyperparathyroidism had detectable PTH-like activity[120] in their serum and the point remains controversial. The various other factors postulated include vitamin D sterols, prostaglandin E_1,[9,10,124,130,164,165,173] and osteoclast-stimulating factors.[20,109] In one case report, indomethacin, an inhibitor of prostaglandin synthesis, produced amelioration of the hypercalcemia associated with a hypernephroma.[19] Subsequent clinical experience and investigation will be required for further clarification of this phenomenon.

ADRENAL TUMORS[44,69,77,98,100,125]

The clinical syndromes produced by adrenal tumors are a heterogeneous group. This heterogeneity is a reflection of several factors such as the division of the adrenal gland into cortex and medulla, the presence of both functioning and nonfunctioning tumors, and the ability of the adrenal cortex to secrete a variety of steroids with different actions. In turn, diagnostic procedures applicable to each of the syndromes differ one from another because of the different hormones involved and the physiological control mechanisms related to various hormonal actions. Also, some of the problems in management are specific to each of the syndromes as a reflection of the differing effects of the hormones on target tissues. The salient features of each syndrome will be presented in the following sections.

Nonfunctioning Adrenocortical Tumors[94]

Because nonfunctioning tumors do not produce characteristic clinical stigmata, these tumors usually grow to a fairly large size before becoming evident. Abdominal pain and a flank mass are the two most common modes of presentation for the nonfunctioning tumors. Intravenous pyelography and arteriography are the two diagnostic procedures of choice for establishing the presence of an adrenal tumor. The size of the tumor is some indication of the probability of malignancy since, as a rule, most tumors weighing over 100 gm are malignant. The majority of nonfunctioning tumors are malignant and should be considered so when they are approached therapeutically. The tumors should be approached transabdominally in order to allow the option of the wide local resection sometimes required of the diaphragm, pancreas, and other structures. Confirmation of malignancy in these neoplasms by means other than direct extension into surrounding tissues is sometimes difficult. The well-differentiated cortical carcinomas are virtually impossible to distinguish histologically from adenomas, and the appearance of subsequent metastases may be the first evidence of the malignant nature of the tumor. Metastases from these carcinomas go to the lymph nodes (30 percent), liver (50 percent), lungs (50 percent), and bones (25 percent). These neoplasms are in general radioresistant and the only effective chemotherapy is that of ortho-para-dichlorodiphenyldichloroethane (o,p'-DDD). Nonfunctioning tumors respond to this agent at a rate of approximately 20 percent. The mean survival time of untreated patients with nonfunctioning tumors is approximately 2.2 months. When radical excision for a cure is possible, the survival rate is approximately 40 percent at 5 years. The rate of appearance of metastases after removal of an adrenal carcinoma is quite high, and the patient must be followed at regular intervals for long periods of time after surgical exploration.

Cushing's Syndrome (Glucocorticoid Excess)[72,74,115,145,158,161]

Cushing's syndrome is caused by excessive secretion of cortisol by the adrenal cortex. The pathology involved can be hyperplasia of the cortex owing to an increased secretion of pituitary (rarely, nonpituitary) ACTH, a benign adrenal cortical adenoma, or an adrenal carcinoma. Approximately 75 percent of the cases in this syndrome are due to an excess of pituitary ACTH and the consequent hyperplasia of the cortex. A small percentage of the cases are owing to ectopically produced ACTH and the hyperplasia of the cortex. About 25 percent of the cases are caused by functioning adrenal neoplasms, and approximately 40 percent of these neoplasms are adrenal carcinomas.

The clinical picture produced is characteristic, and the only difficulty lies in detecting the subtle changes of early cases. Patients may manifest headaches, fullness of the face, weight gain, abdominal striae, and easy bruisability. Acne or menstrual irregularities may be present also. Evidence of androgen excess (virilization) can occur in the benign forms of

Cushing's syndrome but is almost always present in cases of adrenal carcinoma. Virilization is usually appreciated only in the female with such complaints as coarsening of the hair, deepening of the voice, and clitoral hypertrophy. Some carcinomas produce feminization.[58]

The first step in diagnosis of this syndrome should be the collection of urine for measurement of 17-hydroxycorticosteroids (17-OHCS) and 17-ketosteroids (17-KS).[43] Adrenocortical hyperactivity should be expected if the 17-OHCS are greater than 15 mg/day or 17-KS values are above 6 mg/day (female) or 12 mg/day (male). With adrenal carcinomas the 17-KS excretion is almost always at least in the range of 50–200 mg/day. Accuracy in diagnosis using 17-OHCS excretion can be increased by correction for grams of creatinine.[163] The normal range is 3–10 mg/gm creatinine.

The dexamethasone suppression test[95] is a very useful maneuver in differentiating normal obesity from Cushing's disease and in differentiating adrenal hyperplasia from adrenal tumor. Figure 14-3 illustrates the ACTH-cortisol relationships in each of the three situations. A low-dose administration of dexamethasone, 0.5 mg every 6 hours, will result in a depression of urinary excretion of steroids in simple obesity, whereas in adrenocortical hyperactivity the suppression of steroid secretion by this dose of dexamethasone is minimal. In hyperplasia of hypothalamic-pituitary origin, more dexamethasone than usual is required to "shut off" ACTH secretion. The high dose of dexamethasone, 2 mg every 6 hours, will result in a suppression of ACTH and steroid secretion in the form of Cushing's syndrome because of hyperplasia of the cortex; whereas with an autonomously functioning adrenal tumor, no decrease in steroid secretion is seen because ACTH is already suppressed by endogenous cortisol excess. Unfortunately, in the case of ACTH production by a nonpituitary neoplasm, the results of dexamethasone administration erroneously

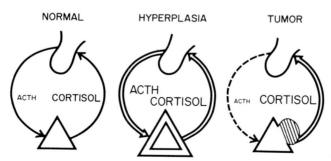

Fig. 14-3. Relationships of cortisol (adrenal) and ACTH (pituitary) during normal states, adrenal hyperplasia, and adrenal tumor.

suggest an adrenal tumor because the neoplasm's ACTH secretion is not suppressed by dexamethasone. The use of a reliable assay for plasma ACTH, when it becomes widely available, will go far in differentiating the various possibilities for Cushing's syndrome one from another.[126]

Should a tumor be diagnosed, the preferred treatment is surgical extirpation. With adrenal hyperplasia it is generally agreed that pituitary irradiation or ablation is the treatment of choice unless the clinical situation is particularly fulminant in terms of cardiovascular and infectious complications. Before surgery for a tumor, intravenous pyelography and arteriography are useful to lateralize the tumor. Adrenal scanning using radioiodinated cholesterol may be a promising technique.[2] For small tumors with low or absent 17-KS excretion, the flank approach is recommended. This is especially useful in the usual patient with truncal obesity, poor wound healing, and a propensity for infections. However, should the tumor be large and/or associated with elevated 17-KS excretion, the abdominal approach should be considered, since the flank incision is a difficult one through which to do a large radical excision.

Postoperative complications are mainly related to the consequences of long-term cortisol excess. Complications such as wound infections, septicemia, pancreatitis, splenic injury, and pulmonary infections are especially common in adrenal surgery for Cushing's syndrome.[44,119] Postoperative administration of steroids is necessary. In the case of adrenal hyperplasia with total adrenalectomy, of course, the replacement therapy is permanent. In the case of a functioning adrenal tumor, steroid replacement may be necessary for a number of weeks or months because of the atrophy produced in the contralateral gland by the steroid-suppressed plasma ACTH. It is sometimes difficult to wean these patients off steroids. A series of daily ACTH injections or infusions may be helpful in restoring the responsiveness of the contralateral gland to endogenous ACTH. Some of the above considerations are outlined in Table 14-4.

For advanced carcinoma, the most efficacious agent presently available is o,p''DDD, a derivative of the commercial insecticide DDT.[13,76,99]

Table 14-4
Surgical Management of Cushing's Syndrome

1. For hyperplasia if rapid progression, severe hypertension, frequent infections, children
2. For all tumors
3. Preoperative localization attempted
4. Flank approach recommended (except for large tumor)
5. Steroid coverage started during case
6. Drains placed
7. Postoperative chest films, amylase determinations, steroid replacement

The starting adult dose of this agent is usually 2–6 gm daily and is increased until toxicity occurs. The maximum dose is usually 10 gm daily. In approximately 80 percent of the patients some combination of symptoms of toxicity such as anorexia, nausea, vomiting, diarrhea, lethargy, somnolence, dizziness, and vertigo occurs. Approximately 70 percent of the patients show some response to the agent in terms of decrease in urinary excretion of steroids. This response lasts, on the average, 5 months. It is estimated that the clinical response rate is approximately 50 percent. Another agent of potential benefit is aminoglutethimide.[144] It has had limited testing but there is some indication that it may produce an inhibition of steroid secretion by functioning adrenal carcinomas. In contrast to o,p'-DDD, aminoglutethimide is not cytolytic but is simply a competitive inhibitor of steroid biosynthesis.

Primary Aldosteronism[28,59,71,91,129,152]

The syndrome produced by an excess in aldosterone excretion is characterized primarily by hypertension, hypokalemia, polydipsia, polyuria, and muscle weakness.[29] Aldosterone is produced by the zonaglomerulosa of the adrenal cortex. Although nodular hyperplasia of this zone has recently been recognized as a cause of primary aldosteronism, most cases are owing to adenomas. Only single case reports appear in the literature in evidence of the rarity of carcinoma as a cause of this disease.[1,21,32,52,55] The difference in size between carcinomas and benign tumors in this syndrome is even more striking than in the case of tumors with excess glucocorticoid production. The carcinomas reported have tended to be large tumors in the kilogram range, as compared to the usual small adenomas producing primary aldosteronism. Many of the adenomas are less than 2 cm in diameter, and a few have been reported in the millimeter range.

The diagnosis of the syndrome of primary aldosteronism rests on the demonstration of an elevated excretion of aldosterone and a suppression of plasma renin activity. The autonomous production of aldosterone by the tumor results in expansion of the extracellular fluid volume and a consequent suppression of renin secretion by the kidney.[27] Almost all cases are associated with hypokalemia unless the patients have a very mild form and are on a low-sodium intake. It is our practice to collect on an outpatient basis two 24-hour urines for aldosterone and an upright plasma sample for renin. Should these results be suggestive of the syndrome, the patient is then brought into a metabolic ward where dietary sodium and potassium, urine collection, and posture can be carefully controlled. A period of low sodium intake and upright posture is used to demonstrate conclusively the presence of suppressed renin activity. A period of high sodium intake is used to demonstrate the persistence of excess excretion of aldosterone in the urine and to accentuate the hypokalemia through increased sodium-potassium exchange in the renal tubule.

At the present time the treatment of choice for adenomas and carcinomas continues to be surgical extirpation. There is some indication that a significant number of patients have primary aldosteronism because of hyperplasia, which may be treated more appropriately with aldosterone antagonists, such as spironolactone, than with surgery.[22] Carcinoma of the adrenal cortex producing this syndrome will most likely be encountered unexpectedly in the exploration of a patient with a preoperative diagnosis of adenoma. The surgical considerations of wide excision are the same as for the other varieties of adrenal carcinoma.

The postoperative management of these patients is considerably simpler than that of patients with Cushing's syndrome. The most common problem is lingering suppression of the aldosterone secretion from the remaining adrenal tissue. This suppression is usually evidenced by an increase in the serum potassium concentration and a tendency toward hypotension. The treatment is the administration of a mineralocorticoid such as α-fluorohydrocortisone, 0.1 mg/day. An example of such treatment in a patient after removal of an aldosteronoma is shown in Figure 14-4.

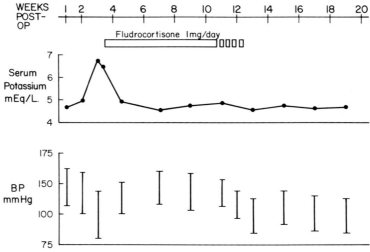

Fig. 14-4. Postoperative course (in weeks) of a patient with a previous aldosteronoma who developed a mineralocorticoid deficiency with hyperkalemia that responded to fludrocortisone.

Pheochromocytoma[74,128,146,155,171,183]

The clinical situation produced by a functioning pheochromocytoma can be quite striking. The tumor arises from the adrenal medulla, a rich source of epinephrine and norepinephrine. During the usual full-blown attack caused by an outpouring of catecholamines, the patient becomes anxious, tremulous, and suffers headaches, palpitations, excessive perspiration, blanching of the skin, and even premonition of impending doom. Actually the syndrome has many presentations and a patient with any sort of episodic "attack" should be suspected of harboring a pheochromocytoma. Some of the possible symptoms and signs encountered are given in Table 14-5. The blood pressure pattern may be that of sustained hypertension with occasional sudden increases in blood pressure, paroxysmal hypertension with intervening periods of normal blood pressure, or, in a few patients, long periods of normotension with only infrequent, brief episodes of hypertension. As in primary aldosteronism (and in contrast to Cushing's syndrome), physical findings may be absent in patients with pheochromocytoma. In a few of the patients nonendocrine findings such as neuroectodermal dysplasias may be present. These manifestations may be seen more frequently in the familial variety of pheochromocytoma and other endocrinopathies, which are discussed later.

The diagnosis of a functioning pheochromocytoma is established primarily by demonstration of an elevation in excretory products from the tumor. The most commonly measured substances are the catecholamines or their metabolic products. In Table 14-6 is given a list of these substances with the normal upper limit of their daily urinary excretion. The stimulation tests (tyramine, glucagon, or histamine) or the blocking tests (regitine) should be used only in borderline cases where the pattern of urinary excretion is unclear. Aortography has been suggested in order to delineate clearly the location of the tumor or discover the possible

Table 14-5
Signs and Symptoms of
Pheochromocytoma

Headache	Premonitions of doom
Palpitations	Psychoses
Tremulousness	Hyperglycemia
Pallor	Weight loss
Sweating	Tachycardia
Syncope	Episodic weakness
Anxiety	Agitation

Table 14-6
Pheochromocytoma: Excretory Products and
Provocative Tests

Urinary excretion (24 hr)		
Catecholamines	100	μg
Epinephrine	20	μg
Norepinephrine	80	μg
Vanillylmandelic acid	6–7	mg
Metanephrines	1–2	mg

[Note if patient is taking methyldopa (Aldomet®), monoamine oxidase inhibitors, neg gram or clofibrate (Atromid-S®)]
Provocative tests
    Tyramine, glucagon, histamine, regitine (blocking)
    Aortogram

extra-adrenal sites for the tumor. It is a potentially dangerous procedure and should be undertaken only with the appropriate precautions.

In preparing the patient for surgery, consideration should be given to the use of alpha- and beta-adrenergic blocking agents.[31,65,121,133] Although the effectiveness of these agents has not been established by randomized trials, a clear clinical impression of most experienced surgeons is that these agents have a beneficial effect in dampening the fluctuations in blood pressure and decreasing the frequency of arrhythmias during surgery. Phenoxybenzamine (starting dose of 20 mg/day) is the drug of choice for alpha-adrenergic blockage. Propranolol (10–30 mg/day) is used for beta blockade. During induction of anesthesia and during the operation itself, a continuous drip of phentolamine has been found useful for smooth control of the hypertensive episodes. Phentolamine and propranolol should also be available in syringes ready for particularly severe spikes in blood pressure or severe arrhythmias. The third type of drug, norepinephrine or phenylephrine, should be available for immediate use after removal of pheochromocytoma. Usually these hypotensive episodes will respond to vigorous fluid and blood replacement alone.

The preferred surgical approach is through a bilateral subcostal incision. This approach affords good visualization of the adrenal glands and also permits the surgeon to explore the entire abdominal cavity for extra-adrenal tumors. Great care should be exercised in handling the tumor in order to avoid a burst of catecholamines into the circulation and the subsequent cardiovascular sequelae. If at all possible, the adrenal vein should be ligated at an early stage of dissection. In sporadic cases of pheochromocytoma the tumor is located bilaterally in 10 percent so both adrenals must be inspected. Also, extra-adrenal locations such as the paravertebral ganglia, mesentery, preaortic area, and urinary bladder should be examined if no adrenal tumor is present. Another 10 percent are malignant in sporadic cases. Unless the carcinoma is growing into surrounding tissues, it is almost impossible to establish the diagnosis of malignancy either by gross inspection of the tumor or by microscopic examination. Unfortunately, many times the first evidence of malignancy is local recurrence of tumor or appearance of distant metastases in the postoperative period.[68] In the familial types of pheochromocytoma the incidence of bilaterality may approach 60 percent, and the incidence of malignancy is somewhat higher also (15–20 percent). Some of the above points on management are reiterated in Table 14-7.

In advanced disease the patient is usually markedly hypertensive and the immediate problem is that of pharmacological control of the blood pressure. Long-term control by alpha-adrenergic blockage has been reported.[49,140] The use of alpha-methyltyrosine has also been reported as showing striking effects in patients with pheochromocytoma.[154] This drug inhibits catecholamine synthesis at its rate-limiting step.[48] Only random reports of radiotherapy are available and the results have been variable. A few cases have responded to cyclophosphamide therapy.

MEDULLARY THYROID CARCINOMA[26,42,107]

Medullary carcinoma deserves special mention among the types of thyroid carcinomas (discussed in another chapter) because of several interesting features. It arises from the thyroidal parafollicular cells, which are thought to originate from the neural crest. Phylogenetically, they originated in the ultimobranchial (UB) body, which later fused with the thyroid gland, and the UB cells ultimately dispersed among the thyroid follicular cells in higher species. The UB body in the lowest species and the parafollicular cells in mammals have been shown to con-

Table 14-7
Surgical Management of Pheochromocytoma

1. Preoperative alpha (phenoxybenzamine) and beta (propranolol) blockade
2. Intraoperative regitine drip; stand by with regitine, propranolol, and norepinephrine in syringe
3. Transverse upper abdominal incision
4. Explore both sides and extra-adrenal sites
5. Tie off adrenal vein first
6. Look for second pheochromocytoma if blood pressure does not fall after tumor removal
7. Liberal whole blood infusion and/or norepinephrine if shock follows tumor removal

tain calcitonin, a peptide hormone with hypocalcemic activity. Since parafollicular cells are also part of the amine precursor uptake and decarboxylation (APUD) family of cells,[118] medullary carcinomas may also produce serotonin, histamine, and catecholamines. Even prostaglandins have been demonstrated in these tumors. Another feature of these tumors is their familial association. Although sporadic cases occur, both the familial syndromes of medullary carcinoma only and syndromes of multiple endocrine adenomatosis are well recognized. In view of the tumors' common APUD origins, it is not surprising that both sporadic and familial cases may be associated with pheochromocytomas, parathyroid disease, mucosal neuromas, and carcinoid tumors.

Diagnosis

The sporadic case of medullary carcinoma is usually diagnosed during the thyroid operation for a cold nodule. In spite of elevated concentrations of plasma calcitonin demonstrable in many of these cases, hypocalcemia is an unusual clinical feature. In fact, there are few specific clinical features. Diarrhea is prominent in some cases and suggests the diagnosis of this carcinoma in a patient with a thyroid nodule. Some "sporadic" cases will subsequently develop other glandular tumors, and a careful post-facto examination of family members will reveal a familial type of situation. Calcitonin assays in plasma have proved to be extremely useful in the diagnosis of occult medullary carcinoma in family members.[15,37,38,79,106] These assays may represent the best means to diagnosis the disease preoperatively and to follow the patient's progress after surgery.[62] Histaminase is another tumor marker and may be used in a manner similar to that for calcitonin.[83]

Treatment

Surgical treatment of the disease consists of total thyroidectomy because of the high incidence of bilaterality and of radical neck dissection because of the high incidence of lymph node metastases. The 5-year survival is considerably less than that for papillary carcinoma, approaching 50 percent in some series, and because of the high degree of malignancy of the lymph metastases, prophylactic neck dissection is indicated. It is especially important to examine the parathyroid glands in cases of medullary carcinoma because of the associated parathyroid disease in the familial form. The question is currently unresolved as to whether or not removal of enlarged parathyroid glands in the normocalcemic patient is justified. No large series are available in this uncommon disease, but some investigators have advocated removal of all enlarged glands (leaving behind 30–50 mg of tissue if all four glands are enlarged).[14]

CARCINOID TUMORS AND SYNDROME[36,156,160,180]

Carcinoid tumors are typically found in the intestinal tract and are small, yellowish submucosal nodules. Occasional carcinoid tumors are found in the ovary and the bronchus. The tumors arise from the enterochromaffin cell which belongs to the family of APUD cells mentioned in the discussion of medullary carcinoma. This family of cells secretes small polypeptide and amine hormones. Serotonin can usually be isolated from these tumors in the intestinal tract, and those located in the stomach are often rich in histamine as well. Bradykinin, a polypeptide with hypotensive effects, is also secreted by the tumor. Approximately 45 percent of the carcinoids are located in the appendix, with another 20 percent in the ileum. They are described as argentaffin tumors because of their ability to reduce silver salts to black metallic silver. Carcinoids of the large bowel do not have this property and seldom produce any manifestations of the carcinoid syndrome. The tumors in any location show a definite relationship of size to malignant potential. Only about 3 percent of the tumors less than 1 cm in diameter demonstrate metastases, whereas virtually all of the tumors over 2 cm are clinically malignant. Regional lymph nodes and the liver are the primary sites for metastases.

Diagnosis of Carcinoid Syndrome

Only a small portion (3 percent) of carcinoid tumors develop the carcinoid syndrome, which is almost always associated with liver metastases. Occasionally primary tumors are located with direct access to the systemic circulation (ovarian carcinoids, bronchial carcinoids), and the carcinoid syndrome may occur without liver metastases. It is speculated that primary carcinoid tumors located within the portal venous drainage system do not produce the syndrome because the vasoactive substances formed in these tumors are inactivated by the liver. The carcinoid syndrome is manifested by bronchoconstriction, cyanosis, peripheral vascular symptoms, and valvular diseases of the right side of the heart. The so-called carcinoid flush is characterized by a sudden light reddening of the upper trunk and is usually precipitated by exertion, emotion, or ethanol intake. These flushes are thought to be due to bradykinin and not to serotonin as originally postulated. Diarrhea is another important part of the syndrome complex and is present in approximately 75 percent of the cases. Serotonin is a sufficient explanation for this feature, but the role of prostaglandins and vasoactive intestinal peptide may be etiologic also. Diagnosis of the carcinoid is confirmed by the measurement in the urine of 5-hydroxyindoleacetic acid, a metabolite of serotonin. The excretion of more than 9 mg/day in a patient without malabsorption indicates the strong likelihood of the carcinoid syndrome. Drugs such as phenothiazines and foods containing phenolic acids such as bananas should be avoided during urine collection because they interfere with the assay. When the urinary excretion tests are equivocal, the diagnosis may be obtained with use of the epinephrine-provocative test. Stimulation of hormones from the carcinoid by epinephrine produces a flush as a positive test.

Treatment

The extent of surgical resection of the tumor depends on the circumstances. For these tumors of the appendix, simple appendectomy will suffice. Metastases from these lesions are extremely rare. Only those tumors greater than 2 cm in diameter or those that have a combination of features such as location at the base of the appendix, invasion of the mesoappendix, and microscopic lymphatic invasion should be treated by radical right colectomy. With the tumor in the small bowel it is advisable to do a segmental resection including the pertinent segment of mesentery. Rectal and large bowel carcinoids can be handled by either simple or radical excision along the guidelines of lesser or greater than 2 cm in diameter and extent of bowel wall invasion. In surgery on patients with the carcinoid syndrome, care should be taken with anesthesia to avoid some of the consequences of vasomotor instability and stimulation of the tumor by elevated endogenous catecholamine levels. Chlorpromazine is a useful antiserotonin drug. Trasylol, a bradykinin antagonist, may be useful for hypotension and bronchospasm.

Advanced disease is treated primarily on a symptomatic basis. There is no clear-cut best combination of chemotherapy, although cyclophosphamide, methotrexate, and regionally infused 5-fluorouracil have been used. Flushing can be controlled with phenoxybenzamine or phenothiazines. The serotonin antagonist methylsergide has been useful in controlling diarrhea. Because of the stimulatory effects of epinephrine on carcinoid tumors, caution should be observed in treating the asthmatic episodes with epinephrine as a bronchodilator. Small doses of isoproterenol inhalation are probably the best treatment for the asthma. The prognosis of patients with carcinoid syndrome is better than that of patients with many other tumors. According to a large series from the Mayo Clinic, 68 percent of patients with resectable tumors survived 5 years, whereas 21 percent of those with liver metastases survived 5 years.

MULTIPLE ENDOCRINE ADENOMATOSIS[7,83,114,160]

Brief mention should be made of the coexistence in a given patient of several endocrine tumors, both of the sporadic variety and those in a familial setting. In any given patient with multiple involvement of the endocrine glands, the case can be termed sporadic only after a systematic,

careful search of family members has been done. It is becoming apparent, for example, that medullary carcinomas and/or pheochromocytomas
can develop in family members many years after the original patient has
his "sporadic" medullary carcinoma removed.

Wermer's syndrome[176] is the familial association of the combination
of pituitary, parathyroid, and pancreatic islet cell tumors. The parathyroids are involved in about 85 percent of the cases with this syndrome.
There is a high incidence (40 percent) of multiple parathyroid adenomas,
and the hyperplasia seen is usually of the chief cell variety. The islet cells
of the pancreas are involved in 75 percent of the cases with 65 percent of
these being the non-beta cell gastrin type and 35 percent being beta cell
insulin-producing tumors. The pituitary is involved in approximately 65
percent of the cases; of these, acromegaly is seen in 30 percent, whereas
45 percent have chromophobe adenomas and present with signs of hypopituitarism. Only a few have Cushing's syndrome. Occasionally carcinoid tumors, thyroid adenomas, and adrenal adenomas are seen with
this syndrome.

Sipple's syndrome[153] consists of medullary carcinoma of the thyroid,
pheochromocytoma, and hyperparathyroidism. Although these three entities are usually present in each patient, familial associations of only one
of these three diseases can be seen as any combination of the three is possible.[102] It should be emphasized again, however, that medullary carcinoma can exist in the occult form with only elevated serum calcitonin as
an indicator of its presence. An even more difficult situation can exist in
familial medullary carcinoma when the presence of a nonfunctioning
pheochromocytoma does not result in hypertension and urinary catecholamines may not be elevated. Familial medullary carcinomas are bilateral in approximately 80 percent of the cases as compared to a 30-percent
incidence in sporadic ones. Pheochromocytomas are bilateral in 60 percent of familial cases as compared to 10 percent in the sporadic cases.
Although both the parafollicular cells of the thyroid and the adrenal medullary cells have the same origin (APUD), a similar origin of the parathyroid glands is difficult to substantiate and the reason for the involvement
of these glands in one syndrome is less clear. It is postulated that the increase in calcitonin may secondarily stimulate the parathyroid glands by
the tendency to lower serum calcium, but elevated parathyroid hormone
concentrations in plasma have been reported with this syndrome in the
presence of normal concentrations of calcitonin. The parathyroids are
most likely involved in some way in the genetic defect.

ECTOPIC PRODUCTION OF HORMONES[132]

Neoplasms of an almost endless variety have been reported as producing peptide and biogenic amine hormones either singly or in combinations.[6,88,92,105,127,131,135] One explanation for this phenomenon is similar to

that concerning the origin of multiple endocrine adenomatoses. Even though most of the cells in the endocrine glands are ectodermal, entodermal, and mesodermal in origin, a hypothesis has been put forth that certain cells derived from neutral ectoderm and which can be described histologically as argentaffin cells are scattered throughout the body including the endocrine glands, the lungs, and gastrointestinal tract.[118] From this cell of common origin it is postulated that even benign tumors in many diverse locations can produce peptide and amine hormones.[175] Furthermore, two main theories have been proposed which explain why carcinomas may produce hormones either singly or in multiple combinations. It is thought that perhaps the totipotentiality of the primordial cell becomes uncovered by gene derepression.[54] This anomaly of nuclear genetic material is consistent with the already present nuclear anomaly of "uncontrolled" cell division. The other hypothesis is simply that the cancer cell can produce an endless array of polypeptide and biogenic amines, some of which just happen to possess biological activity that we can measure or observe clinically.

REFERENCES

1. Alterman SL, Dominguez C, Lopez-Gomez A, Lieber AL: Primary adrenocortical carcinoma causing aldosteronism. Cancer 24:602, 1969
2. Anderson, BG, Beierwaltes, WH: Adrenal imaging with radioiodocholesterol in the diagnosis of adrenal disorders. Adv Intern Med 19:327, 1974
3. Ariyan S, Farber LR, Hamilton, BP, Papac, RJ: Pseudohyperparathyroidism in head and neck tumors. Cancer 33:159, 1974
4. Arnaud CD, Goldsmith RS, Bordier PJ, Sizemore GW et al: Influence of Immunoheterogeneity of circulating parathyroid hormone on results of radioimmunoassays of serum in man. Am J Med 56:785, 1974
5. Aurbach GD, Mallette LE, Patten BM, et al: Hyperparathyroidism: Recent studies. Ann Intern Med 79:566, 1973
6. Azzopardi JG, Williams ED: Pathology of 'nonendocrine' tumors associated with Cushing's syndrome. Cancer 22:274, 1968
7. Ballard HS, Frame B, Hartsock, RJ: Familial Multiple endocrine adenoma-Peptic ulcer complex. Medicine 43:481, 1964
8. Basso N, Passaro E Jr: Calcium-stimulated gastric secretion in the Zollinger-Ellison syndrome. Arch Surg 101:339, 1970
9. Beliel OM, Singer FR, Coburn JW: Prostaglandins: Effect on plasma calcium concentration. Cancer 3:237, 1973
10. Bennett A, Simpson JS, McDonald AM, Stamford IF: Breast cancer, prostaglandins, and bone metastases. Lancet 1:1218, 1975
11. Benson RC Jr, Riggs BL, Pickard BM, Arnaud CD: Immunoreactive forms of circulating parathyroid hormone in primary and ectopic hyperparathyroidism. J Clin Invest 54:175, 1974
12. Benson RC, Riggs BL, Pickard BM, Arnaud CD: Radioimmunoassay of

parathyroid hormone in hypercalcemic patients with malignant disease. Am J Med 56:821, 1974

13. Bergenstal DM, Hertz R, Lipsett MB, Moy RH: Chemotherapy of adreno-cortical cancer with o,p'DDD. Ann Intern Med 53:672, 1960

14. Block MA, Jackson CE, Tashjian AH Jr: Management of parathyroid glands in surgery for medullary thyroid carcinoma. Arch Surg 110:617, 1975

15. Block MA, Jackson CE, Tashjian AH Jr: Medullary thyroid cardinoma detected by serum calcitonin assay. Arch Surg 104:579, 1972

16. Bloom SR, Polack JM, Pearse AGE: Vasoactive intestinal peptide and watery-diarrhea syndrome. Lancet 2:14, 1973

17. Bradley EL, Galambos JT, Lobley CR, Chan YK: Secretin-gastrin relationship in Zollinger-Ellison syndrome. Surgery 73:550, 1973

18. Bradley EL, McGarity WC: Surgical evaluation of parathyroid arteriography. Am J Surg 128:67, 1973

19. Brereton HD, Halushka PV, Alexander RW, et al: Indomethacin-responsive hypercalcemia in a patient with renal-cell adenocarcinoma. Cancer 291:83, 1974

20. Brewer HB: Osteoclastic bone resorption and the hypercalcemia of cancer.

21. Brooks RV, Felix-Davies D, Lee MR, Robertson PW: Hyperaldosteronism from adrenal carcinoma. Br Med J 1:220, 1972

22. Brown JJ, Davies DL, Ferriss JB, et al: Comparison of surgery and prolonged spironolactone therapy in patients with hypertension, aldosterone excess, and low plasma renin. Br Med J 2:729, 1972

23. Cady B: Neck exploration for hyperparathyroidism. Surg Clin North Am 53:301, 1973

24. Chandalia HB, Boshell BR: Hypoglycemia associated with extrapancreatic tumors: Report of two cases with studies on its pathogenesis. Arch Intern Med 129:447, 1972

25. Charters AC, Odell WD, Davidson WD, Thompson JC: Gastrin: immunochemical properties and measurement by radioimmunoassay. Surgery 66:104, 1969

26. Chong GC, Beahrs OH, Sizemore GW, Woolner LH: Medullary carcinoma of the thyroid gland. Cancer 35:695, 1975

27. Conn JW: Plasma renin activity in primary aldosteronism. JAMA 190:222, 1964

28. Conn JW, Knopf RF, Nesbit RM: Clinical characteristics of primary aldosteronism from an analysis of 145 cases. Am J Surg 107:159, 1964

29. Conn JW, Louis LH: Primary aldosteronism: A new clinical entity. Trans Assoc Am Physicians 68:215, 1955

30. Cope O, Keynes WM, Roth SI, Castleman B: Primary chief-cell hyperplasia of the parathyroid glands: A new entity in the surgery of hyperparathyroidism. Ann Surg 148:375, 1958.

31. Crago RM, Eckholdt JW, Wiswell JG: Pheochromocytoma. Treatment with α- and β-adrenergic blocking drugs. JAMA 202:104, 1967

32. Crane MG, Harris JJ, Herber R: Primary aldosteronism due to an adrenal carcinoma. Ann Intern Med 63:494, 1965

33. Croughs RJM, Hulsmans HA, Israel DE, Hackeng WHL, Schopman W:

Glucagonoma as part of the polyglandular adenoma syndrome. Am J Med 52:690, 1972

34. Davies DR, Dent CE, Ives DR: Successful removal of single metastasis in recurrent parathyroid carcinoma. Br Med J 1:397, 1973

35. Davies E Rhys: The radiological and scintigraphic investigation of spontaneous hypoglycaemia. Clin Radio 24:177–184, 1973

36. Davis Z, Moertel CG, McIlrath DC: The malignant carcinoid syndrome. Surg Gynecol Obstet 137:637, 1973

37. Deftos LJ: Radioimmunoassay for calcitonin in medullary thyroid carcinoma. JAMA 227:403, 1974

38. Deftos LJ, Goodman AD, Engelman K, Potts JT Jr: Suppression and stimulation of calcitonin secretion in medullary thyroid carcinoma. Metabolism 20:428, 1971

39. DePeyster FA: Planning the appropriate operations for islet cell tumors of the pancreas. Surg Clin North Am 50:133, 1970

40. DiGiulio W, Morales JO: The value of the selenomethionine Se-75 scan in preoperative localization of parathyroid adenomas. JAMA 209:1873, 1969

41. Dunegan LJ, Watson CG, Kaufman SS, et al: Primary hyperparathyroidism. Preoperative evaluation and correlation with surgical findings. Am J Surg 128:471, 1974

42. Dunn EL, Nishiyama RH, Thompson NW: Medullary carcinoma of the thyroid gland. Surgery 73:848, 1973

43. Eddy RL, Jones AL, Gilliland PF, et al: Cushing's syndrome: A prospective study of diagnostic methods. Am J Med 55:621, 1973

44. Egdahl RH: Surgery of the adrenal gland. N Engl J Med 278:939, 1968

45. Elias E, Bloom SR, Welbourn RB, et al: Pancreatic cholera due to production of gastric inhibitory polypeptide. Lancet 2:719, 1972

46. Ellison EH, Wilson SD: The Zollinger-Ellison syndrome: reappraisal and evaluation of 260 registered cases. Ann Surg 160:512, 1964

47. Ellison EH, Wilson SD: The Zollinger-Ellison syndrome updated. Surg Clin North Am 47:1115, 1967

48. Engelman K, Horwitz D, Jequier E, Sjoerdsma A: Biochemical and pharmacologic effects of α-methyltyrosine in man. J Clin Invest 47:577, 1968

49. Engelman K, Sjoerdsma A: Chronic medical therapy for pheochromocytoma. A report of four cases. Ann Intern Med 61:229, 1964

50. Epstein HY, Abrams RM, Berenbaum ER, et al: Angiographic localization of insulinomas: high reported success rate and two additional cases. Ann Surg 169:349, 1969

51. Ferris DW, Molnar GD, Schnelle N, et al: Recent advances in management of functioning islet cell tumor. Arch Surg 104:443, 1972

52. Filipecki S, Feltynowski T, Poplawska W: Carcinoma of the adrenal cortex with hyperaldosteronism. J Clin Endocrinol Metab 35:225, 1972

53. Fonkelsrud EW, Dilley RB, Longmire WP Jr: Insulin secreting tumors of the pancreas. Ann Surg 159:730, 1964

54. Frenster JH, Herstein PR: Gene de-repression. N Engl J Med 288:1224, 1973

55. Foye LV, Feightmeir TV: Adrenal cortical carcinoma producing solely

mineralocorticoid effect. Am J Med 19:966, 1955

56. Friesen S: The Zollinger-Ellison syndrome. Curr Probl Surg 3–52, 1972

57. Friesen SR: Effect of total gastrectomy on the Zollinger-Ellison tumors: observations by second-look procedures. Surgery 62:609, 1967

58. Gabrilove JL, Sharma DC, Wotiz HH, Dorfman RI: Feminizing adrenocortical tumors in the male. Medicine 44:37, 1965

59. George JM, Wright L, Bell NH, et al: The syndrome of primary aldosteronism. Am J Med 48:345, 1970

60. Gittler RD, Maier H: Carcinoma of the parathyroid. Arch Intern Med 130:413, 1972

61. Goldman L, Gordan GS, Roof BS: The parathyroid: progress, problems and practice. Curr Probl Surg 3:57, 1971

62. Goltzman D, Potts JT, Ridgway EC, Maloof F: Calcitonin as a tumor marker. Use of the radioimmunoassay for calcitonin in the postoperative evaluation of patients with medullary thyroid carcinoma. N Engl J Med 290:1036, 1974

63. Gray RK, Rosch J, Grollman JH: Arteriography in the diagnosis of islet-cell tumors. Radiology 97:39, 1970

64. Greider MH, Rosai J, McGuigan JE: The human pancreatic islet cells and their tumors. II. Ulcerogenic and diarrheogenic tumors. Cancer 33:1423, 1974

65. Gupta S, Ternberg JL, Weldon VV, Pagliara AS: Alphaadrenergic blocking agent in childhood pheochromocytoma. Surgery 74:545, 1973

66. Haff RC, Ballinger WF: Causes of recurrent hypercalcemia after parathyroidectomy for primary hyperparathyroidism. Ann Surg 173:884, 1971

67. Haff RC, Black WC, Ballinger WF: Primary hyperparathyroidism: Changing clinical, surgical and pathological aspects. Ann Surg 171:85, 1970

68. Harrison TS, Freier DT, Cohen EL: Recurrent pheochromocytoma. Arch Surg 108:450, 1974

69. Hayles AB, Hahn HB, Sprague RG, et al: Hormone-secreting tumors of the adrenal cortex in children. Pediatrics 37:19, 1966

70. Heath DA, Wills MR: Normocalcaemic primary hyperparathyroidism with osteitis fibrosa. Postgrad Med J 47:815, 1971

71. Horton R: Aldosterone: Review of its physiology and diagnostic aspects of primary aldosteronism. Metabolism 22:1525, 1973

72. Horwith M, Stokes E: Cushing's syndrome. Experience with total adrenalectomy. Adv Intern Med 10:259, 1960

73. Howard JM, Moss NH, Rhoads ME: Collective review: hyperinsulinism and islet cell tumors of the pancreas with 398 recorded tumors. Surg Gynecol Obstet 90:417, 1950

74. Hume DM: Pheochromocytoma in the adult and in the child. Am J Surg 99:458, 1960

75. Hutter AM, Kayhoe DE: Adrenal cortical carcinoma. Clinical features of 138 patients. Am J Med 41:572, 1966

76. Hutter AM, Kayhoe DE: Adrenal cortical carcinoma. Results of treatment with o,p'DDD in 138 patients. Am J Med 41:581, 1966

77. Huvos AG, Hajdu SI, Brasfield RD, Foote FW Jr: Adrenal cortical car-
     cinoma. Clinicopathologic study of 34 cases. Cancer 25:354, 1970
78. Irvin GL III, Cohen MS, Moebus R, Mintz DH: Primary hyperparathy-
     roidism. Arch Surg 105:738, 1972
79. Jackson CE, Tashjian AH Jr, Block MA: Detection of medullary thyroid
     cancer by calcitonin assay in families. Ann Intern Med 78:845, 1973
80. Kavlie H, White TT: Non-beta hormone-producing islet cell tumors of the
     pancreas. Surg 38:601–7, 1972
81. Kavlie H, White TT: Pancreatic islet beta cell tumors and hyperplasia:
     Experience in 14 Seattle hospitals. Ann Surg 175:326, 1972
82. Kay S, Hume DM: Carcinoma of the parathyroid gland. Arch Pathol
     96:316, 1973
83. Keiser HR, Beaven MA, Doppman J, Wells S Jr, Buja LM: Sipple's syn-
     drome: Medullary thyroid carcinoma, pheochromocytoma, and parathyroid
     disease. Studies in a large family. Ann Intern Med 78:561, 1973
84. Kirwan AO: Parathyroid cyst. Br J Surg 61:365, 1974
85. Kolts BE, Herbst CA, McGuigan JE: Calcium and secretin-stimulated
     gastrin release in the Zollinger-Ellison syndrome. Ann Intern Med 81:758,
     1974
86. Koutras P, White RR: Insulin-secreting tumors of the pancreas. A diag-
     nostic and therapeutic challenge. Surg Clin North Am 52:299, 1972
87. Krementz ET, Yeager R, Hawley W, Weichert R: The first 100 cases of
     parathyroid tumor from Charity Hospital of Louisiana. Ann Surg 173:872,
     1971
88. Kukreja SC, Hargis GK, Rosenthal IM, Williams GA: Pheochromocy-
     toma causing excessive parathyroid hormone production and hypercal-
     cemia. Ann Int Med 79:838, 1973
89. Kumar D, Mehtalia SD, Miller LV: Diagnostic use of glucagon-induced in-
     sulin response. Studies in patients with insulinoma or other hypoglycemic
     conditions. Ann Intern Med 80:697, 1974
90. Laroche GP, Ferris DO, Priestly JT, Scholz DA, Dockerty MB: Hyperin-
     sulinism: Surgical results and management of occult functioning islet cell
     tumor. Review of 154 cases. Arch Surg 96:763, 1968
91. Lauler DP: Preoperative diagnosis of primary aldosteronism. Am J Med
     41:855, 1966
92. Law DH, Liddle GW, Scott HW Jr, Tauber SD: Ectopic production of
     multiple hormones (ACTH, MSH, and gastrin) by a single malignant tumor.
     N Engl J Med 273:292, 1965
93. Lewin MR, Stagg BH, Clark CG: Gastric acid secretion and diagnosis of
     Zollinger-Ellison syndrome. Br Med J 2:139, 1973
94. Lewinsky BS, Grigor KM, Symington T, Neville AM: The clinical and
     pathologic features of "non-hormonal" adrenocortical tumors. Cancer
     33:778, 1974
95. Liddle GW: Tests of pituitary-adrenal suppressibility in the diagnosis of
     Cushing's syndrome. J Clin Endocrinol Metab 20:1539, 1960
96. Liechty RD, Alsever RN, Burrington J: Islet cell hyperinsulinism in adults
     and children. JAMA 230:1538, 1974
97. Lightman SL, Bloom SR: Cure of insulin-dependent diabetes mellitus by

removal of a glucagonoma. Br Med J 1:367, 1974

98. Lipsett MB, Hertz R, Ross GT: Clinical and pathophysiologic aspects of adrenocortical carcinoma. Am J Med 35:374, 1963

99. Lubitz JA, Freeman L, Okun R: Mitotane use in inoperable adrenal cortical carcinoma. JAMA 223:1109, 1973

100. Macfarlane A: Cancer of the adrenal cortex. The natural history, prognosis and treatment in a study of fifty-five cases. Ann Coll Surg Engl 23:155, 1958

101. Mallinson CN, Bloom SR, Warin AP, Salmon PR, Cox B: A glucagonoma syndrome. Lancet 2(7871): 1–5, 1974

102. Markey WS, Ryan WG, Economou SG, et al: Familial medullary carcinoma and parathyroid adenoma without pheochromocytoma. Ann Intern Med 78:898, 1973

103. Marks V: Spontaneous hypoglycaemia. Br Med J 1:430, 1972

104. McGuigan JE: Antibodies to the carboxyl-terminal tetrapeptide of gastrin. Gastroenterology 53:697, 1967

105. Meador CK, Liddle GW, Island DP, et al: Cause of Cushing's syndrome in patients with tumors arising from "nonendocrine" tissue. J Clin Endocrinol 22:293, 1962

106. Melvin KEW, Miller HH, Tashjian AH Jr: Early diagnosis of medullary carcinoma of the thyroid gland by means of calcitonin assay. N Engl J Med 285:1115, 1971

107. Melvin KEW, Tashjian AH Jr, Miller HH: Studies in familial (medullary) thyroid carcinoma. Recent prog Horm Res 28:399, 1972

108. Miller HH, Melvin KEW, Gibson JM, Tashjian AH Jr: Surgical approach to early familial medullary carcinoma of the thyroid gland. Am J Surg 123:438, 1972

109. Mundy GR, Raisz LG, Cooper RA, Schecter GP, Salmon SE: Evidence for the secretion of an osteoclast stimulating factor in Myeloma. N Engl J Med 291:1042, 1974

110. Murad F, Pak CYC: Urinary excretion of adenosine 3',5'-monophosphate and guanosine 3',5'-monophosphate. N Engl J Med 286:1382, 1972

111. Myers RT: Followup study of surgically-treated primary hyperparathyroidism. Ann Surg 179:729, 1974

112. Neelon FA, Lebovitz HE, Drezner M, et al: Urinary cyclic adenosine monophosphate as an aid in the diagnosis of hyperparathyroidism. Lancet 1:24, 1973

113. Neiman RS, Li HC: Hypercalcemia in undifferentiated leukemia. Cancer 30:942, 1972

114. Newsome HH: Multiple endocrine adenomatosis. Surg Clin North Am 54:387, 1974

115. Orth DN, Liddle GW: Results of treatment in 108 patients with Cushing's syndrome. N Engl J Med 285:243, 1971

116. Pak CYC, Ohata M, Lawrence EC, Snyder W: The hypercalciurias. J Clin Invest 54:387–400, 1974

117. Passaro E Jr, Basso N, Walsh JH: Calcium challenge in the Zollinger-Ellison syndrome. Surgery 72:60, 1972

118. Pearse AGE: The cytochemistry and ultrastructure of polypeptide

hormone-producing cells of the APUD series and the embryologic, physiologic, and pathologic implications of this concept. J Histochem Cytochem 17:303, 1969

119. Pezzulich RA, Mannix H Jr: Immediate complications of adrenal surgery 172:125, 1970

120. Powell D, Singer FR, Murray TM, et al: Nonparathyroid humoral hypercalcemia in patients with neoplastic diseases. N Engl J Med 289:176, 1973

121. Prichard BN, Ross EJ: Use of propranolol in conjunction with alpha receptor blocking drugs in pheochromocytoma. Am J Cardiol 18:394, 1966

122. Ptak T, Kirsner JB: The Zollinger-Ellison syndrome, polyendocrine adenomatosis and other endocrine associations with peptic ulcer. Adv Intern Med 16:213, 1970

123. Purnell DC, Scholz DA, Smith LH, et al: Treatment of primary hyperparathyroidism. Am J Med 56:800, 1974

124. Raiz LG: Prostaglandins and the hypercalcemia of cancer. N Engl J Med 289:214, 1973

125. Rapaport E, Goldberg MB, Gordan GS, Hinman F Jr: Mortality in surgically treated adrenocortical tumors. II. Review of cases reported for the 20 year period 1930–1949, inclusive. Postgrad Med 11–12:325–353, 1952

126. Raux MC, Binoux M, Luton JP, et al: Studies of ACTH secretion control in 116 cases of Cushing's syndrome. J Clin Endocrinol Metab 40:186, 1975

127. Rees LH, Bloomfirld GA, Rees GM, et al: Multiple hormones in a bronchial tumor. J Clin Endocrinol Metab 38:1090, 1974

128. Remine WH, Chong GC, Van Heerden JA, et al: Current management of pheochromocytoma. Ann Surg 179:740, 1974

129. Rhamy RK, McCoy RM, Scott HW Jr, et al: Primary aldosteronism: Experience with current diagnostic criteria and surgical treatment in fourteen patients. Ann Surg 167:718, 1968

130. Robertson RP, Baylink DJ, Marini JJ, Adkison HW: Elevated prostaglandins and suppressed parathyroid hormone associated with hypercalcemia and renal cell carcinoma. J Clin Endocrinol Metab 41:164, 1975

131. Rosen SW, Weintraub BD: Ectopic production of the isolated alpha subunit of the glycoprotein hormones. N Engl J Med 290:1442, 1974

132. Ross EJ: Endocrine and metabolic manifestations of cancer. Br Med J 1:735, 1972

133. Ross EJ, Prichard BNC, Kautman L, et al: Preoperative and operative management of patients with phaeochromocytoma. Br Med J 1:191, 1967

134. Said SI, Faloona GR: Elevated plasma and tissue levels of vasoactive intestinal polypeptide in the watery-diarrhea syndrome. N Engl J Med 293:155, 1975

135. Salama F, Luke RG, Hellebusch AA: Carcinoma of the kidney producing multiple hormones. J Urol 106:820, 1971

136. Sanzenbacher LJ, King Denis R, Zollinger RM: Prognostic implications of calcium-mediated gastrin levels in the ulcerogenic syndrome. Am J Surg 125:116, 1973

137. Satava RM, Beahrs OH, Scholz DA: Success rate of cervical exploration for hyperparathyroidism. Arch Surg 110:625, 1975

138. Sato Yoshio, Komatsu Kanji: Diarrheogenic tumor of the pancreas. Am J Surg 126:425, 1973

139. Schantz A, Castleman BJ: Parathyroid carcinoma. A study of 70 cases. Cancer 31:600, 1973

140. Scharf Y, Nahir AM, Better OS, et al: Prolonged survival in malignant pheochromocytoma of the organ of Zuckerkandl with pharmacological treatment. Cancer 31:746, 1973

141. Schein PS, DeLellis RA, Kahn CR, et al: Islet cell tumors: Current concepts and management Ann Intern Med 79:239, 1973

142. Schmitt MG, Soergel KH, Hensley GT, Chey WY: Watery diarrhea associated with pancreatic islet cell carcinoma. Gastroenterology 69:206, 1975

143. Scholz DA, ReMine WH, Priestly JT: Hyperinsulinism: Review of 95 cases of functioning pancreatic islet cell tumors. Mayo Clin Proc 35:545, 1960

144. Schteingart DE, Cash R, Conn JW: Amino-glutethimide and metastatic adrenal cancer. JAMA 198:143, 1966

145. Scott HW, Jr, Foster JH, Rhamy RK, et al: Surgical management of adrenocortical tumors with Cushing's syndrome. Ann Surg 173:892, 1971

146. Scott HW, Jr, Riddell DH, Brockman SK: Surgical management of pheochromocytoma. Surg Gynecol & Obstet 129:707, 1965

147. Seldinger SL: Localization of parathyroid adenomata by arteriography. Acta Radiol 42:353, 1954

148. Shatney CH, Grage TB: Diagnostic and surgical aspects of insulinoma. A review of twenty-seven cases. Am J Surg 127:174, 1974

149. Shieber W, Birge SJ, Avioli LV Teitelbaum SL: Normocalcemic hyperparathyroidism with "normal" parathyroid glands. Arch Surg 103:299, 1971

150. Shield CF III, Haff RC, Murray HM: Islet cell tumors of the pancreas. Am J Surg 128:709, 1974

151. Siegel Hano A: The radiology corner. Insulin-producing tumors of the pancreas. Am J Gastroenterol 61:394, 1974

152. Silen W, Biglieri EG, Slaton P, Galante M: Management of primary aldosteronism: Evaluation of potassium and sodium balance, technic of adrenalectomy, and operative results in 24 cases. Ann Surg 164:600, 1966

153. Sipple JH: The association of pheochromocytoma with carcinoma of the thyroid gland. Am J Med 31:163, 1961

154. Sjoerdsma A, Engelman K, Spector S, Udenfriend S: Inhibition of catecholamine synthesis in man with alpha-methyl-tyrosine, an inhibitor of tyrosine hydroxylase. Lancet 2:1092, 1965

155. Sjoerdsma A, Engleman K, Waldmann TA: Pheochromocytoma: Current concepts of diagnosis and treatment. Ann Intern Med 65:1302, 1966

156. Sjoerdsma A, Melmon KL: Carcinoid spectrum. Gastroent 47:104, 1964

157. Soergel KH: Hormonally mediated diarrhea. N Engl J Med 292:970, 1975

158. Soffer LJ, Iannaccone A, Gabrilove JL: Cushing's syndrome. A study of fifty patients. Am J Med 30:129, 1961

159. Stefanini S, Carboni M, Patrassi N, et al: Beta-islet cell tumors of the pancreas: Results of study on 1,067 cases. Surgery 25:597, 1974

160. Steiner AL, Goodman AD, Powers SR: Study of a kindred with pheochromocytoma, medullary thyroid carcinoma, hyperparathyroidism and Cushing's disease: Multiple endocrine neoplasia, type 2. Medicine 47:371, 1968

161. Stewart DR, Jones PHM, Jolleys A: Carcinoma of the adrenal gland in children. J Pediatr Surg 9:59, 1974

162. Straus FH II, Paloyan E: The pathology of hyperparathyroidism. Surg Clin North Am 49:27, 1969

163. Streeten DHP, Stevenson CT, Dalakos TG, et al: The diagnosis of hypercortisolism. Biochemical criteria differentiating patients from lean and obese normal subjects and from females on oral contraceptives. J Clin Endocrinol 29:1191, 1969

164. Tashjian AH, Jr, Voelkel EF, Goldhaber P, Levine L: Prostaglandins, calcium metabolism and cancer. Fed Proc 33:81, 1974

165. Tashjian AH Jr, Voelkel EF, Levine L, Goldhaber P: Evidence that the bone resorption-stimulating factor produced by mouse fibrosarcoma cells is prostaglandin E_2. A new model for the hypercalcemia of cancer. J Exp Med 136:1329, 1972

166. Terz JJ, Estep H, Bright R, et al: Primary oropharyngeal cancer and hypercalcemia. Cancer 33:334, 1974

167. Thompson JC, Reeder DD, Bunchman HH: Clinical role of serum gastrin measurements in the Zollinger-Ellison syndrome. Am J Surg 124:250, 1972

168. Tilson MD: Carcinoid syndrome. Surg Clin North Am 54:409, 1974

169. Trudeau WL, McGuigan JE: Effects of calcium on serum gastrin levels in the Zollinger-Ellison syndrome. N Engl J Med 281:862, 1969

170. Turner RC, Harris E: Diagnosis of insulinomas by suppression tests. Lancet 2:188, 1974

171. VanWay CW III, Scott HW Jr, Page DL, Rhamy RK: Pheochromocytoma. Curr Probl Surg 4–53 1974

172. Verner JV, Morrison AB: Endocrine pancreatic islet disease with diarrhea. Report of a case due to diffuse hyperplasia of nonbeta islet tissue with a review of 54 additional cases. Arch Intern Med 133:492, 1974

173. Voelkel EF, Tashjian AH Jr, Franklin R, et al: Hypercalcemia and tumor-prostaglandins: The VX_2 carcinoma model in the rabbit. Metabolism 24:973, 1975

174. Wang Chiu-An, Vickery AL Jr, Maloof F: Large parathyroid cysts mimicking thyroid nodules. Ann Surg 175:448, 1972

175. Weichert RF III: The neural ectodermal origin of the peptide-secreting endocrine glands. Am J Med 49232, 1970

176. Wermer Paul: Genetic aspects of adenomatosis of endocrine glands. Am J Med 16:363, 1954

177. Whipple AO, Frantz VK: Adenoma of islet cells with hyperinsulinism. A review. Ann Surg 101:1299, 1935

178. Williams C Jr, Bryson GH, Hume DH: Islet-cell tumors and hypoglycemia. Ann Surg 169:757, 1969

179. Wills MR: Normocalcaemic primary hyperparathyroidism. Lancet 1:849, 1971

180. Wilson H, Cheek RC, Sherman RT, et al: Carcinoid tumors. Curr Probl Surg 1–51, 1970

181. Wilson SD, Ellison EH: Survival in patients with the Zollinger-Ellison syndrome treated by total gastrectomy. Am J Surg 111:786, 1966

182. Wilson SD, Schulte WJ, Meade RC: Longevity studies following total gastrectomy in children with the Zollinger-Ellison syndrome. Arch Surg 103:108, 1971

183. Wolf RL, Mendlowitz M, Fruchter A: Diagnosis and treatment of pheochromocytoma. Mt Sinai J Med 37:549, 1970

184. Wolfe WG, Mullen DC, Silver D: Insulinoma of the pancreas. Use of the tolbutamide test, arteriography, and selenium scan in modern diagnosis. Arch Surg 104:56, 1972

185. Yalow RS, Berson SA: Radioimmunoassay for gastrin. Gastroenterology 58:1, 1970

186. Zollinger RM: Diarrhoeogenic tumours of the pancreas. Aust NZ J Surg 45:129, 1975

187. Zollinger RM, Ellison EH: Primary peptic ulcerations of the jejunum associated with islet cell tumors of the pancreas. Ann Surg 142:709–728, 1955

15

The Advanced Cancer Patient

Advanced cancer and terminal cancer are not synonymous terms. A terminal cancer patient is not expected to survive more than a few weeks and heroic treatment measures are certainly not indicated. In contrast, advanced cancer denotes disease that is usually beyond reasonable hope of long cancer patient survival but is still responsive to therapeutic efforts: palliative bypass operation, radiotherapy to a painful recurrence, palliative surgical resection of a symptomatic mass, or systemic chemotherapy. Pain relief, if this is the problem, demands our attention, but this approach alone is not enough. The incurable patient with advanced disease must be thoroughly evaluated to determine if there are any anticancer treatments that may improve the quality or duration of life. Many of these therapeutic decisions require careful assessment of the cost-benefit ratio in human terms and are the most difficult ones in cancer management. As the disease progresses, supportive measures designed only for comfort then become our major concern.[24]

MANAGEMENT OF NEOPLASIA-RELATED PROBLEMS

Metastases from primary cancers of many sites require therapeutic planning if the patient is in a clinical state that may benefit from these efforts. The most frequent types of metastatic disease requiring such palliative planning are those affecting the bones, central nervous system, liver, lungs, and pleural and peritoneal spaces (with effusion). Specific problems have been referred to in other chapters, but our general approach to these metastatic sites deserves comment.

Bone Metastases

The skeleton in one of the most frequent sites of distant metastasis of solid tumors, particularly from neoplasms originating in the breast, lung, prostate, kidney, and thyroid. These metastases are seldom life threatening but are the cause of both anguish and disability as a result of either severe pain or pathological fractures secondary to bone destruction. The proper management of these symptomatic areas, through radiation therapy, orthopedic intervention, or both, will accomplish relief of symptoms as well as allow effective use of specific antineoplastic agents for overall disease control.

DIAGNOSIS

The axial skeleton, pelvis, proximal long bones, and skull are the most frequent sites of involvement. Pain in these areas of metastasis is the cardinal symptom. However, bone metastases may be asymptomatic initially and are frequently discovered during the workup or follow-up of a patient suspected or known to have a malignant neoplasm. Also, a pathological fracture may precede the clinical diagnosis of cancer and be the first indication of its presence.

The introduction of bone scanning with technetium-labeled polyphosphate (^{99m}Tc) allows earlier and more accurate diagnosis of skeletal metastasis than conventional radiographs.[11] Practically all patients with demonstrable bone metastasis on x-ray will also have a positive bone scan, but 50 percent of the patients suspected clinically of having bone matastasis, despite normal x-rays, will have an abnormal scan compatible with metastasis. Bone scans have also proved to be an accurate staging approach in the workup of patients with apparently localized cancer. One-third of the patients who have breast cancer with clinically positive axillary nodes will have positive bone scans that will be proven clinically positive on subsequent follow-up.[13,24,32,48] The same is true for one-third of the patients with clinically operable lung cancer.

The apparent superiority of the bone scan does not necessarily exclude the value of radiographic diagnosis. A positive bone scan reflects active bone turnover (destruction and formation) and a bone scan in a patient with osteoarthritis may be read as "positive," whereas that of the patient with multiple myeloma may be read as "negative." In both circumstances the radiological examination will clarify the diagnosis. Radiological monitoring is also useful in the follow-up of bone lesions as an index of the response of the lesion to specific treatment. The bone scan will usually remain positive and radiographs will be a better indicator of the progression or regression of the lesion.

TREATMENT

The objective of the "local" treatment of the bone metastasis in the axial skeleton is to relieve pain and either prevent or improve symptoms of cord compression that may be present. In the extremities the objective is to maintain or restore function, either by localized irradiation of the metastasis or by orthopedic intervention to provide internal support for an impending fracture or a pathological fracture that has already occurred. Currently methylmethacrylate[21,54] is used adjunctively in the operative fixation of pathological fractures. The use of this compound allows effective fixation and stabilization of the bone fragments, regardless of the extent of intramedullary destruction. Relief of pain and functional improvement have been accomplished in 90 percent of the patients treated in such a fashion for metastatic disease in bones of the extremities. In most patients the appropriate choice of systemic palliative treatment will be employed concurrently with these local measures.

Central Nervous System Metastases

BRAIN

Cerebral metastases are a frequent complication of systemic cancer, particularly carcinoma of the lung, breast cancer, and melanoma.[19] The brain may be affected as a result of skull metastasis eroding the inner table and producing an epidural mass with secondary brain compression, or by hematogenous spread to the dura or brain parenchyma as single or multiple lesions. The most frequent symptoms of brain metastasis are headache, focal weakness, behavorial and mental changes, seizures, ataxia, and aphasia. The neurological deficit is usually manifested by hemiparesis, impaired cognitive function, unilateral sensory loss and/or papilledema. The possibility of primary brain tumor, cerebral hemorrhage, cerebral infarct, or cerebral abscess should be considered in the differential diagnosis.

The approach to the diagnosis of metastatic brain disease is based first on the history and physical examination, followed by noninvasive laboratory methods (electroencephalogram, brain scan, computerized transaxial tomogram),[1] and finally by invasive contrast studies (arteriogram, pneumoencephalogram). Lumbar puncture usually demonstrates increased intracranial pressure, but cytology on cerebrospinal fluid is positive only if the leptomeninges are involved by tumor. In any event, lumbar puncture has usually been considered dangerous under these clinical circumstances because it could precipitate herniation of the brain.

Therefore, it is never performed as part of the initial workup of the patient with suspected cerebral metastasis. If the noninvasive methods confirm the diagnosis of multifocal metastatic disease, the laboratory investigation is terminated and appropriate treatment instituted. If these studies are not conclusive, the contrast studies are carried out to clarify the diagnosis. Detailed investigation for CNS metastasis should be carried out only in patients with history and physical findings suggestive of brain involvement since extensive laboratory studies in neurologically normal individuals are usually unrewarding.

The plan of management of cerebral metastasis must be based on the diagnosis of single or multiple metastases and the neurologic state.[26] If the patient is deteriorating rapidly, he or she should be immediately treated with mannitol (1.5–2.0 mg/kg body weight) intravenously over 30–60 minutes (20-percent solution); this is followed by dexamethasone 10 mg intravenously and 4 mg every 6 hours. Radiation therapy to the entire cranium should then be instituted. If the patient is neurologically stable but has multiple cerebral metastases, he should receive radiation therapy (after 72 hours of initiation of dexamethasone) at a dosage of 300 rads × 10 over a 2-week period (total dose 3000 rads).[43]

If a solitary metastasis is demonstrated, treatment can be planned as described above or surgical resection may also be considered. If performed, surgical resection should be followed by radiation therapy. Operation is particularly indicated if the diagnosis is uncertain (primary tumor, abscess, hematoma) or if there is progressive increase in intracranial pressure and persistent seizures in spite of the initial therapy with steroids and radiation. Some surgeons advocate operation for all solitary cerebral lesions,[21] but it is difficult to demonstrate an advantage of operative over nonoperative treatment. The 30-day mortality for this clinical problem is approximately 20 percent after operation compared to 16 percent after primary irradiation. The median survival is similar with both modalities (4 months), but the 1-year survival figures are higher in the patients undergoing operation (21 percent) compared with those treated by radiation (10 percent). These results may well be owing to patient selection; but a few patients have survived 5–10 years after resection of solitary brain metastasis, a result that has not been seen after radiation therapy alone.[46]

Metastatic brain tumors have been notoriously resistant to systemic chemotherapy in the past. With the recent introduction of the nitrosourea derivatives that do cross the blood-brain barrier, encouraging results are being observed.[53]

SPINAL CORD

Impending compression of the spinal cord is one of the most pressing emergencies in oncology.[34,41] The spinal cord is contained within a rigid bony canal, and a small compressing tumor mass (less than 10 gm) will produce progressive and irreversible damage if there is undue delay in the diagnosis and treatment. Metastatic tumors account for nearly one-half of these cord compression syndromes, and primary neoplasms,[4,9] either benign or malignant, constitute the remaining half. The initial symptoms of cord compression range from well-localized pain, if the tumor is compressing a nerve root in the epidural space, to motor and sensory loss below the level of the lesion. A Brown-Sequard syndrome will eventually develop if the compression is lateral. These neurologic changes will become permanent if decompression is not carried out immediately.

A high index of suspicion is necessary to establish an early diagnosis of the spinal cord compression. Any patient with a recent onset of neurological dysfunction suggesting involvement of the spinal canal should have an emergency myelogram, which invariably will establish the diagnosis. A lumbar puncture may yield information indicating a spinal block (elevated pressure, high protein, positive cytology), but this procedure should be performed only at the time of the contrast study.

The primary treatment usually consists of operative decompression of the spinal cord by partial resection of the tumor, and this procedure is followed by radiation therapy. This not only will reverse the neurological deficit but also will establish the histological diagnosis, particularly in the absence of other metastasis. Radiation therapy may serve as the only treatment of this complication, particularly if cord involvement is minimal, the tumor is radiosensitive, and there is firm evidence of metastatic disease elsewhere. However, the patient should be followed carefully during this radiation treatment in case the neurological deficit deteriorates, as operative decompression may then be required.

Liver Metastasis

The diagnosis and management of metastatic liver cancer are described in detail in Chapter 8. The overall treatment plan for this problem must be considered palliative and is based primarily on the appropriate chemotherapeutic regimen for the primary cancer. Our use of regional intra-arterial chemotherapy did not prove to offer significant advantages over well-planned systemic drug regimens, but this regional approach still has its proponents. In selected cases, the presence of a solitary liver metastasis should encourage the surgeon to perform a resection of the involved segment as survival has been prolonged under these circumstances, particularly in patients with primary cancer of the colon and rectum.

Lung Metastasis

Metastatic carcinoma to the lungs is a frequent finding in patients with advanced cancer. In most clinical circumstances the lesions are either multiple or associated with pleural effusion, or there is evidence of uncontrolled cancer in other sites. The specific treatment for these patients is systemic chemotherapy. The lung metastasis can appear as a solitary lesion without evidence of other metastatic disease. This clinical condition is no longer considered as unmanageable a problem as multiple metastasis. With proper selection of patients, pulmonary resection has often resulted in prolonged disease control.[12]

Metastatic lung tumors potentially suitable for pulmonary resection include those from soft tissue sarcomas, colorectal cancer, and osteogenic sarcoma. Occasional cases of lung metastasis from renal, testis, uterine, and breast carcinoma have been treated by resection with success. Often the metastasis suitable for resection is discovered during a routine chest x-ray in an asymptomatic patient whose primary tumor is either clinically controlled or recently discovered. In any event, an extensive investigation should be undertaken to rule out other metastatic sites before recommending thoracotomy. This workup should include tomograms of the lung to evaluate the presence of other lung lesions and scanning of the brain, liver, and bones. Thoracotomy will provide the ultimate indication for resection if preoperative workup shows gross disease limited to the lung, particularly a solitary lesion.[27]

The surgical resection should be limited to the lung parenchyma involved (segmentectomy or lobectomy), but occasionally a pneumonectomy is indicated because of the hilar location of the lesion. Several surgeons have suggested that multiple lung metastases from some cancers are suitable for resection, even if bilateral, but this clinical presentation is less appealing than the solitary lesion. Those patients with apparent benefit from resection of more than one lung metastasis appear to have lesions with longer doubling times (>40 days) when serial chest x-rays are available for this determination.

In the case of simultaneous discovery of a localized primary neoplasm and a single lung metastasis, the primary lesion should be removed first. If the operative findings and pathological features of the primary neoplasm seem to indicate a fair probability of local control (lack of lymph node or blood vessel involvement, tumor well localized to the organ of origin, degree of differentiation, etc.), the lung metastasis may be resected in the early postoperative period. If a waiting period is decided on to see if new metastasis will become apparent, the patient should probably undergo systemic chemotherapy and/or immunotherapy in the interim period.

The overall 5-year survival of patients suitable for this approach to lung metastasis is between 40 and 60 percent. Among the factors indicating a favorable prognosis, the type of tumor (colon cancer, soft tissue sarcoma), a long interval between treatment of the primary cancer and development of metastases, and a long tumor doubling time (>40 days) seem to be the most important. This is clearly a clinical approach suitable only for "selected" cases.[39,48]

Malignant Effusions

The accumulation of fluid as a result of tumor involvement in the pleural or peritoneal cavity is frequently seen during the clinical course of patients with advanced solid tumors. It occurs rarely in the pericardial sac. Effusions owing to cancer usually result in a significant compromise of cardiopulmonary and gastrointestinal function and often pose difficult decisions regarding choice of therapy.

Only 40 percent of serosal effusions seen in clinical medicine are the result of cancer implants, so it is mandatory that pathological confirmation of the diagnosis be obtained before therapy unless the diagnosis of advanced cancer has already been well established. The cytological analysis of the aspirated fluid is diagnostic in 60 percent of malignant effusions. In the remaining 40 percent, the diagnosis is made either by needle biopsy of the serosal wall or by open surgical biopsy.[51] In selected patients peritoneoscopy (or laparoscopy) will also provide information helpful in the diagnosis of the etiology of ascites.

Treatment of malignant effusions consists of relieving the mechanical compression from the fluid and, hopefully, preventing its recurrence through the instillation of agents that either have a cytotoxic effect or produce a chemical irritation of the serosal surface that leads to obliteration of the serosal space. These agents include radioisotopes (radioactive gold or phosphorus), alkylating agents, and other chemotherapeutic agents that may or may not have an anticancer effect.

RADIOISOTOPES

Radioactive gold (^{198}Au) has a half-life of 2.7 days and has been widely used in the past in the treatment of malignant effusions. Because this isotope emits both beta and gamma particles, patients must have a reasonable life expectancy to justify this agent. Its administration requires strict radiation safety precautions. The dose of ^{198}Au used ranges from 100–200 mc, and its administration is associated with nausea, vomiting, and low-grade fever. This isotope has proved to be effective in 60 percent of patients with pleural effusions and 27 percent of those treated for malignant ascites.[49]

Radioactive phosphorus (^{32}P) has largely replaced ^{198}Au in the management of malignant effusions because of its safety (it lacks gamma particles and has a half-life of 14 days). This makes it safe for use in ambulatory patients as well. The dose is 10–20 mc, and the side effects and response rates with this isotope are similar to those observed with ^{198}Au.

ALKYLATING AGENTS

The most effective alkylating agents are nitrogen mustard[36] (0.2–0.4 mg/kg) and triethylenethiophosphoramide (thio-TEPA)(0.8–1 mg/kg). They are effective in approximately 40 percent of patients, and drug administration is usually associated with nausea, vomiting, and mild leukopenia.

OTHER AGENTS

5-Fluorouracil (2.5–3.0 mg/kg) and quinacrine in doses of 50–100 mg initially followed by 200–400 mg daily for 4 days produce significant control of pleural effusions in roughly half of the cases. Patients with ascites require a double dose.[56]

If pleural effusion is refractory to the above approaches, the insertion of a chest tube that is connected to water-seal drainage may offer significant relief of the mechanical problems associated with fluid in the chest.[30] This may also lead to partial obliteration of the pleural space and inhibit further fluid accumulation.

COMPLICATIONS OF CANCER

Although most problems in the management of the advanced cancer patient are "elective" in view of the chronic nature of this disease, medical emergencies commonly associated with cancer require prompt and effective action. Hemorrhage, infection, and renal failure are urgent problems that are more frequent in cancer patients than in other patients because of the unique features of the disease or its treatment. Specific local effects of cancer on the nervous system, gastrointestinal tract, genitourinary system, or the vascular system also produce emergency problems requiring a prompt response. Many of these problems have been discussed with the management of specific organ sites, but a brief summary of management approach is indicated to emphasize the occasional need for emergency treatment of these cancer complications.

Hemorrhage

The advanced cancer patient may have either external or internal bleeding as a complication of necrosis of tumor tissue, and local measures or volume replacement may be required depending on the specific problem. Systemic hematologic problems leading to coagulation abnormalities can also occur because of involvement of the bone marrow or the liver by metastatic disease, or marrow suppression due to the chemotherapy employed.[16,36,52] Disseminated intravascular coagulation (DIC) is another acute complication of cancer, or of sepsis related to complications of its treatment. Prompt diagnostic measures are required to allow appropriate therapy by specific blood product components (red cells, fresh frozen plasma, or platelet concentrates), antibiotics, or even heparin in selected circumstances (DIC). Aggressive therapy is usually indicated since many of these emergency problems are reversible situations caused by the anticancer therapy itself.

Infection

Patients with advanced cancer are particularly vulnerable to infections of various sorts including opportunistic infections owing to agents not ordinarily pathogenic in patients with other diseases.[5,6,8] The suppression of immune function frequently observed in advanced cancer patients is a major factor contributing to infectious complications, and most chemotherapeutic agents add to the susceptibility to infection by virtue of associated bone marrow suppression.[23,58-60] Aggressive treatment requires identification of the offending agent, correction of mechanical obstructions contributing to the process (particularly in the respiratory and genitourinary tracts), and appropriate antimicrobial therapy. Protected environments have been employed for aggressive chemotherapeutic treatment of some advanced cancers in the hope of reducing these infectious complications,[5] but the value of this approach is not well established.

Renal Failure

Renal failure in the cancer patient may be due to mechanical obstruction of the genitourinary tract or to systemic complications affecting the renal parenchyma. The former can be managed operatively by nephrostomy, but this is usually considered inappropriate unless there is a reasonable hope of remission of the obstructing pelvic disease by other forms of therapy. The cause of primary renal failure in cancer patients may be reversible, as with hypercalcemia, hyperuricemia, or drug toxicity, or it may be insoluble (such as with amyloidosis). Hypercalcemia may respond to hydration, corticosteroids, kelating agents, or mithramycin, whereas hyperuricemia is probably best prevented with allopurinol in those patients expected to have a rapid breakdown of neoplastic tissue as a result of treatment. In some patients this complication may even require renal dialysis as it is a reversible complication.

Airway Obstruction

Obstruction of the major airway in the head and neck region is an emergency problem that may be caused by a reasonably early cancer of the glottis or a massive recurrent cancer of the pharynx, larynx, or oral cavity. In either case, the institution of an adequate airway by tracheostomy is mandatory as this is an unacceptable way to die.

Superior Vena Caval Syndrome

Obstruction of the superior vena cava by cancer[17,33] in the mediastinum may produce striking physical findings, including swelling of the upper torso and face, a prominent venous pattern over the upper torso, distended jugular veins, and an altered sensorium. Papilledema may also occur as a result of increased intracranial pressure. Prompt therapy is required, initially steroids and diuretics, and then prompt administration of mediastinal irradiation and appropriate chemotherapy. Dramatic reversal of symptoms and physical findings may result, and future treatment can then be planned in a less hurried fashion. The clinical situation with this complication is analogous to the urgency described earlier for patients with metastases involving the central nervous system.

Acute Gastrointestinal Problems

The general surgeon is often called on to deal with obstruction of, or bleeding from, the gastrointestinal tract in patients with advanced cancer involving the peritoneal cavity. The primary cancer may have arisen from the gastrointestinal tract, may be another form of intra-abdominal cancer (such as ovarian or bladder cancer), or may represent a metastatic process from a distant site (particularly lung cancer). Considerable clinical judgment is required in the management of such patients, but it should be stressed at the outset that it must not be assumed that the complication is necessarily a neoplastic one. Many patients with known cancer are subject to intestinal obstruction from adhesions, and peptic ulceration is one of the most frequent causes of gastrointestinal bleeding in all patients, whether cancer is present or not. The cause of the complication may clearly be neoplastic on the basis of physical findings or prior operative findings, but some cancer patients require a more thorough diagnostic evaluation before assuming this.

If the gastrointestinal complication is owing to advanced cancer, there may be indications for interceding by operation, particularly when the patient has a reasonable opportunity for meaningful survival if the complication is successfully treated.[37] This is a difficult decision based on a combination of factors, including the general status of the patient prior to the complication, the extent of disease present, and the potential for other palliative therapy of the primary cancer if the complication is successfully overcome. The risk of emergency celiotomy is high in this clinical situation, but the alternatives are also bleak. It is generally wise to intercede operatively for complete obstruction or for hemorrhage that cannot be managed effectively by transfusions if the intra-abdominal disease is not massive on clinical examination. There is a reasonable chance of achieving worthwhile palliation under these circumstances. This is particularly true of patients with "recurrent" colon or ovarian cancer. However, patients with these or other cancers who have had prior abdominal surgery for a similar complication experience limited or no gain and have a prohibitive operative mortality. Data from our own series support an operative approach the first time that a patient experiences one of these intra-abdominal complications, although we rarely operate for a subsequent episode.

Adrenal Insufficiency

The major group of cancer patients experiencing this type of complication are those who have undergone adrenalectomy or hypophysectomy, usually for breast cancer, and then suffer some form of stress requiring more replacement therapy than they are receiving. A similar problem may occur in some patients who have suppression of adrenal function by a course of steroids that has not been maintained. Replacement of the adrenal glands by metastatic cancer is a theoretical basis for this complication, but this is rarely the cause due to the minimal residual adrenal tissue required for adequate normal adrenal function. The diagnosis of acute adrenal insufficiency, whatever the cause, is a clinical one since there are no classic serum electrolyte changes associated with this acute problem, in contrast to the signs of chronic adrenal insufficiency (Addison's disease). Therapy by adrenal steroid medication must be immediate.

NUTRITIONAL PROBLEMS IN
THE CANCER PATIENT

Nutritional deficiencies and other dietary factors undoubtedly play a role in the etiology of many cancers, but carcinogenesis is beyond the scope of this volume. However, the nutritional effects induced by cancer (or treatment) are of major importance to the practical management of the patient with cancer.

The nutritional defects that have been observed in patients with advanced cancer are complex. They may be owing to specific organ system problems, including primary impairment of food intake because of obstruction or fistulas in the gastrointestinal tract, malabsorption caused by deficiency of enzymes or infiltration of the intestinal tract by the neoplasm itself, or a protein-losing enteropathy that occurs in some neoplastic conditions. Some of these problems may actually be secondary to hormonal effects from the neoplasm itself. Fluid, electrolyte, and vitamin deficiencies are often associated with these nutritional problems also.

Anorexia and cachexia are often associated with advanced cancer and may have no obvious cause in terms of malfunction of specific organ systems. Taste aversion for meat protein and amino acids has been observed, and this undoubtedly contributes to the anorexia. Increased energy requirements in the face of reduced food intake certainly play a role in the development of this common clinical state, but a more specific explanation of the metabolic abnormality is currently unavailable. There are considerable data on the depletion of the protein and glucose compartments, but there is a major need for some specific answers as to the mechanism of this depletion. One attractive hypothesis is the concept of the cancer as a "nitrogen trap," but the application of this theory to cancer patients is still questionable. In spite of the lack of clear answers to our questions regarding the cachexia of cancer, it is clear that the nutritional management of the cancer patient is both an important and practical aspect of overall care.

In addition to the effect of the cancer on the host, the treatments employed for cancer management are all capable of compounding preexisting nutritional problems as well as producing some of their own. Esophagectomy, gastrectomy, pancreatectomy, major intestinal resection, and radical head and neck surgery all produce nutritional problems because of malabsorption and/or decreased capacities for ingested foodstuff. Radiotherapy and chemotherapy are also capable of producing or expanding nutritional problems in patients who already have nutritional defects. The overall role of nutritional management in the cancer patient, be he "early" or advanced, has often been overlooked, but it is a vital aspect of care.

Nutritional Management of the Cancer Patient

In recent years, the study of nutritional needs of surgical patients, and the development of a practical method for conducting intravenous hyperalimentation with central venous catheters, has led to major contributions to the management of cancer patients. Intravenous hyperalimentation may not induce adequate nutrient retention and weight gain in some cancer patients, but it has proven to be an effective way to reverse severe nutritional deficiency in many of these patients.[14] In addition, this approach has frequently corrected the immune deficiency that has been noted in many patients with extensive cancer. The importance of this observation is shown by the fact that immunocompetent cancer patients respond better and live longer than those who are immunosuppressed.

Aggressive nutritional support has certainly made it possible to be more aggressive in the application of regimens of systemic chemotherapy and radiotherapy. Whether this approach actually improves the response of patients to these modalities may be questionable, but the increase in tolerance to the therapy has certainly led to major treatment benefits as shown so well by Copeland and Dudrick.[14] They have demonstrated a positive correlation between nutritional status and the response to chemotherapy as well as tolerance of a larger total dosage of agent.

Chemically defined (elemental) oral diets or tube feedings have proven to be an ideal means of nutritional support for many clinical conditions. These diets are often rejected by the cancer patients, however, because of taste, and this problem is compounded by the anorexia that often occurs in cancer patients. For this reason as well as for other mechanical or functional reasons, the gastrointestinal tract may not be as effective in cancer patients as in other patients. Therefore, the use of intravenous hyperalimentation is generally preferable as it avoids some of these problems of the enteral route for nutritional support.

As a result of these advances in hyperalimentation, nutritional preparation of some depleted cancer patients for whom major surgery is planned has lessened morbidity and mortality and speeded the rate of postoperative recovery. It is actually impractical to carry out protracted nutritional preparation of patients for whom surgery is either the primary or the palliative treatment, but 1 or 2 weeks of intravenous hyperalimentation has been shown to be a useful adjunct in malnourished patients. The effects are more dramatic from this treatment when it is given preoperatively rather than in the postoperative period. However, fistulas and other complications in the postoperative period may well be managed by this approach.

It would be misleading to give the impression that all malnourished patients can be effectively benefited by aggressive nutritional measures. It has been observed that slow-growing cancers are more likely to be responsive to this nutritional approach than more rapidly growing cancers, but the benefit observed has been frequent enough to encourage exploitation of this approach. Future investigation of this highly controlled approach for nutritional support will even allow specific dietary alterations that may assist in the specific anticancer aspects of the treatment itself.

NEUROMUSCULAR SYNDROMES ASSOCIATED
WITH ADVANCED CANCER

A series of neuromuscular disorders that are independent of the actual extent of disease has been described in cancer patients. These neuromuscular manifestations are associated with carcinomas of the lung, ovary, stomach, and, less frequently, prostate, breast, and colon. This class of neuromuscular disorders has also been described in patients with multiple myeloma, Hodgkin's disease, and chronic lymphocytic leukemia. Approximately 6 percent of all patients with cancer will have one of these neuromuscular manifestations.

Based on the classification of Brain and Adams,[7] these syndromes can be grouped as follows:

Neuromuscular disorder. This is characterized by weakness and wasting of the extremities manifested by difficulties in walking and raising the extremities and a decrease in deep tendon reflexes without sensory loss. These changes seem to be directly related to the degree of weight loss and cannot be correlated with any specific muscular or neurological defect.

Carcinomatous myopathy. Two different skeletal muscle disorders are identified. The first is dermatomyositis, which is clinically similar to the same syndrome described in patients without cancer. Usually the onset of myositis precedes the neoplastic diagnosis. Serum levels of LDH and CPK are characteristically elevated, and there are electromyographic and histologic changes compatible with nonspecific myopathy. The second skeletal muscle disorder is a myasthenic syndrome that is clinically similar to myasthenia gravis but has a different pharmacologic and electromyographic pattern. This syndrome is commonly associated with oat cell cancer of the lung[30] and is usually manifested by weakness of the muscles of the pelvic girdle and lower extremities. In contrast to the patient with myasthenia gravis, the cancer patient has a poor response to neostigmine, is very sensitive to neuromuscular blocking agents of the curare type, and shows a significant delay and an increase in amplitude of muscle potentials after repeated stimuli to a muscle through its motor nerve. Guanidine improves muscle strength, which may indicate a defect in acetylcholine release similar to that seen in botulism. These neurologic findings revert to normal if the primary neoplasm is controlled by surgery or radiation.

Carcinomatous neuropathy. Clinically this resembles nonneoplastic polyneuropathy with impairment in both the sensation and the strength of the distal portions of the extremities.[15,55] The histopathological changes observed are disintegration of the axons and demyelinization. These changes are more pronounced in the sensory type of neuropathy, which is manifested by pain and paresthesias in the extremities. There is significant delay in the nerve conduction as well. These neurological changes are progressive and usually irreversible.

Carcinomatous myelopathy. This has been described in association with cancer of the lung. It is manifested clinically as a rapidly evolving flaccid paralysis with significant sensory and sphincteric reflex changes. Histologically, there are noninflammatory necrotic changes in the cord, involving both the white and gray matter, which resemble the changes of poliomyelitis. Prognosis of this syndrome is very poor.

Cerebellar degeneration. One of the most common and easily recognized neurological syndromes associated with neoplasms, cerebellar degeneration is characterized by rapid and progressive instability of gait, ataxia of limb movement, dysarthria, and the absence of an intracranial mass. These neurological changes usually develop over a very short period in contrast with the rather slow course of the familial sporadic cerebellar degeneration that is unrelated to neoplasms. Also, about 50 percent of these patients have significant and permanent impairment of the intellect and memory with associated nystagmus, a finding not seen in the other type of cerebellar atrophy. Examination of the cerebrospinal fluid usually shows a marked increase in lymphocytes and protein. This syndrome may infrequently appear before diagnosis of the primary cancer. Pathologic study reveals a diffuse loss of the Purkinje cells in the entire cerebellum. This type of loss is not seen in other cerebellar syndromes, which are more localized to specific regions in the cerebellar hemispheres.

Progressive multifocal leukoencephalopathy. This rather rare syndrome is associated with lymphatic and reticuloendothelial system neoplasms, but it has also been observed with other cancers.[47] At the beginning, the patient has an asymmetric neurologic abnormality and an abnormal EEG without specific features. Usually the CSF and both radiological and isotope studies of the brain are within normal limits. Histopathologically, there are foci of demyelination with changes found particularly in the oligodendroglia. These strongly suggest a virus etiology of this syndrome that is characteristically associated with neoplastic disease.[22]

MANAGEMENT OF PAIN IN
THE CANCER PATIENT

The management of pain in the patient with advanced cancer plays a major role in total patient care, particularly when the neoplasm is no longer responsive to specific treatment. It is important to know the specific anatomic areas as well as the etiology of the pain because treatment can often be specifically directed. Infections associated with necrotic soft tissues or poorly drained cavities (bladder or maxillary sinuses) are frequently the cause of a persisting throbbing ache and discomfort. Antibiotics, debridement, daily irrigations, and wound care together with proper surgical drainage often relieve the discomfort. Incomplete intestinal obstruction as a result of intra-abdominal carcinomatosis may produce constant cramping abdominal pain that is associated with intermittent nausea and vomiting. These discomforts may be relieved partially over long periods of time with gastrointestinal intubation, liquid diet, and daily mild laxatives; such procedures are used instead of a celiotomy, which seldom provides long-lasting benefits. Bone pain secondary to metastatic bone disease responds well to radiation therapy as described earlier.

As the disease progresses the specific pain may become less responsive to the locally directed measures described above. We must then resort to neuropharmacologic and/or neurosurgical control of the pain, depending on its location and its severity. Fortunately, pain control by unusual means is required in only a minority of advanced cancer patients.

Analgesic Drugs

The effectiveness of neuropharmacological control of pain is sometimes obscured by a host of factors that may lead to widespread use of drugs of different mechanisms of action and rather unpredictable effectiveness. Lim,[31] in a summary of neuropharmacology of pain therapy, concluded that: (a) aspirin and the non-narcotic antipyretic analgesics act peripherally by blocking the generation of impulses at the chemoceptors for pain; (b) morphine and the non-narcotic analgesics probably block synaptic transmission in the central pathways for pain; and (c) amphetamine and other non-narcotic, antiappetite analgesics also act centrally, possibly causing analgesia in the same way they suppress appetite, that is, by inhibiting the perception of pain. Also, Moertel,[37] in a controlled trial, concluded that aspirin was distinctly superior and cheaper than any of the other drugs he tested, including propoxyphene, ethoheptazine, promazine, acetaminophen, and codeine.

For more severe pain, narcotics such as morphine (and the synthetic counterparts in the form of meperidine, methadone, oxymorphone hydrochloride, and oxycodone hydrochloride) are metabolized in the liver, and oral administration is less effective than the parenteral route. The prolonged use of narcotics for pain control leads inevitably to depression and addiction. Combinations of drugs or the alternating use of several different drugs may delay the onset of these problems. As the patient becomes terminally ill it is crucial both for him and for those caring for him that constant relief of pain and discomfort be accomplished. For this purpose the appropriate dose and frequency of administration must be given regardless of some of the side effects noted.

Neurosurgical Control of Pain

The surgical interruption of nerve pathways may be a useful and effective approach to pain control in the patient with advanced cancer and should be instituted early when these approaches are indicated to provide maximum comfort for the remaining life span. Candidates for this procedure should be in an early stage of intractable pain, have a life expectancy of at least 3 months, and have pain in a location amenable to surgical interruption of its pathways. These procedures can be performed at the level of the peripheral nerve (nerve block), dorsal nerve root (rhizotomy), spinothalamic tract (cordotomy) or by a direct approach to the thalamus. Procedures above the thalamus (lobotomy, leukotomy, cingulumotomy) are specifically directed to relieve the anxiety related to pain rather than the sensation of pain itself.

SPINOTHALAMIC TRACTOTOMY (CORDOTOMY)

Interruption of the spinothalamic tract is the most frequently employed neurosurgical procedure for pain and is performed at the level of the cervical spinal cord for control of pain in the upper trunk (down to the xiphoid) and the upper extremities. For abdominal, pelvic, and lower extremity pain, this tract is severed at the level of the upper thoracic spinal cord. Satisfactory results are achieved in 70–80 percent of cases. It is not unusual for pain on the opposite side to become "unmasked" after control of the pain at the site of the lesion, thereby requiring bilateral cordotomy. This should probably not be done simultaneously because of associated complications.[2]

Urinary bladder dysfunction may lead to the permanent need for an indwelling bladder catheter after bilateral cordotomy (20 percent). Impairment in pulmonary ventilation and postural hypotension are associated with cervical cordotomy which may be life threatening if bilateral sections are performed in one stage. Impotency, loss of libido, and bilateral muscle weakness are also potential complications of this procedure and should be considered in the selection of candidates.

More recently, a technique for percutaneous interruption of the spinothalamic tracts under stereotactic control has been refined and has gained wide acceptance.[18,40,50] This procedure can be performed under local anesthesia and the desired lesion can be induced with radiofrequency waves. This approach can be performed in patients considered to be high risks for general anesthesia.

RHIZOTOMY

Rhizotomy results in effective sensory denervation, but section of the roots located above and below the specific root is required because of overlap of dermatomes. This procedure can be useful in the control of pain in the trunk when cordotomy is contraindicated. If performed for painful extremities, it will be effective, but its usefulness is significantly reduced by the resulting denervated limb without proprioceptive discrimination. This loss may result in severe injuries (burns, lacerations, etc.). Also, with extensive rhizotomy of the trunk, the patient loses sensation from intrathoracic and intra-abdominal viscera with subsequent masking of cardiopulmonary and abdominal symptoms. The value of sacral rhizotomy is reduced by significant alterations of sexual, rectal, and bladder function that may occur. For this reason it is recommended that a preliminary sacral nerve block with evaluation of bladder sensation be performed before surgical section of these roots.

The intrathecal administration of phenol blocks the posterior sacral and lumbar roots. This procedure is performed under fluoroscopy with radiopaque material added to the phenol. The x-ray table is tilted into appropriate position to guide the material appropriately. Bladder dysfunction may also be seen after phenol rhizotomy.[42]

Pain in patients with advanced head and neck cancer involving the maxillofacial complex can be controlled by the percutaneous block of the trigeminal nerve, by intracranial medullary tractectomy, or by cranial nerve rhizotomy.

INTRACEREBRAL PAIN CONTROL

An intracerebral procedure alters the emotional reaction to pain and is not associated with many of the complications seen with tractectomy and rhizotomy. The current techniques consist of selected lesions produced by electrocoagulation, radiofrequency, or fine wire leukotomy. The use of stereotactic control has the added refinement of a procedure with minimal complications and extends its use to a wide variety of patients. The dreaded personality deterioration observed with classic frontal lobotomy is not seen with the current methods.[3]

When properly selected, the neurosurgical control of intractable pain is a very rewarding procedure. It has improved the outlook for the patient with advanced cancer and has alleviated the anxiety of both the patient and his family.

PSYCHOSOCIAL ASPECTS OF MANAGEMENT OF THE ADVANCED CANCER PATIENT

The difficulty for the physician in telling patients that they have cancer depends on the magnitude of the presenting problem and the ultimate prognosis of the individual patient. The physician must always give correct information to the patients under his care, however, both to ensure cooperation in the treatment plan and to reduce the anxiety and fear associated with a lack of knowledge of what is going on. In addition, the patient who has advanced cancer must, in most instances, know the complete truth about his or her disease as there are numerous personal decisions and plans that must be considered, pondered, and finally formalized if there is a real risk of early death with cancer.

This whole area of concern has received much more emphasis in recent years from the standpoint of the so-called dying patient, but the concepts are just as applicable to the patients who are at an earlier stage but threatened, nevertheless, by a serious disease that is likely to lead to death in the not too distant future. Knowledge of the extent and nature of the cancer problem must be transmitted to the patient in a slow, clear, and unhurried fashion, and, preferably, in a quiet room with some degree of privacy. Including an immediate family member in this discussion, rather than appearing to carry out separate explanations, is frequently helpful as the patient is less likely to feel that the physician and his own family are talking about the real truth at another time and place. This approach also assists in the development of a positive role for the family in the management of this severe illness. Frank discussions are mandatory since avoiding these will only lead to more anxiety and fear on the part of the patient. Many studies have shown that patients from whom the facts are withheld are actually aware of their diagnosis and may, in addition, have unfounded fears that have not been resolved because of the secrecy of those around them.

At the time of the discussion of a patient's problem, questions from the patient concerning the diagnosis and management should be encouraged, rather than avoided, for the reasons mentioned above. Interestingly enough, patients with cancer often avoid a direct line of questioning into specific details of long-term prognosis as they undoubtedly repress those queries for which they have an unconscious fear of the answers. Allowing the patient to express the concerns and fears he feels able to deal with is a convenient way to communicate effectively and to reduce the anxiety produced by the diagnosis.

It is our experience that the patient with advanced cancer finds it much easier to focus on the problems of his immediate future. He welcomes a positive plan of action to deal with both his physical and emotional problems as he perceives them. He desperately needs to know that some hope remains regarding possible improvement of his situation, even if the chosen goals for improvement are limited in scope. He also needs to know that he will not be abandoned, nor will efforts to help be discontinued. The message from the physician that there is "nothing more that he can do" is a truly damaging one to the patient's psyche since there *is* something the physician can do for every patient to help him deal with his problems as he sees them. The effectiveness of the physician in this role is obviously strengthened by his continuing willingness to communicate honestly in a two-way fashion.

Response to "Bad News"

Kubler-Ross[28] has described a sequence of psychological stages of reactions usually observed when a person is given news that a serious health problem exists that will probably lead to early death. Simply stated these five stages of reaction are denial (and shock over the news), depression, anger (why me?), bargaining, and acceptance of the situation as it is. Kubler-Ross described these reactions after objective observations of the grief process in a large number of patients. An appreciation of these normal psychodynamics will help the physician in his attempt to assist the patient through this difficult emotional process. The concepts she outlined apply as well to immediate family members, although they often progress more slowly through these stages than the patient. The optimal situation is that of the patient and the family progressing together through these various steps at a similar rate. As stated earlier, the physician in charge must be able to allay the anxiety produced by these realizations by obtaining information from the patients and their families regarding both their reactions and their understanding of the specific cancer problem.

It has often been the practice among physicians and other health care personnel to avoid an immediate involvement in the grief process described above, but it is clearly a major role for the physician who has assumed responsibility for the patient with advanced cancer. All of us are aware that our own death is certain, but we consider it a distant event and thereby tend to deny it. Many cancer patients function with sufficient hope of long-term control of their disease that they basically deny or suppress concern over their ultimate death in a quite similar fashion. For this reason, these stages of psychological reaction or response may well be protracted, depending on the medical status of the patient, but the concepts are undoubtedly operative in one fashion or another as governed by the course of the disease.

The personal involvement of the physician and his communication with the patient throughout his illness are major aspects of treatment, no matter in what form or at what rate these reactions proceed. Willingness to spend time with the patient, in terms of expressing genuine interest as well as assisting in the solution of his many varied problems, is a crucial aspect of his care. The patient must not feel isolated and abandoned during this terminal process. Hope, whether it is for a limited life of high quality with freedom from pain or for a satisfactory death process, must also be sustained during this phase. The physician is the leader of this group consisting of nurses and other health care personnel, counsellors, and the patient's family. They all play important roles in the psychologic approach to this catastrophic illness.

REFERENCES

1. Baker HL Jr, Campbell JK, Houser OW, Reese DF, Sheedy PF, Holman CB: Computer assisted tomography of the head: An early evaluation. Mayo Clin Proc 49:17–27, 1974
2. Belmusto L, Brown E, Owens G: Clinical observance on respiratory and vasomotor disturbances as related to cervical cordotomies. J. Neurosurg 20:225–232, 1963
3. Bertrand C, Martinez N, Hardy J: Frontothalamic section for intractable pain, in Knighton RS, Dumke PR, (eds): Pain. Henry Ford Hospital International Symposium. Boston, Little, Brown and Co, 1966, p 531
4. Bhalla SK: Metastatic disease of the spine. Clin Orthop 73:52–60, 1970
5. Bodey GP, Rodriguez V, Freireich EJ, Frei E III: Protected environment—prophylactic antibiotics and cancer chemotherapy. Recent Results Cancer Res 29:15–23, 1970
6. Bodey GP, Rodriguez V, Smith JP: Serratia species infections in cancer patients. Cancer 25:199–205, 1970
7. Brain WR, Adams RD: Epilogue: A guide to the classification and investigation of neurological disorders associated with neoplasms, in Brain WR, Norris FH Jr (eds): The Remote Effects of Cancer on the Nervous System. New York, Grune & Stratton, 1965, pp. 216–221
8. Browder AA, Huff JW, Petersdorf RD: The significance of fever in neoplastic disease. Ann Intern Med 55:932–942, 1961
9. Bruce J, McKissock W: Surgical treatment of malignant extradural spinal tumors. Br Med J 1:1341–1344, 1965
10. Cahan WG, Gastro EB: Significance of a solitary lung shadow in patients with breast cancer. Ann Surg 181:137–143, 1975

11. Charkes ND, Malmud LS, Caswell T, Goldman L, et al: Preoperative bone scans. JAMA 233:516–518, 1975

12. Choksi LB, Takita H, Vincent RG: The surgical management of solitary pulmonary metastasis. Surg Gynecol Obstet 134:279–482, 1972

13. Citrin DL, Bessent RG, Greig WR, et al: The application of the ^{99m}Tc phosphate bone scan to the study of breast cancer. BR J Surg 62:201–204, 1975.

14. Copeland EM, Dudrick SJ: Cancer nutritional concepts. Semin Oncol 2:329–335, 1975

15. Croft PB, Wilkinson M: The course and prognosis in some types of carcinomatous neuromyopathy. Brain 92:1–8, 1969

16. Davis RB, Theologides A, Kennedy BJ: Comparative studies of blood coagulation and platelet aggregation in patients with cancer and non-malignant diseases. Ann Intern Med 71:67–80, 1969

17. Failor HJ, Edwards JE, Hodgson CH: Etiologic factors in obstruction of the superior vena cava: A pathologic study. Mayo Clin Proc 33:671–678, 1958

18. Gildenberg PL, Zanes C, Flitter M, Lin PM, Lautsch EV, Truex RC: Impedance measuring device for detection of penetration of the spinal cord in anterior percutaneous cervical cordotomy. J Neurosurg 30:87–92, 1969

19. Gottlieb JA, Frei E III, Luce JK: An evaluation of the management of patients with cerebral metastases from malignant melanoma. Cancer 29:701–705, 1972

20. Haar F, Patterson RH Jr: Surgery for metastatic intracranial neoplasm. Cancer 30:1241–1245, 1972

21. Harrington KD, Johnston JO, Turner RH, Green DL: The use of methyl-methacrylate as an adjunct in the internal fixation of malignant neoplastic fractures. J Bone Joint Surg 54-A:1665–1676, 1972

22. Henson RA, Hoffman HL, Urich H: Encephalomyelitis with carcinoma. Brain 88:449–464, 1965

23. Hersh EM, Freireich EJ: Host defense mechanisms and their modification by cancer chemotherapy. Meth Cancer Res 4:355–451, 1968

24. Hickey RC: Palliative Care of the Cancer Patient. Boston, Little, Brown and Co, 1967

25. Hoffman HC, Marty R: Bone scanning: Its value in the preoperative evaluation of patients with suspicious breast masses. Am J Surg 124:194–199, 1972

26. Horton J, Baxter DH, Olson KB: The management of metastases to the brain by irradiation and corticosteroids. Am J Roentgenol Radium Ther Nucl Med 111:334–336, 1971

27. Joseph WL: Criteria for resection of sarcoma metastatic to the lung. Cancer Chemother Re 58:285–290, 1974

28. Kubler-Ross E: On Death and Dying. New York, Macmillan, 1969

29. Lambert CJ, Shah HH, Urschel HC Jr, et al: The treatment of malignant pleural effusions by closed trocar tube drainage. Ann Thorac Surg 3:1–5, 1967

30. Lambert EH, Rooke ED: Myasthenic state and lung cancer, in Brain WR, Norris FH Jr (eds): The Remote Effects of Cancer of the Nervous System.

New York, Grune & Stratton, 1965, pp 67–80

31. Lim RKS: Neuropharmacology of pain and analgesia, in Lim RKS (ed): Pharmacology of Pain. Third International Pharmacological Meeting, vol. 9. London, Pergamon Press Ltd, 1968, pp 183–217

32. Lentle BC, Burns PE, Dicrich H, Jackson FI: Bone scintiscanning in the initial assessment of carcinoma of the breast. Surg Gynecol Obstet 141:43–47, 1975

33. Lokich JJ, Goodman R: Superior vena cava syndrome: Clinical management. JAMA 231:58–61, 1975

34. Long DM: Spinal cord compression secondary to neoplasm. Minn Med 51:2139–2144, 1968

35. Mark JBD, Goldenberg IS, Montague ACW: Intrapleural mechlorethamine hydrochloride therapy for malignant pleural effusion. JAMA 187:858–860, 1964

36. Miller SP, Sanchez-Avalos J, Stefanski T, Zuckerman L: Coagulation disorders in cancer. I. Clinical and laboratory studies. Cancer 20:1452–1465, 1967

37. Moertel CG: Advanced gastrointestinal cancer: Clinical management and chemotherapy. New York, Paul B Hoeber Publishing Co, 1969

38. Moertel CG, Ahmann DL, Taylor WF, Schwartan N: A comparative evaluation of marketed analgesic drugs. N Engl J Med 286:813–815, 1972

39. Morton DL, Joseph WL, Ketcham AS, et al: Surgical resection and adjunctive immunotherapy for selected patients with multiple pulmonary metastases. Ann Surg 178:360–366, 1973

40. Mullan S, Harper PV, Hekmatpanah J, Torres H, Dobbin G: Percutaneous interruption of the spinal pain tracts by means of a strontium-90 needle. J Neurosurg 20:931–939, 1963

41. Mullins GM, Flynn JP, Mahdi AM, McQueen JD, Owen AH Jr: Malignant lymphoma of the spinal epidural space. Ann Intern Med 74:416–423, 1971

42. Nathan PW: Treatment of intractable pain by chemical rhizotomy with phenol solutions, in Gillingham FJ (ed): Neurosurgery. Philadelphia, JB Lippincott Co, 1970, p 304

43. Nisce LZ, Hilaris BS, Chu FCH: A review of experience with radiation of brain metastasis. Am J Roentgenol Radium Ther Nucl Med 111:329–333, 1971

44. Payne WS, Clagett T, Harrison EG: Surgical management of bilateral malignant lesions of the lung. J Thorac Cardiovasc Surg 43:279–290, 1962

45. Perryman CR, Pavasek EJ, McAllister JD: Clinical evaluation of radioactive chrome phosphate in the control of malignant pleural and ascitic effusions. Radiology 73:865–870, 1959

46. Raskind R, Weiss SR, Manning JJ, Wermuth RE: Survival after surgical excision of single metastatic brain tumors. Am J Roentgenol Radium Ther Nucl Med III:323–328, 1971

47. Richardson EP Jr: Progressive Multifocal Leukoencephalopathy, in Vinken PJ, Gruyn GW (eds): Handbook of Clinical Neurology, vol. 9. Amsterdam, North-Holland Publishing Co, 1970, pp 485–499

48. Robbins GF, Knapper WH, Barrie J, et al: Metastatic bone disease devel-

oping in patients with potentially curable breast cancer. Cancer 29:1702–1704, 1972

49. Rose RG: Intracavitary radioactive collodial gold; result in 257 cancer patients. J Nucl Med 3:323–331, 1962

50. Rososmoff HL: Bilateral percutaneous cervical radiofrequency cordotomy. J Neurosurg 31:41–46, 1969

51. Samuels ML, Olds JW, Howe CD: Needle biopsy of pleura; an evaluation in patients with pleural effusion of neoplastic origin. Cancer 11:980–983, 1958

52. Sanchez-Avalos J, Soong BCF, Miller SP: Coagulation disorders in cancer. II. Multiple myeloma. Cancer 23:1388–1398, 1969

53. Shapiro WR: Malignant brain tumor chemotherapy: Part II. Clinical studies. Clin Bull 3:90–93, 1973

54. Sim FH, Daugherty TW, Ivins JC: The adjunctive use of methylmethacrylate in fixation of pathological fractures. J Bone Joint Surg 56-A:40–48, 1974

55. Trojaborg W, Frantzen E, Anderson I: Peripheral neuropathy and myopathy associated with carcinoma of the lung. Brain 92:71–82, 1969

56. Ultmann JE, Gellhorn A, Osnos M, Hirschberg E: The effect of quinacrine on neoplastic effusions and certain of their enzymes. Cancer 16:283–288, 1963

57. Vietzke WM, Gelderman AH, Grimley PM, Valsamis MP: Toxoplasmosis complicating malignancy—experience at the National Cancer Institute. Cancer 21:816–827, 1968

58. Vogel CL, Cohen MH, Powell RD Jr, DeVita VT: Pneumocystis carinii pneumonia. Ann Intern Med 68:97–108, 1968

59. Western KA, Perera DR, Schultz MG: Pentamidine isethionate in the treatment of pneumocystis carinii pneumonia. Ann Intern Med 73:695–702, 1970

60. Whitecar JP Jr, Bodey GP, Luna M: Pseudomonas bacteremia in cancer patients. Am J Med Sci 260:216–223, 1970

16

Cancer Management—Future Prospects

For many years both the health professions and the general public have been anxiously awaiting a "breakthrough" of some sort that would alleviate the cancer problem. Many envisaged a major advance as a result of research as has occurred in recent years in the treatment of tuberculosis, the prevention of poliomyelitis, and the development of organ transplantation and open heart surgery. One of our major advances in the field of cancer, however, has been the ultimate realization by the scientific community that cancer in man is a multifaceted problem and will not be modified significantly by a single research finding. The problems of cancer appear to be as complex and varied as life itself, but progress is being made. The outlook for patients with some forms of cancer has improved as a result of many new observations in both basic and clinical research, while many of our common forms of cancer continue to be a major challenge.

Currently the significant advances in clinical cancer management relate to the widespread appreciation of the contributions of the various disciplines to the evaluation and treatment of the cancer patient. Improvement in diagnostic measures, an appreciation of the importance of accurate diagnosis in the staging of disease, multiple technical improvements in therapeutic procedures, the rational use of systemic methods of therapy (particularly as adjuvants to regional treatment), and the importance of rehabilitation in overall cancer patient management are all clear-cut gains. These advances, coupled with recently improved attitudes of all health care personnel and the public toward cancer, have led to positive benefits for the cancer patient.

In what areas can we expect future progress? The answer to this question must be speculative, but it is quite clear that a major investigative effort must be placed on prevention in view of our present ineffectiveness in this area. The expansion of research in viral and chemical carcinoma is essential. The epidemiology of human cancer is another major area for investigation. The participation of the practicing physician will be as essential to this overall project of prevention as it has been to the therapeutic arena.

The continued application of the scientific method to treatment planning is essential, as has been demonstrated by our gains in recent prospective clinical trials. Chemotherapy shows promise of becoming a more rewarding treatment in view of recent clinical experiences demonstrating major benefits from drugs. The most exciting aspect of this approach has been the use of drugs as adjuvants to other forms of treatment. Progress in adjuvant chemotherapy for our more common cancers has been slow thus far, but the clinical examples of major benefit are convincing models that establish the validity of the concept. It is now only a matter of time before these adjuvant principles are successfully applied to a broader range of cancer patients.

The role of the cancer-bearing host has received more attention with the growth of new knowledge in both transplantation immunology and tumor immunology. This field has been explored only superficially, but many of the therapeutic limitations of these mechanisms have already been identified. The possibility of harnessing immune mechanisms for therapy would appear to be limited to adjuvant therapy, but exploitation of these immune mechanisms for prevention and treatment of cancer has great promise.

Many investigators continue working to expand on the progress that has been made, but the clinician's cooperation, continued interest, and willingness to exploit their findings is essential for this new knowledge to be of benefit to the cancer patient.

Index

a
b
c
d
7 e
8 f
9 g
0 h
1 i
8 2 j